SILENT VICTORIES

*The History and Practice of Public Health
in Twentieth-Century America*

Edited by

John W. Ward

and

Christian Warren

OXFORD
UNIVERSITY PRESS
2007

OXFORD
UNIVERSITY PRESS

Oxford University Press, Inc., publishes works that further
Oxford University's objective of excellence
in research, scholarship, and education.

Oxford   New York
Auckland   Cape Town   Dar es Salaam   Hong Kong   Karachi
Kuala Lumpur   Madrid   Melbourne   Mexico City   Nairobi
New Delhi   Shanghai   Taipei   Toronto

With offices in
Argentina   Austria   Brazil   Chile   Czech Republic   France   Greece
Guatemala   Hungary   Italy   Japan   Poland   Portugal   Singapore
South Korea   Switzerland   Thailand   Turkey   Ukraine   Vietnam

Copyright © 2007 by Oxford University Press, Inc.

Published by Oxford University Press, Inc.
198 Madison Avenue, New York, New York 10016
www.oup.com

Oxford is a registered trademark of Oxford University Press

ISBN-13: 978-0-19-515069-8
ISBN-10: 0-19-515069-4

CIP information available online from the Library of Congress

9   8   7   6   5   4   3   2   1

Printed in the United States of America
on acid-free paper

Preface

At the beginning of the twentieth century, the crude death rate in the United States stood at 17.2 per 1000 population, infant mortality was around 120 per 1000, and life expectancy was less than 50 years.[1,-3] Respiratory infections and diarrheal diseases were responsible for the majority of deaths. To many health experts, simply comparing health-oriented public activities and expenditures in healthy and unhealthy communities pointed to the solution. In 1895, Hermann M. Biggs, director of the Department of Pathology and Bacteriology in the New York City Health Department, made such a comparison. His conclusion that, "with certain limitations, . . . the inhabitants of any city have it largely within their power to determine what degree of healthfulness their city shall have . . . " constituted an early expression of what would become Biggs's oft-repeated motto: "Public Health is Purchasable".[4] In 1913, the newly christened U.S. Public Health Service (PHS) had a budget of $200,000.[5] At the century's end, the budget for the Department of Health and Human Services stood at $375.5 billion.[6] In 2000, the mortality rate had fallen to 8.7 per 1000; infant mortality stood at 6.9 per 1000; life expectancy nationwide had risen to 77 years; and infectious diseases had given way to cardiovascular disease and cancer as the great cullers of human life.[3,7] Although public health interventions could not account for all of the progress, a good deal of health had been purchased.

And so it was natural, at the end of the century, to reflect on the progress and prospects for continuing to improve the nation's health. Accordingly, in 1999, the *Morbidity and Mortality Weekly Report* (*MMWR*), the nation's health bulletin, published a series of reports highlighting 10 public health advances that had contributed to the dramatic improvements in America's health over the previous century.[8–19] With the encouragement and support of Jeff Koplan, then Director of CDC, the *MMWR* editor invited senior academicians, scientists, and other health leaders to nominate the public health advances that had the greatest impact on death, illness, and disability in the United States in the previous 100 years. Based on these nominations, the *MMWR* commissioned 10 brief reports, written by epidemiologists at the Centers for Disease

Control and Prevention (CDC) and other public health institutions that described, primarily in quantitative terms, the improvements in health resulting from public health interventions. The reports' favorable reception encouraged expansion of the project into a book-length exploration of the history and practice of public health in the twentieth century.

The book comprises 10 parts, each focusing on a particular area of public health. Every section opens with a review by senior scientists of the discoveries, medical advances, and programs that framed the public health response to the problem, and the subsequent impact on morbidity and mortality. An accompanying chapter, written by an academic historian or social scientist, focuses on a key moment or specific theme in the history of the section's topic. The historical chapters highlight the contributions of individuals and of local or regional programs. Often, they address the social, professional, and cultural conflicts involved at nearly every stage of a public health intervention—those shaping their creation as well as those arising during implementation of an intervention. The book ends with an assessment of some of the public health challenges for the twenty-first century. The unique architecture of the volume presents viewpoints on both the scientific and sociocultural contexts at work in many settings, permitting a nuanced understanding of how public health contributed to the country's progress in the twentieth century.

The book's deliberate focus is on major advances in public health; it is not intended to be comprehensive. Some worthy topics, such as gains in environmental protection or the global response to the AIDS pandemic, are not featured. No chapters focus specifically on controversies such as the Tuskegee syphilis study or the swine flu vaccination program. But neither does the book ignore or deny failures and controversies. It argues, in fact, that tremendous progress resulted despite setbacks, scandals, and the emergence of new diseases and other unforeseen health threats.

Again and again, these chapters make clear that America's nascent public health system had to contend at nearly every turn with long-standing obstacles, such as the tendency of a free society to resist constraints on personal freedom and privacy, even in the name of the "greater good"; economic interests that resisted or sought to manipulate public health interventions to their benefit; inequitable distribution of economic and social capital and disparate access to health care; and the constant political tensions between national and local leaders over efficiency, authority, and autonomy.

Controversies and failures become lessons learned—reminders of the risks of unchecked hubris and hidden cultural biases. These examples are correctly raised in program planning and human subject review panels as red flags of caution. Public health's successes, in contrast, become the fabric of everyday life. It is good, as Charles-Edward Amory Winslow pronounced in a 1923 lecture series at Yale University, to keep the successes fresh in mind. After citing salient statistics from 1900 to 1920, he mused: "If we had but the gift of second sight to transmute abstract figures into flesh and blood, so that as we walk along the street we could say 'That man would be dead of typhoid fever,' 'That woman would have succumbed to tuberculosis,' 'That rosy infant would be in its coffin,'—then only should we have a faint conception of the meaning of the silent victories of public health."[20]

A number of important historical factors pervade the book's chapters, and although no chapter fully addresses the history of any one of these, readers will see them at work and trace their development through the volume. Five factors merit brief highlight here: (1) changes in the social demographics of the U.S. population; (2) dramatic shifts in longevity and the burden of disease; (3) the impact of social reform movements (with the ebb and flow of eras in which reform thrived, giving way to years when the spirit of the times hardened against change); (4) the accelerating efficacy of biomedical technology; and (5) the century-long growth of an infrastructure comprising private and public organizations, led by specialists trained in schools of public health and administered through an empowered system of coordinated local, state, and federal public health agencies.

In the twentieth century, the size, distribution, wealth, and ethnic makeup of the American population changed dramatically. From 1900 to 2000, the U.S. population tripled, growing from 76 million to more than 281 million, and the migration from the country to the cities early in the century, followed by the subsequent migration to suburban communities, produced an increasingly metropolitan populace.[21] The level of education—a positive health predictor—rose throughout the century; by 1998, 83% of Americans had graduated from high school, compared with only 13% in 1910. Americans also grew in affluence: except for the years of the Great Depression, average incomes rose throughout the century, another important determinant of good health.[22] The proportion of income spent on life's necessities such as food and clothing also declined, leaving more resources for discretionary spending and other expenses. One of these expenses was health care: little more than an incidental expense in 1900, by 1997 health costs accounted for an average of 17% of personal income. The proportion of Americans living in poverty, first measured in 1959, also declined. However, at century's end more than one in 10 (12%) Americans remained in poverty.[22]

Immigration contributed to this shifting demographic picture, especially at the beginning and end of the century. From 1900 to 1920, a 40-year surge in immigration crested, with more than 14.5 million new arrivals crowding into America's cities. Federal restrictions through much of the mid-century kept immigration rates comparatively low. After the Immigration Act of 1965 lifted most restrictions, immigration rates began climbing once again, rising dramatically in the late 1980s and early 1990s, with many of the most recent immigrants arriving from Asia and Latin America. By 2000, census figures counted one quarter of the U.S. population as "nonwhite." The waves of immigration fueled social movements to accommodate the new arrivals. Public health institutions likewise evolved.[21]

Large social movements and major political and military events spurred the development of public health in America. Public health programs by their nature are deeply enmeshed in the contemporary social and political milieu; hence, the emphasis on social services for the poor during the Progressive Era (1890–1920) provided a rich ferment for efforts to improve the health of children and mothers through programs for better sanitation, hygiene, and maternal education and care. Progressive Era pioneers such as Alice Hamilton studied the health risks of workers, ushering in the field of occupational medicine. Muckraking journalists exposed unsafe and unsanitary industrial practices that threatened both workers and consumers, and pushed lawmakers to pass legislation to improve food safety. In response to the Great Depression of the 1930s, the federal government increased its support of public health at the local level and provided support for medical services for children crippled by polio. During the Great Society movement of the 1960s, public health advocates urged public health agencies to redouble their efforts to reduce health disparities among the poor and to expand into new areas, from environmental health to motor vehicle safety and smoking prevention.

In a different fashion, the nation's preparation for war revealed the country's poor health conditions and spurred the development of new public health programs. In the twentieth century, the Public Health Service often acted as a health-based extension of the American military, especially in times of war. Domestically, medical examinations of men drafted to enter the armed services during two world wars revealed the need for public health programs to combat nutritional deficiencies and venereal diseases. Conversely, medical and health agencies were quick to adopt insights and technologies developed in wartime, from industrial hygiene and toxicology to venereal disease prevention.

As the social demographics of the American population transformed, so too did its basic health statistics: in 2000, Americans lived longer and experienced a very different disease burden than did their counterparts a century earlier. Life expectancy at birth rose from 47.3 to 77.3 years, reflecting the dramatic improvements in infant survival resulting from infectious disease control and improved nutrition; average family size decreased through reproductive planning; and mortality from injuries and cardiovascular diseases fell.[23]

One consequence of these improvements, noted as early as the 1940s, was an aging population: the average age of a person in the United States increased from 23 years in 1900 to 35 years in 2000.[21] Much of this improvement was due to the success in prevention and treatment of acute and infectious diseases, leading to the so-called *epidemiologic transition*—a fundamental shift in the prevalent burden of disease from acute and infectious conditions to chronic and complex conditions and syndromes. Consequently, public health's mission adapted, largely by expansion, to embrace behavioral factors such as smoking and diet and technological factors such as automobile safety.

Although this book focuses on public health activities more than on advances in science and medicine, the application of new scientific knowledge and technology shaped public health and contributed to its success. The germ theory of disease, conceived by Robert Koch and Louis Pasteur in the late nineteenth century, led to the discovery of an infectious cause of many diseases and formed the basis of the movement for milk pasteurization, water treatment, and food inspection—and later, to the discovery of new vaccines and antibiotics. The vitamins and minerals absent in dietary deficiency diseases were identified and used to fortify commonly used food items. New understanding of the ovulatory cycle, first described in the early twentieth century, led to technologies that public health programs used to promote family planning.

While medical improvements often yielded new opportunities for public health, they also often added new responsibilities: for example, new pharmaceutical and surgical interventions to treat cardiovascular disease were incorporated into public health strategies. The development of highly effective therapies to slow the almost invariable progression of HIV infection to AIDS and death expanded public health activities from their previous single focus on prevention to include referral for medical evaluation and treatment with expensive and long-term regimens. Ironically, the adoption of new technologies in health care also led to new health risks. Blood banking and the increased use of injections improved the care of many health conditions while also contributing to infectious disease problems such hepatitis B and hepatitis C. The hospital environment promoted the growth of microorganisms resistant to multiple antibiotics.

Over the twentieth century, a complex public health infrastructure—comprising academic centers, privately funded organizations, and government agencies—evolved to conduct research, train professionals, and implement policies. In 1916, the first U.S. school of public health was established at The Johns Hopkins University; within six years, Columbia, Harvard, and Yale had followed suit. By 2005, a total of 36 universities had accredited schools of public health.[24-26] Reflecting the expanding role of public health, these schools' curricula grew from an initial emphasis on hygiene and sanitation to a multidisciplinary scope that embraces such diverse fields as biostatistics, health services administration, and environmental science.[24,26]

At the beginning of the century, the work of public health was supported primarily by nongovernmental organizations. In 1910–1920, the Rockefeller Foundation supported hookworm eradication projects, one of the earliest campaigns for a specific disease,[27] which led to the foundation's subsequent support of county health departments. Other early efforts to promote community health included support by the National Consumers League of maternal and infant health in the 1920s, sponsorship by the American Red Cross of nutrition programs in the 1930s, and support by the March of Dimes of research in the 1940s and 1950s that led to a successful polio vaccine. Since early in the century, labor organizations worked for safer workplaces.[11] More recently, community-based organizations promoted social activism to counter new health threats such as AIDS and to make established behaviors such as drunk driving no longer socially or legally tolerated. These organizations have also taken on the broader role of providing prevention services to the community, particularly to populations such as injecting drug users and immigrant communities that lack access to government services because of cultural, logistic, or political constraints.

Although the contributions of nongovernment organizations and academic centers were vital to public health's success, government—particularly the federal government—incrementally assumed greater responsibility for public health. The U.S. Constitution vests states with most of the power to protect public health. In 1900, 40 of the 45 states had health departments, concentrating for the most part on sanitation and the microbial sciences. As the system evolved, states took on other public health activities such as laboratory services, personal health services (e.g., sexually transmitted disease treatment), and health resource activities (e.g., health statistics, regulation of health-care services).[28] In 1911, the successful control of typhoid by sanitation measures implemented by health authorities in rural Yakima County Washngton resulted in civic leaders establishing a full-time county health department. This action served as a model for other counties. [27] By 1950, 86% of the U.S. population was served by a local health department.[29] In 1945, the American Public Health Association enumerated minimum functions of local health departments.[30] In 1988, the Institute of Medicine defined these functions as assessment, policy development, and assurance.[31]

A century ago, the federal government's involvement in public health was largely limited to the quarantine duties carried out by Public Health and Marine Hospital Service, renamed the Public Health Service (PHS) in 1912. With the passage of the 16th Amendment to the Constitution in 1913, and the subsequent creation of a federal income tax, federal resources became available to address health problems. In 1917, PHS awarded the first federal funds to support state and local public health programs,[28] and the Social Security Act of 1935 expanded this support.[29] In 1939, PHS, together with health, education, and welfare agencies, joined the Federal Security Agency, forerunner of the Department of Health and Human Services. In 1930, Congress established the National Institutes of Health (formerly the Hygiene Laboratories of the Public Health Service) and the Food and Drug Administration. The Centers for Disease Control and Prevention (CDC) was established in 1946. To provide minimum health-care coverage for low-income and elderly Americans, Congress enacted legislation to begin Medicare and Medicaid in 1965. In 1970, the Occupational Safety and Health Administration and the Environmental Protection Agency joined the federal public health establishment.[19]

Although public health agencies and services increased throughout the century, these resources represented a small proportion of overall health-care costs. In 1993, federal, state, and local health agencies spent an estimated $14.4 billion on core public health functions, representing only 1–2% of the $903 billion in total health-care expenditures.[32] Hermann Biggs would no doubt be shocked at the dollar amounts, but in terms of its share of total health expenditures, the cost of prevention still purchases a great deal of health.

Fairly early in this book's long gestation came the attacks on the World Trade Center and the Pentagon. In the months that followed, the threats of bioterrorism and the dictates of homeland security appeared to be transforming again the nation's public health agenda and shoring up the federal level as the seat of centralized authority. History may well mark September 11, 2001, as the defining moment in public health for the twenty-first century. If so, it little diminishes the record of struggle and accomplishment that is this book's subject. In fact, the power of the public health infrastructure to affect health outcomes—the power that makes public health an essential partner in providing security against bioterrorism (and in eliminating the global health disparities that exacerbate global tensions)—is a power developed through ongoing efforts on the part of public health professionals and their organizations to meet the health challenges of the twentieth century.

References

1. National Office of Vital Statistics. Death rates in the United States by age, sex, and race, 1900–1953. Vital Statistics Reports No. 43 (1–7, 10, 21), 1956.
2. Guyer B, Freedman MA, Strobino DM, Sondik EJ. Annual summary of vital statistics: trends in the health of Americans during the 20th century. *Pediatrics* 2000:106: 1307–17.

3. National Center for Health Statistics. Health, United States, 2004. Hyattsville, MD: Public Health Service, 2004.

4. Biggs HM. The health of the city of New York: Wesley M. Carpenter lecture, 1895. New York Academy of Medicine Pamphlet 16701, 421.

5. Etheridge EW. The Butterfly Caste: A Social History of Pellagra in the South. Westport, CT: Greenwood Press, 1972.

6. HHS. FY 2000 President's Budget for HHS. Washington, DC: Available at: http://www.os.dhhs.gov/budget/fy01budget/hhs2000.pdf. Accessed 15 March 2005.

7. MacDorman MF, Minino AM, Strobino DM, Guyer B. Annual summary of vital statistics—2001. *Pediatrics* 2002:110:1037–52.

8. Centers for Disease Control and Prevention. Ten great public health achievements—United States, 1900–1999. *MMWR* 1999:48:241–43.

9. Centers for Disease Control and Prevention. Impact of vaccines universally recommended for children—United States, 1990–1998. *MMWR* 1999:48:243–48.

10. Centers for Disease Control and Prevention. Motor-vehicle safety: a 20th century public health achievement. *MMWR* 1999:48:369–74.

11. Centers for Disease Control and Prevention. Improvements in workplace safety—United States, 1900–1999. *MMWR* 1999:48:461–69.

12. Centers for Disease Control and Prevention. Control of infectious diseases. *MMWR* 1999:48:621–29.

13. Centers for Disease Control and Prevention. Decline in deaths from heart disease and stroke—United States, 1900–1999. *MMWR* 1999:48:649–56.

14. Centers for Disease Control and Prevention. Healthier mothers and babies. *MMWR* 1999: 48:849–57.

15. Centers for Disease Control and Prevention. Safer and healthier foods. *MMWR* 1999: 48:905–13.

16. Centers for Disease Control and Prevention. Fluoridation of drinking water to prevent dental caries. *MMWR* 1999:48:933–40.

17. Centers for Disease Control and Prevention. Tobacco use—United States, 1900–1999. *MMWR* 1999:48:986–93.

18. Centers for Disease Control and Prevention. Family planning. *MMWR* 1999:48:1073–80.

19. Centers for Disease Control and Prevention. Changes in the public health system. *MMWR* 1999:48:1141–47.

20. Winslow CEA. The Evolution and Significance of the Modern Public Health Campaign. New Haven, CT: Yale University Press, 1923, 64–65.

21. Caplow T, Hicks L, Wattenberg BJ. The First Measured Century: An Illustrated Guide to Trends in America, 1900–2000. Washington, DC: AEI Press. Available at: http://www.pbs.org/fmc/book.htm. Accessed 15 January 2005.

22. Hobbs F, Stoops N. Demographic trends in the 20th century. U.S. Census Bureau. Census 2000 Special Reports, Series CENSR-4. 2002.

23. National Center for Health Statistics. Health, United States, 2004. Hyattsville, MD: Public Health Service, 2004. Available at: http://www.cdc.gov/nchs/data/hus/hus04trend.pdf#027. Accessed 15 January 2005.

24. Roemer MI. Preparing public health leaders for the 1990s. *Public Health Rep* 1988: 103:443–51.

25. Winkelstein W, French FE. The training of epidemiologists in schools of public health in the United States: a historical note. *Int J Epidemiol* 1973:2:415–16.

26. Association of Schools of Public Health. Available at: http://www.asph.org/index.cfm. Accessed 15 January 2005.

27. U.S. Treasury Department/Public Health Service. History of county health organizations

in the United States 1908–1933. In: Public health bulletin no. 222. Washington, DC: Public Health Service, 1936.

28. Altman D, Morgan DH. The role of state and local government in health. *Health Affairs* 1983:2:7–31.

29. Mountin JW, Flook E. Guide to health organization in the United States, 1951. PHS publication no. 196. Washington, DC: Public Health Service, 1951.

30. Emerson H, Luginbuhl M. 1200 local public school departments for the United States. *Am J Public Health* 1945:35:898–904.

31. Institute of Medicine. The Future of Public Health. Washington, DC: National Academy Press, 1988.

32. Centers for Disease Control and Prevention. Estimated expenditures for core public health functions—selected states, October 1992–September 1993. *MMWR* 1995:44:421, 427–29.

Contents

Contributors

Daniel M. Albert, Ph.D.
Curator of Transport
National Museum of Science and
    Industry
London, England

Rima D. Apple, Ph.D.
Professor
Women's Studies Program
School of Human Ecology
University of Wisconsin-Madison
Madison, WI.

Allan M. Brandt, Ph.D.
Amalie Moses Kass Professor of the
    History of Medicine
Division of Medical Ethics
Harvard University Medical School
Cambridge, MA

Brian A. Burt, Ph.D., M.P.H., B.D.Sc.
Professor Emeritus, School of
    Dentistry
Professor Emeritus
Department of Epidemiology
School of Public Health
University of Michigan
Ann Arbor, MI

Michele L. Casper, Ph.D.
Epidemiologist
Division for Heart Disease and Stroke
    Prevention
National Center for Chronic Disease
    Prevention and Health Promotion
Centers for Disease Control and
    Prevention
Atlanta, GA

Jill E. Cooper, Ph.D.
Faculty
Rutgers Preparatory School
Somerset, NJ

Janet B. Croft, Ph.D., M.P.H.
Chief, Epidemiology and Surveillance
    Branch
Division for Heart Disease and Stroke
    Prevention
National Center for Chronic Disease
    Prevention and Health Promotion
Centers for Disease Control and
    Prevention
Atlanta, GA

Jacqueline E. Darroch, Ph.D.
Associate Director, Reproductive
    Health Program

HIV, TB & Reproductive Health
Global Health Program
Bill & Melinda Gates Foundation
Seattle, WA

Ann M. Dellinger, Ph.D., M.P.H.
Team Leader, Motor Vehicle Injury
   Prevention Team
Division of Unintentional Injury
   Prevention
National Center for Injury Prevention
   and Control
Centers for Disease Control and
   Prevention
Atlanta, GA

Peter Drotman, M.D., M.P.H.
Editor-in-Chief, *Emerging Infectious
   Diseases*
National Center for Infectious
   Diseases
Centers for Disease Control and
   Prevention
Atlanta, GA

Michael P. Eriksen, D.Sc.
Director
Institute of Public Health
Georgia State University
Atlanta, GA.
Former Director
Office of Smoking and Health
Centers for Disease Control and
   Prevention

**Emilio J. Esteban, D.V.M., M.B.A.,
   M.P.V.M., Ph.D.**
Director, Western Laboratory
Office of Public Health and Science
Food Safety and Inspection Service
United States Department of
   Agriculture
Alameda, CA

Karin Garrety, Ph.D.
Senior Lecturer
Department of Management

University of Wollongong
New South Wales, Australia.

Wayne H. Giles, M.D., M.S.
Acting Director, Division of Adult and
   Community Health
National Center for Chronic
   Disease Prevention and Health
   Promotion
Centers for Disease Control and
   Prevention
Atlanta, GA

Lawrence W. Green, M.D.
Office on Smoking and Health
National Center for Chronic Disease
   Prevention and Health Promotion
Centers for Disease Control and
   Prevention
Atlanta, GA

Kurt J. Greenlund, Ph.D.
Acting Associate Director for
   Science
Division for Heart Disease and Stroke
   Prevention
National Center for Chronic Disease
   Prevention and Health Promotion
Centers for Disease Control and
   Prevention
Atlanta, GA

Gregory W. Heath, D.H.Sc., M.P.H.
Guerry Professor and Head
Department of Health and Human
   Performance
The University of Tennessee at Chat-
   tanooga
Chattanooga, TN

Alan R. Hinman, M.D., M.P.H.
Senior Public Health Scientist
Task Force on Child Survival and
   Development
Emory University
Atlanta, GA

Former Director, Immunization
  Division and National Center
for Prevention Services, Centers for
  Disease Control and Prevention,
  Atlanta GA

Corinne G. Husten, M.D., M.P.H.
Acting Director
Office on Smoking and Health
National Center for Chronic Disease
  Prevention and Health Promotion
Centers for Disease Control and
  Prevention
Atlanta, GA

Bruce H. Jones, M.D., M.P.H.
Injury Prevention Program Manager
Directorate of Epidemiology and
  Disease Surveillance
U.S. Army Center for Health Promo-
  tion and Preventive Medicine
Aberdeen Proving Ground, MD

Nora L. Keenan, Ph.D.
Epidemiologist
Division for Heart Disease and Stroke
  Prevention
National Center for Chronic Disease
  Prevention and Health Promotion
Centers for Disease Control and Pre-
  vention
Atlanta, GA

Jeffrey P. Koplan, M.D., M.P.H.
Vice President for Academic Health
  Affairs
Woodruff Health Science Center
Emory University
Atlanta, GA
Former Director
Centers for Disease Control and
  Prevention

Milton Kotelchuck, Ph.D., M.P.H.
Chairman and Professor
Department of Maternal and Child
  Health

School of Public Health
Boston University
Boston, MA

Philip J. Landrigan, M.D., DIH, M.Sc.
Professor and Chair
Department of Community and
  Preventive Medicine
Mt. Sinai School of Medicine
New York, NY

Alexandra M. Levitt, Ph.D.
Health Scientist
Office of the Director
National Center for Infectious
  Diseases
Centers for Disease Control and
  Prevention
Atlanta, GA

Ann Marie Malarcher, Ph.D.
Acting Chief, Epidemiology
Office on Smoking and Health
National Center for Chronic Disease
  Prevention and Health Promotion
Centers for Disease Control and
  Prevention
Atlanta, GA

Walter Orenstein, M.D.
Professor of Medicine and Pediatrics
Director of the Program for Vaccine
  Policy and Development
Emory University School of Medicine
Atlanta, GA
Former Director National Immuniza-
  tion Program
Centers for Disease Control and
  Prevention
Atlanta, GA

Stephen Ostroff, M.D.
HHS Representative to the Pacific
  Islands
Office of Global Health Affairs
U.S. Department of Health & Human
  Services

Honolulu, HI
Former Deputy Director
National Center for Infectious
  Diseases (NCID)
Centers for Disease Control and
  Prevention
Atlanta, GA

Terry F. Pechacek, M.D.
Associate Director for Science
Office on Smoking and Health
National Center for Chronic Disease
  Prevention and Health Promotion
Centers for Disease Control and
  Prevention
Atlanta, GA

Linda Pederson, M.D.
Consultant
Business Computer Associates
Northrop Grumman Information
  Technology
Office on Smoking and Health,
National Center for Chronic
  Disease Prevention and Health
  Promotion
Centers for Disease Control and
  Prevention
Atlanta, GA

Gretchen Ann Reilly, Ph.D.
Instructor of History
Temple College
Temple, TX

Anthony Robbins, M.D.
Professor
Public Health and Family Medicine
Tufts University School
  of Medicine
Boston, MA
Former Director, National
  Institute for Occupational Safety
  and Health,
Centers for Disease Control and
  Prevention, Atlanta GA

Naomi Rogers, Ph.D.
Associate Professor
Women's, Gender, and Sexuality
  Studies
Section of the History of Medicine
Yale University
New Haven, CT

Johanna Schoen, Ph.D.
Assistant Professor
Departments of Women's Studies
  and History
The University of Iowa
Iowa City, IA

Christopher Sellers, M.D., Ph.D.
Associate Professor
Department of History
State University of New York
Stony Brook, NY

Richard D. Semba, M.D., M.P.H.
Associate Professor
Department of Ophthalmology ,
  School of Medicine
Center for Human Nutrition
Department of International Health
Bloomberg School of Public Health
Johns Hopkins University
Baltimore, MD

David A. Sleet, Ph.D.
Associate Director for Science
Division of Unintentional Injury
  Prevention
National Center for Injury Prevention
  and Control (NCIPC)
Centers for Disease Control and
  Prevention
Atlanta, GA

Robert V. Tauxe, M.D., M.P.H.
Chief, Foodborne and Diarrheal
  Diseases Branch
Division of Bacterial and Mycotic
  Diseases

National Center for Infectious
  Diseases (NCID)
Centers for Disease Control and
  Prevention
Atlanta, GA

Stephen B. Thacker, M.D., M.Sc.
Director
Office of Workforce and Career
  Development
Centers for Disease Control and
  Prevention
Atlanta GA

Scott L. Tomar, D.M.D., D.P.H.
Associate Professor
Division of Public Health Services
  and Research
College of Dentistry
University of Florida
Gainesville, FL

John W. Ward, M.D.
Director, Division of Viral Hepatitis
National Center for Infectious Dis-
  eases

Centers for Disease Control and
  Prevention
Atlanta, GA
Former Editor, *Morbidity and Mortal-
  ity Weekly Report (MMWR)*

Christian Warren, Ph.D.
Historian
The New York Academy of
  Medicine
New York, NY

Jacqueline H. Wolf, Ph.D.
Associate Professor of the History of
  Medicine
Department of Social Medicine
College of Osteopathic Medicine
Ohio University
Athens, OH

Zhi Jie Zheng, M.D., Ph.D.
Office of Prevention, Education, and
  Control
National Heart, Lung, and Blood
  Institute
National Institutes of Health
Bethesda, MD

PART I

CONTROL OF
INFECTIOUS DISEASES

1

Control of Infectious Diseases: A Twentieth-Century Public Health Achievement

ALEXANDRA M. LEVITT
D. PETER DROTMAN
STEPHEN OSTROFF

The marked decline in infectious-disease-associated mortality that took place in the United States during the first half of the twentieth century (Fig. 1.1) contributed to the sharp drop in infant and child mortality[1,2] and the more than 30-year average increase in life expectancy[3] over the past 100 years. In 1900, the three leading causes of death were pneumonia, tuberculosis (TB), and diarrhea and enteritis, which (together with diphtheria) were responsible for one third of all deaths (Fig. 1.2). Of these deaths, 40% occurred among children aged less than 5 years[1] Cancer accounted for only 3.7% of deaths because few people lived long enough for the disease to develop. By the end of the twentieth century, cancers and heart disease accounted for almost three-fourths of all deaths.*

Despite this overall progress, one of the most devastating disease outbreaks in human history occurred during the twentieth century. The 1918 influenza pandemic killed 20 million people, including 500,000 Americans, in less than a year—more deaths during a comparable time period than have resulted from any war or famine.[4] The last decades of the century were marked by the recognition and pandemic spread of the human immunodeficiency virus (HIV), resulting in an estimated 22 million deaths worldwide by the year 2000. These episodes illustrate the volatility of infectious-disease–associated death rates and the unpredictability of disease emergence. This chapter reviews major twentieth-century achievements in the control of infectious diseases in the United States and ends with a discussion of challenges for the twenty-first century.

3

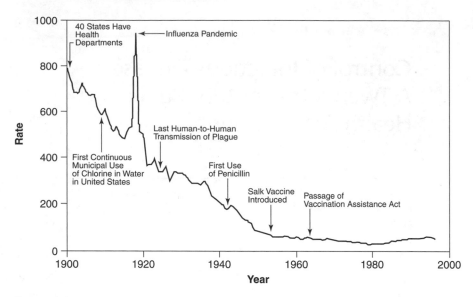

Figure 1.1. Crude death rate (per 100,000 population per year) for infectious diseases—United States, 1900–1996. (Adapted from Armstrong GL, Conn LA, Pinner RW. Trends in infectious disease mortality in the United States during the 20th century. *JAMA* 1999:281:61–66. Data on chlorine in water from: American Water Works Association. Water chlorination principles and practices. AWWA manual no. M20. Denver, CO: American Water Works Association, 1973.)

Landmarks in the Control of Infectious Diseases

Public health activities to control infectious diseases in the 1900s were stimulated by the nineteenth-century discovery that microorganisms are the cause of many diseases (e.g., typhoid fever, cholera, tuberculosis, malaria, tetanus, plague, and leprosy). Landmarks in disease control during the twentieth century included substantial improvements in sanitation and hygiene, the implementation of universal childhood-vaccination programs, and the introduction of antibiotics. Scientific and technological advances (Box 1.1) played a major role in each of these landmarks and provided the underpinning for today's disease surveillance and control systems. Scientific findings also have contributed to a new understanding of the evolving relationships between human beings and microbes.

Sanitation and Hygiene

The nineteenth-century population shift from rural to urban areas that accompanied industrialization, along with successive waves of immigration, led to overcrowding and inadequate housing. Municipal water supplies and rudimentary waste-disposal systems were quickly overwhelmed and set the stage for the emergence and spread

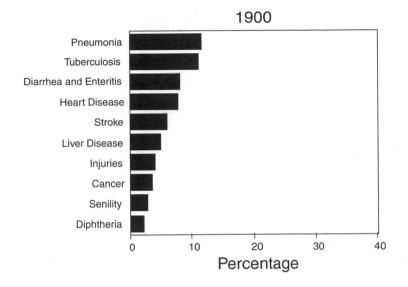

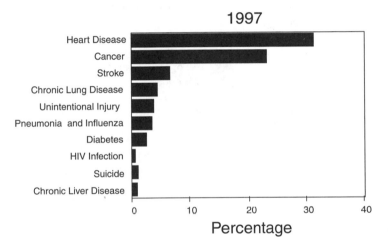

Figure 1.2. The 10 leading causes of death as a percentage of all deaths in the United States, 1900 and 1997.

of infectious illnesses (including repeated outbreaks of cholera, TB, typhoid fever, influenza, yellow fever, and foodborne illnesses).

By 1900, however, the incidence of many of these infectious diseases had begun to decline as a result of public health improvements, which continued into the twentieth century. Sanitation departments were established for garbage removal, and outhouses were gradually replaced by indoor plumbing, sewer systems, and public systems for solid-waste disposal and treatment. The incidence of cholera, which

Infectious diseases and immunology have been an intense focus of medical research throughout the twentieth century, as indicated by this list of Nobel Prize Winners in Physiology and Medicine:*

1901	Emil A. von Behring	Serum therapy used in the treatment of diphtheria
1902	Sir Ronald Ross	Malaria
1905	Robert Koch	Tuberculosis
1907	Charles Louis Alphonse Laveran	Protozoa as agents of disease
1908	Paul Ehrlich Elie Metchnikoff	Immunity
1913	Charles Richet	Anaphylaxis
1919	Jules Bordet	Immunity
1927	Julius Wagner-Jauregg	Malaria inoculation in the treatment of dementia paralytica
1928	Charles Nicolle	Typhus
1939	Gerhard Domagk	Antibacterial effects of prontosil
1945	Alexander Fleming Ernst Boris Chain Howard Walter Florey	Penicillin
1948	Paul Hermann Muller	Use of DDT against disease-carrying arthropods
1951	Max Theiler	Yellow fever
1952	Selman Abraham Waksman	Streptomycin and its use against tuberculosis
1954	John Franklin Enders Frederick Chapman Robbins Thomas Huckle Weller	Growth of polio viruses in tissue culture
1958	Joshua Lederberg	Genetic recombination in bacteria
1960	Frank Macfarlane Burnet Peter Brian Medawar	Acquired immunological tolerance
1966	Francis Peyton Rous	Tumor viruses
1969	Max Delbrück Alfred D. Hershey Salvador E. Luria	Replication and genetic structure of viruses
1972	Gerald M. Edelman Rodney R. Porter	Chemical structure of antibodies
1976	Baruch S. Blumberg	Viral hepatitis and cancer of the liver
	Daniel Carelton Gajdusek	Person-to-person transmissability of kuru, a progressive neurodegenerative disease
1980	Baruj Benacerraf Jean Dausset George D. Snell	Genetically-determined cell surface structures that regulate immunologic reactions (the major histocompatibility complex)
1984	Cesar Milstein Georges J.F. Koehler Niels K. Jerne	Monoclonal antibodies

1987	Susumu Tonegawa	Generation of antibody diversity
1990	Joseph E. Murray	Reducing the risk of immune-system
	E. Donnall Thomas	rejection of transplanted organs
1996	Peter C. Doherty	
	Rolf M. Zinkernagel.	Mechanism of cell-mediated immunity
1997	Stanley B. Prusiner	Prions

Several other Nobel Prizes have been awarded for discoveries that have facilitated the development of tools and strategies for detecting and controlling infectious diseases. These include prizes given for work on gene regulation (e.g., Beadle and Tatum, 1959; Jacob, Lwoff, and Monod, 1965; and Gilman and Rodbell, 1994); nucleic acid structure and replication (e.g., Kornberg and Ochoa, 1959; Crick, Watson, and Wilkins, 1962; and Nathans, Smith, and Arber, 1978) and retroviral replication and evolution (e.g., Baltimore, Temin, Dulbecco, 1975; and Bishop and Varmus, 1989).

* Of 91 Nobel Prizes in Physiology and Medicine awarded during 1901–2000, 27 were for discoveries related to infectious diseases and immunology. No prizes in Physiology and Medicine were awarded in 1915–18, 1921, 1925, or 1940–42.

reached its peak during 1830–1896, when Eurasia and North America experienced four pandemics, began to fall as water supplies were insulated from human waste by sanitary disposal systems. Chlorination and other drinking-water treatments began in the early 1900s and became a widespread public health practice, sharply decreasing the incidence of cholera, typhoid fever, and other waterborne diseases. The incidence of TB also declined as improvements in housing reduced crowding, and TB-control programs were put in place. In 1900, TB killed 200 of every 100,000 Americans, most of them city residents. By 1940 (before the introduction of antibiotic therapy), TB remained a leading killer, but its mortality rate had decreased to 60 per 100,000 persons.[5]

Substantial advances in animal and pest control also were made in the twentieth century. Nationally sponsored, state-coordinated vaccination and animal-control programs eliminated dog-to-dog transmission of rabies. Malaria, which had been endemic throughout the Southeast, was reduced to negligible levels by the late 1940s through regional mosquito-control programs that drained swamps and killed mosquito larvae on bodies of water.

The threat of pandemic and uncontrolled plague epidemics also was greatly diminished by the end of the century as a result of efforts by the U.S. Marine Hospital Service. During the early 1900s, infected rats and fleas were introduced via shipping into port cities along the Pacific and Gulf coasts (e.g., San Francisco, Seattle, New Orleans, Pensacola, and Galveston), as well as into Hawaii, Cuba, and Puerto Rico. The largest outbreaks occurred in San Francisco in 1900–1904 (121 cases, 118 deaths) and in 1907–1908 (167 cases, 89 deaths). The U.S. Marine Hospital Service engaged in laboratory diagnosis, epidemiologic investigations, quarantine and ship inspection activities, environmental sanitation measures, and rodent- and vector-control operations. The last rat-associated outbreak of plague in the United States occurred in 1924–1925 in Los Angeles. That outbreak, which was characterized by a high percentage of pneumonic plague cases, represented the last identified instance of human-to-human transmission of plague in the United States.

After plague was introduced into San Francisco, it spread quickly to various wild rodent species and their fleas, where it still persists throughout much of the western third of the United States. Today, these wild-rodent foci of infection are direct or indirect sources of infection for approximately 10–15 cases of human plague per year (mostly bubonic), which occur in New Mexico, Arizona, Colorado, and California.[†]

Twentieth-century advances in sanitation and hygiene transformed city life and reinforced the idea that collective public health action (e.g., providing clean drinking water) should be a routine function of government. Cities such as Philadelphia and Boston had established health offices as early as the 1790s[6] in response to repeated outbreaks of yellow fever and other infectious diseases.[‡] About 70 years later, Massachusetts and California founded the first state health departments (in 1869 and 1870, respectively), and by the turn of the century, 38 states had followed suit. The first county health departments began to appear in 1908[7] and often identified disease prevention as a major goal. During 1920–1950, state and local health departments, which had benefited from scientific discoveries and increased staffing, were able to make substantial progress in disease-prevention activities related to sewage disposal, water treatment, food safety, and public education regarding hygienic practices.

One of the disease-control duties assumed by state and local health departments in large cities was the regulation of food-handling practices (see Chapter 2) at food-processing plants, restaurants, and retail food stores. The need for such regulation was illustrated by the famous story of Typhoid Mary (see Chapter 2), which underscored not only the growing expectation among Americans that government should promote public health but also a tendency to associate infectious-disease problems with immigrants or other populations, rather than with specific risk factors or behaviors—a trend that has persisted into the twenty-first century. During the 1980s, for example, the gay community was blamed for the AIDS epidemic, and in the early 1990s, the Navajo Nation was stigmatized when an outbreak of hantavirus pulmonary syndrome occurred in their community.[8]

Twentieth-century Americans placed an increasing emphasis on public health action at the federal as well as the local levels. In 1902, Congress changed the name of the Marine Hospital Service to the Public Health and Marine Hospital Service. Ten years later, it became the U.S. Public Health Service (PHS) and it assumed broadened responsibilities for the control of infectious disease. Currently, PHS includes the National Institutes of Health (NIH), the Centers for Disease Control and Prevention (CDC), and the Food and Drug Administration (FDA). The NIH was founded in 1887 as a one-room laboratory of hygiene. The forerunner of NIH's National Institute for Allergy and Infectious Diseases (NIAID)—the National Microbiological Institute—began in 1948 when the PHS Rocky Mountain and Biologics Control Laboratories merged with the NIH Division of Infectious Diseases and Division of Tropical Diseases. The forerunner of CDC—the PHS Communicable Disease Center—opened in downtown Atlanta in 1946. The center was charged with assisting state and local health officials in the fight against malaria, typhus, and other infectious diseases. The forerunner of FDA—the U.S. Bureau of Chemistry[§]—was founded in 1906 to ensure that food and drugs were unadulterated and properly labeled. During the second half of the century, the FDA's mandate was expanded to include responsibility for ensuring the safety and efficacy of medical products, including vaccines and pharmaceuticals used to treat and prevent infectious diseases.

Interest in public health, and the fledgling disciplines of microbiology and infectious diseases, also led to the formation of several nongovernmental organizations, including the American Public Health Association (1872) and the American Society for Microbiology (1899). In addition, the *Journal of Infectious Diseases* was first published in 1904. In 1916, Johns Hopkins University in Baltimore, Maryland, created the first U.S. school of public health with a grant from the Rockefeller Foundation.

Although twentieth-century improvements in sanitation and hygiene have had tremendous societal benefits, foodborne and waterborne diseases remain significant public health concerns. Illness caused by nontyphoidal *Salmonella* species increased during the second half of the century, and other novel foodborne and waterborne agents began to appear, including *Escherichia coli* O157:H7, *Campylobacter* spp., *Cryptosporidium parvum*, *Listeria monocytogenes*, *Legionella* spp., and caliciviruses. A 1999 report estimated an annual burden that year of 76 million foodborne illnesses that resulted in 325,000 hospitalizations and 5000 fatalities.[9] In 1993, the largest outbreak of waterborne illness in U.S. history occurred when an estimated 400,000 persons in Milwaukee, Wisconsin, were infected with the parasite *Cryptosporidium*. Factors associated with the challenges of foodborne and waterborne illnesses that likely will persist into the twenty-first century include (1) changing dietary habits that favor foods more likely to transmit infection (e.g., raw seafood, sprouts, unpasteurized milk and juice, and fresh fruits and vegetables); (2) globalization of the food supply; (3) mass-production practices; and (4) aging and inadequately-maintained water supply systems. Although mass food production and distribution have resulted in an abundant and generally safe food supply, they have also increased the potential for large and geographically dispersed outbreaks of illness.

Immunization

Immunization is a critical intervention to prevent infectious diseases (see also Chapter 4). Strategic vaccination campaigns have virtually eliminated diseases that were common in the United States during the beginning and middle decades of the century (e.g., diphtheria, tetanus, whooping cough, polio, smallpox, measles, mumps, rubella, and *Haemophilus influenzae* type b meningitis).[10] Starting with the licensure of the combined diphtheria-pertussis-tetanus (DPT) vaccine in 1949, state and local health departments began providing childhood vaccines on a regular basis, primarily to poor children. In 1955, the introduction of the Salk polio vaccine led to the federal appropriation of funds to support childhood-vaccination programs initiated by states and local communities. In 1962, a federally-coordinated vaccination program was established through the passage of the Vaccination Assistance Act—a landmark piece of legislation that has been continuously renewed and now supports the purchase and administration of a full range of childhood vaccines.

The success of vaccination programs in the United States and Europe gave rise to the twentieth-century concept of *disease eradication*—the idea that a selected disease could be eliminated from all human populations through global cooperation. In

1980, after an 11-year campaign (1967–1977) involving 33 nations, the World Health Organization declared that smallpox had been eradicated worldwide—about a decade after it had been eliminated from the United States and the rest of the Western Hemisphere. Polio and dracunculiasis (a non-vaccine-preventable disease)** are currently targeted for eradication, and many other infectious diseases may be targeted in the twenty-first century, including measles, *Haemophilus influenzae* type b infections, filariasis, onchocerciasis, rubella, and hepatitis B.

Antibiotics and Other Antimicrobial Drugs

The discovery of the antibiotic penicillin and its development into a widely available medical treatment were other major landmarks in the control of infectious diseases. Penicillin and other antibiotics allowed quick and complete treatment of previously incurable bacterial diseases (see also Chapter 3). In addition, the new antibiotics targeted more organisms and caused fewer side effects than the sulfa drugs that became available in the late 1930s. Discovered fortuitously in 1928, penicillin was not developed for medical use until the 1940s, when it was produced in significant quantities and used by the United States and allied military forces to treat sick and wounded soldiers.

Antibiotics have been in civilian use for nearly six decades (Box 1.2) and have saved the lives and improved the health of millions of persons infected with typhoid fever, diphtheria, bacterial pneumonia, bacterial meningitis, plague, tuberculosis, and streptococcal and staphylococcal infections. During the twentieth century, drugs also were developed to treat viral diseases (e.g., ribavirin, zidovudine, and acyclovir), fungal diseases (e.g., nystatin, ketoconazole, and amphotericin B), and parasitic diseases (e.g., chloroquine, mebendazole, and metronidazole).

Unfortunately, the therapeutic advances that characterized the second half of the twentieth century are being swiftly reversed by the emergence of drug resistance in bacteria, parasites, viruses, and fungi.[11] Whether this phenomenon would eventually

---

Box 1.2. The First American Civilian Saved by Penicillin.

Antibiotics are so widely relied on in the United States that Americans have come to take them for granted after a only a few generations of use. The first U.S. civilian whose life was saved by penicillin died in June 1999 at the age of 90. In March 1942, a 33-year-old woman named Anne Sheafe was hospitalized for a month with a life-threatening streptococcal infection at New Haven Hospital in New Haven, Connecticut. She was delirious and her temperature spiked at almost 107° F. Treatments with sulfa drugs, blood transfusions, and surgery had no effect. As a last resort, Anne Sheafe's doctors injected her with a tiny amount of an obscure experimental drug called penicillin. Her hospital chart, now at the Smithsonian Institution, recorded a sharp overnight drop in temperature, and by the next day she was no longer delirious. Anne Sheafe survived to marry, raise a family, and enjoy another 57 years of life.

occur was debated during the early years of the antibiotic era, but the debate ended rapidly after penicillin was used to treat staphylococcal infections. However, within several years, many strains of *Staphylococcus aureus* had become penicillin-resistant, requiring changes in recommended therapy. Since the 1950s, this organism has developed resistance to each of the drug types that have replaced penicillin, and over the last several years, strains of *S. aureus* with reduced susceptibility to the last remaining antibiotic (vancomycin) have been appearing. Other diseases that have been substantially impacted by antibiotic resistance include gonorrhea, tuberculosis, pneumococcal infection, typhoid fever, bacterial dysentery, malaria, and HIV. A primary reason for the swift development of antibiotic resistance is the natural tendency of organisms to mutate and share genetic material. However, this process has been facilitated by injudicious prescribing of antibiotics by the medical, veterinary, and agricultural industries; unrealistic patient expectations; the economics of pharmaceutical sales; and the growing sophistication of medical interventions (e.g., transplant surgery and chemotherapy) that require the administration of large quantities of antibiotics.[12] Growing antibiotic resistance poses a substantial threat to the gains in infectious-disease control made over the last five decades and warrants fresh approaches to promoting wise antibiotic stewardship by prescribers, patients, and industry to ensure the effectiveness of these drugs in future generations.

Technological Advances in Detecting and Monitoring Infectious Diseases

Technological change was a major theme of twentieth-century public health, particularly in the area of infectious disease. Twentieth-century techniques that increased the capacity for detecting, diagnosing, and monitoring infectious diseases included the development of serologic testing (at the beginning of the century) and molecular assays (at the end of the century). Computers and electronic forms of communication have also had an impact on epidemiology, greatly enhancing the nation's ability to gather, analyze, and disseminate disease-surveillance data.

Serologic Testing

Serologic testing, which came into use in the 1910s, provided one of the cornerstones for laboratory-based (as opposed to clinical) diagnosis. It remains a useful diagnostic and epidemiologic tool. The impact of serologic testing can be illustrated by reviewing early twentieth-century efforts to control sexually transmitted diseases (STDs).[13,14] Syphilis and gonorrhea were widespread by 1900, with transmission rates rising with the increasing urbanization of the United States. Gonorrhea contracted from infected mothers during delivery accounted for a substantial proportion of cases of congenital blindness, giving rise to the practice of treating the eyes of newborn babies with silver nitrate. However, gathering data on the incidence of these diseases was difficult, not only because infected persons were unwilling to discuss their sexual activities or ask for treatment but also because syphilis and gonorrhea were difficult to diagnose (especially during the latent stages of disease). Thus,

STDs were not only unmentionable in polite society but also largely invisible from an epidemiologic perspective.

This situation began to change when serologic testing became available. During World War I, blood tests for syphilis were given to young men before their induction into the army. The Surgeon General reported that in 1917 and 1918, infection with STDs was the most frequent cause for rejection of draftees;[13] the next highest cause was heart disease. The high incidence of venereal disease documented among young men during World War I stimulated the initiation of the first (though short-lived) national syphilis control program via the Chamberlain-Kahn Act of 1918.[14]

Viral Isolation and Tissue Culture

The first virus isolation techniques also came into use at the turn of the twentieth century. They involved straining infected material through successively smaller sieves and inoculating test animals or plants to show that the purified substance retained disease-causing activity. The first "filtered" viruses were tobacco mosaic virus (1886);[15] and the virus that causes foot-and-mouth disease in cattle (1897).[16] The U.S. Army Command under Major Walter Reed filtered yellow fever virus in 1900.[17] The development of techniques for growing monolayers of cells in culture dishes allowed viral growth *in vitro* and paved the way for large-scale production of live or heat-killed viral vaccines. Negative staining techniques for the visualization of viruses under the scanning electron microscope (which was invented in the late 1930s) were available by the early 1960s.

Molecular Techniques

During the last quarter of the twentieth century, molecular biology provided powerful new tools for detecting and characterizing infectious pathogens. Antibody-based assays and nucleic acid hybridization and sequencing techniques[18] rendered possible the characterization of the causative agents of previously unknown diseases (e.g., hepatitis C, Lyme disease, human ehrlichiosis, hantavirus pulmonary syndrome, AIDS, Ebola and Marburg hemorrhagic fevers, new variant Creutzfeldt-Jakob disease, and Nipah virus disease).

Molecular tools have greatly enhanced capacity for tracking the transmission of new threats and for finding new ways to prevent and treat them. The HIV virus (formerly also called LAV, for lymphadenopathy-associated virus) was identified in 1983, within a few years of the recognition of AIDS by Western scientists as a new human disease,[19] and serologic AIDS tests came into widespread use before the end of the decade.[20] Had AIDS emerged 100 years ago, when laboratory-based diagnostic methods were in their infancy, it might have remained a mysterious syndrome of unknown cause for many decades. Moreover, the development of the drugs currently used to treat HIV-infected persons and prevent perinatal transmission of the virus (e.g., replication analogs and protease inhibitors) required an understanding of retroviral replication at the molecular level, a knowledge base that is only a few decades old.

Future advances in molecular biology, bioinformatics, and other areas are likely to revolutionize the detection, treatment, control, and prevention of infectious diseases in the twenty-first century. Advances in microbial genomics will enable epidemiologists to identify any microbial species, subtype, or strain within hours or minutes. A detailed understanding of human genetics will help physicians target vaccines and prophylactic drugs to the most susceptible persons, and improved knowledge of human immunology will stimulate the development of vaccines that not only prevent disease but also boost the immunity of people who are already infected with HIV or other pathogens (see Chapter 2). Over the next century, infectious diseases may be found to cause many chronic cardiovascular, intestinal, and pulmonary diseases (Box 1.3), which could lead to profound changes in the way these diseases are treated and prevented.[21–27] Moreover, in-depth knowledge of climatic and environmental factors that influence the emergence of animal- and insect-borne diseases (facilitated by the availability of remote-sensing technologies) will inform public health policy and allow public health authorities to predict outbreaks and institute preventive measures months in advance.

Although the technology revolution has been beneficial in the control and diagnosis of infectious diseases, the increase in genetic knowledge may have negative consequences in terms of personal privacy, autonomy, and safety. Special protections may be needed, for example, to ensure that individuals control access to information about their genetic make-up (e.g., by physicians, medical insurers, employers, public health workers, and researchers). Even more alarming, microorganisms can be intentionally manipulated or "weaponized" to cause harm—as we know from the events of October 2001, when highly-purified anthrax spores sent through the U.S. mail killed five people.

Box 1.3. Infectious Agents May Cause Chronic Diseases.

The two leading causes of death in the United States as we enter the twenty-first century are cancer and cardiovascular disease, rather than the infectious diseases that afflicted our forebears 100 years ago (see Fig. 1.2). However, the distinction between chronic and infectious diseases has begun to blur.

Current research suggests that some chronic diseases formerly attributed to lifestyle or environmental factors are actually caused by or intensified by infectious agents. For example, most peptic ulcers—long thought to be due to stress and diet—are now known to be caused by the bacterium *Helicobacter pylori*.[21] Several types of cancers, including some liver[22,23] and cervical cancers,[24] are linked to infectious agents. *Chlamydia pneumoniae* infection has been proposed as a contributor to coronary artery disease,[25,26] and enteroviruses appear to be associated with type 1 diabetes melitus in some children.[27]

Thus, in the twenty-first century, it is possible that some forms of cancer, heart disease, and diabetes, may be treated with antimicrobial drugs or prevented by vaccines.

Challenges for the Twenty-first Century

The success in reducing morbidity and mortality from infectious diseases during the first three quarters of the twentieth century led many medical and public health experts to become complacent about the need for continued research into treatment and control of infectious microbes.[11] However, subsequent developments—including the appearance of new diseases such as AIDS and severe acute respiratory syndrome (SARS), the reemergence of tuberculosis (including multidrug-resistant strains), the spread of cholera and West Nile encephalitis to the Americas, and an overall increase in U.S. infectious-disease mortality during 1980–1998 (Fig. 1.1)—have reinforced the realization that as long as microbes can evolve, new diseases will arise.

Molecular genetics provides a new appreciation of the remarkable ability of microbes to evolve, adapt, and develop drug resistance in an unpredictable and dynamic fashion (Box 1.4). Scientists now understand the way in which (1) resistance genes are transmitted from one bacterium to another on plasmids and (2) viruses evolve through replication errors, through the reassortment of gene segments, and by jumping species barriers. Recent examples of microbial evolution include the emergence and intercontinental spread of a virulent strain of avian influenza H5N1 first identified

---

Box 1.4. New Modes of Disease Transmission Created by Twenty-first-century Technology.

Although the impact of technology on the control of infectious diseases has been overwhelmingly positive, certain twentieth-century technological advances have created the following new niches and modes of transmission for particular pathogens:

- The bacteria that cause Legionnaire's disease have been spread through modern ventilation systems.
- HIV and hepatitis B and C viruses have been spread through unscreened blood donations.
- Foodborne diseases (e.g., Salmonellosis and *E. coli* O157 infection) have been transmitted by centrally processed food products that are distributed simultaneously to many states or countries.
- Airplanes have replaced ships as major vehicles of international disease spread, carrying not only infected people (e.g., individuals with SARS or influenza) but also disease-carrying animals and insects (e.g., mosquitoes that carry malaria parasites or West Nile virus).
- As a result of economic development (e.g., mining, forestry, and agriculture) and an expanded tourist trade that caters to persons who wish to visit undeveloped areas, more people are traveling to tropical rain forests and other wilderness habitats that are reservoirs for insects and animals that harbor unknown infectious agents.
- In the United States, increasing suburbanization, coupled with the reversion of agricultural land to secondary growth forest, has brought people into contact with deer that carry ticks infected with *Borrelia burgdorferi*, the causative agent of Lyme disease, and has brought household pets into contact with rabies-infected raccoons.

in Hong Kong, the multidrug-resistant W strain of tuberculosis in the United States, and strains of *Staphylococcus aureus* with reduced susceptibility to vancomycin in the United States and Japan.[11,28]

Although twentieth-century achievements in the control of infectious disease have been effective, the public health community cannot rest. The United States must be prepared to address the unexpected, whether it be an influenza pandemic, a disease caused by a novel or unrecognized organism, a drug-resistant disease, a foodborne outbreak, or an outbreak of smallpox caused by a bioterrorist. Continued protection of U.S. health requires improved capacity for disease surveillance and outbreak response at the state, local, and federal levels; the development and dissemination of new laboratory and epidemiologic methods; and ongoing research into environmental factors that facilitate disease emergence.[11,28,29]

Acknowledgments

We thank Drs. Heidi Davidson and Robert Pinner for allowing us to reprint their graph on infectious disease mortality rates during the twentieth century (Fig. 1.1). We also thank Carol Snarey for editing the manuscript.

Notes

* Some proportion of cancer and heart disease may be caused or exacerbated by infectious agents (see Box 1.3).
† Epidemiologic investigations since 1970 indicate that most cases are acquired through infectious flea bites (78% of total), direct contact with infected animals (20%) or, rarely, inhalation of infectious respiratory droplets or other airborne materials (2%). The only identified sources of infection for the cases acquired through inhalation were exposures to infected cats with cough or oral lesions.
‡ The first Philadelphia health office opened in 1794. Paul Revere was the first president of the Boston board of health, which was founded in 1796.
§ In 1927, the Bureau of Chemistry was reorganized into two agencies: the Food, Drug, and Insecticide Administration and the Bureau of Chemistry and Soils. In 1930, the name of the Food, Drug, and Insecticide Administration was shortened to the Food and Drug Administration.
** Dracunculiais, or guinea worm disease, is a waterborne parasitic illness that in past years caused acute illness and permanent disabilities in millions of people in India, Pakistan, and several African countries. Its eradication depends on environmental and behavioral interventions that reduce exposure to contaminated water rather than on vaccination.

References

1. Department of Commerce and Labor, Bureau of the Census. Mortality Statistics, 1900 to 1904. Washington, DC: Government Printing Office, 1906.
2. Hoyert DL, Kochanek KD, Murphy SL. Deaths: Final Data for 1997. National Vital Statistics Reports:47,19. Hyattsville, MD: National Center for Health Statistics, 1999.
3. Bunker JP, Frazier HS, Mosteller F. Improving health: measuring effects of medical care. *Milbank Q* 1994:72:225–58.
4. Crosby AW, Jr. Epidemic and Peace, 1918. Westport, CT: Greenwood Press, 1976, 311.
5. U.S. Congress, House Select Committee on Population. 1978. World Population: Myths and Realities; Fertility and Contraception in the United States; Legal and Illegal Immigration to

the United States; Population and Development Assistance; Domestic Consequences of United States Population Change; Final Report:5, 4 (December 1979),720–21.

6. Smillie WG. Public Health: Its Promise for the Future. New York: Macmillan, 1955.

7. Hinman A. 1889 to 1989: A century of health and disease. *Public Health Rep* 1990: 105:374–80.

8. Centers for Disease Control. Update: outbreak of hantavirus infection—southwestern United States, 1993. *MMWR* 1993:42:477–79.

9. Mead PS, Slutsker L, Dietz V, et al. Food-related illness and death in the United States. *Emerg Infect Dis* 1999:5:607–25.

10. Centers for Disease Control. Status report on the Childhood Immunization Initiative: reported cases of selected vaccine-preventable diseases—United States, 1996. *MMWR* 1997:46:665–71.

11. Institute of Medicine. Emerging Infections: Microbial Threats to Health in the United States. Washington, DC: National Academy Press,1994.

12. DM Bell. Promoting appropriate antimicrobial drug use: perspective from the Centers for Disease Control and Prevention. *Clin Infect Dis* 2001:33(suppl 3):S245–50.

13. Selvin M. Changing medical and societal attitudes toward sexually transmitted diseases: a historical overview. In: Holmes KK, Mardh P-A, Sparling PF, Wiesner PJ, eds. Sexually Transmitted Diseases. New York: McGraw-Hill, 1984, 3–19.

14. Fleming WL. The sexually transmitted diseases. In: Last JM, ed. Maxcy-Rosenau Public Health and Preventive Medicine, 11th ed. New York: Appleton-Century-Crofts, 1980, 251–73.

15. Mayer, A. Über die Mosaikkrankheit des Tabaks. *Landwn. Vers-Stnen.* 1886:32:451–67. (Translation published in English as Phytopathological Classics No. 7 [1942], American Phytopathological Society, St. Paul, MN).

16. Brown F. Stepping stones in foot-and-mouth disease research: a personal view. In: Sobrino F, Domingo E, eds. Foot and Mouth Disease: Current Perspectives.. Madrid: Horizon Bioscience and CRC Press, 2004, 1–18.

17. Reed W, Carroll J, Agramonte A. Experimental yellow fever, 1901. *Mil Med.* 2001 Sep;166(9 Suppl):55–60.

18. Dumler JS, Valsamakis A. Molecular diagnostics for existing and emerging infections. Complementary tools for a new era of clinical microbiology. *Am J Clin Pathol* 1999;112(suppl 1):S33–39.

19. Karpas A. Human retroviruses in leukaemia and AIDS: reflections on their discovery, biology and epidemiology. *Biol Rev Camb Philos Soc* 2004: 79:911–33.

20. Schochetman G, Epstein JS, Zuck TF. Serodiagnosis of infection with the AIDS virus and other human retroviruses. *Annu Rev Microbiol* 1989:43:629–59.

21. Dunn BE, Cohen H, Blaser MJ. Helicobacter pylori: a review. *Clin Microbiol Rev* 1997: 10:720–41.

22. Montesano R, Hainaut P, Wild CP. Hepatocellular carcinoma: from gene to public health. *J Natl Cancer Inst* 1997:89:1844–51.

23. Di Bisceglie AM. Hepatitis C and hepatocellular carcinoma. *Hepatology* 1997:26(suppl 1):34S–38S.

24. Muñoz N, Bosch FX. The causal link between HPV and cervical cancer and its implications for prevention of cervical cancer. *Bull PAHO* 1996: 30:362–77.

25. Danesh, J, Collins R, Peto R. Chronic infections and coronary heart disease: is there a link? *Lancet* 1997:350:430–36.

26. Mattila KJ, Valtonen VV, Nieminen MS, Asikainen S. Role of infection as a risk factor for atherosclerosis, myocardial infarction, and stroke. *Clin Infect Dis* 1998:26:719–34.

27. Haverkos HW, Haverkos LM, Drotman DP, Battula N, Rennert OM. Enteroviruses and type 1 diabetes melitus. In: Quinn T, ed. Infectious Agents in Chronic Diseases (in press).
28. Preventing Emerging Infectious Diseases: A Strategy for the 21st Century. Atlanta, GA: Centers for Disease Control, U.S. Department of Health and Human Services, 1998.
29. Binder S, Levitt AM, Sacks JJ, Hughes JM. Emerging infectious diseases: public health issues for the 21st century. *Science.* 1999;284(5418):1311–3.

Suggested Reading

Hinman A. 1889 to 1989: a century of health and disease. *Public Health Rep* 1990: 105:374–80.
Selvin M. Changing medical and societal attitudes toward sexually transmitted diseases: a historical overview. In: Holmes KK, Mardh P-A, Sparling PF, Wiesner PJ, eds. Sexually Transmitted Diseases. New York: McGraw-Hill, 1984, 3–19.

2

Advances in Food Safety to Prevent Foodborne Diseases in the United States

ROBERT V. TAUXE
EMILIO J. ESTEBAN

In the United States, the food supply is both broader and far safer than it was 100 years ago. At the start of the twentieth century, contaminated foods frequently caused typhoid fever, septic sore throat, and trichinosis—diseases that now rarely occur. Along with the treatment of drinking water and sewage sanitation, food-safety measures have become routine; these measures have been developed and initiated in response to specific public health threats and are continually evolving. At the same time, the shift of the U.S. food supply from small, local farms to huge, global agribusinesses has opened new niches for pathogens, as well as the potential for more systematic disease prevention. The methods public health authorities use to detect, investigate, and understand these public health threats have also advanced over the last century. This chapter, which addresses the progress achieved in the field of food safety, serves to support the continuing effort to make food safer.

The Social Setting of the Food Supply in 1900

In 1900, the United States was predominantly rural. The census conducted that year found 60% of the population living in rural areas, and another 14% living in towns of fewer than 25,000 persons.[1] Farmers constituted 38% of the labor force. Whereas grain milling and meatpacking industries were centralized in the Midwest, most other foods were produced in dairies, truck farms, and other local food industries located near the consumer. Many foods were available only seasonally, and domestic iceboxes provided limited refrigeration. Fresh foods were supplemented by canned goods, which had become available after the Civil War, though concerns about their safety and quality limited their general acceptance.[2] Kitchen gardens supplied produce, and much food processing occurred in the home, from slaughter and plucking of live fowl to making sausages and preserves. A popular cookbook from 1871, written for a general homemaking audience, gave instructions for making pickles, preserves, catsup, ginger beer, and dehydrated soup at home in addition to providing recipes for the principal meals.[3] Because of the substantial effort required to provide food at the household level, middle-class households in that era required a staff. The 1900 census revealed that 9% of the nonagricultural working population reported their occupation as housekeeper or servant.[1]

Cities with increasing populations were just beginning to appreciate the benefits of treated municipal water supplies and sewage collection systems at the turn of the century,[4,5] although sewer systems still poured waste into lakes and rivers that served as the water supply. In 1900, only 6% of the population had access to water that was filtered, and 24.5% of the urban population had sewerage.[5]

The Impact of Foodborne Diseases Early in the Twentieth Century and the Public Health Response

In 1900, American life expectancy at birth was 47 years. In Massachusetts, where vital statistics records were maintained, the infant mortality rate was 141 per 1000 live births.[6] Fifteen years later, when national infant mortality was first reported, the rate was 100 per 1000 live births.[6] Foodborne and waterborne diseases were substantial contributors to mortality. In 1900, the annual rate for death caused by gastroenteritis was 142 per 100,000 persons and that for typhoid fever was 31.3 per 100,000.[6] Contaminated food and water likely were the primary sources of both illnesses. In 1928, the standard public health textbook covered only a fraction of the foodborne diseases discussed in today's texts; these diseases included typhoid fever, bovine tuberculosis, septic sore throat (a severe streptococcal infection due to *Streptococcus zooepidemicus* and related strains), scarlet fever, trichinosis, botulism, and salmonellosis (see Table 2.1).[7]

Severe outbreaks of illness involving substantial numbers of cases captured public attention early in the twentieth century, when the cases were traced to seemingly safe food supplies. For instance, in 1911, one Boston dairy that operated with state-of-the-art cleanliness but without pasteurization caused 2000 cases of septic sore throat and 48 deaths.[7] In 1919, a multistate botulism outbreak was recognized in Alliance, Ohio, where a luncheon at a country club made 14 attendees ill, killing seven.[18] A detailed investigation implicated a glass jar of olives that had been commercially bottled in California. Though no statistical tests were applied, the link to the olives was clear from the food histories of the cohort of luncheon attendees and was confirmed by feeding laboratory animals the leftover olives. Within a few months, olives from the same bottling plant caused at least eight more deaths in similar outbreaks in Michigan and Tennessee; a botulism outbreak in Montana was traced to similar olives from a second California firm.[19] Investigators at the Bureau of Chem-

Table 2.1. Principal foodborne infectious threats identified in standard textbooks of 1928 and 1939, ranked by number of citations in index.

1928: Rosenau [7]	1939: Shrader [30]
Typhoid fever (*Bacillus typhosus*, now *Salmonella* Typhi)	Botulism
	Salmonellosis
Botulism	Bovine tuberculosis
Salmonellosis (*Bacillus enteritidis*, now *Salmonella*)	Brucellosis
	Typhoid fever (*Eberthella typhosa*, now *Salmonella* Typhi)
Trichinosis	
Brucellosis, Malta fever	Trichinosis
Tuberculosis (foodborne)	Tapeworm
Septic sore throat (*Streptococcus epidemicus*, now *Streptococcus zooepidemicus*)	Septic sore throat
	Staphylococcal food poisoning
Streptococcal scarlet fever	Amebiasis
Tapeworm	

istry, forerunner of today's Food and Drug Administration, discovered that the jars were not heated sufficiently at the packing plant to kill the botulism spores. However, the Bureau of Chemistry lacked authority to halt a food processor even after it was shown to produce unsafe food. It could only seize batches of processed food that were proved to be contaminated by laboratory testing. The bureau could only warn the public that if they wished to reduce their risk of dying of botulism, they should avoid eating olives packed in glass.[19]

In 1924, raw oysters caused a nationwide outbreak of typhoid fever. A team of public health officials documented 1500 cases and 150 deaths in 12 cities, from New York to San Francisco. The investigators gathered food-consumption histories from patients, surveyed large numbers of healthy persons about their eating habits, and interviewed cohorts of persons who had eaten the oysters.[20] Although no statistics were applied, the investigation exemplified the case-control method. Investigators reported that in New York City, 176 of 246 typhoid fever victims had eaten raw oysters within 30 days of illness, while only 28 of 275 healthy persons living in the same area had done so; both ill and well persons ate tomatoes and lettuce with the same frequency. One New York company was determined to be the source of the implicated oysters; this company stored the harvested oysters in freshwater pens, a practice known as floating. The pens were located near a wharf where boats dumped sewage into the water. As a result of this outbreak, many consumers lost confidence in eating oysters, leading to the formation of the National Shellfish Sanitation Program in 1925. The program encouraged standard regulations and industry practices that would keep oysters away from human sewage by monitoring shellfish-growing waters for sewage contamination and prohibiting the floating of oysters and other dangerous practices.[21] This program continues to operate into the twenty-first century as the Interstate Shellfish Sanitation Conference.

Microbial Investigations of Foodborne Pathogens

By the start of the twentieth century, European bacteriologists had identified the microbial cause of some foodborne infections by using newly developed laboratory methods. Diagnosis of specific infections replaced the pre-microbiological concept of *ptomaines*, which were injurious substances believed to form spontaneously in spoiled food. In 1884, Georg Gaffky first cultivated the causative agent of typhoid fever, now called *Salmonella* Typhi, making possible the bacteriologic diagnosis of that common disease.[8] In 1886, August A. H. Gaertner investigated an outbreak of 54 enteric illnesses among people who ate raw ground beef. The meat had come from a cow that died with severe diarrhea and was pronounced safe to eat after visual inspection. Gaertner isolated a bacterial pathogen, now called *Salmonella* Enteritidis, from the meat itself and from the spleen of a young man who had died following the consumption of the notorious meal, which first linked human salmonellosis to animal infection.[9] In 1894, Emile-Pierre van Ermengem first isolated the bacterium *Clostridium botulinum* from suspect cured meat and from autopsy specimens during an investigation of a botulism outbreak.[10] This discovery underlined the need for scientific evaluation of food processing and opened the door to many investigations of the impact of variations in food processing on the safety of food.

In the United States, the first public health laboratories were established at the end of the nineteenth century to perform basic analyses of milk and water and to diagnose typhoid fever and other communicable diseases.[11] Massachusetts established a State Hygiene Laboratory in 1886; Providence, Rhode Island, did so in 1888, and California in 1905. State boards of health, initially staffed by volunteers, grew in size and professionalism; by 1915 these boards of health had been established in some form in every state.[11] Outbreak investigations were coordinated through these departments. For instance, the first typhoid carrier was identified by the New York City Board of Health through use of epidemiologic and laboratory techniques.[12] The carrier, who became known as Typhoid Mary, was a private cook who worked for several families in New York. In 1906, a familial outbreak of typhoid fever brought this cook to the attention of local public health authorities, who documented through bacteriologic testing that she was a chronic carrier. She was detained, but later was allowed to return to work as a cook, causing another outbreak of typhoid fever among hospital staff. Typhoid Mary ultimately was confined for life in a city hospital after causing at least 51 cases in 10 separate outbreaks of typhoid fever.

Local and state public health resources were supplemented by the federal Public Health and Marine Hospital Service (now called the U.S. Public Health Service). Founded in 1798 to provide medical care for sailors as part of the Department of Treasury, this uniformed service had grown in responsibility by the end of the nineteenth century. The Commissioned Corps of the service detected and treated communicable illness in immigrants and prevented interstate spread of epidemic disease. The first bacteriology laboratory of the Public Health and Marine Hospital Service opened on Staten Island in 1887. This laboratory was moved to Washington, D.C., in 1903, then known as the Hygienic Laboratory. Under Dr. Milton Rosenau, it became a premier research institution on milk safety and was the nucleus for the National Institutes of Health.[13]

Food Safety Regulation in the Nineteenth and Twentieth Centuries

From the nineteenth century through the start of the twentieth century, regulatory control of food was driven by consumer health concerns and the partnership of local medical societies with honest businessmen and trade associations. Milk was one of the greatest concerns for regulators and consumers. Cows fed with cheap by-products of other industries (e.g., waste from cotton gins) gave bad-flavored milk. Producers could stretch supplies and improve the look and taste of inferior "swill milk" by adding water of dubious origin, magnesia, and chalk.[14] In 1862, after 40 years of effort, the New York State Legislature passed an act that levied a fine on anyone selling impure or adulterated milk.[14]

The first law applying to food in general was passed by Illinois in 1874, and in 1879, the first federal bill to prevent food adulteration was introduced. By 1895, a total of 27 states had passed some type of food regulation.[15] In 1883, because of concern about unsafe substances used to disguise spoiled foods, the Bureau of Chemistry within the Department of Agriculture, led by Harvey W. Wiley, began testing for such contaminants.

In 1906, two new regulations created the current federal food-regulatory system. Upton Sinclair's novel *The Jungle*, published earlier that year, highlighted poor working conditions in slaughter plants and focused national attention on the meat supply. The Meat Inspection Act mandated that a federal inspector be present at slaughter to examine each carcass for visible signs of disease and to reject grossly diseased animals.[16] The logic behind this law was that disease or carcass contamination that was visible to a trained inspector threatened the consumer. Also in 1906, the Meat Inspection Service was formed as an agency within the U.S. Department of Agriculture's Bureau of Animal Industry to fulfill the requirements of the Act. Though public confidence was restored, the efficacy of these meat inspections in preventing disease was not established, and doubts were soon expressed. For example, in 1912, Charles Chapin, a public health leader from Rhode Island, voiced the opinion that visual inspection did nothing to prevent trichinosis and thought it "doubtful whether any sickness among consumers has been prevented."[17] The Pure Food and Drug Act, passed on the same day as the Meat Inspection Act, addressed growing concern over toxic food additives and quack patent medicines. The act made the Bureau of Chemistry responsible for testing and regulating foods for the presence of adulterants and for regulating the misbranding of foods, drinks, and drugs transported via interstate commerce.[16] The logic behind this law was that laboratory tests would accurately identify unsafe levels of contamination in foods and that the threat of court actions based on these tests would prevent contamination. The Meat Inspection Act and the Pure Food and Drug Act established separate regulatory strategies for meat and for other foods, a duality that continues to this day.

Changes in the Food Supply

Over the course of the twentieth century, food preparation practices changed dramatically, as new technologies transformed the kitchen. The electric refrigerator became available during World War I, followed by gas and electric stoves, frozen foods, the precooked convenience dinner, and most recently, the microwave oven.[2] As illustrated by a wartime cookbook published in 1942, which included a chapter titled "Entertaining Without a Maid,"[22] the family cook was disappearing from middle-class homes. Food became increasingly processed before purchase, and the kitchen changed into a place for food storage and final meal assembly. In addition, more meals were outsourced to restaurants: by 1998, 38% of the family food budget was spent on food prepared and eaten outside the home.[23] The art of cooking disappeared from school curricula, and with the increasing popularity and availability of restaurants, cooking became optional for young adults living independently. Restaurants also increasingly provided employment opportunities. In 1997, the growing restaurant industry employed 6% of the nonfarm workers.[24]

As the United States became more urban and populous, food production became industrialized and involved larger and more centralized food-processing factories. Farms grew larger, crop yields and animal production-efficiency increased, and large agribusinesses replaced small family farms. Interstate transport of perishable foods began with refrigerated railroad cars in the 1870s and later largely switched to refrigerated trucks. Currently, refrigerated cargo jets transport highly perishable foods internationally, making fresh produce available year-round. The supermarket stocked with foods from around the world has become an icon of modern life. Availability of a wide variety of foods has helped spark changes in patterns of eating. U.S. consumers now eat more fruit and chicken than they used to and fewer eggs and less milk.[25] Health-conscious consumers seek foods that are lower in fat, salt, and cholesterol. Consumers also are increasingly seeking foods that contain fewer preservatives, and thus have fewer barriers to microbial growth.

Evolving Control of Pesticides and Other Chemicals in Foods

Insecticides and herbicides have increased crop yield, decreased food cost, and enhanced the appearance of food throughout the twentieth century.[26] However, residues of these pesticides remaining on foods also create potential health risks. During the 1950s and 1960s, the first pesticide regulations established maximum residue levels allowable on foods (the so-called residue tolerances) and established an approval process for pesticide use. In 1970, the new Environmental Protection Agency (EPA) took over the administration of many environmental regulations, including most of the regulation of pesticides used in food production. Propelled by public concern about the environmental impact of pesticides, the EPA removed dichlorodiphenyl-trichloroethane (DDT) and several other persistent pesticides from the U.S. marketplace, although they continue to be exported for use in other countries. In 1996, the Food Quality Protection Act focused on (1) the protection of children from pesticides, (2) the consumer's right to know the results of pesticide monitoring, and (3) the use of a single, health-based standard for all pesticide residues in food.

Currently, four agencies play major roles in protecting the public from pesticides and other chemical residues in food. The EPA approves and sets tolerances on pesticides used in food production and on other industrial chemicals that could contaminate food. The FDA determines which animal drugs can be used and establishes tolerances for residues of animal drugs in meat. The USDA tests meat and poultry for concentrations of residues that exceed tolerances set by the EPA and FDA. The health impact of pesticide exposure typically is chronic in nature and more difficult to estimate than the health effects of acute infections. However, the actual human exposure to pesticides can be measured with precision. In 1999, the CDC began monitoring this exposure by testing blood samples for residual pesticides.[27]

Improving Prevention Technologies

During the twentieth century, new prevention technologies were developed by scientists in industry, public health, and regulatory agencies for the most severe food-safety threats. The history of retort canning and of milk pasteurization illustrates the tenacious efforts that translated that research into universal protection.

Retort Food Canning

Canning was widely practiced in the nineteenth century, but was not well standardized at that time. Spores of the bacterium *Clostridium botulinum,* present in dirt and dust, survive boiling, so they may still be in vegetables that have been simply boiled as they are canned. The spores germinate and grow in conditions that are sufficiently moist and warm and that have minimal amounts of oxygen, such as the interior of a sealed can or jar. As they germinate, the bacteria can produce botulism toxin in the canned food. This potent toxin paralyzes muscles, including the muscles involved in respiration.

Before the development of modern intensive-care medicine, half of the persons affected by botulism died of respiratory paralysis. Even now, botulism often leads to many weeks in the intensive care unit.[28] During and after World War I, outbreaks of botulism focused attention on the public health hazard of poorly canned foods. These outbreaks, culminating in the dramatic 1919 multistate olive outbreaks described above, led state health departments to begin surveillance for botulism cases and drove the canning industry to fund research on safe canning methods. From this research evolved the standard *botulism retort cook* method of 1923. A retort is a large pressure cooker that uses steam under pressure to reach temperatures above 212° F. The new industry standard defined the higher temperature and length of time required to completely eliminate botulinum spores from canned food. This process reliably reduced botulinum spore counts from one trillion per gram—the highest conceivable level of contamination—to zero, a 12-log kill.[29] Thereafter, this standard retort cook method was enthusiastically and widely adopted by the canning industry.

In 1930, because of concern that canners were using vegetables of inferior quality, a federal quality standard was developed and titled the McNary-Mapes Amendment to the Pure Food and Drugs Act.[30] However, there were still concerns that defective can seams could allow spores to enter a can after heat treatment. In 1973, after an outbreak of botulism was traced to commercially canned vichyssoise soup that was adequately heated during canning but apparently became contaminated afterwards because of defects in the can, additional regulation was created to address that gap.[31]

Pasteurization of Milk

Milk pasteurization, another fundamental foodborne-disease prevention technology, was also slowly adopted in the twentieth century. In the early 1900s, tainted cows' milk was known to be a source of many infections, including typhoid fever, tuberculosis, diphtheria, and severe streptococcal infections; many families chose to routinely boil milk for infants.[7] The first commercial pasteurizing equipment was manufactured in Germany in 1882.[32] Pasteurization began in the United States as early as 1893, when private charity milk stations in New York City began to provide pasteurized milk to poor children through the city health department,[14] a movement that spread to other cities. In 1902, an estimated 5% of the New York City milk supply underwent heat treatment.[32]

By 1900, standard pasteurization was defined as 140° F for 20 minutes on the basis of the time and temperature required to inactivate *Mycobacterium tuberculosis*, the most heat-resistant pathogen known to affect milk at that time. These standards were confirmed by investigations of Dr. Milton Rosenau that were published in 1909.[33] Experiments conducted in a dairy plant in Endicott, New York, evaluated the effectiveness of commercial pasteurization equipment in killing *M. tuberculosis* in milk and led to a public health ordinance that defined pasteurization as heating to 142° F for 30 minutes in approved equipment. However, the technology was slow to be applied. Pasteurization was opposed by some who thought it might be used to market dirtier milk and that it might affect the nutritional value of milk.[34] Some persons concerned about recontamination during distribution maintained that the only way to guarantee the safety of milk was to boil it in the home just before drinking it.[32] In addition, many thought the best way to prevent milk-associated diseases was through scrupulous attention to animal health and to clean milk production, which could be supported by an on-farm inspection and certification system. While the subsequent certification movement led to substantial improvements in dairy conditions, outbreaks of illness caused by "certified" milk showed that dairy hygiene alone was not enough; pasteurization was also needed as a final processing step to guarantee milk safety.

Despite the evidence suggesting the importance of pasteurization in the milk production process, differing milk-safety strategies were adopted by different jurisdictions. Not until 1923 did a public health expert combine the two processes of pasteurization and certification. This expert, a U.S. Public Health Service officer in Alabama, used both a standard definition for milk that was clean enough to be pasteurized and a standard definition of the pasteurization process itself.[13] As other states signed on one by one, this standard became the national Public Health Service Standard Milk Ordinance of 1927. Under this ordinance, milk was first graded on the basis of the sanitation measures used in its production, and then only Grade A milk could be pasteurized.[35] By the end of the 1940s, pasteurization was heavily promoted and had become the norm. In 1950, after several cases of Q fever were attributed to raw-milk consumption, the issue was raised of whether *Coxiella burnetti*, the causative organism of Q fever, could survive pasteurization.[36] Research showed that this organism was even more resistant to heat than *M. tuberculosis*, so the temperature for pasteurization was raised to 145° F. Though regulation occurred at the local and state level, the Conference of Interstate Milk Shippers developed reciprocal inspection agreements in 1950, analogous to the function of the Interstate Shellfish Sanitation Conference. This body set standards for dairies of any size.[13] As a result, 99% of the fresh milk consumed in the United States is pasteurized Grade A.[37]

Universal acceptance of the practices of canning and pasteurization was not achieved for decades. For both technologies, time was needed to overcome concerns that these methods were unreliable, that they decreased nutritional value, and that they would mask poor food quality and sanitation. These concerns were ultimately addressed by formal grading processes that helped assure the public that milk would be clean enough to be pasteurized and that vegetables would be of high enough quality to be canned. Concerns about nutrient loss were found to be largely unwarranted, and were countered by fortifying milk with vitamins. Both processes were ultimately defined by clear microbial target endpoints so that *milk pasteurization* and a *botulism retort cook* were given standard meanings in all jurisdictions. The concern about equipment reliability was addressed through industry efforts and approval processes. The industry developed quality grading standards and pathogen-reduction processes and these were formally adopted via federal regulation.

As a result of these efforts, outbreaks of botulism caused by commercially canned foods and outbreaks of illness caused by pasteurized milk have become extremely rare. Foodborne botulism now affects approximately 25 persons a year, almost always those who have consumed home-canned vegetables or home-preserved meats and fish.[28] Although outbreaks of infections associated with unpasteurized milk still occur with some frequency, outbreaks caused by pasteurized milk are exceedingly rare, and are usually the result of post-pasteurization contamination.[37]

The Evolution of Surveillance and the Elimination of Other Foodborne Threats

Over the course of the twentieth century, public health surveillance grew from a local process, which was administered by individual counties and cities, to a nationwide network involving all states and the CDC. Since 1951, the Council of State and Territorial Epidemiologists (CSTE) has determined which conditions should be reported nationally; and since 1961, the CDC has published national surveillance data in the *Morbidity and Mortality Weekly Report* (*MMWR*). The list of notifiable diseases has changed over time, reflecting public health priorities and the availability of useful data. Notifiable disease surveillance is possible only for those conditions that are routinely diagnosed in clinical practice. Among foodborne diseases, typhoid fever and botulism surveillance data began to be collected early in the twentieth century, and collection of national statistics regarding non-typhoid salmonellosis began in 1942. In 1964, after a large multistate outbreak of *Salmonella* serotype Derby infections that affected many hospitals, reports of diagnosed cases of salmonellosis were supplemented by serotyping data from public health laboratories to create the national Salmonella Surveillance System.[38] State public health laboratories began serotyping strains of *Salmonella* sent to them from clinical laboratories, and the CDC began collecting weekly information on *Salmonella* that was serotyped. Since then, public health surveillance based on laboratory subtyping of infectious organisms has proved vital in detecting and investigating countless outbreaks of salmonellosis and many other diseases.

The federal regulatory apparatus also has evolved over the last 100 years.[16] (See Box 2.1.) The Bureau of Chemistry and the Meat Inspection Service have now become the Food and Drug Administration (FDA) and the Food Safety and Inspection Service (FSIS), respectively. The U.S. Public Health Service was moved from the Department of Treasury to become part of the new Federal Safety Agency, a precursor to the Department of Health and Human Services. In 1938, following a catastrophic outbreak of poisoning from an untested sulfanilamide elixir, passage of the Food, Drug, and Cosmetic Act gave the FDA authority to require pre-market testing of drugs and authority over food labeling and quality control. The act currently serves as the central authority for the FDA. Shortly after the passage of the act, the FDA was moved from the Department of Agriculture to the Federal Safety Agency because of the apparent conflict in mission between promoting the agriculture industry and maintaining food safety. In 1968, the FDA was added to the Public Health Service. As a vestige of its origin, the FDA is still funded through the congressional agriculture committees rather than through the health committees. The FSIS remains an agency within the U.S. Department of Agriculture.

Few statistics on foodborne disease morbidity were collected consistently throughout the twentieth century. However, the food supply is far safer by the twenty-first century than it was at the beginning of the 1900s. One index of the prevalence of food- and waterborne diseases is the infant mortality rate. From 1900 through 1950, this rate decreased rapidly from 141 per 1000 live births (for Massachusetts) to 29.2 per 1000 nationwide; life expectancy at birth increased from 47 to 68.2 years.[6] In 1950, deaths caused by gastroenteritis and typhoid fever had fallen to a rate of 5.1 and 0.1 per 100,000 population, respectively. National surveillance data are available for typhoid fever beginning in 1912, making it a useful marker. The incidence of typhoid fever fell precipitously with municipal water treatment, milk pasteurization, and shellfish-bed sanitation long before vaccines or antibiotics were commonly used (Fig. 2.1). Trichinosis, caused by eating pork infested with parasitic cysts, has become exceedingly rare. During the 1940s, an estimated 16% of persons in the United States had trichinosis, most of which was asymptomatic; 3,000–4,000 clinical cases were diagnosed every year, and 10–20 deaths occurred.[39] This disease was controlled by improving the safety of the foods consumed by pigs themselves and by breaking the cycle of transmission through garbage and swill. The rate of infection declined markedly as a result of these measures; from 1991 through 1996, only three deaths and an average of 38 cases were reported per year.[40] The spread of other serious zoonotic infections among animals also was controlled, virtually eliminating animal anthrax, tuberculosis, and brucellosis in herds. By the 1960s, foodborne infections, like many other infectious diseases, were believed to be under control.

Box 2.1. Landmark Events in the Evolution of Food-Safety Regulation in the United States, 1900–1999. (Adapted from Refs. 84, 121–27.)

1906   Pure Food and Drug Act. Regulates foods other than meat by prohibiting the interstate sale of food that is adulterated or misbranded.

1906   Meat Inspection Act. Sets sanitary standards for animal slaughter and for meat. Federal in-plant inspection began with power to condemn meat instantly.

1924   National Milk Safety Ordinance. Sets national standards for milk hygiene, microbial standards for milk grading, and uniform definition of pasteurization process.

1927   The Bureau of Chemistry reorganized. Regulatory functions are assigned to the new Food, Drug and Insecticide Administration (within the USDA), and nonregulatory functions are assigned to the Bureau of Chemistry and Soils.

1938   Federal Food, Drug and Cosmetic Act. This replaces the 1906 Pure Food and Drug Act and defines the process of regulatory approval for medicines, food additives, and drugs used in agriculture.

1939   The Federal Security Agency (FSA) created (precursor of the Department of Health and Human Services). The Public Health Service is moved into FSA from the Department of Treasury.

1940   The Food and Drug Administration moves into FSA from the Department of Agriculture.

1946   The National Communicable Disease Center organized in Atlanta, Georgia. Except for tuberculosis and venereal diseases, which had separate units in Washington, the CDC is given responsibility for national strategies for controlling all communicable disease, and for national reference laboratory functions. The Enteric Reference laboratory opens at CDC in 1949.

1950   The Epidemic Intelligence Service established at CDC. This provides emergency national response to outbreaks.

1951   Council of State and Territorial Epidemiologists. This is authorized to determine what diseases should be reported by states to the Public Health Service (see Ref. 85).

1953   The FSA becomes the Department of Health, Education and Welfare (HEW).

1958   Food Additives Amendment (the Delaney clause) passes. Regulates food additives thought to be potential carcinogens.

1961   CDC gains responsibility for publishing weekly reported human disease surveillance data.

1968   The FDA moves to be part of the Public Health Service.

1970   Presidential Reorganization Plan #3. Creates the Environmental Protection Agency, consolidating some pesticide regulations.

1996   Food Quality Protection Act. This eliminates the application of Delaney clause to pesticides.

1996   Pathogen Reduction Rule published by USDA. Changes meat inspection from manual and visual inspection of each carcass to supervised process monitoring, with national microbial standards for meat.

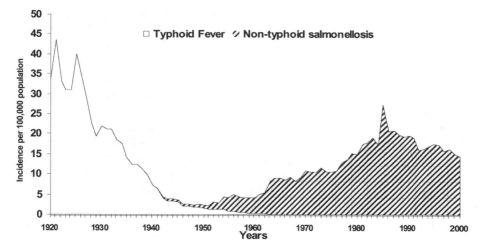

Figure 2.1. The fall of typhoid fever and the rise of nontyphoidal salmonellosis in the United States, 1920–2000. (CDC. National surveillance data.)

Emerging Challenges

An array of newly recognized pathogens illustrates the dynamic nature of foodborne disease. Although some pathogens (e.g., caliciviruses) have a human reservoir, most of these emerging foodborne pathogens are transmitted from animals; modern, industrialized food supply fosters the spread of pathogens through larger, more concentrated animal populations. Unlike typhoid fever, dysentery, and cholera, these infections are not associated with human sewage, but rather with animal manure. They often circulate among food animals without causing illness in them. Many nontyphoidal *Salmonella* strains have reservoirs in our food animals and serve as indicators of this phenomenon. Reports of these infections increased steadily from 1942, when reporting began, through 1990 (see Fig. 2.1). Healthy animals serve as reservoirs for other pathogens, including *Campylobacter* (endemic in healthy chickens), *E. coli* O157 (in cattle), and *Vibrio vulnificus* (in oysters). These pathogens are not detected by visual inspection of the animal. Because *V. vulnificus* is found naturally in warm brackish water, monitoring shellfish beds for human sewage contamination does not eliminate the risk of these pathogens. Even *Vibrio cholerae* O1, the great killer of the nineteenth century, was found to have an established natural niche in the bayous of the Gulf of Mexico, where it persists independent of human sewage contamination.[41] For some bacteria, antimicrobial resistance has emerged because of the use of antibiotics in agriculture (causing resistance in the pathogens *Salmonella* and *Campylobacter*) and human medicine (causing resistance in *Shigella*).[42]

Given the complexity of the U.S. food supply and the growing appetite for diverse cuisines in this country, the emergence of new challenges in the field of foodborne illness is not surprising. At least 13 pathogens have been identified or newly recognized as foodborne challenges since 1976, appearing at the rate of about one every

2 years (Table 2.2)[45] These emerging infections account for 82% of the estimated 13.8 million cases and 61% of the 1800 deaths attributable to known foodborne pathogens each year in the United States.[46] In contrast, five pathogens that were common before 1900 (i.e., *Brucella*, *Clostridium botulinum*, *Salmonella* Typhi, *Trichinella*, and toxigenic *Vibrio cholerae*) only caused an estimated 1500 cases and 13 deaths in 1997, many of which were associated with travel abroad. The preponderance of recently identified pathogens in the total burden reflects the progress that occurs in controlling pathogens once they are identified and studied.

Foodborne disease has been linked to an expanding variety of foods. Perishable foods increasingly are being imported into the United States from around the world, sometimes bringing pathogens with them. Immigrants, who tend to retain their native food habits and tastes, also can help introduce novel combinations of pathogens and foods.[47] Into the twenty-first century, outbreaks increasingly are being associated with fresh fruits and vegetables and less with foods historically implicated in foodborne disease.[48] Produce items are a particular concern because often they are eaten raw. Microbes can move to the interior of fruits and vegetables, where they cannot be washed off or killed by light cooking, as has been demonstrated experimentally with *E. coli* O157:H7 in apples and alfalfa sprouts.[49–51] Even growing vegetables in soil fertilized with manure containing *E. coli* O157:H7 can lead to internal contamination.[52]

Safety breakdowns in large, modern food-processing plants can result in outbreaks involving substantial numbers of persons. In 1986, post-pasteurization contamination of milk at a single dairy led to an estimated 150,000 infections with multidrug-resistant salmonellosis in seven states.[53] In 1995, a nationwide epidemic of *Salmonella* Enteritidis infections traced to a nationally distributed brand of ice cream caused illness in an estimated 250,000 persons.[54] That epidemic was caused by the use of the same refrigerated trucks to transport contaminated raw eggs and pasteurized ice cream ingredients, leading to post-pasteurization contamination of the ice cream products.

As new pesticides are developed and new food-production uses are authorized for existing compounds, unsuspected chemical contamination of food may occur.

Table 2.2. New and emerging foodborne pathogens identified since 1977, or whose connection with food was established since 1977.

Campylobacter jejuni
Campylobacter fetus ssp fetus
Cryptosporidium parvum
Cyclospora cayetanensis
Escherichia coli O157:H7 and other Shiga-toxin producing *E. coli*
Listeria monocytogenes
Norwalk-like viruses
Nitzchia pungens (the cause of amnesic shellfish poisoning)
Spongiform encephalopathy prions
Vibrio cholerae O1
Vibrio vulnificus
Vibrio parahaemolyticus
Yersinia enterocolitica

Unlike infectious exposures that cause disease quickly, toxic chemical exposures may take many years to be detected. These exposures may affect many persons at once. For example, in January 1999, a total of 500 tons of chicken feed contaminated with polychlorinated biphenyls (PCBs) and dioxins were distributed to farms in Belgium, leading to withdrawal of Belgian chickens from the market for several weeks. Estimates of the total number of human cancer cases that may ultimately result from this incident range between 40 and 8000.[55]

Three foodborne disease outbreaks in the United States shook the complacency of food safety professionals near the end of the twentieth century. In 1986, an estimated 3200 persons in eight states were infected with *Salmonella* Enteritidis after they ate a commercially packaged stuffed pasta (CDC, unpublished data). Although the product was labeled "fully cooked," the stuffing contained raw eggs, and the farm where the eggs originated harbored the same strains of *Salmonella* Enteritidis as were found in the ill case-patients and the pasta. This outbreak investigation led to the discovery that *S.* Enteritidis outbreaks were generally associated with egg-containing foods and explained a massive increase in infections caused by this type of *Salmonella*.[56] Eggs had previously been associated with salmonellosis in the 1960s, but contamination at that time occurred on the outside of the shell and therefore could be eliminated by routine disinfection. Following egg-associated outbreaks in the 1960s, egg grading, washing, and disinfection became the standard for the egg industry. However, the eggs in these new *S.* Enteritidis outbreaks all involved grade A disinfected eggs, suggesting that these *Salmonella* were on the inside of the shell. Researchers at the Department of Agriculture showed that hens fed *Salmonella* Enteritidis developed chronic, asymptomatic infections of their reproductive tracts and laid normal-looking eggs that contained *Salmonella* within their shells.[57] The pasta outbreak was the herald event in an epidemic of *S.* Enteridis infections among egg-laying chickens that began in the Northeast and spread across the nation.[58] As the epidemic spread to new states, tracing the eggs implicated in the outbreaks back to their source farms was crucial in showing each local egg industry that they, too, were affected by the epidemic. In response, new control measures are being implemented from farm to table, including better farm-management practices, refrigeration of eggs, education for cooks, and pasteurization of eggs while they are still in the shell.[59]

In 1993, an outbreak of *E. coli* O157:H7 infections on the West Coast caused 732 recognized illnesses, 55 cases of hemolytic uremic syndrome, and four deaths.[60, 61] This outbreak, caused by undercooked ground beef from one fast-food chain, had wide-reaching impact. The severity of the illness, the size of the outbreak, and the feeling of helplessness among parents of affected children shifted the prevailing notion that food safety was primarily an issue of consumer education and that consumers were responsible for cooking their food properly. After the hamburger outbreak in 1993, responsibility became redistributed to each link of the food-production chain. This outbreak brought food safety to the top of the nation's policy agenda, leading to substantial changes in the approach to both meat safety and the safety of food in general.

Following the 1993 outbreak, many states made *E. coli* O157:H7 infection and hemolytic uremic syndrome notifiable diseases. Molecular methods for characterizing strains were pilot-tested in that outbreak and subsequently become the basis for a new surveillance technology called PulseNet (vide infra). Food safety became an issue of public policy, and a new consumer action group (Safe Tables Our Priority, or STOP), consisting of parents of children harmed or killed in the outbreak, lobbied for change. Many restaurants and meat grinders put new emphasis on food-safety measures, and the meat supplier to the implicated fast-food restaurant chain became the industry leader in making meat safer. The Department of Agriculture declared *E. coli* O157:H7 to be an adulterant in raw ground beef, meaning that raw meat contaminated with *E. coli* O157:H7 should be withheld from trade. Perhaps most important, the strategy for meat inspections shifted from direct visual and manual carcass inspection, as had been done since 1906, to a new system, called Hazard Analysis and Critical Control Point (HACCP) monitoring. The HACCP monitoring relies on process controls (e.g., more careful slaughter, steam scalding, and more cleansing of equipment to reduce pathogens) and on testing the finished meat for microbial contamination to ensure that the process meets national standards.[62]

In the spring of 1996, a total of 1465 persons in 20 states, the District of Columbia, and two Canadian provinces became ill with a distinctive combination of recurrent diarrhea and extreme fatigue. The organism implicated in this outbreak was the newly recognized parasite *Cyclospora cayetanensis*.[63] Illnesses were linked to eating fresh raspberries imported from Guatemala, where this crop had been recently introduced; the way in which the berries became contaminated, however, remains unknown. Investigators in Guatemala found that the same organism caused a springtime wave of diarrhea in the children of agricultural workers, who became ill after drinking untreated water.[64] After procedural changes on raspberry farms and in the living conditions of Guatemalan workers, limited raspberry imports resumed, though with recurrent outbreaks, production of raspberries for export was greatly reduced.[75] The epidemic, which brought the obscure *Cyclospora* organism to the fore, demonstrates how foodborne pathogens considered to occur only rarely can suddenly appear, and it illustrates the potential hazards associated with growing fresh produce in the developing world, flying it to the developed world, and eating it after only a quick rinse. The incident illustrates the close connection between the poor conditions of workers' lives in the developing world and the casual treatment of U.S. dinner plates.

Now, at the beginning of the twenty-first century, foodborne disease remains unconquered. The burden of foodborne diseases in the United States, newly estimated using the most recent and improved surveillance data, is 76 million cases of foodborne infections each year; one in four Americans are affected annually, leading to 323,000 hospitalizations and 5000 deaths.[46] An increasing array of pathogens are being recognized as being foodborne (Table 2.3), and much of the foodborne disease burden is not accounted for by known pathogens, indicating that many more are yet to be identified. The previously idiopathic Guillain Barre syndrome and hemolytic uremic syndrome are now known to be postinfectious complications of *Campylobacter* and *E. coli* O157:H7 infections, respectively. Other apparently idiopathic syndromes also may prove in the future to follow foodborne infections.

Table 2.3. Principal foodborne infections in 1997, ranked
by estimated annual number of cases caused by foodborne transmission, United States [46]. (Values over 1,000 are rounded to
the nearest 1000.)

Norwalk-like viruses	9,200,000
Campylobacter	1,963,000
Salmonella (nontyphoid)	1,342,000
Clostridium perfringens	249,000
Giardia lamblia	200,000
Staphylococcus food poisoning	185,000
Toxoplasma gondii	112,000
E. coli O157:H7 and other Shiga-toxin producing *E. coli*	92,000
Shigella	90,000
Yersinia enterocolitica	87,000
Enterotoxigenic *E. coli*	56,000
Streptococci	51,000
Astrovirus	39,000
Rotavirus	39,000
Cryptosporidium parvum	30,000
Bacillus cereus	27,000
Other *E. coli*	23,000
Cyclospora cayetanensis	14,000
Vibrio (non cholera)	5000
Hepatitis A	4000
Listeria monocytogenes	2000
Brucella	777
Salmonella Typhi (typhoid fever)	659
Botulism	56
Trichinella	52
Vibrio cholerae, toxigenic	49

The Lessons of Prevention

Although no vaccine exists for most emerging foodborne pathogens, the progress in food safety in the twentieth century shows that other strategies of prevention can be highly effective, including controlling the pathogens at the food-animal reservoir, preventing the pathogens from contaminating foods, stopping the multiplication of pathogens that get into food, and killing pathogens already present on food (Table 2.4). Success has often depended on understanding the precise mechanisms of transmission well enough to interrupt them with targeted control measures and new technologies.

Early in the twentieth century, the stream of human sewage was separated from the human food and water supplies, controlling many infections for which humans are the primary reservoir. More recent advances have prevented animal manure from contaminating human food and water supplies. Now, control of some foodborne diseases depends on improving the safety of the food and water that the animals themselves consume.

Table 2.4. Generalized schema of foodborne disease prevention.

Production Stage	Sources or Multipliers of Contamination	Control Strategies in	
		Current Use	Future
Growing or rearing	Contaminated feed and water, manure, wildlife, other animals	Feed sterility, animal disease control, rodent control, biosecurity, competitive exclusion	Water treatment, manure treatment, feed security, vaccination, probiotics
Slaughter or harvest and processing	Water baths and sprays, fecal contamination, cross-contamination	HACCP,* plant sanitation, inspection, microbial testing, water disinfection, steam scalding, pasteurization, irradiation	Irradiation, high pressure, intense light, new additives
Distribution	Contaminated ice, poor refrigeration, dirty trucks	Ice regulation, refrigeration, vehicle disinfection	Dedicated vehicles
Cooking	Cross-contamination, time/ temperature abuse, ill food handler	Food handler education, handwashing, facility inspection and licensing	Food handler certification, paid sick leave, automated handwashing

*Hazard analysis and critical control point programs, which apply safety engineering principles to food production.

Despite recent advances, ill humans still can contaminate the foods they prepare in the kitchen, and the increase in food preparation outside of the home sparks concern for the health and hygiene of restaurant workers. Infections with caliciviruses, *Shigella* and hepatitis A can easily spread from ill food handlers to consumers via food. The unwary cook also can easily transfer microbes from raw meat to other foods being prepared or make other food-handling errors that can lead to illness in the consumer. Such problems will persist until food handlers are routinely educated in food safety, have clear incentives for hand washing and other hygiene practices, and can take paid leave for illness.

For some foods, especially those that are the pooled products of many animals, even meticulous sanitation may not prevent contamination of the final product, and a definitive pathogen elimination technology is critical. The history of pasteurization is a model for other efforts. The shift in public health strategy for milk from advising homemakers to boil their infant's milk to requiring the dairy industry to provide pathogen-free milk for all consumers is a model to be followed for other high-risk foods.

Disease prevention is a cyclical process (Fig. 2.2). First, surveillance of an infection is conducted to measure the burden of the problem, track the success or failure

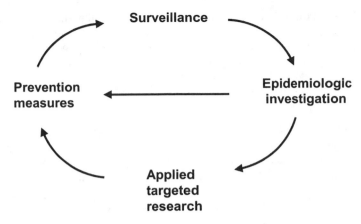

Figure 2.2. The cycle of prevention in public health (as proposed by Dr. Paul Mead).

of control measures, and detect outbreaks. Outbreak investigations then are initiated to discover new pathogens, new food sources of infection, and gaps in the food-safety system. These investigations can link a specific pathogen to a particular food, identify the likely point of contamination, and therefore define the point at which better control is needed. The investigation may lead directly to control or may identify the type of applied research needed; applied research conducted by industry, academic scientists, and government researchers can lead to successful prevention measures. New regulatory approaches may be suggested or endorsed by industry, consumer groups, and regulatory agencies. Once short-term control and long-term prevention measures are applied, continued surveillance defines whether they are successful. For major public health threats, ultimate control may require repeated turns of this cycle.

Improving Surveillance, Improving Prevention

Improvements in public health surveillance can propel improved disease prevention. In the United States, several developments made in the last 5 years of the twentieth century are increasing the scope and the sensitivity of public health surveillance. National surveillance was begun for several of the newly recognized conditions, including *E. coli* O157:H7 in 1993, *Cyclospora* in 1996, and *Listeria monocytogenes* in 1998. *Salmonella* serotype-specific surveillance data sent electronically from state public health laboratories to the CDC began to be routinely analyzed for state, regional, and national surges in the incidence of specific serotypes using the Surveillance Outbreak Detection Algorithm (SODA).[65] In addition to enhanced nationwide surveillance, a new active surveillance effort, called FoodNet, began in 1996 in five participating state health departments (*www.cdc.gov/foodnet*). Growing to eight participating sites by 2000, FoodNet's active surveillance has provided accurate, detailed information about diagnosed infections with pathogens that are likely to be foodborne as well as surveys of laboratory practices and of the general population.[76]

Standardized subtyping of foodborne pathogens increases the ability of public health surveillance to detect and investigate outbreaks.[66] Just as standardized serotyping revolutionized *Salmonella* surveillance in the 1960s, PulseNet now provides molecular DNA "fingerprints" to enhance surveillance for several bacterial foodborne pathogens. PulseNet is the national network for molecular subtyping of these pathogens, connecting all state public health laboratories, federal food regulatory agency laboratories, and Canadian health authorities. Through PulseNet, participating laboratories use a standardized pulsed-field gel electrophoresis (PFGE) method to produce a molecular DNA fingerprint of bacterial strains isolated from ill persons. Although knowing the fingerprint does not influence patient care, it can be critical for public health surveillance. The fingerprints from various state laboratories can be compared online with each other and with a national database maintained at the CDC. The appearance of a pattern in many states at once may be the first indication of a widespread outbreak, for which a detailed epidemiologic investigation could be implemented to determine the source. Because laboratories at the FDA and FSIS participate in PulseNet, strains of bacteria isolated from foods can be compared with strains that affect humans.

Better surveillance in the twentieth century increasingly unveiled widespread outbreaks involving many jurisdictions. Before modern surveillance technologies were available, recognized foodborne outbreaks typically fit the textbook pattern of a sharp local increase in cases following a local common exposure (e.g., a catered event). Disease-control efforts were handled by local health departments and would commonly entail closure of a restaurant, destruction of a batch of food, and/or education of a food handler. Occasionally, a link would be observed between outbreaks occurring in several places at once, such as the botulism outbreak of 1919 or the typhoid fever outbreak of 1924, but such recognition was rare.

Currently, geographically dispersed outbreaks are being recognized more frequently because of serotyping and the PulseNet system. Dispersed outbreaks do not cause a sharp local increase in cases, but instead cause a few apparently sporadic cases in many jurisdictions concurrently. In addition, they often are caused by foods contaminated at a low level and shipped to many places. The increase in cases in any one place may not be sufficient to attract notice from public health professionals; therefore, widespread outbreaks are detected only when the bacterial strains are subtyped in public health laboratories and are then compared with strains from many jurisdictions. Subsequent investigation can identify a systematic problem in food production or processing that can have implications for the entire industry.

In recent years, PulseNet has revealed many dispersed outbreaks that follow this new scenario, and the investigations have led to substantial advances in prevention. In 1997, shortly after the state health department in Colorado began testing *E. coli* O157:H7 isolates with PulseNet, 16 cases of infection with the same unusual pattern were detected in Colorado and in a neighboring state.[67] These cases were linked to ground beef produced at a large factory. Because that plant worked leftover beef from one production lot into subsequent days' production, the volume of potentially contaminated meat was an astounding 25 million pounds of meat. This meat was recalled, and the re-work practice was discouraged throughout the industry. In 1998, an increase in apparently sporadic *Listeria* cases occurred in several states, just as the PulseNet method for *Listeria* was first being implemented. A total of 101 cases in 22 states were identified as having the same DNA fingerprint and were associated with the consumption of cooked hot dogs from one production plant.[68] In response to this finding, the company instituted a recall of the hot dog products. Investigation suggested that further measures were needed to control recontamination of hot dogs after processing. Such measures are now being considered by the entire industry. In 1999, a cluster of 78 *Salmonella* Newport infections in 13 states was detected by SODA and PFGE subtyping.[69] Epidemiologic investigation linked these cases to consumption of fresh imported mangoes. The mangoes had been treated with a new hot-water dip process that had been developed to replace methyl bromide fumigation for the elimination of fruit flies before export. As a result of the investigation, this process is being modified as it is introduced worldwide. In 2000, a cluster of *Salmonella* Enteritidis infections with the same unusual PFGE pattern was detected by SODA in western states; 88 infections in eight states were associated with drinking unpasteurized orange juice that had been treated with an alternative to pasteurization.[70] Following this outbreak, the federal regulations for juice were revised to make contamination less likely to recur.[71]

Monitoring of the frequency of contamination with pathogens and toxins in foods has been expanded. The new meat safety and inspection rule, published in 1996 by USDA, includes routine monitoring of ground beef for *E. coli* O157:H7 and of meat and poultry for the prevalence of *Salmonella*. In addition, limits are set on the frequency with which *Salmonella* is permitted on raw meat products.[62] Since 1967, the FSIS National Residue Program has monitored chemical residues in meat, poultry, and egg products, enforcing the safe limits set by the FDA and EPA and focusing on those residues most likely to have the greatest impact on public health.[72] Similarly, since 1991, the Agricultural Marketing Service monitors pesticide residues in fresh produce.[73] The systematic monitoring of the food supply for pathogens opens the door for tracking and quantifying the flow of pathogens by comparing the distribution of serotypes and subtypes in both food and case-patients.

The recent focus on the safety of many foods, including meat and poultry, eggs, seafood, and fresh produce, may be leading to fewer infections. In the early 1990s, industry efforts to reduce post-cooking contamination of hot dogs and other ready-to-eat meats were followed by a decline in *Listeria* infections of approximately 44%.[74] Egg safety efforts from farm to table also appear to be working, as the incidence of *Salmonella* Enteritidis infections has also declined 44% since the peak in 1995.[59] *Cyclospora* appears to have been controlled by Guatemalan raspberry farm sanitation and limitations on Guatemalan raspberry imports.[75] From 1996 through 2000, the total incidence of the principal bacterial foodborne infections under surveillance at FoodNet declined 13%.[76] These modest but sustained declines indicate some success in recent efforts to reduce *Campylobacter*, *Salmonella*, and *Listeria* infections. However, the incidence of *E. coli* O157:H7 infections remained stable during this four-year period, indicating a need for further investigations into the spread of this pathogen and for further prevention efforts (e.g., the irradiation of ground beef).

Expectations for the Twenty-First Century

We should expect the unexpected in the future.[77] More novel pathogens will be recognized, and established pathogens will appear in new food vehicles. In addition, as the population of the United States ages and becomes more subject to immunocompromising conditions and treatments, the number of persons at higher risk for foodborne infections grows. The continued globalization of food production and increasing international travel will result in new food sources, cuisines, and food-processing methods to create more challenges for the control of foodborne diseases. We can meet these challenges with a flexible and responsive public health system and a commitment to the surveillance, investigation, and research needed to find solutions. Collaborative international efforts will be critical to increase cooperation across international borders. The spectre of bioterrorism forces consideration of the security of our food supply as well as its safety. A strong and flexible public health infrastructure with enhanced surveillance and investigative capacity is a critical bulwark against foodborne bioterrorism.[78]

The philosophic shift that places responsibility for food safety within each link of the food chain will continue. The entire food industry will be increasingly involved in developing food-safety plans and standards, as each link in the chain imposes them on their suppliers. Microbial standards will increasingly be written into purchase contracts. Increasing consumer food-safety education will mean that more consumers demand safer food to begin with. The scope of the shift in food-safety responsibility is illustrated in Europe, where the consumer perspective now governs food-safety policy after the bovine spongiform encephalopathy epidemic led to a collapse in public confidence.

Preventing contamination before food reaches the consumer will be increasingly important. For many zoonotic pathogens, this means bringing elements of the human urban sanitary revolution to animal production, including reliable disinfection of drinking water and disposal of collected feces. For example, *Campylobacter* in chicken flocks and *E. coli* O157 in dairy herds may be spread among the animals through contaminated drinking water and perhaps through multiplication in feedstuffs.[79,80] Feed and water hygiene on farms may play a key role in the spread of virulent *Salmonella* strains like Typhimurium DT104 and multidrug-resistant *Salmonella* Newport. The importance of such hygiene is illustrated by the European epidemic of bovine spongiform encephalopathy that became foodborne in cattle when they were fed brain tissue from cattle with the disease; it subsequently spread to people who presumably consumed beef. Control will depend on complete elimination of unsafe cattle by-products from cattle feed.[81,82]

New regulatory approaches can orchestrate the work of many partners in disease prevention. Pathogen reduction can be achieved by setting specific targets, or food-safety objectives, similar to tolerance limits that are set for pesticides. However, because microbes multiply, the process will not be as simple. Risk-assessment modeling can help account for biologic complexity and can indicate which critical processes must be monitored to achieve the goal.

New prevention technologies are critical to progress in food safety, including vaccinating animals against zoonotic foodborne pathogens and feeding them nonpathogenic enteric organisms to prevent the colonization of harmful microbes. Composting treatments that reliably rid animal manure of pathogens have not yet been standardized. Treating foods with ionizing radiation, an important process that is now being adopted, can eliminate many pathogens from foods and would substantially reduce the burden of bacterial foodborne illness.[83] Other pathogen elimination technologies may be useful, including high-pressure treatment, ultrasound, and high-intensity light. The successes of the twentieth century and the new challenges faced mean that public health surveillance, scientific investigation of new problems, responsible attention to food safety from farm to table, and partnerships to bring about new control measures will be crucial to the control and prevention of foodborne disease into the foreseeable future.

Acknowledgments

We gratefully acknowledge the thoughtful reviews of Jose Rigau, Ellen Koch, Balasubramanian Swaminathan, Patricia Griffin, Cynthia Tauxe, and the advice of many others.

References

1. Abstract of the Twelfth Census of the United States, 1900. Washington, DC: Census Office, Government Printing Office, 1902.
2. Ierley M. Open House: A Guided Tour of the American Home, 1637–Present. New York: Henry Holt, 1999.
3. Porter M. Mrs. Porter's new Southern cookery book. In: Szathmary LI ed. Cookery Americana. Philadelphia: John E Potter, 1871.
4. Sixth Annual Report of the State Board of Health of Ohio. Columbus, OH: State Board of Health, 1890.
5. Melosi M. The Sanitary City: Urban Infrastructure in America from Colonial Times to the Present. Baltimore: Johns Hopkins University Press, 2000.
6. Historical Statistics of the United States. Colonial Times to 1970, Part 1, Bicentennial ed. Washington, DC: Bureau of the Census, U.S. Department of Commerce, 1975.
7. Rosenau MJ. Preventative Medicine and Hygiene, 5th ed. New York: D Appleton, 1928.
8. Gaffky G. Zur aetiologie des abdominaltyphus. *Mittheilungen aus den Kaiserlichen Gesundheitsamte* 1884:2:372–420.
9. Karlinski J. Zur kenntnis des *Bacillus enteritidis* gaertner. *Zentralbl Bakteriol Mikrobiol Hyg [B]* 1889:6:289–92.
10. van Ermengem E. Ueber einen neuen anaeroben Bacillus und seine Beziehungen zum Botulismus. *Z Hyg Infek* 1897:26:1–56.
11. Duffy J. The Sanitarians: A History of American Public Health. Chicago: University of Chicago Press, 1990.
12. Soper G. Typhoid Mary. *The Military Surgeon* 1919:45:1–15.
13. Williams R. The United States Public Health Service: 1798–1950, vol. 2. Washington, DC: Commissioned Officers Association of the United States Public Health Service, 1951.
14. Duffy J. Public Health in New York City 1866–1966. New York: Russell Sage Foundation, 1974.
15. Okun M. Fair Play in the Marketplace: The First Battle for Pure Food and Drugs. Dekalb, IL: Northern Illinois University Press, 1986.
16. Merrill R, Francer J. Organizing federal food safety regulation. *Seton Hall Law Review* 2000:31:61–173.

17. Chapin C. Sources and Modes of Infection. New York: John Wiley, 1912.
18. Armstrong C. Botulism from eating canned ripe olives. *Public Health Rep* 1919:34: 2877–905.
19. Botulism: protective measures and cautions from the U. S. Bureau of Chemistry, Department of Agriculture. *Public Health Rep* 1920:35:327–30.
20. Lumsden L, Hasseltine H, Veldee M. A typhoid fever epidemic caused by oyster-borne infections (1924–1925). *Public Health Rep* 1925:50(suppl):1–102.
21. History of the National Shellfish Sanitation Program. Interstate Shellfish Sanitation Conference, 2000 Refer to:http://www.issc.org/issc/NSSP/Background/history_nssp.htm. Accessed January 27, 2001.
22. Berolzheimer R. The American Woman's Cook Book. Chicago: Consolidated Book Publishers, 1942.
23. Manchester A. Food consumption: household food expenditures. U.S. Department of Agriculture, Economic Research Service, 2000. Refer to: www.ers.usda.gov/briefing/consumption/Expenditures.htm. Accessed January 30, 2001.
24. Statistical Abstract of the United States, 1998. Washington, DC: Bureau of the Census, Government Printing Office, 1998.
25. Putnam J. Major trends in the U.S. food supply, 1909–99. *Food Rev* 2000:23:8–15.
26. History of American agriculture 1776–1990. In: Farm Machinery and Technology 2001. Economic Research Service, U.S. Department of Agriculture. Refer to: www.usda.gov/history2/text4.htm. Accessed June 15, 2001.
27. National Report on Human Exposure to Environmental Chemicals. Atlanta: Centers for Disease Control and Prevention, 2001.
28. Botulism in the United States, 1899–1996. In: Handbook for Epidemiologists, Clinicians and Laboratory Workers. Atlanta: Centers for Disease Control and Prevention, 1998.
29. Esty J, Meyer K. The heat resistance of spores of *B. botulinus* and allied anaerobes. *J Infect Dis* 1922:31:434.
30. Shrader JH. Food Control: Its Public Health Aspects. New York: John Wiley, 1939.
31. Thermally-processed low acid foods packaged in hermetically sealed containers. *Federal Register* 1973:38:2398.
32. Westhoff D. Heating milk for microbial destruction: a historical outline and update. *J Food Protect* 1978:41:122–30.
33. Rosenau M. The Thermal Death Time of Pathogenic Micro-organisms in Milk. [Hygienic Laboratory Bulletin #56]. Washington, DC: United States Public Health and Marine Hospital Service, 1909.
34. Potter M, Kaufmann A, Blake P, Feldman R. Unpasteurized milk: the hazards of a health fetish. *JAMA* 1984:252:2048–54.
35. Milk investigations: preparation of a standard milk-control code. In: Annual Report of the Surgeon General of the Public Health Service of the United States for the Fiscal Year 1928. Washington, DC: United States Public Health Service, 1928, 53.
36. Bell J, Beck M, Huebner R. Epidemiological studies of Q fever in southern California. *JAMA* 1950:142:868–72.
37. Headrick M, Korangy S, Bean N, Angulo F, Altekruse S, Potter M, Klontz K. The epidemiology of raw milk-associated foodborne disease outbreaks reported in the United States, 1973 through 1992. *Am J Public Health* 1998:88:1219–21.
38. Proceedings of the National Conference on Salmonellosis. In: National Conference on Salmonellosis. Atlanta: Centers for Disease Control, 1964.
39. Schantz P. Trichinosis in the United States—1947–1981. *Food Tech* 1983:83–86.
40. Moorhead A. Trichinellosis in the United States, 1991–1996: declining but not gone. *Am J Trop Med Hyg* 1999:60:66–9.

41. Blake PA. Endemic cholera in Australia and the United States. In: Wachsmuth IK, Blake PA, Olsvik O eds. *Vibrio cholerae* and Cholera. Washington, DC: American Society for Microbiology, 1994:309–19.

42. Lee LA, Puhr ND, Maloney EK, Bean NH, Tauxe RV. Increase in antimicrobial-resistant Salmonella infections in the United States. *J Infect Dis* 1994:170:128–34.

43. Smith K, Besser J, Hedberg C, et al. Quinolone-resistant infections of *Campylobacter jejuni* in Minnesota, 1992–1998. *N Engl J Med* 1999:340:1525–32.

44. Tauxe R, Puhr N, Wells JG, Hargrett-Bean N, Blake P. Antimicrobial resistance of Shigella isolates in the USA: The importance of international travelers. *J Infect Dis* 1990:162:1107–11.

45. Tauxe RV. Emerging foodborne diseases: an evolving public health challenge. *Emerg Infect Dis* 1997:3:425–34.

46. Mead P, Slutsker L, Dietz V, et al. Food-related illness and death in the United States. *Emerg Infect Dis* 1999:5:607–25.

47. Mead PS, Mintz ED. Ethnic eating: foodborne disease in the global village. *Infect Dis Clin Pract* 1996:5:319–23.

48. Tauxe RV, Kruse H, Hedberg C, Potter M, Madden J, Wachsmuth. Microbial hazards and emerging issues associated with produce: a preliminary report to the National Advisory Committee on Microbiologic Criteria for Foods. *J Food Protect* 1997:60:1400–8.

49. Buchanan R, Edelson S, Miller R, Sapers G. Contamination of intact apples after immersion in an aqueous environment containing Escherichia coli O157:H7. *J Food Protect* 1999:62:444–50.

50. Taormina P, Beuchat L, Slutsker L. Infections associated with eating seed sprouts: an international concern. *Emerg Infect Dis* 1999:5:626–34.

51. Burnett S, Chen J, Beuchat L. Attachment of *Escherichia coli* O157:H7 to the surfaces and internal structures of apples as detected by confocal scanning laser microscopy. *Appl Environ Microbiol* 2000:66:4679–87.

52. Solomon E, Yaron S, Matthews K. T 31 Transmission and internalization of *Escherichia coli* O157:H7 from contaminated cow manure into lettuce tissue as monitored by laser scanning confocal microscopy. In: International Association for Food Protection, 88th Annual Meeting. Minneapolis, MN, 2001.

53. Ryan C, Nickels M, Hargrett-Bean N, et al. Massive outbreak of antimicrobial-resistant salmonellosis traced to pasteurized milk. *JAMA* 1987:258:3269–74.

54. Hennessy TW, Hedberg CW, Slutsker L, et al. A national outbreak of *Salmonella* Enteritidis infections from ice cream. *N Engl J Med* 1996:334:1281–86.

55. van Larebeke N, Hens L, Schepens P, et al. The Belgian PCB and dioxin incident of January-June 1999: exposure data and potential impact on health. *Environ Health Perspect* 2001:109:265–73.

56. St. Louis ME, Morse DL, Potter ME, et al. The emergence of Grade A eggs as a major source of *Salmonella* Enteritidis infections: implications for the control of salmonellosis. *JAMA* 1988:259:2103–7.

57. Gast R. Applying experimental infection models to understand the pathogenesis, detection and control of *Salmonella enterica* serovar Enteritidis in poultry. In: Saeed A, Gast R, Potter M, Wall P, eds. *Salmonella enterica* serovar Enteritidis in Humans and Animals: Epidemiology, Pathogenesis, and Control. Ames, IA: Iowa State University Press, 1999, chap. 2, 233–43.

58. Angulo FJ, Swerdlow DL. Epidemiology of human *Salmonella enterica* Serovar Enteritidis infections in the United States. In: Saeed AM, Gast RK, Potter ME, Wall PG, eds. *Salmonella enterica* serovar Enteritidis in Humans and Animals: Epidemiology, Pathogenesis, and Control. Ames, IA: Iowa State University Press, 1999, 33–41.

59. Outbreaks of *Salmonella* serotype Enteritidis infections associated with eating raw or undercooked shell eggs—United States, 1996–1998. *MMWR* 2000:49:73–79.
60. Bell BP, Goldoft M, Griffin PM, et al. A multistate outbreak of *Escherichia coli* O157:H7-associated bloody diarrhea and hemolytic uremic syndrome from hamburgers: the Washington experience. *JAMA* 1994:272:1349–53.
61. Griffin P, Bell B, Cieslak P, et al. Large outbreak of *Escherichia coli* O157:H7 infections in the Western United States: The big picture. In: Karmali M, Goglio A, eds. Recent Advances in Verotoxin-producing *Escherichia coli* Infections. Amsterdam: Elsevier, 1994:7–12.
62. Pathogen reduction: hazard analysis and critical control point (HACCP) systems; the final rule. *Federal Register* 1996:61:38805–989.
63. Herwaldt B, Ackers M, the Cyclospora Working Group. An outbreak in 1996 of cyclosporiasis associated with imported raspberries. *N Engl J Med* 1997:336:1548–56.
64. Bern C, Hernandez B, Lopez M, et al. Epidemiologic studies of *Cyclospora cayetanensis* in Guatemala. *Emerg Infect Dis* 1999:5:766–74.
65. Hutwagner LC, Maloney EK, Bean NH, Slutsker L, Martin SM. Using laboratory-based surveillance data for prevention: an algorithm for detecting *Salmonella* outbreaks. *Emerg Infect Dis* 1997:3:395–400.
66. Swaminathan B, Barrett T, Hunter S, Tauxe R, and the CDC PulseNet Task Force. PulseNet, the molecular subtyping network for foodborne bacterial disease surveillance, United States. *Emerg Infect Dis* 2001:7:382–89.
67. Centers for Disease Control and Prevention. *Escherichia coli* O157:H7 infections associated with eating a nationally distributed commercial brand of frozen ground beef patties and burgers—Colorado, 1997. *MMWR* 1997:46:777–78.
68. Centers for Disease Control and Prevention. Update: Multistate outbreak of listeriosis—United States. *MMWR* 1999:47:1085–86.
69. Sivapalasingam S, Barrett E, Kimura A, et al. A multistate outbreak of *Salmonella enterica* serotype Newport infections linked to mango consumption: Impact of water-dip disinfestation technology. *Clin Infect Dis* 2003:37:1585–90.
70. Rangel J, Kimura A, Palumbo M, et al. Multistate outbreak of *Salmonella* Enteritidis infections linked to consumption of unpasteurized orange juice. Abstract no. 650 In: 38th Annual Meeting, Infectious Diseases Society of America, New Orleans, LA, 2000.
71. Food and Drug Adminstration. FDA publishes final rule to increase safety of fruit and vegetable juices, 2001. Available at: www.fda.gov/bbs/topics/NEWS/2001/NEW00749.html Accessed on June 15, 2001.
72. 2000 FSIS National Residue Program. Washington, DC: Food Safety and Inspection Service, 2000.
73. Pesticide Data Program: Annual Summary, Calendar Year 1999. Washington, DC: Agricultural Marketing Service, Department of Agriculture, 2001.
74. Tappero J, Schuchat A, Deaver K, Mascola L, Wenger J. Reduction in the incidence of human listeriosis in the United States: effectiveness of prevention efforts? *JAMA* 1995:273:1118–22.
75. Herwaldt B. *Cyclospora cayetanensis*: a review, focusing on the outbreaks of cyclosporiasis in the 1990s. *Clin Infect Dis* 2000:31:1040–57.
76. Centers for Disease Control. Preliminary Foodnet data on the incidence of foodborne illnesses—selected sites, United States, 2000. *MMWR* 2001:50:241–46.
77. Swerdlow D, Altekruse S. Foodborne diseases in the global village: what's on the plate for the 21st century. In: Scheld W, Craig W, Hughes J, eds. Emerging Infections 2. Washington, DC: ASM Press, 1998,273–94.
78. Sobel J, Khan AS, Swerdlow DL. Threat of a biological terrorist attack on the US food supply. *Lancet* 2002: 359:874–80.

79. Kapperud G, Skjerve E, Vik L, et al. Epidemiological investigations of risk factors for *Campylobacter* colonization in Norwegian broiler flocks. *Epidemiol Infect* 1993:111: 245–55.
80. Hancock D, Besser T, Rice D. Ecology of *Escherichia coli* O157:H7 in cattle and impact of management practices. In: Kaper J, O'Brien A (eds.), *Escherichia coli* O157:H7 and other Shiga toxin-producing *E. coli strains*. Washington, DC: American Society for Microbiology Press, 1998, 85–91.
81. Taylor D, Woodgate S. Bovine spongiform encephalopathy: the causal role of ruminant-derived protein in cattle diets. *RevSciTech* 1997:16:187–98.
82. Will R, Ironside J, Zeidler M, et al. A new variant of Creutzfeld-Jakob disease in the UK. *Lancet* 1996:347:921–25.
83. Tauxe R. Food safety and irradiation: protecting the public health from foodborne infections. *Emerg Infect Dis* 2001:7:516–21.
84. Ensuring Safe Food, from Production to Consumption. Washington, DC: National Academy Press, 1998.
85. Thacker S. Historical development. In: Teutsch S, Churchill R, eds. Principles and Practice of Public Health Surveillance. New York: Oxford University Press, 1994, 3–17.

Suggested Reading

Duffy J. The Sanitarians: A History of American Public Health. Chicago: University of Chicago Press, 1990.
Melosi M. The Sanitary City: Urban Infrastructure in America from Colonial Times to the Present. Baltimore: Johns Hopkins University Press, 2000.
Tauxe RV. Molecular subtyping and the transformation of public health. Foodborne Pathogens and Diseases. 2006:3:4–8.

3

A Brief Romance with Magic Bullets: René Dubos at the Dawn of the Antibiotic Era

JILL E. COOPER

On September 8, 1939, René Jules Dubos, an attendee at the International Congress in Soil Science, climbed the stairs to the podium at the glamorous Waldorf-Astoria Hotel in New York City. Dubos, a little-known yet promising scientist from the nearby Rockefeller Institute for Medical Research, carried with him a bottle containing 500 g of a potent new bactericide he and a colleague had isolated from soil bacteria. He was about to introduce the world to tyrothricin, the first clinically useful antibiotic. Dubos shook the small bottle of gray powder in front of his audience, announcing to his colleagues and the assembled media that it contained enough powder to protect 5 trillion mice against pneumonia and streptococcus-induced blood poisoning.[1]

This dramatic gesture launched a revolution in medicine. The ensuing decade witnessed the introduction of antibiotic therapy as modern science's triumphant response to infectious disease. The tables turned as the bacteria responsible for devastating illnesses like tuberculosis and pneumonia suddenly seemed completely controllable by the wonder drugs of the era. Countless thousands of people who would have died as a result of infection finally had hope for survival. Perhaps no treatment contributed more to the hubris of twentieth-century medical science than the development of antibiotics. A revolution in medicine had begun and it originated from an unlikely source.

When René Jules Dubos joined the staff at the Rockefeller Institute for Medical Research (RIMR) in 1927, the 26-year-old Frenchman brought unusual skills and expertise to his new position. Trained first as an *ingenieur agronome* in Paris and then later as a doctoral candidate in soil microbiology at the New Jersey Agricultural

Station, Dubos was a unique addition to the laboratory of the internationally known immunochemist Oswald T. Avery. Anxious to leave what he perceived as the moribund field of soil science for the more promising and fulfilling disciplines of biochemistry and medical immunology, the young agricultural scientist jumped at the rare opportunity to join the medical researchers at the prestigious Rockefeller Institute.

Although he eagerly accepted the fellowship to work with Avery, his concerns about the relevance of his own educational background caused him some trepidation. Serendipity, not medical research or respected biochemical training, linked his doctoral thesis to Avery's research interests. Avery was trying to degrade the cellulose capsule responsible for lobar pneumonia at the same time as Dubos concluded a project investigating cellulose-decomposing microorganisms in the soil. Dubos pointed out to Avery the potential applicability of his skills in this area, and Avery gave the ambitious new Ph.D. a chance. Dubos realized that he had little preparation for medical research at the Rockefeller Institute. In fact, before his interview with Avery a few months earlier, he knew nothing at all about the Institute or its research.[2] He suspected his transition might be difficult, but convinced himself that the benefits accompanying this opportunity to change the trajectory of his career outweighed any temporary discomfort.

Against considerable odds, the young research Fellow in the department of Respiratory Diseases found rapid success in the Avery laboratory. Once focused on the task Avery originally hired him to address, Dubos solved in a few months the problem that had vexed his researchers for over a decade. Using soil-enrichment techniques and the isolation of specific enzymes—the methods Dubos learned as a soil microbiologist—he designed and implemented a protocol to strip the pneumococcus of its protective polysaccharide coating without causing harm to the host organism. This discovery, broadcast to the international scientific community in the pages of *Science*, marked a noteworthy advance in the efforts to address the devastating effects of lobar pneumonia.[3] It also laid the groundwork for Dubos's next great scientific achievement: the development of the world's first clinically useful antibiotic.

René Dubos occupies a critical and yet surprising role in the history of antibiotics research. In the late 1930s, Dubos used the techniques that brought him success in his lobar pneumonia investigations to isolate bacterial enzymes with new clinical applications. After a few projects with limited but promising results, he sought a bacterial enzyme with wider applicability than his very specific polysaccharide-decomposing enzyme of five years earlier. He isolated tyrothricin and introduced it to the public in September of 1939. Tyrothricin became the first clinically useful antibiotic—a category of substances named by Selman Waksman to denote compounds produced by one living organism that are specifically harmful to another living organism. Decades earlier, Paul Ehrlich, 1908 Nobel Laureate for his work on immunity, predicted that substances like tyrothricin existed. He suggested that chemical "magic bullets" could target disease-causing microorganisms and destroy them without damaging the host. Tyrothricin became Dubos's magic bullet. While artificial substances like sulfa drugs and Ehrlich's Salvorsan had been used previously with some success, tyrothricin represented the first naturally occurring substance with antimicrobial powers. This discovery earned him international acclaim and numerous awards from physicians and scientists. Temporarily seduced by the promise of treating bacterial diseases with magic bullets, he advocated the search for more. Within a very brief time, however, the limitations of this approach became apparent to Dubos. Long before most of his contemporaries in science, or the public at large, called for the cautious and responsible use of antibiotics, René Dubos issued public criticisms of the very drugs that had made him famous. Therefore, his was but a brief romance with magic bullets.

The Road to Antibiotic Therapy

A few years after Dubos and Avery introduced their pneumonia-fighting enzyme to the scientific community, another discovery stole the spotlight from their efforts. In early 1935, an article in a German medical journal announced Gerhard Domagk's discovery of Prontosil, a drug that would reorient the international medical community's approach to bacterial disease.[4] Prontosil's active ingredient, sulfanilamide, had long been manufactured by German dye industries. Before 1935, however, no one had tested sulfanilamide for its antibacterial properties. The early sulfa drugs showed exceptional promise against a variety of infective organisms, particularly streptococcus.

Even though promising results from clinical trials accompanied Domagk's initial paper, American physicians were slow to prescribe Prontosil to their patients. In the mid-1930s, physicians on both sides of the Atlantic had serious misgivings about treating diseases chemotherapeutically. Although Paul Ehrlich enjoyed modest success with his 1910 discovery of Salvarsan, his search for magic bullets that would selectively eradicate microbial pathogens proved overwhelmingly fruitless.[5] Thus most medical authorities in the age of Prontosil had little hope for its application. Only a few American clinicians used the drug, and then only as a last resort for their most desperate patients. When it proved successful, they often attributed the patients' recovery to some other therapeutic measure. Attitudes changed in December 1936, when newspapers worldwide credited Prontosil with the dramatic recovery of President Franklin D. Roosevelt's son. Suffering from a severe streptococcal infection, Franklin D. Roosevelt, Jr., lay near death when physicians commenced treatment with Prontosil. Soon after his rapid and full recovery, headlines in the December 20 edition of the *New York Times* hailed the "New Control of Infections."[6] Public demand stimulated wider use and increased confidence in sulfa drugs.

The demonstration of the efficacy of Prontosil devastated Oswald Avery. Prontosil defeated a wide variety of Gram-positive bacteria, including the pneumococcus, under investigation by Avery and his researchers. Because it successfully attacked pneumococci regardless of their immunological type, Prontosil proved more broadly useful than Dubos's and Avery's soil enzyme.[7] As Dubos remembered, "sulfonamides came into use for the treatment of pneumococcus pneumonia and somehow or other removed the social pressure for the discovery of new ways of treating pneumococcus infection by serum therapy. That after all was one of the great potentials of Dr. Avery's work."[8] Avery had searched for decades for a successful medical approach to lobar pneumonia. Once sulfa drugs appeared, Avery's search for a pneumonia vaccine appeared out of date and useless. Dubos recalled the intense depression that Avery experienced as a result of the development of sulfa drugs. For the two or three years that followed the confirmation of Domagk's achievement, Avery was a "dispirited man."[9]

Fortunately, Dubos proved less devastated by the advent of sulfa drugs. He quickly recognized that the opportunity to make significant contributions in the field still existed. Sulfa drugs, lauded by the press, public, and an increasing number of physicians, were beginning to reveal a number of limitations. When given in adequate doses, sulfonamides frequently proved toxic. Other times, they were rendered powerless by pus or other necrotic tissue products.[10] All of these faults became apparent within 5 years of Domagk's initial introduction of Prontosil. Dubos believed it would be more fruitful to seek a gentler alternative to what he perceived as chemically modified poisons.[11] Sulfa drugs had reinvigorated the world medical community's interest in the chemotherapeutic treatment of bacterial disease, but they did not successfully treat all bacterial infections. Apparently, there was still opportunity to make meaningful contributions to the field of infectious bacterial disease.

In his return to the study of pneumonia, Dubos split his efforts between the search for a vaccine against pneumococcal infection and the isolation of a new soil enzyme with broader bactericidal properties. To produce an anti-pneumonia vaccine, Dubos experimented with ways to make the pneumococcus into a better antigen. "What I did was work out a fairly practical technique whereby the pneumococcus could be killed under conditions that very rapidly inactivated their autolytic enzymes. This actually prevented the enzymatic deterioration of the structure of the pneumococcus cell. We found that such pneumococci were far more effective antigens than the pneumococci that were killed by the usual techniques of heating or adding phenol or other poisons to them."[8] Meanwhile, Walter Goebel labored in Avery's laboratory on what was billed as the first synthetic vaccine against pneumonia.[1] Dubos wrestled with his vaccine project for over two years but admitted in retrospect that this work had no significant consequences.

Meanwhile, Dubos also sought a bacterial enzyme with broader applicability than the one he isolated in 1930. Sulfa drugs had eclipsed the enzyme that ate away the polysaccharide coating of the type III pneumococcus responsible for lobar pneumonia. So this time Dubos sought an enzyme with a less specific appetite. He thought it possible "that there also exist microorganisms capable of attacking not only soluble, isolated substances, but also the intact living cells of other unrelated microbial species. Specifically, an attempt was made to recover from soil the microorganisms that could attack the living cells of pathogenic Gram-positive cocci."[12] He hypothesized that since pathogenic cells like pneumococcus, streptococcus, and staphylococcus all retained the Gram stain, their cell walls shared a similar architecture.[13] This structural similarity, he believed, could be the Achilles' heel for Gram-positive bacteria. Thus, he began his quest for a microorganism able to attack the cell wall of the Gram-positive staphylococcus, pneumococcus, and streptococcus bacteria. This was the beginning of the investigation that would make him famous.

Dubos utilized laboratory techniques similar to the ones he practiced during his early days in the Avery laboratory a decade prior. "Suspensions of living streptococci and staphylococci were added to soil in the hope that there would develop in these soil preparations a microbial flora capable of attacking the Gram positive cocci."[13]

His sustained faith in the validity of this approach proved reasonable when, countless soil samples later, Dubos isolated an aerobic sporulating soil microbe, *Bacillus brevis*, capable of destroying his Gram-positive bacterial species.

> Soon after adding the suspensions of living staphylococcus to the soil samples, I observed that they were being decomposed. To clinch the demonstration that something in the soil was attacking staphylococci, I made a suspension of these staphylococci in a liquid medium and added to it a small amount of the soil in which the staphylococci were disappearing. Stained preparations revealed a new bacterium, long and very different from the staphylococcus. Whenever it came in contact with the staphylococci, they lost their staining character and disintegrated. I thought that I had in fact obtained a bacterium that attacked staphylococcus. Through standard bacteriological technique I isolated a bacterium which belonged to the species of *Bacillus brevis*. Pure culture of this bacterium added to a suspension of staphylococci grew in contact with them and caused their disintegration.[8]

Dubos was encouraged by these results. He immediately wrote a scientific paper announcing his isolation of the antagonistic *Bacillus brevis*.[14] His July article regarding the bactericidal properties of his soil microbe earned him a brief mention in the *New York Times* column "Reported from the Fields of Research." The article noted that "the preliminary results, described as 'startling' in *The Journal of the American Medical Association*, indicate that medicine may be on the trail of a substance promising to be even more useful than sulfanilamide and sulfapyridine."[15] In the words of one of his colleagues, Dubos had once again "dipped his hand into the soil—for him that cornucopia of nature—to find a microbe that could break down the cellular integrity of the Gram-positive bacteria. The isolations, from so-called enrichment cultures, were rather delicate ones requiring who knows how much artistry, for the predator bacteria benefit only indirectly from their ability to inhibit or destroy others."[11]

Based on his experience with previous projects in the Avery laboratory, Dubos pursued as his next step the isolation of a bacteriolytic enzyme from *Bacillus brevis*. He extracted what he believed to be the enzyme responsible for the bactericidal activity of *Bacillus brevis*. The extract proved effective against streptococcus and pneumococcus infection in protection tests in mice performed by Dubos.[16] With the assistance of Carlo Cattaneo, an Italian chemist on fellowship in the Avery laboratory, he "found that the active principle could be separated in solution in acid acetone. Further study demonstrated that the purified preparation was soluble and stable in alcohol, acetone, dioxane, and glacial acetic acid, but insoluble in water, chloroform, sulfuric ether and benzol. It was obvious that my substance was not an enzyme."[17] Additional work revealed that "*Bacillus brevis* owes its antagonistic activity not to the activity of an enzyme selectively directed against the Gram positive structure, but rather to the production of a toxic principle which causes the death of the susceptible bacterial cells."[13] Contrary to what Dubos originally hypothesized, the cell walls of Gram-positive bacteria disintegrated as a result of cell death. They were not the cause of the cell's demise.

Dubos named the active substance responsible for the lysis of the deadly bacteria tyrothricin because its morphology and bactericidal properties resembled those of the *Tyrothrix* (meaning "threads from cheese") bacteria studied and named many

years earlier by one of Pasteur's early associates, the great French agricultural bacteriologist Emile Duclaux. Dubos single-handedly purified several hundred grams of
tyrothricin at what he considered "a tremendous expenditure of labor."[8] Fortunately,
Rollin Hotchkiss, a young organic chemist in Avery's laboratory, showed interest in
Dubos's project and came forward with an offer to assist him in the purification of
tyrothricin. Dubos recalled that in the middle of 1939, Hotchkiss asked him for a
sample of tyrothricin and then, "in his typical mysterious way (because he's a person
who often likes to work alone) he disappeared for a few weeks or months. One day
he came back and in his peculiar way asked me to look at something through his microscope. I saw some crystals and knew almost immediately that they were crystals
isolated from the tyrothricin I had given him. Together we promised to test these
crystals against bacteria."[8]

Despite encouraging preliminary findings regarding tyrothricin and Dubos's
proven ability to isolate useful bacterial enzymes, administrators at the Rockefeller
Institute were reluctant to permit Hotchkiss to join the tyrothricin work. Hotchkiss
recalled that "my adventure did not have the sanction or encouragement of my administrative superiors—not until I had made some progress and we were deeper into
World War II."[11] With or without the encouragement of their superiors, Dubos and
Hotchkiss "contrived to commandeer some lab help and some large equipment for a
summer of growing gallons of the soil organisms *Bacillus brevis* and preparing the
raw material Dubos had isolated. The crude brownish material was practically in-
compatible with water and, under organic solvents, congealed into a sticky mass as
unpleasant as so much uncouth earwax. But it was powerful wax all right."[11] Even
when greatly diluted, the substance exhibited strong antibacterial properties both in
the test tube and in the peritoneal cavity of mice.

The transformation from sticky brown wax to an effective liquid required the use
of large quantities of hot organic solvents including ether. At the request of several
of their Rockefeller colleagues, Hotchkiss and Dubos were banished from their laboratory space in the Rockefeller Hospital to the roof of the power house, where there
was no risk of endangering the patients or their co-workers. Soon thereafter, Hotchkiss
remembered, "the admirable traditions of The Rockefeller Institute administration to
ease the toil of honest research came to our aid. Soon I was granted my first technical assistant, and we were given keys to unlock and work in the lavish mouse dormi-
tory and surgery which Alexis Carrel had built and abandoned when he moved to
Europe."[11] There, the soil microbiologist and organic chemist worked side-by-side to
conduct fractionation experiments and mouse assays. Dubos found through his animal protection tests that the substance Hotchkiss helped him purify was extremely
potent, with as little as seven-billionths of an ounce adequate to kill 1 billion pneumococci or virulent streptococci in only two hours.

Scientific papers published by Dubos a few months before the Third International
Congress of Microbiologists about this discovery, coupled with his presentation at
the meeting in New York, proved pivotal in the history of antibiotics research. Dubos's search for tyrothricin marked the first deliberate pursuit of a bacterial antago-
nist with chemotherapeutic potential. His successful investigations in 1939 yielded
the first clinically useful antibiotic. Moreover, it also suggested to medical researchers
the clinical potential of other soil microorganisms. The *New York Times* made explicit

the connection between Dubos's success with tyrothricin and his agricultural heritage. They reported, "it was no mere 'hunch' that led Dr. Dubos to examine the soil for germ-killing agencies. Ever since Pasteur's time it has been known that bacteria play their part in rendering the soil a fit medium for the growth of plant and trees. In other words, the combat waged in the blood between disease germs and their enemies has its counterpart in the soil."[18] Thus, agricultural scientists dating back to Pasteur had chronicled the phenomenon of bacterial antagonism. Dubos, however, was the first to apply it and introduce it to medical science.

Some scientists followed Dubos's example further and faster than others. Immediately after finishing his presentation at the Waldorf-Astoria, Dubos shared an observation with Alexander Fleming, a fellow conference attendee. He said to Fleming, "the substance I have reported on has some of the activity of an extract of a fungus which you described in a paper almost ten years ago."[8] The organism to which Dubos referred was *Penicillium notatum*. When Fleming first observed and reported the anti-staphylococcal properties of the fungus on a contaminated Petri dish in 1929, he believed that a better understanding of the phenomenon was in order. He spent the next few years studying the life history of his fascinating mold and testing its toxicity in rabbits in mice. By 1932, however, Fleming decided that penicillin (the extract from *Penicillium notatum*) would not be of use therapeutically because it lost most of its potency within 10 to 14 days. Researchers at the London School of Hygiene and Tropical Medicine confirmed Fleming's prediction. Harold Raistrick, one of the world's foremost authorities on molds, argued that penicillin "could apparently be produced only in minute quantities, it was unstable as Fleming had already discovered, and it appeared to have no practical value."[19] Thus, Fleming abandoned penicillin research. When Dubos hinted at its usefulness in September 1939, Fleming simply responded saying "well that substance of the mold has no interest. It is very unstable. It really doesn't amount to much and if I were a chemist I would not follow that substance."[8] At the time of the International Congress, Fleming instead promoted the combination of vaccines and sulfa drugs.[20]

Dubos's work on tyrothricin had a more productive impact on the researchers at Oxford University's Sir William Dunn School of Pathology. Howard Florey, the School of Pathology's new director, also attended the congress in New York. However, since England and France declared war on Germany the same day the conference opened, Florey hurried back to Oxford soon after the meeting began. It is unclear whether Florey remained long enough in New York to attend Dubos's presentation on September 9. Nevertheless, evidence points to the influence of Dubos's tyrothricin work on Florey and the researchers in his laboratory.

Howard Florey and Ernst Chain, a German chemist who joined the Florey laboratory in 1935, decided in early 1939 to conduct a survey of naturally occurring antibacterial substances. During his subsequent literature search on the subject at the Radcliffe Library at Oxford University, Chain unearthed more than 200 references, including Fleming's 1929 report on penicillin.[21] Florey and Chain selected penicillin as one of a number of substances worth further investigation. Chain admitted, however, that at the time they thought it unlikely that penicillin offered therapeutic promise. He remarked that "as far as I am concerned the problem of reinvestigating penicillin was a biochemical one. . . . I was interested to find out the reasons for [the] extraordinary instability of the active principle. . . . It never struck me for a fraction of a second that this substance could be used from the chemotherapeutic point of view because, evidently, a substance which is so unstable that it goes off while you look at it, does not give very great promise with regard to practical applicability."[19]

It was only after Dubos published his July 1939 paper on tyrothricin that Florey and Chain recognized the potential chemotherapeutic value of the extract. In fact, the inquiries into penicillin at Oxford did not begin in earnest until September 1939.[19] A few days after the opening of the Microbiological Congress in New York, Florey wrote a letter in which he acknowledged "there has been some prominence to soil bacteria given in U.S. medical journals."[21] It was in this same letter that Florey spelled out "his hopes for a substance that would defeat an enemy more powerful than Hitler and which, in the end, would save more lives than were ever taken in all the wars and all the plagues in human history" and announced that their work on penicillin had actually begun.[21] The juxtaposition of Florey's citation of the American soil bacteriology work with his proclamation of hopes for penicillin makes a strong case for the influence of Dubos on the Oxford group's pursuit of clinically useful antibiotics. His influence is again documented in November 1939 when Florey cited Dubos's work on tyrothricin in his application to the Rockefeller Foundation for funds to support their antibacterial research.[22] Although it is unclear at which major scientific meeting it occurred, both Dubos and Hotchkiss recalled "a conference at which, after René had spoken about our antibacterial agent, a person identified as Professor Florey arose to say that Dubos's first reports had helped encourage the Oxford group to reconsider penicillin."[11]

Selman Waksman also attended the International Congress in New York. He, too, used Dubos's work with tyrothricin as a springboard to exciting new lines of research. Waksman knew of Dubos's work on this subject over a year before the Congress because of the "many discussion of this and similar ideas" between Dubos and Waksman during 1938 and 1939, the years in which Dubos toiled at the Rockefeller Institute on tyrothricin. Since 1936, Waksman himself had been working with and writing about antagonistic and associative phenomena among microbes. However, he did not pursue the study of these microbial relationships in the hope of contributing to modern therapeutics. He was, after all, still an agricultural scientist at the New Jersey Agricultural Experiment Station. His response to a 1932 research grant proves he was little interested in chemotherapeutic studies before tyrothricin. When William H. White of the National Tuberculosis Association and Stanhope Bayne-Jones of the National Research Council urged Waksman in the early thirties to study the destruction of the tubercle bacillus in the soil, he lacked the interest to pursue the project himself so he simply passed it on to one of his graduate students. Nothing of consequence came of the research.[23]

Dubos suggested that before 1940 "Dr. Waksman had never thought at all of obtaining from soil microorganisms drug-like agents that might be useful in combating infectious disease. However, my discovery of tyrothricin and the successful development of penicillin made him aware of the immense source of potential drugs that existed in the microorganisms of the soil that he knew so well how to handle."[8] Years later, Waksman pointed to Dubos's work on these substances as the "beginning of an epoch." Waksman, convinced of the possibilities of the investigative approach to soil, returned from the International Congress ready to search the soil for bacteria, fungi, and actinomycetes with bactericidal properties. He enlisted the help of his research associates at the New Jersey Agricultural Experiment Station and the pharmacologists and chemists of Merck & Co. in his search for what the public would know as "antibiotics."[24] Streptomycin, one of many antibiotics developed under Waksman's research program, ultimately earned him the Nobel Prize for Medicine.

Colleagues at the Rockefeller Institute also recognized the potential that tyrothricin represented. Avery urged Dubos to "use the rest of the department to push your work because it is the most important work now going on in the department."[8] Dubos recounted that "Dr. Avery was very interested in the development of the work on tyrothricin, yet I think that what he found most interesting was the excitement of finding under such unorthodox conditions . . . something that had such enormous activity in bacteria."[8] Oswald Robertson, a clinical researcher in the Rockefeller Institute laboratory of Peyton Rous, wrote to Avery that "I am glad to know that you and Dr. Dubos are going ahead with the effects of the enzyme in experimental pneumonia. I am awaiting eagerly the result of the further development of this most exciting work."[25]

During the months following the Microbiological Congress in New York, Dubos and Hotchkiss discovered that tyrothricin was actually a mixture of two biologically active substances. They named the first substance Hotchkiss crystalized tyrocidine. While effective *in vitro*, it proved ineffective in animal models. Gramicidin, the second and more hopeful substance, was effective against Gram-positive bacteria both in the test tube and in animals.[8] Hotchkiss and Dubos took this more specific and refined information about gramicidin to the annual Society of American Bacteriologists (SAB) meeting held that December in New Haven. By this time, "considerable excitement had been aroused in biochemical and biomedical colleagues and in industry."[11] Letters flooded into the Rockefeller Institute asking permission and advice for the production of tyrothricin and its products. The directors at the Rockefeller Institute, sensing the potential usefulness of tyrothricin, asked Dubos and Hotchkiss to patent the process of its production "which they hoped would save the elixir for the general good, as required by the Rockefeller charter."[11] Then, within a week after the SAB meeting, Hotchkiss and Dubos "released, to all drug companies and colleagues who requested it, the special *B. brevis* culture, together with full instructions for making the crude and purified extracts."[11]

Tyrothricin's demonstrated efficacy in mice encouraged Dubos to search for practical applications for his new drug. One of its earliest uses suggests Dubos's close connection with the animal pathology group at the Rockefeller Institute in Princeton. Ralph Little, a veterinarian there, encouraged Dubos to send samples of tyrocidine and gramicidin for use against bovine mastitis, an infection of cow udders. Veterinarians used gramicidin at the 1939–40 World's Fair when an outbreak of bovine mastitis infected a number of the cows on display at the Borden pavilion. Elsie, the famous Borden cow, was among the earliest subjects to benefit from gramicidin.[8]

As a result of his work on gramicidin, René Dubos became a subject of great interest to his fellow scientists, physicians, and the public. Medical and biological researchers in New York City invited Dubos to deliver a lecture on gramicidin to the Harvey Society in March 1940.[12] That same month, the *New York Times* reported

Dubos's discovery as one that offered new hope in the fight against tuberculosis.[26] The American Academy of Pediatrics awarded Dubos its Mead Johnson Award.[27] At their annual meeting in 1940, the American College of Physicians awarded Dubos its John Phillips Memorial Award in recognition of his success in antibiotics research.[28] Dubos "was hailed by many distinguished physicians attending the meeting as a worthy successor of his countryman, Pasteur," a comparison Dubos both enjoyed and encouraged by his frequent references to Pasteur in his public addresses.

The public was clearly seduced by the notion of magic bullets in this period before penicillin and streptomycin. Warner Brothers capitalized on this fascination when it released a feature film in 1940 celebrating Paul Ehrlich's search for microbe killers. Dubos only fueled the public's enthusiasm. In these early months of 1940, Dubos spoke repeatedly about the great therapeutic agents that undoubtedly awaited medical scientists in the soil. He argued that the method he used to isolate gramicidin had a distinguished past in bacteriological chemistry and deserved the consideration of physiologists and biochemists. After all, he noted, "it can be stated that one can find in nature, in soil or water for instance, microorganisms capable of performing almost every possible type of biochemical reaction."[12] He promised his audience at the American College of Physicians meeting that "the bacteria present in the soil possess an adaptive mechanism which enables them to develop powerful specific chemicals against the deadly bacterial enemies of man, promising to open up an inexhaustible treasure house of nature containing a specific antidote against any specific hostile microbe."[28] The *New York Times* quoted him in September 1940 as saying that "steps were being taken at several institutions to breed a species of soil bacteria with a particular appetite for germs of tuberculosis."[29] Gramicidin, he implied, was only the beginning.

In April 1940, reports from Selman Waksman at the New Jersey Agricultural Experiment Station about successes against gram-negative bacteria, and from Howard Florey's group at Oxford regarding the efficacy of penicillin as a chemotherapeutic agent later that same year, appeared to substantiate Dubos's claims.[30] That scientific research along these lines garnered the interest of a large and increasing scientific community was demonstrated as 200 bacteriologists attended a roundtable discussion on antibacterial agents at the December 1940 SAB meeting convened by Dubos.[23] The race for magic bullets was on and René Dubos was leading the charge. Textbooks and clinical manuals credited Dubos with having "stimulated renewed interest in the study of antibacterial agents of biologic origin."[31] The press acknowledged him as the leader of the back-to-the-soil movement witnessed in the world's laboratories as they tried to explain why scientists had been inspired "to pack dirty earth into their shining, sterile laboratory glassware as part of the effort to better human health."[32]

The recognition that resulted both directly and indirectly from the tyrothricin work gained Dubos a secure position within the Rockefeller Institute, and in the American scientific community. In 1941, Rochester University granted Dubos the first of his many honorary degrees and he received notification that he was one of the 15 scientists elected that year to the National Academy of Sciences. He became a full member at the Rockefeller Institute, and a number of leading research universities broached new employment opportunities. Harvard University, in particular, demonstrated an earnest desire to attract Dubos to join their faculty. In 1941, it would have been diffi-cult to find a scientist anywhere in the United States with a more celebrated and promising scientific career.

Magic Bullets Reconsidered

However, at precisely the time René Dubos reached the heights in his profession, he began to question the use of the antibiotic wonder drugs that put him there. In 1941, the darker side of gramicidin became apparent to Dubos and others who cared to see it. Researchers at the Mayo Clinic reported a strong hemolytic effect on rabbit and sheep erythrocytes suspended in tissue culture medium to which tyrothricin had been added. Further studies revealed that both tyrocidine and its more gentle coun-terpart, gramicidin, caused rapid hemolysis. Attempts made to nullify the hemolytic effect resulted in a total loss of the substance's antibacterial activity.[33] Meanwhile, research at the Rockefeller Institute painted a similarly discouraging picture. Al-though tests on bovine mastitis and mouse peritonitis demonstrated tyrothricin's great promise, experimental studies carried out in rabbits and dogs at the Rockefeller Institute revealed that it was ineffective, not to mention toxic, when administered in-travenously. "While it was obvious that tyrothricin and gramicidin could not be used for the treatment of systemic infections . . . the lack of toxic effects by routes other than intravenous—left open the possibility that the substances might be useful in the treatment of certain local infections in man."[34] Nevertheless, Dubos was terribly dis-appointed at tyrothricin's severe limitations.

Surprisingly, for years after researchers demonstrated tyrothricin's hemolytic ef-fects, the press still lauded Dubos's discovery as praiseworthy. It was billed as "one of the most romantic stories in modern research, a story of shrewd detective work and clearheaded thinking."[35] Tyrothricin, argued journalists, deserved recognition of the same degree as that accorded sulfa drugs and penicillin, despite its internal toxi-city. The wonders it worked in body cavities and upon superficial wounds (particu-larly those of soldiers) earned Dubos gratitude and respect from the American public. That Dubos "found tyrothricin in a set of dime-store tumblers at the Rocke-feller Institute for Medical Research" only added to the story's popular appeal.[35]

Physicians also exhibited notable enthusiasm for gramicidin after its hemolytic effects became known. Audiences at medical conventions where the story of grami-cidin was told marveled as much at the story of how the Rockefeller Institute's token soil microbiologist unearthed the magical substance as they did at its potential med-ical applications. At the 1941 annual clinical congress of the American College of Surgeons, Doctors Charles H. Rammelkamp and Chester Keefer of the Boston Uni-versity School of Medicine presented the clinical implications of gramicidin to their colleagues. They reported the effective use of gramicidin in the treatment of many serious infections, including skin ulcers, pleurisy, and pus-ridden wounds. However, "these and other important results were not all that aroused the interest of the United States' foremost surgeons. For the discovery of gramicidin itself was even more of a sensation that its chemical effects."[36] The story held such wide interest that it was re-counted in the pages of *Harper's Magazine* after the College of Surgeons meeting.

At this point, René Dubos faced a potentially career-altering decision. Clinical studies verified that gramicidin provided effective treatment for a number of previously stubborn conditions. He could have continued to champion the cause of antibiotic wonder drugs even though gramicidin could not yet be administered intravenously or by mouth. Recognizing its shortcomings, his peers in scientific research, the medical profession, and the public embraced the drug and the scientist who discovered it. Dubos believed that another return to his soil-enrichment techniques might yield a different chemotherapeutic agent useful in the bloodstream. Instead, he chose to search no further for new antibiotics. He remembered the early 1940s as a period in which many became intoxicated with the possibilities of antibiotics. "I guess I was one of the few who didn't. As a matter of fact, because I didn't find the problem of searching for such substances intellectually stimulating, I removed myself from the field."[8]

In 1942, Dubos not only left the field of antibiotic research, he also left the Rockefeller Institute—the place that had been his scientific home since 1927. At the same time his professional career was reaching exciting new levels, a very personal tragedy was unfolding at home. While René Dubos was isolating tyrothricin, his wife suffered a devastating relapse of tuberculosis. Marie Louise first contracted tuberculosis from her father as a young child in Limoges, but quickly recuperated. Although initially puzzled how a woman who lived as comfortably as Marie Louise could develop tuberculosis, her husband ultimately became convinced that the stress and anguish over her family's safety in war-torn France reactivated the tuberculosis that to all appearances had been cured many years earlier when she was a child.[9] Her illness progressed rapidly and, as a result, her physicians prescribed bed rest and care at the Raybrook Sanatorium in the Adirondack Mountains of New York. Hence, René Dubos worked feverishly during the week on his research and traveled upstate every weekend to the sanatorium to visit his desperately ill wife.[6] Over the next three years, her health improved and deteriorated unpredictably, causing her husband immeasurable concern. When, in 1941, her health improved to the point that she could return home to New York City, René Dubos worried that the fast-paced life of the city might not suit her. He began to consider seriously offers to leave New York City and the Rockefeller Institute, where he had so recently experienced such overwhelming professional success.

In the spring of 1942, Dubos agreed to join the faculty of the Harvard University School of Medicine. Harvard offered him the George Fabyan Professorship of Comparative Pathology and Tropical Medicine made vacant with the June retirement of Ernest Tyzzer. Dubos doubted his suitability for the appointment. "I remember saying to the dean of the Medical School and the director of the Massachusetts General Hospital that I had never been in the tropics, let alone not being a physician. This was absolutely irrelevant, they replied immediately, for their interest was in having somebody who could organize scientific programs around these problems and did not demand a medical degree."[37] In fact, there was not a clinician on staff in the department. "That combined chair was offered to me with the understanding that since I was not a pathologist, and knew little or nothing about Tropical Medicine, I would take advantage of the chair to become a professor of research."[8] Dubos accepted the research professorship with the intention of redirecting his professional focus to the physiology and immunology of the tubercle bacillus and tuberculosis infection.

Dubos revealed the great difficulty with which he made his decision to leave the Rockefeller Institute in a letter to one of the men who lobbied most enthusiastically for Dubos's invitation to join the Harvard faculty—the chairman of the physiology department, Walter B. Cannon. "I need not tell you how much I shall regret the Rockefeller Institute, where I have lived and worked in such happy and stimulating surroundings. I know however, that I shall find at Harvard University, a new and even richer atmosphere—in fact the very word 'University' has almost a romantic appeal for me."[38] Therefore, Dubos set plans in motion for his move to Cambridge, Massachusetts. Unfortunately, Marie Louise would not accompany him northward. She died nine days after her husband had accepted the position at Harvard University.

Although administrative duties and war-related research projects delayed his undistracted foray into tuberculosis studies until his 1944 return to the Rockefeller Institute, his time at Harvard proved invaluable to the formation of his new ecological model of disease. During his two years in Cambridge he was exposed to like-minded individuals who understood disease as a complex phenomenon that defied simple solutions. He exchanged his ideas about bacteria and disease with the public and with his colleagues in science and medicine. Soon after his arrival at Harvard, the Lowell Institute invited Dubos to participate in their time-honored public lecture series. Dubos accepted the invitation and chose to discuss immunity in terms of the individual constituents and properties of the bacterial cell. The series of eight lectures that he delivered formed the basis of his first book, *The Bacterial Cell in its Relation to Problems of Virulence, Immunity and Chemotherapy*.[39]

At the heart of this book was an attack on the notion of bacterial fixity dominant among medical bacteriologists. Dubos, referring repeatedly to the works of nineteenth- and very early twentieth-century agricultural bacteriologists, reminded his contemporaries that "bacteria are more striking in their variability and plasticity than in the fixity of their morphological, biochemical and physiological characteristics. . . . Transformation—permanent or transient —not only of a quantitative, but often of a qualitative nature—appear in an unpredictable manner under conditions where the 'purity' of the culture cannot be doubted."[39] Dubos pointed to the rapidity with which bacteria can adapt to changing environments as just cause for questioning the wisdom of overzealous chemotherapeutic treatment. This book rapidly became a standard textbook in the field of bacteriology.

Dubos also took the opportunity as a member of the Harvard Medical School faculty to warn the medical students there against the overprescription of antibiotic substances. In the midst of tremendous press coverage of the medical miracles performed by wonder drugs like penicillin, Dubos advised the rising physicians against their excessive use. This was an extremely bold step for a man with no medical degree and who, until a few years earlier, had no affiliation with a medical school. In 1943, he warned a class of incoming pre-medical students not to follow the example of their elder colleagues who practice the wasteful and inconsiderate use of new antiseptics. A year later, in an issue of the *Journal of the American Medical Association* that offered several commentaries promoting the clinical use of penicillin, Dubos cautioned clinicians that most antibiotics are merely "protoplasmic poisons," and reminded them that "although many of these substances of biologic origin exhibit great antiseptic activity *in vitro*, only a few retain this property in the presence of animal tissues; in this respect antiseptics of biologic origin present the same problem as chemical antiseptics."[40] Although Dubos was not entirely alone in voicing his concerns regarding the toxicity of antibiotic wonder drugs and antibiotic-resistant strains of bacteria, his criticism of magic bullets certainly represented a rare perspective in 1944, and a surprising one indeed considering his integral role in their development.[41]

Conclusion

Tyrothricin opened many doors for René Dubos. It earned him more fame and professional recognition than any agricultural scientist since Louis Pasteur. The success tyrothricin and its derivatives bestowed upon Dubos catalyzed a shift in the direction of his thinking. Dubos, newly convinced of the power and efficiency of chemotherapeutic wonder drugs, abandoned his immunological approach to infectious disease in favor of one that privileged cure over prevention. His example inspired scientists to search for antibacterial agents in the soil and encouraged physicians to employ these agents in the treatment of patients.

Antibiotics seduced Dubos, however, for only a short time. By 1941 his enthusiasm waned in light of tyrothricin's unmistakable limitations. Almost overnight, he changed from champion to critic of chemotherapeutic agents. His admonitions against the overzealous use of antibiotics, however, went largely unheeded. As a result, many of his predictions regarding the danger of antibiotic-resistant bacterial strains have been realized in modern medicine. Thus far, little attention has been paid to Dubos's vital contributions to antibiotics research, leaving historians to wonder if his story would not have figured more prominently had his romance with magic bullets not been so brief.

References

1. Vaccines made from chemicals. *New York Times*, 31 August 1938, 17.
2. Benison S. René Dubos and the capsular polysaccharide of pneumococcus. *Bull Hist Med* 1976:50:459–77.
3. Avery OT, Dubos RJ. The specific action of a bacterial enzyme on pneumococcus of Type III. *Science* 1930:72:151–52.
4. Domagk G. Prontosil bei Streptokokkenerkrankungen. *Dtsch Med Wochenschr* 1935:61:250–53.
5. Ehrlich, P. Allegemeines uber Chemotherapie. *Verh Dtsch Ges Inn Med*1910:27:226–34.
6. Ryan F. The Forgotten Plague: How the Battle Against Tuberculosis was Won—and Lost. Boston: Little, Brown, 1992.
7. Corner GW. A History of the Rockefeller Institute: Origins and Growth. New York: St. Martin's, 1985.
8. Benison S. Interview with René Dubos, vol. 1. New York: Columbia University Oral History Research Office, 1955.
9. Dubos RJ, Escande JP. Quest: Reflections on Medicine, Science, and Humanity. New York: Harcourt Brace Jovanovich, 1979.

10. Florey HW, Abraham EP. The work on penicillin at Oxford. *J Hist Med Allied Sci* 1951:6:302–17.
11. Hotchkiss R. From Microbes to Man: Gramicidin, René Dubos, and the Rockefeller. In: Moberg C, Cohn Z. Launching the Antibiotic Era: Personal Accounts of the Discovery and Use of the First Antibiotics. New York: Rockefeller University Press, 1990.
12. Dubos RJ. Utilization of selective microbial agents in the study of biological problems. The Harvey Lectures 1939–1940:35:223–42.
13. Dubos RJ, Hotchkiss R. Origin, nature, and properties of gramicidin and tyrocidine. Transactions and Studies of the College of Physicians of Philadelphia 1942:10:11N19.
14. Dubos RJ. Bactericidal effect of an extract of a soil bacillus on Gram-positive cocci. Proceedings of the Society for Experimental Biology and Medicine 1939:40:311–12.
15. Streptococci destroyed. *New York Times,* 23 July 1939, 4.
16. Dubos RJ. Studies on a bactericidal agent extracted from soil bacillus: II. Protective effect of the bactericidal agent against experimental pneumococcus infections in mice *J Exp Med* 1939:70:11–17.
17. Dubos RJ, Cattaneo C. Studies on a bactericidal agent extracted from a soil bacillus: III. Preparation and activity of a protein-free fraction. *J Exp Med* 1939: 70: 249–256.
18. Sugar coated germs. *New York Times,* 17 September 1939, 8.
19. Clark RW. The Life of Ernst Chain: Penicillin and Beyond. New York: St. Martin's, 1985.
20. Macfarlance G. Alexander Fleming: The Man and the Myth. Cambridge, MA: Harvard University Press, 1984.
21. Bickel L. Rise Up to Life: A Biography of Howard Walter Florey. New York: Scribners, 1972.
22. Hobby G. Penicillin: Meeting the Challenge. New Haven: Yale University Press, 1985.
23. Waksman S. The Antibiotic Era: A History of the Antibiotics and of their Role in the Conquest of Infectious Disease and in Other Fields of Human Endeavor. Tokyo: Waksman Foundation of Japan, 1975.
24. Waksman S. My Life with the Microbes. New York: Simon & Schuster, 1954.
25. Robertson O. Letter to Oswald Avery. Oswald Robertson Papers. Philadelphia: American Philosophical Society.
26. Two new germicides prove powerful. *New York Times,* 22 March 1940, 14.
27. Kone E. Biography of René Jules Dubos. René Dubos Papers. Sleepy Hollow: Rockefeller Archive Center.
28. Laurence WL. Tells how earth grows germ killer. *New York Times,* 5 April 1940, 11.
29. Laurence WL. Chemists extend war on bacteria. *New York Times,* 21 September 1940, 8.
30. Untitled. *New York Times,* 26 April 1940, 20.
31. Herrell WE. Penicillin and Other Antibiotic Agents. Philadelphia: W.B. Saunders Co., 1945.
32. Davis HM. The soil: all things to all men. *New York Times Magazine,* 6 April 1941, 12–28.
33. Heilman D, Herrell WE. Hemolytic effect of gramicidin. *Proc Soc Exper Biol Med* 1941:46:182–84.
34. Dubos RJ. Tyrothricin, gramicidin, and tyrocidine. In: Antibiotics Annual, 1959–1960. New York: Antibiotics, Inc., 1960.
35. Ratcliff JD. The third wonder. *This Week,* 2 July 1944, 5.
36. Pfeiffer J. Germ killers from the earth: the story of gramicidin. *Harpers* 184: March 1942, 431–37.
37. Freese AS. A scientist talks about careers in science. *Today's Health* September 1969 24–27.
38. Dubos RJ. Letter to Walter Cannon, 30 May 1942. Boston: Walter B. Cannon Papers. Countway Medical Library.

39. Dubos RJ. The Bacterial Cell in its Relation to Problems of Virulence, Immunity and Chemotherapy. Cambridge, MA: Harvard University Press, 1945.
40. Dubos RJ. Antimicrobial agents of biologic origin. *JAMA* 1944:124:633–36.
41. Moberg C. René Dubos: a harbinger of microbial resistance to antibiotics. *Antibiot Drug Resist* 1996:2:287–97.

Suggested Reading

Hotchkiss R. From microbes to man: gramicidin, René Dubos, and the Rockefeller. In: Moberg C, Cohn Z. Launching the Antibiotic Era: Personal Accounts of the Discovery and Use of the First Antibiotics. New York: Rockefeller University Press, 1990.
Moberg CL. René Dubos, Friend of the Good Earth: Microbiologist, Medical Scientist, Environmentalist. Washington DC: ASM Press, 2005.

PART II

CONTROL OF DISEASE THROUGH VACCINATION

4

A Shot at Protection: Immunizations Against Infectious Disease

ALAN R. HINMAN
WALTER A. ORENSTEIN

Edward Jenner, an eighteenth-century English physician, observed that milkmaids who had recovered from cowpox, a pustular ailment of cattle, did not have the same facial scars from smallpox as most other people in England did. In 1796, he demonstrated that inoculation of a susceptible individual with material from a cowpox lesion provided protection against subsequent exposure to smallpox. Now, in the early years of the third century of the vaccine era, it is appropriate to consider the successes and failures of immunizations. This chapter will describe some of the progress made as a result of immunization, as well as the challenges remaining to realize the full current and future potential of immunizations. It will concentrate on smallpox, poliomyelitis, and measles, and will briefly address some other vaccine-preventable diseases of childhood. This chapter will focus on the experience in the United States.

The Beginning of the Vaccine Era

Smallpox and measles were introduced to North America with the earliest European colonization, and epidemics of smallpox and measles were responsible for large numbers of deaths among the susceptible indigenous populations. In addition to natural transmission between colonists and natives, there is evidence that blankets and other items containing crusts from smallpox lesions were deliberately given to natives to introduce disease.[1] Recurrent epidemics of smallpox, measles, and diphtheria were reported in the colonies.[2] At the beginning of the twentieth century, infectious diseases were the major killers in the United States. Tuberculosis was the leading cause of death, accounting for 11.3% of all deaths, and diphtheria was the 10th most frequent cause of death, accounting for 2.3% of all deaths.

After introduction of vaccination to protect against smallpox in 1796, it was nearly 100 years before the next vaccination (against rabies) was introduced by Louis Pasteur in 1885. The pace of vaccine introduction then increased, and in the last years of the twentieth century there was a marked acceleration in the introduction of new vaccines (Table 4.1).[3]

The introduction and widespread use of vaccines have had a dramatic impact on the occurrence of infectious diseases in the United States. Table 4.2 summarizes the representative annual morbidity (typically, average morbidity reported in the three years prior to introduction of the vaccine) in the twentieth century for cases reported of diseases against which children have been routinely vaccinated and the number of cases reported in 2000.

Table 4.1. Year of vaccine development or licensure United States, 1798–2000.

Disease	Year	Status
Smallpox*	1798	Developed
Rabies	1885	Developed
Typhoid	1896	Developed
Cholera	1896	Developed
Plague	1897	Developed
Diphtheria*	1923	Developed
Pertussis*	1926	Developed
Tetanus*	1927	Developed
Tuberculosis	1927	Developed
Influenza	1945	Licensed for use in U.S.
Yellow fever	1953	Licensed for use in U.S.
Poliomielitis*	1955	Licensed for use in U.S.
Measles*	1963	Licensed for use in U.S.
Mumps*	1967	Licensed for use in U.S.
Rubella*	1969	Licensed for use in U.S.
Anthrax	1970	Licensed for use in U.S.
Meningoccal	1975	Licensed for use in U.S.
Pneumococcal	1977	Licensed for use in U.S.
Adenovirus	1980	Licensed for use in U.S.
Hepatitis B*	1981	Licensed for use in U.S.
Haemophilus influenzae type b*	1985	Licensed for use in U.S.
Japanese encephalitis	1992	Licensed for use in U.S.
Hepatitis A	1995	Licensed for use in U.S.
Varicella*	1995	Licensed for use in U.S.
Lyme disease	1998	Licensed for use in U.S.
Rotavirus*[†]	1998	Licensed for use in U.S.
Conjugated pneumococcal*	2000	Licensed for use in U.S.

*Recommended for universal use in U.S. children. Smallpox vaccination ended in 1971.
[†]Rotavirus vaccine withdrawn in 1999.

Table 4.2. Comparison of 20th-century annual morbidity* and current morbidity, vaccine-preventable diseases of children, United States.

Disease	20th Century Annual Morbidity	2000**	Percent Decrease
Smallpox	48,164	0	100.00
Diphtheria	175,885	4	99.99
Measles	503,282	81	99.98
Mumps	152,209	323	99.80
Pertussis	147,271	6755	95.40
Polio (paralytic)	16,316	0	100.00
Rubella	47,745	152	99.70
Congenital rubella syndrome	823	7	99.10
Tetanus	1314	26	98.00
Haemophilus influenzae type b and unknown (<5 years)	20,000	167	99.10

*Typically, average during 3 years before vaccine licensure.
**Provisional data.

Smallpox

Smallpox has been recognized as an epidemic disease since before the modern era, and evidence of smallpox scars in mummies has been found in remains more than 3000 years old.[4] Smallpox came to the Americas with the earliest waves of European colonization and, with measles, was a major factor in the collapse of the Aztec and Inca empires.[5] During the eighteenth century, five European monarchs died of smallpox.[6] At the end of the eighteenth century, an estimated 400,000 deaths due to smallpox occurred each year in Europe.

Although there were (and still are) groups opposed to vaccination, vaccination against smallpox became well enough accepted in the United States that, to prevent transmission in schools, in the 1850s Massachusetts enacted a law requiring vaccination prior to school entry.[7] Other states followed suit and by the turn of the twentieth century, nearly half of the states had laws requiring vaccination.

Until the twentieth century, most of the smallpox seen in the United States was variola major, which has a case-fatality rate as high as 20%. During the period 1900–1904, on average more than 48,000 cases and more than 1500 deaths were reported annually in the United States. Early in the twentieth century, variola minor (which has a case-fatality rate of ≤1%) became the predominant form, and the number of deaths due to smallpox declined, leading some to lose enthusiasm for vaccination. Nonetheless, the number of cases continued to decline, from more than 100,000 cases reported in 1921 to approximately 10,000 cases annually during the 1930s. The last case of smallpox in the United States occurred in 1949.

In 1959, the World Health Assembly voted to undertake a global eradication program. At that time an estimated 10–15 million cases were occurring each year around the world, concentrated in 31 countries with endemic transmission. The primary strategy undertaken at first was mass vaccination, attempting to reach at least 80% of the population with vaccine of assured quality. This approach was successful in many countries but did not achieve the desired result in many other areas, particularly Africa and the Indian subcontinent. The surveillance-containment strategy, which focused on detecting cases of smallpox and vaccinating all persons who might have come in contact with patients, resulted in a more focused approach; hence, smallpox transmission was interrupted in several countries with population vaccination levels of only 50–60%.[8]

The last naturally occurring case of smallpox in the world occurred in Somalia in October 1977, and the World Health Organization (WHO) certified the global eradication of smallpox in May 1980. Vaccination against smallpox was discontinued in the United States in the early 1970s (before eradication was achieved) because the risk of importation and subsequent spread was judged to be smaller than the continuing risk of the rare complications of vaccination (disseminated vaccinia, vaccinia encephalitis). It is estimated that the United States recoups its total investment in the global eradication program every 26 days as a result of not having to vaccinate against smallpox.

Stocks of smallpox virus continue to exist in at least two reference laboratories (one at the Centers for Disease Control and Prevention (CDC) in the United States and the other in Russia); they were scheduled to be destroyed by the end of the twentieth century. However, evidence that there might be stocks of smallpox virus in the hands of nations or individuals who might use the virus as an agent of bioterrorism have put plans for destruction of the reference strains on hold.[9]

Poliomyelitis

Paralytic poliomyelitis is caused by one of three types of poliovirus—enteroviruses that are typically spread by fecal-oral or oral-oral means. Most persons infected by polioviruses have no manifestations of infection other than development of life-long immunity to the type of virus causing the infection. Only one in approximately every 200 persons infected develops permanent paralysis.[10]

The first recorded depiction of the effects of what was probably paralytic poliomyelitis is an Egyptian stela more than 3000 years old, which depicts a man with a withered leg. Over the next centuries, paralysis in children was recorded but did not occur in epidemic fashion. This was probably because polioviruses infected virtually every person in the first several months of life, at a time when they were partially protected by maternally derived antibodies. Universal infection at a very early age also meant that there were not the significant accumulations of susceptible populations required to sustain an epidemic. It was only after substantial improvements in sanitary conditions (allowing the development of susceptible populations) that poliomyelitis appeared as an epidemic disease, often affecting adults as well as children.

Small outbreaks of polio were recorded in Europe during the nineteenth century. The first recorded sizable epidemic of paralytic poliomyelitis in the United States occurred in 1894 in Vermont and affected 132 persons.[11] An epidemic in New York City in 1916 resulted in paralysis of more than 9000 persons and was a major cause of panic in the city, as recounted in Chapter 5.[12] In the first half of the twentieth century there were recurring epidemics of polio with increasing numbers of persons affected, reaching a peak in 1952 when more than 20,000 cases of paralytic poliomyelitis were reported (Fig. 4.1). Swimming pools, movie theaters, and other places where children might congregate were closed because of fear of transmission of polio.

Major efforts to develop polio vaccine resulted in large-scale trials of Jonas Salk's inactivated (killed) poliovirus vaccine (IPV). The Francis Field Trials (named after Dr. Thomas Francis, who oversaw them) were perhaps the largest controlled clinical trials ever conducted in the United States. The trials involved more than 1.8 million school children in 44 states: some received vaccine, some received placebo, and some were merely observed.

On April 12, 1955 (exactly 10 years after the death of Franklin Delano Roosevelt, the president who suffered from poliomyelitis), it was announced that the Salk vaccine prevented poliomyelitis (efficacy approximately 79%). This major news event was celebrated throughout the nation. The vaccine was licensed by the Food and Drug Administration within a few days. Several days later it was reported that some recipients of the Salk vaccine had developed paralysis (often in the same limb where the vaccine had been injected). This led to a major investigation coordinated by the Communicable Disease Center (now the CDC in Atlanta, Georgia, which demonstrated that the cases of vaccine-associated paralysis were related to vaccine from a single manufacturer—Cutter Laboratories). It was subsequently shown that this manufacturer had used inadequate procedures for inactivation of the virus. Recall of this vaccine stopped the problem and vaccination recommenced. In total, 260 vaccine-associated cases (192 paralytic) occurred in the Cutter incident: 94 among vaccinated children, 126 among family contacts of vaccinated persons, and 40 among community contacts.[13]

Widespread use of IPV resulted in an immediate and dramatic reduction in the number of cases of paralytic polio reported. However, in the next few years some

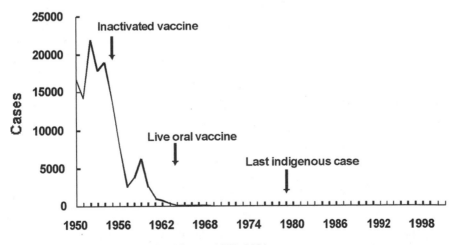

Figure 4.1. Poliomyelitis—United States, 1950–2001.

outbreaks of polio were reported in communities where there had been high uptake of the Salk vaccine. The outbreaks occurred because, although vaccinated individuals were protected, there was still opportunity for circulation of wild polioviruses. Consequently, when the Sabin live, attenuated (oral) poliovirus vaccine (OPV) was introduced in 1961, it rapidly replaced IPV in the United States and in most other countries around the world. The Netherlands and Finland were among the few countries that relied exclusively on IPV.

The OPV has the advantages of simplicity of administration and the induction of gastrointestinal immunity that substantially diminishes the risk of transmission of poliovirus on subsequent exposure and spread to unimmunized close contacts. However, it also carries a slight risk of paralysis in those who receive the vaccine or who are in close contact with a vaccinee. This risk is on the order of one case of paralysis for every 2.6 million doses administered. The principal risk is associated with the first dose administered. Here, the risk is on the order of one case of paralysis for every 750,000 first doses administered.

In the United States, the use of OPV led to a further reduction in reported cases of paralytic poliomyelitis; the last outbreaks of polio in this country occurred in the 1970s, with outbreaks in unimmunized populations along the U.S.–Mexico border (1969) and in groups that opposed immunization (Christian Scientists and Amish, 1972 and 1979, respectively). The last case of paralysis caused by wild poliovirus acquired in the United States occurred in 1979. Nonetheless, there were individual cases of paralysis due to wild poliovirus during the early 1980s resulting from infection acquired in other countries.

Because of the continuing risk of vaccine-associated paralysis in the absence of indigenous or imported cases of paralysis due to wild poliovirus, the relative balance of benefits and risks associated with OPV changed over time and vaccine policy changed with it. In 1997 the Public Health Service Advisory Committee on Immunization Practices (ACIP) and the American Academy of Pediatrics (AAP) recommended a shift from an all-OPV schedule to one in which the child first received two doses of IPV and subsequently received two doses of OPV. Thus, the child would receive the benefit of OPV without undergoing the risk. In 2000, reflecting the continuing downward trend in incidence of polio worldwide with concomitant decrease in the risk of importation of wild poliovirus into the United States, the recommendation shifted to an all-IPV schedule.[14] This approach is increasingly being taken in other industrialized countries.

In 1985, the countries of the American Region of the World Health Organization resolved to eradicate poliomyelitis from the hemisphere. The strategy to eradicate polio had four major elements:

1. High routine immunization coverage (at least three doses of OPV in the first year of life to all children).
2. National Immunization Days (NIDs)—twice-yearly campaigns in which all children less than 5 years of age receive a dose of OPV, regardless of prior immunization status.
3. Effective surveillance to detect all cases of poliomyelitis, focusing on detection of all cases of acute flaccid paralysis (AFP) in children less than 15 years of age.

4. Effective response to continued risk of transmission through "mop-up" campaigns, typically involving house-to-house administration of OPV to all children living in areas at risk of continued transmission.

As a result of a major effort, wild poliovirus transmission has been interrupted in the Western Hemisphere: there has not been a case of wild poliovirus-caused paralysis in the Americas since August 1991 (in Peru).

In 1988, the World Health Assembly adopted a target of global eradication of poliomyelitis by 2000, using the strategy effectively implemented in the Americas. Global efforts have been coordinated by a unique public-private partnership involving the World Health Organization (WHO), the United Nations Childrens Fund (UNICEF), Centers for Disease Control and Prevention (CDC), U.S. Agency for International Development (USAID), Rotary International (which has committed more than $500 million over a 20-year period), and other bilateral and multilateral agencies working with individual countries. The result has been that polio transmission has been interrupted in the Western Pacific Region of WHO (including China, Philippines, Laos, Cambodia, and Vietnam). The European Region of WHO apparently had its last case of indigenous transmission in late 1998, but there were two cases of paralysis in Bulgaria in early 2001, apparently resulting from importation of wild polioviruses from India. At the end of 2000, only 20 countries reported continuing occurrence of poliomyelitis. Most of these countries were in sub-Saharan Africa, but South Asia, including India, Afghanistan, and Pakistan, reported the bulk of the 2880 cases reported to WHO for 2000 (as of August 14, 2001).

The major impediments to global eradication of polio are: (1) internal conflicts in a number of countries including Afghanistan, Angola, Democratic Republic of Congo, Somalia, and Sudan; (2) maintaining political and financial commitments in the face of a disappearing disease; and (3) political actions in the northern state of Kano, Nigeria, in 2004 that resulted in a resurgence of polio in Nigeria and the exportation of polio to 12 other African countries that had been free of polio for up to 7 years. The eradication program is now back on track but it appears that transmission will not be interrupted globally until 2008 or later.

A major issue following successful eradication of wild poliovirus will be how and when to stop vaccination with OPV. An outbreak of Type 1 polio on the island of Hispaniola during 2000 and 2001 was caused by a vaccine virus that had circulated on the island for about 2 years and acquired transmissibility and neurovirulence characteristics similar to wild viruses.[15] Low immunization coverage on the island had allowed the vaccine virus to circulate among inadequately vaccinated children. This outbreak illustrates the need to maintain high immunization levels until it is safe to stop OPV use in order to avoid similar outbreaks in other countries.

Measles

Measles has been recognized as a distinct disease entity at least since the tenth century, when it was first distinguished from smallpox.[16] Soon after the European colonization of the New World, measles began to appear in epidemics in the Americas, with severe impact on indigenous populations that had not previously been exposed.

Outbreaks were reported as early as 1635 in what is now the United States.[2] A major epidemic occurred in the colonies during 1713–1715. For example, clergyman and writer Cotton Mather lost his wife, maid, and three children to measles in a two-week period. The fact that epidemics occurred at irregular intervals, often associated with known importations, and that many of the deaths recorded were in adults, suggests that measles was not an endemic disease throughout the colonies at this time. It was reported that 800–900 children died of measles in Charleston, South Carolina, in 1772 and measles was a leading cause of death in Boston that year. Although most measles cases and deaths occurred in children, adults who had escaped measles infection as children (often because they lived in rural areas) were also affected. During the Civil War, approximately 75,000 soldiers acquired measles and 5000 died.[17] During World War I, 90,000 U.S. soldiers acquired measles and more than 2000 died.[18] In the early decades of the twentieth century, thousands of fatal measles infections were reported each year, most of them in young children.[19]

By the beginning of the twentieth century, the major characteristics of measles had been fully established: it is highly infectious with a predictable 10-day incubation period, no long-term carrier state, and one attack confers lifelong immunity.[20] Isolation had been regarded as highly desirable, but Chapin accurately pointed out in 1910 that "Measles is a disease which in cities it seems impossible to check to any appreciable extent by isolation. . . . It seems in the highest degree probable that the disease prevails because of the unrecognized but infectious prodromal stage. No amount of isolation after the disease is recognized can atone for the harm done before the diagnosis is made."[21]

Measles is so highly contagious that it is essentially a universal disease, in the absence of immunization. In the pre-vaccine era, virtually all U.S. residents had developed antibodies to measles virus by the age of 15. Persons living in isolated communities such as on islands were only affected following importation of the virus from elsewhere, at which time virtually all susceptible persons would become infected, after which the virus would disappear from the population. In larger populations, the virus circulates continuously.

The introduction of measles vaccine in 1963 and its subsequent widespread use led to dramatic declines in the reported incidence of measles (Fig. 4.2), leading to announcement in 1966 that the epidemiologic basis existed to eradicate measles from the United States, using four strategies:[22] (1) routine immunization of infants at 1 year of age; (2) immunization at school entry of children not previously immunized; (3) surveillance; and (4) epidemic control.

During the period 1967–1969, considerable effort and resources were devoted to measles eradication, with the result that reported measles declined to an all-time low level of 22,231 reported cases in 1968. However, in 1969, rubella vaccine was licensed and major program emphasis shifted to its implementation. In consequence, there was an increase in the number of reported measles cases, reaching a peak of 75,290 cases in 1971.[23] Renewed public health efforts led to a resumption in the decline in incidence, reaching a record low of 22,094 cases in 1974. However, the incidence of measles rebounded, reaching a high of 57,345 cases in 1977. At the same time there was evidence of overall declines in immunization status of children in the United States. As a result, a Childhood Immunization Initiative was announced in

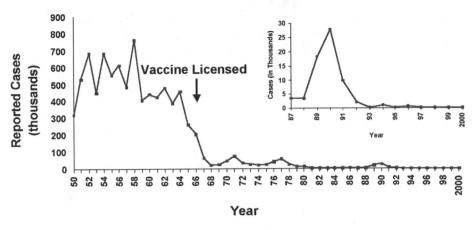

Figure 4.2. Measles Cases, United States—1950–2000.

1977, providing increased governmental support for immunization and undertaking major efforts to identify and immunize schoolchildren who had not been vaccinated. Initial success in this initiative led to the announcement, in October 1978, of a goal to eliminate indigenous measles from the United States by October 1, 1982.

The measles elimination program had three major elements: (1) achieving and maintaining high immunization levels, (2) strong and effective surveillance, and (3) aggressive response to the occurrence of disease.[24] To assure high immunization levels, major emphasis was placed on enactment and enforcement of school immunization requirements. The result was that, by 1981, all 50 states had laws requiring measles immunization (or history of disease) prior to first entry to school. Since the 1981–82 school year, ≥95% of children entering school have had proof of measles immunization. However, levels in preschoolers were not so high. From 1979 to 1985, when the U.S. immunization survey was discontinued, measles immunization coverage of two-year-old children was never greater than 68%.

Application of the measles-elimination strategies led to a further major reduction in reported incidence of measles, to a record low level of 1497 cases in 1983. Nonetheless, the target of elimination was not achieved and measles incidence in the mid-1980s averaged 3500 to 4000 cases per year. Two predominant patterns of transmission were detected—a preschool pattern in which unvaccinated preschool children predominated, particularly in urban areas; and a school-age pattern in which measles was transmitted primarily among school-age children who had not been protected by a single dose of vaccine.[25]

A major resurgence of measles occurred from 1989 to 1991, with 55,685 cases and 123 deaths reported. The primary populations affected were unvaccinated preschool children living in poor urban areas, although many of the early outbreaks involved measles in college students who had previously received a single dose of vaccine.

To overcome the problem of vaccine failure, a second dose of measles-containing vaccine was recommended for all children starting in 1989. Following the 1989–91 resurgence, a new Childhood Immunization Initiative (CII) was launched in 1993 with a massive infusion of funds to support immunization to improve immunization coverage of preschool children. The CII also included a renewed call for elimination of measles. As a result of these efforts, immunization levels in preschool children reached 90% and measles incidence again declined. From 1998 to 2000, 100 cases or fewer were reported each year, an incidence of fewer than one per million population. An expert panel convened in 2000 concluded that measles was no longer an endemic disease in the United States and that the continuing small numbers of cases represented importations or limited spread from importations.[26, 27] In addition to the U.S. target of elimination, elimination targets have been set for the American (2000), Eastern Mediterranean (2010), and European (2007) regions of the World Health Organization, and there is continuing discussion about the feasibility and/or desirability of attempting global eradication of measles.[28]

Other Vaccine-Preventable Diseases

Pertussis (Whooping Cough)

Pertussis is a highly infectious disease caused by the bacterium *Bordetella pertussis* and transmitted by inhalation of droplets aerosolized by sneezing, coughing, and the like. Infection is characterized by a protracted cough illness lasting many weeks and often accompanied by paroxysms of coughing ending in a characteristic inspiratory "whoop." It has primarily been considered a disease of infants, but in recent years it has been recognized that adults also may suffer from pertussis and may play an important role in transmission. The first known description of an outbreak dates from 1578 (in France).[29] The earliest reference to whooping cough in the colonies is from Boston in 1659, but there was no further reference until 1738, when there was an epidemic in South Carolina. Recurrent epidemics occurred in South Carolina in 1759 and 1765.[2]

In the pre-vaccine era, pertussis was responsible for recurrent epidemics of disease, with as many as 265,000 cases (1934) and 9296 deaths (1923) reported in a single year. Although the first pertussis vaccine was licensed in 1926, its use did not become universal until the licensure of combined DTP vaccine in the late 1940s. Widespread use of pertussis vaccines has had a major impact on the occurrence of the disease in the United States (Table 4.2).

Until the 1990s, pertussis vaccines used in the United States consisted of suspensions of killed organisms. These whole-cell vaccines were associated with a number of adverse events. The common events were mild (e.g., inflammation at the site of injection, fever) and occurred in up to 50% of vaccinees. Some, however, were more disturbing (e.g., hypotonic-hyporesponsive episodes, febrile convulsions). These latter occurred with a frequency of approximately·one per 1750 injections each. The Institute of Medicine (IOM) estimated encephalopathy caused by pertussis vaccine occurred in 0–10.5 persons per million vaccinations.[30] In addition, there were a number of rare adverse events (frequency ≤1/100,000) that occurred following vaccination and that were alleged by some to be caused by the vaccine (e.g., sudden infant death syndrome [SIDS], infantile spasms[29]). Careful study revealed that there was not an increased frequency of these events associated with vaccination and that it was extremely unlikely that the vaccine actually caused the events. However, the publicity generated by the claims against the vaccine led to striking reductions in vaccination coverage in the United Kingdom and some other countries, with resultant epidemics of whooping cough a few years later.[31]

Acellular pertussis vaccines, containing purified, selected components of *Bordetella pertussis*, were developed and introduced in the 1980s (Japan) and 1990s (U.S., other industrialized countries). These vaccines are associated with fewer adverse events known to be caused by pertussis vaccine and with similar effectiveness as the whole-cell vaccines.[32] Because of their increased costs, the acellular vaccines have not been introduced in immunization programs in developing countries.

The impact of pertussis vaccines has been substantial, with more than a 95% reduction in reported cases from representative twentieth-century annual morbidity. However, further reductions in pertussis may be difficult with present vaccines and vaccination strategies. Adolescents and adults, for whom there were no pertussis vaccines available in 2000, appear to be a reservoir for continuing transmission of the organism. Improved control may require vaccines that can be used in these older populations.

Diphtheria

Diphtheria is caused by the bacterium *Corynebacterium diphtheriae* and is transmitted by inhalation of droplets of respiratory secretions generated by coughing, sneezing, and so on. Its primary manifestations are: (1) development of a local inflammatory membrane, which, if located on the nasopharynx or larynx, can cause respiratory obstruction; and (2) remote manifestations of the exotoxin elaborated by the bacterium, which can cause damage to the myocardium, nervous system, or kidneys. Case-fatality rates may be as high as 50% in the absence of treatment. Cutaneous diphtheria occurs and is generally a mild disease.

The earliest description of what is probably diphtheria is that of Hippocrates in the fifth century B.C.[33] The first large-scale outbreak in colonial America occurred in 1735, with appearance of the disease in New Hampshire, subsequently spreading throughout New England.[2] A serious outbreak in Massachusetts in 1740 killed the wife of the president of Harvard and caused postponement of commencement exercises.

In the late nineteenth century diphtheria was recognized as a disease with continuing occurrence in the population; peaks in incidence were observed approximately every 10 years. Deaths due to diphtheria declined beginning in the early years of the twentieth century as a result of the use of diphtheria antitoxin and other measures such as intubation and tracheostomy. The maximum number of cases reported in a single year was 206,939 (1921), and as many as 13,000 deaths were recorded in a single year (1920). Diphtheria toxoid was introduced in 1923 and was followed by a decline in incidence. The most dramatic rates of decline occurred following World War II, after DTP vaccine was introduced and widely used. Since the 1980s, diphtheria has become a sporadic or imported disease in the United States, although the causative agent continues to circulate in some populations.

Tetanus

Tetanus is caused by the toxin elaborated by *Clostridium tetani*—anaerobic bacteria widely distributed in soil and animal droppings. Two primary types of tetanus are known—that resulting from inoculation of organisms into a sealed site (as with a puncture wound) and that resulting from inoculation of the organisms into the umbilical stump of an infant born to a susceptible mother (and thereby lacking circulating antitoxic antibodies). Both forms of the disease are characterized by the occurrence of convulsive muscle spasms that may result in fractures of bones and inability to eat or breathe. Untreated tetanus has a high case-fatality rate. Tetanus was first described by Hippocrates. It is unique among the vaccine-preventable diseases against which children and adults are routinely vaccinated in that it is not transmitted from one person to another.[34]

Reductions in tetanus mortality occurred first from improving conditions of childbirth and care of wounds, then from use of tetanus antitoxin to treat individuals who had developed tetanus, and finally from active immunization with tetanus toxoid, which was introduced in the 1920s but did not gain universal use in children until the introduction of combined DTP in the years following World War II. Routine immunization of military recruits resulted in a striking reduction in the incidence of tetanus in U.S. military personnel during the war compared to the experience in World War I.

The maximum number of reported deaths from tetanus in the United States was 1560 in 1923. With widespread use of tetanus toxoid, tetanus has become an uncommon disease in the United States, with an average of 47 cases reported each year in the period 1990–1999. Virtually all of these cases occurred in elderly persons who had grown up before tetanus toxoid came into wide use. Neonatal tetanus is rare in the United States, but in 1998 it accounted for an estimated 215,000 neonatal deaths, primarily in developing countries.

Haemophilus Influenzae Type B (Hib)

Hib disease, a bacterial infection, was first described at the end of the nineteenth century and has since come to be recognized as one of the leading causes of bacterial meningitis and other invasive bacterial diseases among preschool-age children. In the pre-vaccine era, approximately one in 200 US. children developed invasive Hib disease before the age of 5 years, and two out of three cases were in children less than 88 months of age.[35] The first Hib vaccines were introduced in the 1980s and had an appreciable impact on the occurrence of disease. However, they were not effective in young infants, and it was not until the introduction of the conjugated Hib vaccines effective in infants and young children in the late 1980s that the incidence plummeted. Hib disease has virtually disappeared from the United States in a period of less than 10 years.[36]

Mumps

Mumps is a viral disease first described by Hippocrates. It is spread through respiratory contact and was virtually a universal disease in the pre-vaccine era. Attesting to its somewhat lower infectiousness than conditions such as measles, sufficient numbers of children escaped infection to allow epidemics of mumps to occur during periods when young adults were brought together, as in military mobilization. Mumps was the leading cause of days lost from active duty in the U.S. Army in France during World War I. Although mumps commonly causes orchitis when it occurs in adult males (and oophoritis in females), it rarely results in sterility. In the United States, it was primarily considered a nuisance illness and consequently there was not immediate adoption of universal vaccination when the first attenuated mumps vaccine was introduced in 1967. However, when mumps vaccine was combined with measles and rubella in 1971, it rapidly gained wide acceptance in the United States. As a consequence, the reported incidence of mumps has declined dramatically compared to the pre-vaccine era.[37]

Rubella

Rubella is a viral disease spread by respiratory contact. First recognized as a distinct entity in the late eighteenth century, rubella was not considered a serious threat to human health until 1941, when an Australian ophthalmologist described a number of cases of congenital cataracts (often associated with congenital heart defects or deafness) in children born to women who had suffered rubella during early pregnancy. Subsequent investigations demonstrated that rubella infection in early pregnancy was a major cause of severe birth defects. An epidemic of rubella in 1963–1964 resulted in 20,000 infants being born in the United States with congenital deformities and an additional 12,000+ pregnancies terminated by stillbirth or spontaneous or induced abortion. The most common major defect was deafness; however, rubella infection in pregnancy can cause serious abnormalities in many organ systems, including the heart, eyes, brain, and endocrine system. Since rubella epidemics occurred at intervals of 6 to 9 years, there was concern about the impact of another epidemic, anticipated in 1970 or soon thereafter. Consequently, there was great relief when live, attenuated rubella vaccines were introduced in 1969.

The vaccine was immediately introduced into universal use for children in the United States. The reasons for vaccination of children when the population primarily affected was women of childbearing age were that children were responsible for primary transmission of the virus (particularly schoolchildren), and there was concern that the vaccine itself might result in congenital abnormalities if injected into a woman who was unknowingly pregnant or conceived shortly after immunization. Subsequent experience has not documented a risk to infants born to women who had received vaccine before they knew they were pregnant. Although the risk measured to date is zero, there is a maximum theoretical risk of congenital rubella syndrome following vaccination of a pregnant woman of 1%. Consequently, the vaccine is not recommended for women known to be pregnant.[38]

Widespread use of rubella vaccine in the United States has resulted in major declines in the incidence of rubella and has prevented the recurrence of major epidemics. However, because of incomplete protection of women of childbearing age, cases of congenital rubella syndrome (CRS) continue to occur on a sporadic basis or in limited outbreaks. Ultimate control and/or elimination of CRS will require assuring protection of women of childbearing age as well as controlling and/or interrupting transmission by continued vaccination of young children. In the United States, the major issue in 2000 is the susceptible adult not born in the United States, particularly persons of Hispanic ethnicity who were raised in countries that did not have rubella vaccination programs.

Immunization Delivery in the United States

Childhood immunizations in the United States are given in both the private and public sectors. Until the mid-1950s, there was no specific governmental support for immunizations. With the introduction of IPV, funds were specifically appropriated by Congress to support polio vaccination. However, general federal support for immunization did not occur until the passage of the Vaccination Assistance Act in 1962, which has been in effect ever since, periodically renewed and modified. This act authorized grants to states and other governmental agencies to support purchase of vaccine for free administration at local health departments and to support surveillance and communication/education. Since 1992, the grants have also supported immunization delivery activities.

Historically, parents who had effective health insurance coverage (or who could afford the cost of vaccines) took their children to private providers for immunization and well-child care. Those who did not took their children to public health clinics for free immunization, which often was provided as a single, categorical service. With a growing number of vaccines (which were increasingly expensive), vaccine cost became an even more important issue. At 2006 prices, the cost for vaccines (irrespective of physician administration fees) is approximately $1000 in the private sector (CDC, unpublished data). Consequently, the passage of the Vaccines For Children (VFC) Act in 1992 was pivotal in changing the balance of public- and private-sector immunizations. VFC provides free vaccines to providers for use with children who are covered by Medicaid or the Children's Health Plan. Whereas before the passage of VFC it was estimated that approximately 50% of children received immunizations (free) in the public sector, it is now estimated that more than 70% of children receive immunizations in the private sector, where they are also receiving other preventive and curative services (in a "medical home").

Immunization efforts in the United States have been significantly helped by enactment and enforcement of state laws that require immunization before first entry into school (or day care). The first school laws date to the mid-nineteenth century. Since 1980 all states have had school immunization laws in place, and since the 1981–1982 school year, at least 96% of children entering school have provided proof of immunization. Although these laws have ensured that school-age children are fully immunized, they have not ensured that preschool-age children received vaccine on schedule. This was amply demonstrated by the measles epidemic of 1989–1991. In response to this epidemic, another major national Childhood Immunization Initiative was announced, with massive infusions of funds to support immunization delivery as well as the traditional support for vaccine purchase and surveillance. In addition, local immunization coalitions were formed to improve immunization services. The result was an unprecedented increase in immunization coverage among young children.[39]

Table 4.3 summarizes current immunization levels in 19- to 35-month-old children, which are now at historic high levels.[40] Although the situation in the United States is now better than ever before, there is continuing cause for concern because:

- There are 11,000 births each day in the United States, and each child needs to be immunized.
- At least 25% of children receive immunizations from more than one provider.
- The immunization schedule is complex and getting even more so—in 2003 children should receive 16–20 injections of 11 different vaccine antigens before age two.
- Both parents and providers overestimate the level of protection in their children. Most parents support immunization and feel their children are fully immunized. Most physicians feels likewise, but studies have shown that pediatricians typically overestimate coverage in their patients by *more than* 20%.
- Few physicians use reminder or recall systems to notify their patients of immunizations due (reminder) or overdue (recall).

To deal with these issues, the National Vaccine Advisory Committee (NVAC) has called for development of a nationwide network of population-based immunization registries (confidential, computerized information systems that contain information about children and immunizations).[41] The Healthy People 2010 objectives call for 95% of children ages zero to six to be enrolled in population-based immunization registries by 2010.[42]

Table 4.3. Vaccination coverage among children aged 19–35 months, United States, 2003.

Vaccine (# Doses)	Coverage (%)
DTP/DTaP* 3+	96.0
DTP/DTaP 4+	84.8
Poliovirus 3+	91.6
Hib** 3+	93.9
Measles 1+	93.0
Hepatitis B 3+	92.4
Varicella 1+	84.8
PCV*** 3+	68.1
Series	
4+ DTP/3+ Polio/1+ Measles	82.2
4/3/1/3+ Hib	81.3
4/3/1/3/3+ Hepatitis B	79.4
4/3/1/3/3/1+ Varicella	72.5

*Diphtheria and tetanus toxoids and pertussis vaccine/diphtheria and tetanus toxoids and acellular pertussis vaccine.
**Haemophilus influenzae* type b vaccine.
***Pneumococcal conjugate vaccine.

Challenges and Future Prospects

In the twenty-first century, one of the most important challenges to continued success with immunizations is the very success of the program to date. Today's parents (and today's physicians) no longer see and fear the diseases against which we are immunizing children. Most of today's parents did not themselves suffer (or see their siblings or friends suffer) from diphtheria, polio, measles, or Hib disease. Consequently it is difficult for them to appreciate the benefits of immunization, and they are increasingly likely to be influenced by the real (or alleged) risks associated with immunization.

The biotechnology revolution will give us an increasing number of vaccines in the next several years. Some of the first candidates probably will be conjugated meningococcal vaccines and live-attenuated influenza vaccines for children. Along with the promise of even greater protection will come a number of new challenges, including how to deliver these new vaccines (increased use of combination vaccines and novel means of delivery will clearly be important). Additionally, newer vaccines may address problems that are not as universal and catastrophic as, for example, measles, and this will necessitate further assessments of benefits and risks. On the other hand, new vaccines may well address noninfectious conditions such as cancer or heart disease. This may bring in new target groups for vaccination.

In all the enthusiasm for new vaccines, it must be recalled that we currently do not do a very good job in protecting adults with vaccines. Although annual influenza vaccination and once-in-a-lifetime immunization with pneumococcal vaccine have been recommended for decades for all persons *over* 65 years of age, in 1999 only 66.7% of these persons had received influenza vaccine in the preceding 12 months and only 54.1% had ever received pneumococcal vaccine.[43]

Thus, although there has been great progress and there is great promise for the future, there remain significant challenges if we are to realize the full benefits that vaccines can offer.

References

1. Fenner F, Henderson DA, Arita I, et al. Smallpox and its eradication. Geneva, Switzerland: World Health Organization, 1988, 239.
2. Duffy J. Epidemics in Colonial America. Baton Rouge, LA: Louisiana State University Press, 1953.
3. Centers for Disease Control and Prevention. Impact of vaccines universally recommended for children—United States, 1900–1998. *MMWR* 1999:48:243–48.
4. Fenner F, Henderson DA, Arita I, et al. Smallpox and its Eradication. Geneva, Switzerland: World Health Organization, 1988.
5. Henderson DA, Moss B. Smallpox and vaccinia. In: Plotkin S, Orenstein WA, eds. Vaccines, 3d ed. Philadelphia: WB Saunders, 1999, 97.
6. Hopkins DR. Peasants and Princes. Chicago: University of Chicago Press, 1983.
7. Orenstein WA, Hinman AR. The immunization system in the Untied States—the role of school immunization laws. *Vaccine* 1999:17:S19–S24.
8. Foege WH, Millar JD, Henderson DA. Smallpox eradication in West and Central Africa. *Bull WHO* 1975:52:209–22.

9. World Health Organization Executive Board Resolution EB109/17. Smallpox eradication: destruction of smallpox virus stocks. January 2002. Available at http://policy.who.int/cgi-bin/om_isapi.dll?infobase=WHA&softpage=Browse_Frame_Pg42, accessed April 30, 2006.
10. Sutter W, Cochi S, Melnick J. Live attenuated poliovirus vaccines. In: Plotkin S, Orenstein WA, eds. Vaccines, 3d ed. Philadelphia: WB Saunders, 1999, 364–408.
11. Cavery CS. Preliminary report of an epidemic of paralytic disease, occurring in Vermont, in the summer of 1894. *Yale Med J* 1894:1:1. Cited in Paul JR. A History of Poliomyelitis. New Haven: Yale University Press, 1971.
12. Rogers N. Dirt and Disease: Polio before FDR. New Brunswick, NJ: Rutgers University Press, 1992.
13. Nathanson N, Langmuir AD. The Cutter incident: poliomyelitis following formaldehyde-inactivated poliovirus vaccination in the United states during the spring of 1995. II. Relationship of poliomyelitis to Cutter vaccine. *Am J Hyg* 1963:78:29–60.
14. Centers for Disease Control and Prevention. Poliomyelitis prevention in the United States: updated recommendations of the Advisory Committee on Immunization Practices (ACIP), 2000. *MMWR* 2000:49(RR05):1–22.
15. Centers for Disease Control and Prevention. Outbreak of poliomyelitis—Dominican Republic and Haiti, 2000. *MMWR* 2000:49:1094, 1103.
16. Bloch AB, Orenstein WA, Wassilak SG, et al. Epidemiology of measles and its complications. In: Gruenberg EM, Lewis C, Goldston SE, eds. Vaccinating Against Brain Syndromes: The Campaign Against Measles and Rubella. New York: Oxford University Press, 1986, 5–20.
17. U.S. Army. The Medical and Surgical History of the War of the Rebellion (1861–1865), medical vol., 1st part. Washington, DC: Government Printing Office, 1870, 637, 710.
18. U.S. Army. The Medical Department of the United States Army in the World War, Vol. 15. Washington, DC: Government Printing Office, 1925, 576.
19. Bureau of the Census. Historical Statistics of the United States: Colonial Times to 1970. Washington, DC: U.S. Dept of Commerce, Bureau of the Census, 1975.
20. Hinman AR, Bart KJ, Orenstein WA, et al. History of measles control efforts. In: Gruenberg EM, Lewis C, Goldston SE, eds. Vaccinating Against Brain Syndromes: The Campaign Against Measles and Rubella. New York: Oxford University Press, 1986, 36–48.
21. Chapin CV. The Sources and Modes of Infection. New York: John Wiley, 1910, 103–4.
22. Sencer DJ, Dull HB, Langmuir AD. Epidemiologic basis for eradication of measles in 1967. *Public Health Rep* 1967:82:253–56.
23. Hinman AR, Brandling-Bennett AD, Nieburg PI. The opportunity and obligation to eliminate measles from the United States. *JAMA* 1979:242:1157–62.
24. Hinman AR, Kirby CED, Eddins DL, et al. Elimination of indigenous measles from the United States. *Rev Inf Dis* 1983:5:538–45.
25. Markowitz LE, Preblud SR, Orenstein WA, et al. Patterns of transmission in measles outbreaks in the U.S., 1985–1986. *N Engl J Med* 1989:320:75–81.
26. Hutchins S, Markowitz L, Atkinson W, et al. Measles outbreaks in the U.S., 1987 through 1990. *Pediatr Infect Dis J* 1996:15:31–38.
27. Centers for Disease Control and Prevention. Measles – United States, 1999. *MMWR* 2000; 49:557–60.
28. Centers for Disease Control and Prevention. Advances in global measles control and elimination: Summary of the 1997 international meeting. *MMWR* 1998:47(RR11):1–23.
29. Edwards KM, Decker MD, Mortimer EA Jr. Pertussis vaccine. In: Plotkin S, Orenstein WA, eds. Vaccines, 3d ed. Philadelphia: WB Saunders, 1999, 293–344.

30. Howson CP, Howe CJ, Fineberg HV, eds. Adverse Effects of Pertussis and Rubella Vaccines. A Report of the Committee to Review Adverse Consequences of Pertussis and Rubella Vaccines, Institute of Medicine. Washington, DC: National Academy Press 1991.
31. Gangarosa EJ, Galazka AM, Wolfe CR, et al. Impact of anti-vaccine movements on pertussis control: the untold story. *Lancet* 1998:351:356–61.
32. Centers for Disease Control and Prevention. Petussis vaccination: use of acellular pertussis vaccines among infants and young children – recommendations of the Advisory Committee on Immunization Practices (ACIP). *MMWR* 1997:46(No. RR-7):1–25.
33. Mortimer EA Jr, Wharton M. Diphtheria toxoid. In: Plotkin S, Orenstein WA, eds. Vaccines, 3d ed. Philadelphia: WB Saunders, 1999, 140–57.
34. Wassilak SGF, Murphy TV, Roper MH, Orenstein WA. Tetanus toxoid. In: Plotkin S, Orenstein WA, eds. Vaccines, 3d ed. Philadelphia: WB Saunders, 1999, 745–82.
35. Ward J, Zangwill KM. Haemophilus influenzae vaccines. In: Plotkin S, Orenstein WA, eds. Vaccines, 3d ed. Philadelphia: WB Saunders, 1999, 183–221.
36. Centers for Disease Control and Prevention. Progress toward eliminating Haemophilus influenzae type b disease among infants and children—United States, 1999. *MMWR* 2000:49:585–89.
37. Plotkin SA. Mumps vaccine. In: Plotkin S, Orenstein WA, eds. Vaccines, 3d ed. Philadelphia: WB Saunders, 1999, 441–70.
38. Plotkin SA, Reef S. Rubella vaccine. In: Plotkin S, Orenstein WA, eds. Vaccines, 3d ed. Philadelphia: WB Saunders, 1999, 707–44.
39. Orenstein WA, Rodewald LA, Hinman AR. Immunization in the United States. In: Plotkin S, Orenstein WA, eds. Vaccines, 3d ed. Philadelphia: WB Saunders, 1999, 1357–86.
40. Centers for Disease Control and Prevention. National, state, and urban area vaccination coverage among children aged 19–35 months—United States, 2003. *MMWR* 2004;53:658–61.
41. National Vaccine Advisory Committee. Development of community and state-based immunization registries, January 12, 1999. Available at: http://www.cdc.gov/nip/registry/pubs/nvac.htm, accessed April 30, 2006.
42. Healthy People 2010. Objective 14–26. Washington, DC: Department of Health and Human Services, 2000.
43. Centers for Disease Control and Prevention. Influenza and pneumococcal vaccination levels among persons >65 years—United States, 1999. *MMWR* 2001:50:532–37.

Suggested Reading

Fenner, F, Henderson DA, Arita I, et al. Small Pox and Its Eradication. Geneva Switzerland: World Health Organization, 1988.
Oshinsky D. Polio: An American Story. New York: Oxford University Press, 2005.

5

Polio Can Be Conquered: Science and Health Propaganda in the United States from Polio Polly to Jonas Salk

NAOMI ROGERS

On December 13, 2002, President George W. Bush announced that, as a result of growing bioterrorist concerns since the September 11 attacks, his administration was "evaluating old threats in a new light." Bush proposed an ambitious new program to vaccinate as many as 10 million Americans, starting with mandatory vaccination for members of the U.S. armed forces, followed by voluntary vaccinations for "first responders" such as police, firefighters and health workers, with access to the vaccine widening to members of the general public.[1]

Questions about possible side effects and contagion immediately consumed the mass media. For many reasons, Americans were not convinced that the Bush administration's new smallpox vaccination program made sense. To soften public resistance, the Bush administration coordinated a media campaign to call to the public's mind the collective fear of infectious disease that had been so widespread in the United States decades earlier. Both the popular press and public health journals retold the story of New York City's 1947 smallpox scare, illustrated with images of patients scarred by smallpox, and photos of long lines of anxious and impatient people waiting for their vaccine shots.[2,3,4,5] Health professionals revisited America's smallpox history to assess likely fatality rates and compliance, the effectiveness of health intervention and education, and potential adverse reactions to the vaccine. For a brief moment, the medical past was alive and contagious.[6,7,8,9]

Despite this effort to revive memories of the "bad old days" of smallpox, even within the context of post-September 11, America did not embrace the Administration's pre-emptive defense against bioterrorism. Many professional organizations and hospital unions resisted implementing the vaccination program.[10] To an already skeptical public, this resistance made sense, and their doubts seemed validated in March 2003 with the deaths of a nurse, a nurse's aide, and a National Guardsman, and reports of numerous cases of medical complications.. The result was the temporary suspension of the vaccine program in some states and the passage of the Smallpox Emergency Compensation Act in April 2003, which provided $42 million for workers and their families harmed by complications from the vaccine.[11,12] By December 2003, only around 39,000 health workers had accepted the vaccine.[13,14]

In the 1940s and early 1950s, health officials in the United States did not have to manufacture fear of infectious disease. Polio, although a minor cause of morbidity and mortality, was visible and frightening, a viral disease that crippled some but not all, and occurred in epidemics that could not be safely predicted or prevented. There was no vaccine or other certain preventive measure, and therapies were varied and controversial.[15,16,17,18] The disease was widely discussed in newspapers, newsreels, and family magazines, and science writers like Paul de Kruif, Roland Berg, and Victor Cohn found eager readers for their reports on polio among both the lay public and health professionals (Fig. 5.1).[19,20,21]

The case of polio prompts us to look at early audiences of popular science, for many sources crossed professional lines and were addressed not only to potential patients and their families but also to health professionals themselves. A didactic and prescriptive literature, this polio material sought to create consumers of science and medicine.[22,23] Anticipating and shaping questions readers might have, polio guides provided information that patients and their families might take to their medical providers, and that nurses and physicians might use to reassure families and neighbors, as well offering optimistic insights into the workings of laboratory scientists and the implications of their research for private and public health practices. There were three main types of popular polio resources: guides to prevention, which suggested practical and reassuring hygiene techniques; therapeutic manuals for the care of paralyzed patients; and inspirational tales of the disabled overcoming social stigma and achieving success in school, the workplace, or romance. By 1940, the health education divisions of medium and large public health departments were regularly publishing and distributing popular polio tracts. During the next decade, however, a new and independent polio propaganda industry arose, spurred by the founding of the National Foundation for Infantile Paralysis (NFIP), a philanthropic organization that raised public funds to pay for medical care, rehabilitation equipment, and scientific research. Popularizing a fervent public faith in scientific research as the best weapon in the fight against disease, writers and designers from the NFIP turned the organization's investment in science into a potent publicity tool. As the title of one NFIP pamphlet proclaimed in 1949, "polio can be conquered."[24,16,17,18]

I will explore several examples of printed polio health literature from the early 1940s to the early 1960s, a period bracketed by the founding of the NFIP in 1938 and the federal government's approval of the Salk polio vaccine in 1955 and the Sabin oral vaccine in 1960. The polio vaccines appeared at a high water mark in the

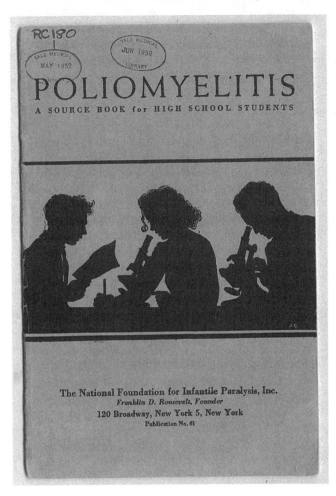

Figure 5.1. This pamphlet from the National Foundation for Infantile Paralysis provided high school students with basic information about what was currently understood about the causes, prevention, and treatment of poliomyelitis, and offered hope for a cure through dedicated research. (From March of Dimes, used by permission.)

history of American biomedical sciences, and they became one of the great symbols of the impressive potential of modern medical research.[25]

Consistently throughout this literature, polio science was personified by two figures: the ordinary clinician and the white-coated scientist (often an MD as well). The popularized polio literature included a little medical theory, a little philosophy, some public health policy, and frequently a commercial message. The audience was urged to consume particular services or products or donate money to continue the process of scientific research and medical care. But the theories and products of science—even its authoritative voice—proved as unpredictable and complicated as polio epidemics themselves. Nonetheless, readers turned to these guides for every kind of information and advice. Following a brief overview of the assumptions and resources shaping the popular conceptions of polio, I will discuss a polio guide distributed by a state health department; two commercial guides produced, respectively, by Metropolitan Life and the manufacturer of Lysol disinfectants; guides representing the popularized science and professional philanthropy of the NFIP; and finally, a children's book about Jonas Salk, the great polio hero.

Crippled Children, Money, and Medicine

By the 1930s, the care and rehabilitation of crippled children had become part of the larger problem of polio.[26,27] Polio epidemics were growing more frequent and more serious, and an accurate understanding of how and where polio affected the body became more crucial for both health professionals and the lay public. By 1940, there had been significant transformations in medical and lay interpretations of polio. In the popular imagination, the typical victim of the disease was no longer an impoverished child marked by the signs of institutional neglect but rather an alert, well-fed, mainstream American child. While elite scientists debated among themselves, ordinary physicians and nurses struggled to provide practical and comforting care, sometimes turning to the products and ideas of the most modern science of their day, sometimes rejecting it. The public, similarly, sought out popularized science, assessing for themselves current therapies and theories. We know something of these dynamics from the letters, oral histories, and photograph albums of families, and from articles, conference papers, and discussion sections in professional journals. From the polio guides themselves we see some of the ways elite and popular science, practical care, and reflective theory came together.

Polio had once been seen as a disease of immigrants and the poor, but with the 1932 presidential election of Franklin Delano Roosevelt—a wealthy lawyer from the Roosevelt clan whose bout with paralytic polio a decade earlier had become part of his admirable battle to return to public, political life—polio gained a new cultural importance. Until Roosevelt's New Deal administration established the 1935 Social Security Act, with its special provision to oversee the care of crippled children, polio care was charity care. Private welfare agencies provided some resources, but children crippled by polio jostled for priority with the agencies' other clients disabled by malnutrition, childbirth complications, tuberculosis, and syphilis. In 1938, however, polio philanthropy was transformed by a new kind of professionalized fund-raising with the organization of the National Foundation for Infantile Paralysis (NFIP), headed by Wall Street lawyer Basil O'Connor, Roosevelt's former law partner. Under O'Connor, the NFIP grew into a centralized and highly sophisticated philanthropic organization. Although local chapters were led by prominent businessmen and society women, O'Connor did not rely solely on well-meaning amateur volunteers. He recruited a national staff of professionals from public relations, health education, and science journalism, and he developed close connections with the elite of the medical profession through his friendship with Morris Fishbein, the powerful secretary of the American Medical Association (AMA) and an outspoken critic of socialized and alternative medicine.[28,29,30] Despite the use of *foundation* in its title, the NFIP had no endowment like the Rockefeller Foundation, and more like the National Tuberculosis Association, it relied on public funds raised through its sophisticated March of Dimes campaigns. In the NFIP's modernized campaigns, polio philanthropy was no longer welfare, the crippled no longer the deserving poor. The propaganda of the NFIP personified polio as a well-dressed poster child, awkwardly leaning on crutches or getting out of a wheelchair. This child appeared defiantly alone—no charity case in an institution surrounded by hovering nurses or physicians, but someone who could be the son or daughter of any ordinary American family.

Until the 1950s, most health officials thought of potential polio victims as children, although epidemiologists had begun to point out the rising numbers of paralyzed adolescents and adults. The NFIP's publicity campaigns identified this fear, exploited it to some extent, and sought to shape it into what were considered appropriate health behaviors. This era of polio research was tumultuous and confusing. As Yale virologist Dorothy Horstmann admitted as late as 1948, "In spite of all the information collected by many investigators in many lands, we still cannot say why poliomyelitis suddenly became epidemic almost 60 years ago, why it is increasing rather than decreasing like other infectious diseases, why it is a summer disease with a preference for certain lands, how it is spread or how it may be prevented."[31] A "filterable virus" had been identified as the specific etiological cause of polio as early as 1909, but the other characteristics of the disease remained puzzling, and different theories of how the virus traveled through the body and the population rose and fell. In the 1910s and 1920s, scientists had believed that polio was a contagious, enteric disease, spread by coughing, spitting, and kissing or perhaps by some asymptomatic "Polio Polly";[20] by 1940, polio was considered a neuro-tropic and unpredictably infectious disease, its virus traveling primarily in central nervous tissue pathways and not in the blood. Only during the late 1940s was polio reconceived as an endemic disease with enteric features, in which blood played a crucial role in developing immunity. According to this new model—one largely accepted by scientists today—the polio virus invaded non-neurological tissues, spreading the disease from person to person by nasal and fecal matter and only rarely causing neurological complications. The theoretical and technical insights of this new model allowed virologists like Jonas Salk to develop a safe vaccine.[15,32]

Polio Politics, Physicians, and the Public

Health departments had long treaded cautiously in order not to alienate local private physicians, a balance made more difficult during the Great Depression, when general practitioners saw free clinics and other government health services as threats to their dwindling paying patient clientele. Yet as municipal and state officials began closing hospital clinics and wards, with no money to pay medical staff or buy drugs and equipment, New Deal agencies in the 1930s began to venture further into medical arenas. In this desperate medical marketplace, federal officials found that some physicians appreciated the government relief checks that enabled patients to pay their medical bills, as well as the federal works programs that cleared mosquito-breeding swamps, renovated school buildings with fly-screens and toilets, and built hospital wings and laboratory buildings.[33]

In their efforts to stretch limited resources, American families facing sickness in the Depression years relied on domestic remedies, patent medicines, and alternative practitioners whose fees were lower than regular physicians.[34] But there were also broader forces behind the public's turning away from organized medicine. Although Roosevelt's New Deal advisors recognized the crucial role of sickness in contributing to a cycle of poverty and unemployment, pressure from the conservative leaders of the AMA kept any kind of government health insurance off the federal political agenda. Progressive physician groups like the Physicians Committee for the Improvement of Medical Care (founded in 1937) and the Physicians Forum (founded in 1941) lobbied in Washington to expand government-funded medical services, but they lacked the resources of Morris Fishbein, editor of both the *Journal of the American Medical Association* and the AMA's popular health magazine *Hygeia*[35,36,37] Americans continued to respect medical science and many of its individual practitioners—nurses had especially high status in many communities—but there was growing anger and resentment among patients in rural areas, patients of color, and the poor, all forced to rely on the goodwill of individual doctors and all facing unequal access to health facilities segregated by class and race.[33]

Recognizing the tense medical politics of the 1930s and 1940s, the NFIP was careful to avoid designing any policies that appeared to value one kind of medical care or practitioner over others. It agreed to pay for any kind of polio care "if recommended by a physician." As some states struggled to determine who should be recognized by law as a licensed physician, the NFIP left the definition deliberately vague. Doctors, nurses, and physical therapists, who appreciated the funding that it provided for medical expenses, hospital bills, and rehabilitative therapy and equipment, extended their loyalty to the NFIP.[38] The NFIP's policies helped to smooth over tensions in the medical marketplace and yet at the same time continued to highlight awareness that polio therapy and research cost money.

The NFIP featured scientists in all their popular guides. Unlike the physicians of the AMA, scientists remained glorious in their white coats, untainted by medical politics and in-fighting, their heroic work dramatized by Hollywood in *The Story of Louis Pasteur* (1936) and *Dr Ehrlich's Magic Bullet* (1940). Insulin, sulfonamide, and later streptomycin and penicillin were hailed as miracle drugs, the products of ever-progressive scientific research. Despite the humanizing writing of science journalists like Paul de Kruif in *Microbe Hunters* (1926), *Men Against Death* (1932), and *The Fight for Life* (1938), scientists remained in the public mind more austere and distant than ordinary clinicians.[25,39,40] Writers did have to balance the exciting and inspiring search for scientific truth with the confused state of polio science, which until the early 1950s was unable to explain how polio spread through the body and through the community, or to offer an effective preventative or assessment of the array of therapeutic options. The public, thus, was expected to care about and admire the intricacies of polio science, to understand why scientists had no clear answers yet, and to contribute its faith through funding. Physicians in this literature were presented as reactive figures—ever hopeful, ever willing to try out the products of scientific research and to reassure their patients that polio science was closer to conquering the disease. Medical theories of polio were not restricted to the complex pages of professional journals, but were freely debated and interpreted in the popular press. Such guides played a crucial role in the development of what historians have called the Golden Age of Medicine. As a topic of popular science polio—so frightening and devastating a disease—had special powers to turn the difficulties of scientific explanation into assets for the consumers of science.

No Doubt the Day Will Come

In 1941 the Department of Public Health of the state of Illinois published a pamphlet, "Things You Want to Know About Infantile Paralysis," and made it "available to Illinois residents without charge." In its opening section, "Facing the Facts," the public's fear of polio was acknowledged and then dismissed as irrational: "many people seem to have an unreasoning fear of anterior poliomyelitis or, as it is commonly called, infantile paralysis." The morbidity statistics for polio were compared to those of other diseases in order to show that deaths from polio were less common than deaths from diphtheria, pulmonary tuberculosis, or pneumonia. Nor, readers were assured, was polio so unusual in eluding the grasp of doctors and scientists; like polio, rheumatic fever, appendicitis, diabetes, and "a host of other illnesses" had no easy preventative.

Following a common trope that a poorly understood disease must be caused by something "invisible," the guide explained the polio virus in a section entitled "The Invisible Enemy." In terms that reflected the scientific consensus of the 1930s, polio was presented as a confusing kind of enteric disease, with its virus found "chiefly" in the nose, throat, and bowels. But this knowledge had not yet produced guidelines for prevention. "Scientists cannot yet say definitely" whether it is spread by direct contact, raw sewage, contaminated water, milk, other food "or even by summer insects." Drawing on the model of New York City's department of health that employed bacteriologists and chemists as researchers, the Illinois guide portrayed scientists working not only in university laboratories but also in public health departments. "Scientists in laboratories and in public health work everywhere are constantly studying this virus," the guide explained, "and no doubt the day will come when they can say with certainty just how it is spread from person to person and how it might practically be kept from spreading."[41]

Families suspecting their children had polio were urged to contact their physicians. The phrasing made clear that many families would hesitate to go to a doctor first, preferring to try other initial remedies. "There is just one good thing about being deathly afraid of infantile paralysis," the guide said bluntly, "and that is that such fear may make people call the physician quickly." Readers were assured that timing was critical, for, according to prevailing theory, muscles in the early stages had not yet developed paralysis, and "the physician can do the most to help the patient and to prevent further trouble." Like appendicitis, cancer, pneumonia, syphilis, tuberculosis, and "the majority of diseases," polio could "usually be 'nipped in the bud,' and often cured, *if the physician is called in time*."[41] Care for polio patients in a hospital was neither assumed nor recommended. Indeed, as many readers may have recognized but this guide left unstated, most American hospitals refused to admit polio cases as they were considered too contagious. They were usually sent first to a contagious disease ward, a facility not available in private community hospitals but as a separate building or wing at the municipal or county public hospital, and later to a crippled children's home or back to their family.[42–45] It was, readers were reminded (perhaps because the authority for such decisions was rarely clear-cut), better "for the patient to remain quietly at home than to be moved to a hospital. *This should be decided by the physician*."[41]

Laboratory science, according to the Illinois pamphlet, could offer some definite hope for both families and practitioners. Although private physicians would probably know "what danger signs to look for, and what special tests to make" they could be assisted, for no additional charge, by a "consultant" from the Illinois Department of Public Health. This official not only had special diagnostic skills but could also give the patient polio serum "without charge."[41] Serum made from the blood of patients who had recovered from the disease, known as "convalescent" serum, had been first developed during the 1910s. Although discredited by elite medical journals, and contradicted by the work of scientists like Simon Flexner at New York's Rockefeller Institute for Medical Research, which suggested that the polio virus did not travel through the blood, such serum continued to be produced and distributed by many health departments during the 1920s and 1930s.[16] Further, drawing on another popular theory of adult immunity based on evidence that adults rarely developed the paralytic form of the disease during an epidemic, Illinois health officials also used "normal adult serum" collected by state officials from "healthy city-bred adults" who have usually "built up, in their own blood serum, a strong degree of resistance to the disease."[41] The use of serum no longer made scientific sense in 1941, but patients and their families could take comfort in the imprimatur of the public health laboratory.

Anticipating the future of a disabled person in 1941, Illinois officials recognized, could be disheartening for both child and parents. Yet should the child recover without paralysis, the pamphlet assured readers, a "single attack" usually conferred "lifetime immunity" to the disease. Even if there was significant paralysis, however, there could still be hope for a "normal" life. Families were urged to turn to the example of the nation's most prominent polio survivor—who had just been re-elected to an unprecedented third term—for comfort and inspiration: "even the unfortunate patient who is left physically handicapped by infantile paralysis may live to be a President of the United States of America."[41] Unconscious of the ironic yet powerful symbolism of a disabled president who hid his disability, these were words that parents and health professionals could use to reassure a child, relatives, and other members of the community.[26,46,47]

Keep Your Home "Hospital Clean"

By the late 1940s, rehabilitation medicine was reinvigorated as a professional specialty as it moved out of crippled children's homes and into veterans' hospitals.[48,49] The war generation was returning to peace and suburbia, having experienced not only the impressive military medicine of skilled surgery and antibiotics, but also the constant propaganda of the Office of War Information's posters, movies, and pamphlets warning against enemy spies, venereal disease, mosquitoes, and mental disease. Both the tactics and personnel of the NFIP's impressive publicity facilities had been harnessed as part of these militarized health campaigns. During the war, Basil O'Connor had taken on an additional role as head of the American Red Cross, and Dorothy Ducas, from the NFIP's Public Relations Department, had run the Magazine Division of the Office of War Information.

In the economic boom of postwar America, more families were buying private health insurance and seeking health care at doctors' offices and hospitals.[50,51] The medical marketplace was infused by the postwar economic boom. Even before the war the production of popular science and medical advice had been expanding beyond the work of health departments to include a mixture of voluntary agencies, commercial manufacturers, disease philanthropies, life insurance companies, and pharmaceutical industries. The first edition of pediatrician Benjamin Spock's best-selling *Baby and Child Care* appeared in 1946, and life insurance companies sought out the same market. In 1946, the Metropolitan Life Insurance Company came out with *Common Childhood Diseases*, a 35-page "reference book, for permanent use in the home" consisting of a compilation of the many health-education pamphlets that Metropolitan Life had been producing "for a long time."[52] Scientific investigation, readers were reminded, was an incontrovertible means of medical progress: "it is comforting to parents to know that many new ways have been found, through recent discoveries in medical science, to protect the life and health of babies and young children."[52] Although this pamphlet appeared 8 years before the development of a polio vaccine, immunization against smallpox and typhoid had become a standard part of middle-class pediatric practice, a crucial part of what historian Nancy Tomes has identified as the growing notion of health as a "luxury good."[22] Urging health consumers to expand their use of physicians for well-baby care and regular pediatric visits, the book included an "Immunization Timetable" and a model "Record of Immunization," as domesticated models of a doctor's office chart.[52]

Fourteen diseases were discussed in the Metropolitan Life guide, with three pages allotted for polio. By 1946 most scientists had rejected the enteric picture of polio, and they saw polio as a disease of the nervous system.[32,16] Polio, readers were told, "is caused by a virus which attacks the central nervous system."[52] The decline of the enteric model, however, left the problem of how to protect a child from infection. There were no "specific means of preventing infantile paralysis," but Metropolitan Life urged parents to take "various precautions" like keeping children away from "movies, parties, crowded trains, and all public gatherings" and "from public beaches and swimming pools" during an epidemic. A brief reference to the enteric model surfaced with a warning to avoid playing in or near streams, lakes, or ditches into which sewage drained, for the virus "as well as the germs of other diseases" had been found in "sewage-contaminated water," a reference to the work of epidemiologist John Paul and his Yale Polio Unit. Most usefully, from a prescriptive standpoint, the neurotropic model of polio had reinvigorated an older view about the danger of focal infection. Thus, children should avoid having tonsil or teeth extractions or other operations "on and about the nose, throat and mouth," lest the polio virus enter the body "and come in contact with nerves."[52] The rest of this advice drew on familiar general arguments about private hygienic behavior. As the mechanism of polio's transmission was "still unknown," parents should, "to be on the safe side," "keep the home as clean as possible. Use plenty of soap and water, fight flies, mice, rats, and other vermin, and protect food from flies." Children should additionally be guarded "from overfatigue and from sudden chilling." This advice, the guide tried to make clear, was not to be taken as a replacement for professional medical care: "do not delay" in consulting a doctor "for even minor upsets."[52]

The Metropolitan Life guide presented the greatest scientific progress as having occurred in the area of polio therapy. The care of paralyzed patients had never been made the subject of any elite scientific research program, so the guide derived its conclusions from an unconventional source, carefully disguised. As a yardstick of progress, parents were first reminded that only 15–20% of those infected by the polio virus developed permanent paralysis, and that many "show a complete and early recovery."[52] The American public had become more optimistic about healing polio's crippling effects with the publicized work of Sister Elizabeth Kenny, an Australian nurse who had set up her own polio institute in Minneapolis in 1942, and who traveled around the country propounding her method of early treatment by "hot packs" and specific physical therapies.[17,26,53–55] By the mid-1940s Kenny's methods were widely adopted by nurses, doctors, and physical therapists, although researchers still disagreed with her theories of the disease, and clinicians were not convinced that her methods must be practiced only by a formally trained Kenny therapist. Kenny's struggles to convince doctors of the worth of her method were dramatized by Hollywood in *Sister Kenny,* a 1946 RKO movie starring Rosalind Russell. Recognizing her popular appeal and the simultaneous controversy among health professionals, the writers of the Metropolitan Life's guide tried to have it both ways, not naming Kenny but nevertheless arguing that recovery would be speedier and that "crippling aftereffects" could be prevented or lessened with "early treatment under a skilled physician, nurse and physical therapist" who understood the importance of "proper controlled rest and motion of the affected muscles."[52]

The commercial implications of preventive techniques practiced at home were clearly spelled out in contemporary guides, such as a *Handbook on Infantile Paralysis* distributed by the manufacturers of Lysol disinfectants, in which advertisement was mixed with a condensed version of a 1950 article on polio by a *Good Housekeeping* science writer. As the manufacturer stated on the front cover—although in small print—the pamphlet's distribution was "a public service with no intention of suggesting that LYSOL will prevent or cure Polio." Nonetheless readers could easily be misled by the smiling family featured on the cover: a husband carrying a toddler and a mother with her hand on a teenage girl's shoulder, relaxed, healthy, and free of anxiety.[56]

At the center of the pamphlet, interrupting the text on polio, were two pages addressed to "MOTHERS!" The idea of scientific motherhood had by the 1940s become a standard part of both public health education and commercial texts, playing on the public's growing "germ consciousness" and rising consumer anxieties.[57,58] "Do this to help keep your home *hygienically* clean—as many health authorities recommend," the explicit advertising section urged women. "No available household germicide—not even LYSOL—will kill the polio virus. Yet LYSOL, the world's largest-selling germicide, will help you keep your home 'hospital clean.' " This call was accompanied by a picture of a modern, safe hospital, reflecting the expanding use of hospital care by middle-class Americans, especially for childbirth,[56,59,61] and using the same arguments hospitals had developed to attract paying patients. And the places that Lysol's "*effective antiseptic* solution" would be especially useful recalled the enteric model of polio: it would clean the bathroom and kitchen, and disinfect baby's bed, playpen, diaper pail, and the sickroom.[56] Laboratory research was also part of what made this product safe and effective (and free from intrusive FDA labeling): "scientific research has developed an amazing new-formula 'Lysol' . . . [so that it] needs no poison label, but it has the same germicidal power it always had."[56]

Despite the Lysol pamphlet's warnings of the dangers of intimate personal contact, towels, bathing, and kissing, the text borrowed from *Good Housekeeping* referred consistently to the neurotropic model of polio. According to *Good Housekeeping*, the virus of infantile paralysis "enters the intestinal tract usually through the mouth or nose," then travels "briefly through the blood stream" and then "attacks the nerve cells."[56] "People are inclined to believe that polio is a mysterious ailment about which very little is known. Actually, doctors do know a great deal about it . . . in the last two decades. . . . Much more has been learned."[56] Unlike the Illinois pamphlet, which had identified "city-bred adults" as the best source of serum, the public was now warned that infection could occur as frequently in the city as in the country. Health officials were starting to reject the most draconian quarantine measures employed during polio epidemics, and the public was assured that it was not necessary during epidemics to close schools, fairs, circuses, and swimming pools, although children should probably avoid the latter "during an outbreak."[56] In another change from the early 1940s, therapy was reconceived as best undertaken in a hospital. Cases with severe paralysis should be taken to a hospital "not because of the risk of contagion but because good care for this type of polio patient requires the services of a team of experts."[56]

The pamphlet did not mention polio serum, but did discuss the blood-concentrate gamma globulin, which had been used during World War II and had been tested as a polio preventive in the late 1940s.[16] Anti-polio gamma globulin "is not and could not be the final answer to the polio problem," for recent scientific evidence suggested "that paralytic polio could probably be prevented by vaccination."[56] Nevertheless, many of the techniques and therapies discussed were clearly intended to be used at home: bed rest to prevent deformities, a firm, hard bed, blanket rolls, pads or sandbags to keep limbs in proper position, and (without using Elizabeth Kenny's name) "intermittent hot packs" for relief from pain in order to "to get the muscles and joints moving as soon as possible."[56]

Polio Can Be Conquered

Polio Can Be Conquered was the bold title of a 1949 pamphlet written by science reporter Alton Blakeslee of the Associated Press (Fig. 5.2).[24] Like most polio writers in the 1940s and 1950s, Blakeslee had written this guide in cooperation with the

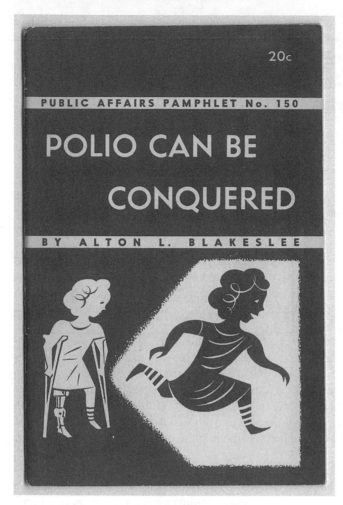

Figure 5.2. Alton Blakeslee's pamphlet "Polio Can be Conquered" exemplifies the NFIP's approach to promoting public confidence that scientific research was the best weapon in the fight against disease. (From March of Dimes, used by permission.)

NFIP, relying on its publicity department for images and scientific information. On the inside and back covers the publisher claimed the additional authority of public service: the New York Public Affairs Committee, which had been established a decade earlier "to make available in summary and inexpensive form the results of research on economic and social problems."

In the 1940s, a new generation of American virologists had begun to find the virus in blood and in non-neurological tissue, thus undermining the picture of polio as primarily a disease of the nervous system. By the end of the decade John Enders's team at the Boston Children's Hospital had published their innovative demonstration of the way the polio virus (and therefore, in theory a vaccine) could be grown in safe, non-neurological tissue. This research won the Boston group a Nobel Prize in 1954, just at the time that Jonas Salk's polio vaccine was being tested in trials organized and funded by the NFIP.[16,18] But while the pamphlet's opening sentence announced that "the conquest of polio now is in sight," Blakeslee's science was seriously outdated and did not reflect the most recent breakthroughs.[24] In Blakeslee's account blood played no role in spreading the polio virus through the body. Scientists knew that "antibodies are in the blood," he explained, but that the virus only "attacks the nerve cells. The two do not come into contact."[3,4,24] "We don't know yet how polio spreads," Blakeslee admitted, pointing to reliable standbys like coughing, sneezing, food, or airborne dust. "Certain kinds of filth flies" had been blamed but there was "no conclusive evidence," nor was there "proof" of the danger of catching polio by swimming in sewage-contaminated waters.[24]

Compared to the old-fashioned, general advice about polio's transmission, the therapy sections of Blakeslee's pamphlet were concrete and optimistic. Drawing on recent research on polio rehabilitation, Blakeslee was able to offer impressive specificity in his assessment of the likely impact of polio infection: 40–60% of cases would recover completely, 25–30% would be mildly affected, 15–25% severely, and 8% would die.[24] (According to the *Good Housekeeping* reporter, 50% of those infected by polio recovered "completely," 30% had a "slight handicap," 12% had "severe aftereffects," and 8% died.[56]) Reflecting the widespread integration of Elizabeth Kenny's methods, Blakeslee argued that affected muscles must be "stretched and exercised, even though the exercising caused mild pain." Kenny had little use for water therapy and believed any splinting was harmful, but Blakeslee suggested using a "warm pool" and bed rest, corsets, and splints.[24] In his discussion of therapy, Blakeslee referred to the heated debate over Kenny's theory of the disease. Polio, she had argued, was systemic rather than solely neurological, and those who employed her therapeutic methods but did not accept her theory would not be successful. Kenny had used these arguments as part of an attack against the monopolistic NFIP, but here Blakeslee relied on the familiar NFIP response to her claims that while "this question of *the nature* of the disease still remains open," irrespective of theory, polio treatment "is essentially the same" and "with trained personnel the results are similar."[24]

Kenny's criticisms of the NFIP had linked poor science to autocratic organization. Perhaps to defuse such attacks, Blakeslee was careful to remind a wary public that polio patients and their families did not receive "charity, in any sense. Rather, the funds from the March of Dimes are a trust fund to restore health, strength, and usefulness to polio victims."[24] These "dimes and dollars given by the American people" are also used to finance researchers who seek "to learn the habits of the polio virus and then to block its march along human nerves. They finance the search for the bullets of drugs or vaccines to end the insidious career of an unseen enemy."[24] In this story, doctors were portrayed as consumers of science like their patients, the simple recipients of scientific tools: "top scientists predict that a safe vaccine for humans will some day be found."[24] The popular fascination with the scientist in white, the drama of the laboratory, and the magical products possible from research were reinforced by new NFIP posters in the late 1940s that featured not only a child discarding braces or a wheelchair but also a scientist holding a test tube.[18,45]

Polio Survivors Tell Their Stories

By the late 1940s, there was an expanding audience for polio literature: the adult polio survivor.[62] Disabled men and women began to play an active part in the polio industry as the writers and designers of polio guides. In 1949, Turnley Walker, a public relations consultant, was paralyzed by polio and entered New York's Hospital for Special Surgery, his care paid for by the NFIP. He had been considering a professional writing career, and while in the hospital he began to write about his experience as a "polio," a newly popular term, usually applied to adults. Walker saw this effort as a way of producing "something for use in the March of Dimes. My only thought was that I might be able to do something to help repay the Foundation for saving me and my family from total financial disaster."[63] When the North American Newspaper Alliance syndicate published Walker's material in newspapers around the country, the great popular response led him to write a book, *Rise Up and Walk*, which was chosen by the Book of the Month Club in 1950.[64,65]

One section in *Rise Up and Walk* describes Walker and other polio survivors reading and responding to popular polio tracts. It was hardly a critical view, as the book was distributed by the NFIP, but Walker conveyed something of the emotional and intellectual appeal of this kind of literature in the late 1940s. For disabled adults, especially men who were the main economic resource for their households, the experience of paralysis was fraught with emotional and financial worries, as few standard private health insurance plans covered polio's extensive therapy and rehabilitation costs. Walker described his own "overpowering worry" about "the costs of the hospital and your treatments," for "the medical equipment and attention which surround you indicate the terrific expense of polio."[64] The financial side was ameliorated first, he recalled, when his wife appeared at his hospital bedside "carrying a miracle in the shape of a brisk white business envelope." As she read it, "gratefulness at what it says makes you weep together." The NFIP pamphlet explained that the organization "will stand behind you, taking care of all your medical and hospital expenses if need be, until you are able to go to work again . . . it lets you *know* that you are not lost forever, but only out of circulation for a while because of a dreadful accident."[64] Walker and his fellow patients discussed the NFIP later among themselves and began to see the organization "suddenly become a personal and powerful friend of yours."[64] They also found the NFIP view of polio as an "accident" that would not necessarily lead to total dependence for disabled adults facing life out of the hospital useful to counter the therapeutic pessimism of hospital staff. "It is strange and interesting how completely the Foundation has become the final authority for all of you. You have come to know that it is your great ally in your fight, stronger than the hospital, as wise as all the doctors."[64]

The second NFIP pamphlet that Walker encountered while in the hospital addressed polio as a puzzle of science. The guide became not just a source of personal revelation but a social tool as other patients asked him read it out loud. "You begin to read, intending to skip along the highlights. But the book holds your attention, line by line . . . polio is no longer simply the strange numbness which grips your leg but a coolly insane murderer crawling through your neighborhood with sub-microscopic stealth. . . . You glance up, and see the other faces riveted upon your own."[64] The book's dark and dramatic presentation of polio had great emotional appeal for these men. "You are reaching some understanding of the terrifying virus which slithers its way into the brains and spinal cords of children and grown men by pathways not yet discovered . . . the sole deadly epidemic still at large."[64]

The book that so riveted Walker and his hospital companions was Roland Berg's *Polio and Its Problems*, funded, published and distributed by the NFIP in 1948.[20] Following the familiar preface, which stated that *"polio is an uncontrolled disease,"* Berg presented scientists as the single source of hope for conquering polio; medical practitioners, by comparison, were weaker men, sometimes diverted from the path of scientific truth by a desire to comfort.[20] Berg explained that the neurological theory of polio made therapies based on blood-borne immunity obsolete. Thus, doctors who still resorted to the use of polio serum ignored "the adverse results of experimental and clinical study" that had shown "virtually no evidence that the virus passes through or remains in the blood stream."[20] "It is often difficult," Berg acknowledged, "for the physician who may not value its use to withhold it. If he should do so, and his patient should develop paralysis or die he may be blamed by the parents or relatives for neglecting to take all measures possible."[20] Such a situation was "unfortunate" for "it is not consistent with medical ideals." Later he reminded both medical and lay readers that "serum has a protective quality but no therapeutic value."[20]

Berg's account of the fight against polio discussed only one practicing physician, the "prominent New York pediatrician" Philip Stimson, who could detect even the smallest signs of illness which "may mean infantile paralysis."[20] Using the NFIP's typically dramatic term for polio, Berg warned "Don't take a chance with the Crippler. Play safe; put the patient to bed and don't delay calling a physician." In an aside that contradicted March of Dimes campaigns, Berg also warned his readers against the "popular misconception . . . that any disease can be conquered if sufficient money and skill are gathered for the purpose"; unfortunately, "progress in medical science cannot always be thus purchased." But some pages later, without irony, he referred to the time when "scientists discover the golden pill for polio that will forever remove the menace." In an effort to counter the popular belief in polio as a disease that baffled scientists, Berg argued that "it is surprising how large a store of knowledge has been built up—especially in the last 10 years of concerted research." His final sentence, with a flourish, made firm the link between polio and science, for "only in the laboratories of medical scientists still seeking the absolute cure or prevention, can the problems of polio finally be answered."[20]

At Home in the Privacy of His Laboratory

With the massive publicity around the Salk vaccine trials of 1954, the clinical professional in popular polio literature was transformed fully into a science consumer. Now, both physicians and nurses were pictured as skilled technicians, applying the new scientific technology developed by great research heroes who had conquered polio. During the 1950s, children became a new audience for this kind of polio literature, which was now framed as a children's science story. In Dorothy and Philip Sterling's *Polio Pioneers: The Story of the Fight Against Polio* (1955), polio history was remade into the story of virus hunters alone. Doctors, when they appeared, gratefully received the insights of scientific researchers who were the ones who actively discovered "how to hunt a germ" and "how to fool a germ."[66]

In 1960, science writer John Rowland, already the author of *Ernest Rutherford: Atom Pioneer* (1955) and *The Penicillin Man: The Story of Sir Alexander Fleming* (1957), turned polio history into the saga of one man, Jonas Salk. In *The Polio Man: The Story of Dr. Jonas Salk,* Rowland ignored the work of Salk's rival Albert Sabin and Sabin's live virus vaccine, which would shortly be approved by the U.S. government as the official American vaccine.[68–69] Salk was the public's favorite, and as an NFIP grant recipient, he had the entire NFIP publicity department behind him. Salk's vaccine had been quickly made a symbol of the culmination of the years of public donations to the March of Dimes. Rowland made Salk's identity as a trained physician part of the story and called him "Dr. Salk" throughout. Working with patients had helped, in this version of his biography, to humanize Salk and distinguish him from chemists and other laboratory researchers distanced from the human consequences of disease. As a boy the young Salk had told his father "I don't really want to be an ordinary doctor. . . . I want to find out something of the causes of the disease."[69] His experience as a "medical research man" at New York's Mount Sinai Medical Center taught him clinical priorities and "gave a sense of urgency to all that was being done, since there was always the knowledge that a research task done in a few days, instead of a few weeks or months, might save lives. . . . The task of the ordinary doctor is to fight disease when it shows itself," Salk learned, but "even more important and even more valuable . . . is the medical research workers who tried to stop the illness from coming at all."[69]

As a scientist Salk was made to embody all the ideal virtues of the Cold War researcher: self-effacing, uncomfortable with the press and publicity, interested not in worldly honor and glory but only in further pursuing his scientific work. In this post-*Sputnik* era, science writers who wrote inspirational stories of great scientists as a means to attracting young people to the scientific professions were conscious that they were performing a distinctly patriotic duty. Character, as the well-publicized travails of Robert Oppenheimer, Julius Rosenberg, and other "atomic science spies" demonstrated, was a crucial element in securing American democracy and global harmony. Thus, according to Rowland's depiction of the famous April 1955 meeting where results of the year-long assessment of the Salk vaccine trials were announced, "the press conference was a trying business for Dr. Salk, who still felt much more at home in the privacy of his laboratory than he did facing a battery of newsreel cameras and a crowd of reporters from newspapers."[69] After the announcement, although reporters pleaded with him, Salk "would give no hint" of his next research projects. As Salk explained it, "The scientist isn't a politician, and isn't a propagandist. He observes and classifies facts, and then he reaches conclusions on the basis of the data at his disposal. He must avoid being influenced by the pressures on him, or even by the bias of his hypotheses."[69] Salk's single breach of scientific ethics occurred in his relationship with the NFIP, "that great charitable body" which had "helped the work with substantial grants—for such a piece of research on such a large scale is an expensive business." Salk had kept NFIP authorities "informed" of the progress of the vaccine trials, for "after all, the Foundation had provided the large sum of money that was necessary to launch the trial, and it was only fair that they should be given what information was available." Nonetheless these officials were "sworn to secrecy."[68] Thus Salk was praised for his awareness of the importance of patronage in the marketplace of science, yet he was also the epitome of the cautious scientific researcher who "would never take all the credit to himself, as many a lesser man would have tried to do" and who "never thought of himself as an inventor, a patentee of something out of which money could be made," replying to reporters, in a widely repeated remark, "Can you patent the sun?"[68,69]

Conclusion

By 1960, as the tone of Rowland's book suggests, the messy horror of epidemic polio was beginning to fade into history, to be replaced by the cleansing certainty of the laboratory. The drama of medical and scientific battles, the dashed hopes of families struggling with a paralyzed child, the desperate effort to keep houses and streets clean enough to halt the unpredictable and unstoppable—these stories now can be captured only in memoirs or in some of the images so useful to American officials in their recent bioterrorism mobilization campaigns. The contradictory therapeutic prescriptions and explanatory versions of the disease were probably visible to an educated public then, as now. But even before the polio vaccines were developed, health experts—especially those employed by the NFIP—made scientific research a public enterprise, in which even obscure scientific questions could be laid out and debated. The assumption that public funding of science was an appropriate civic activity would be developed later in much greater political sophistication by HIV/AIDS and breast cancer activists.

Polio is still a frightening disease. In 2004, global health protests emerged over the Nigerian government's suspension of its vaccination program and the World Health Organization's warning that travelers to West and Central Africa should be fully immunized against the disease. These events may prompt new therapeutic investigations of polio and focus public health policy once again on polio-vaccination education and enforcement.[70] Whatever historical parallels are drawn on in the case of Nigeria, it is clear that the history of disease remains a powerful and constant tool for government officials, medical professionals, the mass media, and the public. During the first SARS outbreaks in 2003, newspapers and television news programs displayed old photos of passengers riding trolley cars and police directing traffic, all in face masks to ward off infection during the 1918–19 influenza pandemic—pictures eerily matched by contemporary images in Hong Kong, Beijing, and Toronto. In both epidemics, health professionals and the lay public were dying; in both epidemics, people wanted scientific tools to predict, prevent, and heal. Calling on history, even when its stories were horrifying and deadly, still in a way had the power to clarify and reassure.

Acknowledgments

My thanks to John Warner, Daniel Wilson, and Chris Warren for their insightful comments and suggestions, and to Meg Hyre for her careful, thoughtful editing.

References

1. Connolly C, Milbank D. U.S. revives smallpox shot. *Washington Post,* 14 December 2002.
2. Connolly C, Milbank D. Smallpox vaccination begins with the military. *Washington Post,* 14 December 2002.
3. Cook R. Smallpox planning vs. polio shot? Associated Press, 2003. Available at: http://www.cbsnews.com/stories/2003/05/07/politics/main552844.shtml. Accessed 28 December 2004.
4. Weinstein I. An outbreak of smallpox in New York City. *Am J Public Health* 1947:37:1381. Available at: http://www.homelandsecurity.org/journal/Articles/OutbreakinNYC1947b.htm. Accessed 28 December 2004.
5. Elliott VS. Smallpox 1947: "people were terrified." *AMNews,* 23 June 2003. Available at: http://www.ama-assn.org/amednews/2003/06/23/hlsa0623.htm. Accessed 13 February 2005.
6. Sepkovitz KA. The 1947 smallpox vaccination campaign in New York City, revisited [letter]. *Emerg Infect Dis* 2004:10:960–61.
7. Cardiac deaths after a mass smallpox vaccination campaign, New York City, 1947. *MMWR* 2003:52:933–36.
8. Leavitt JW. 'Be safe, be sure.' New York City's experience with epidemic smallpox. In: Rosner D (ed.), Hives of Sickness: Public Health Epidemics in New York City. New Brunswick, NJ: Rutgers University Press; 1995, 85–114.
9. Leavitt JW. Public resistance or cooperation? A tale of smallpox in two cities. *Biosecurity and Bioterrorism* 2003:1:185–92.
10. Benin AJ et al. Reasons physicians accepted or declined smallpox vaccine, February through April 2003. *Journal of General Internal Medicine* 2004:19:85–89.
11. CDC. Update: adverse events following civilian smallpox vaccination-United States, 2003. *MMWR* 2004:53:106–7.
12. Drexler M. A pox on America. *The Nation,* April 28, 2003, 276:7–8
13. Johnston RD. Contemporary anti-vaccination movements in historical perspective. In: Johnston RD (ed.), The Politics of Healing: Histories of Alternative Medicine in Twentieth-Century North America. New York: Routledge, 2004, 259–86.
14. For an example of the frustration of the public health establishment, see Connolly C. Bioterror preparedness still lacking, health group concludes. *Washington Post,* 12 December 2003.
15. Rogers N. Dirt and Disease: Polio before FDR. New Brunswick, NJ: Rutgers University Press, 1992.
16. Paul JR. A History of Poliomyelitis. New Haven, CT: Yale University Press, 1971.
17. Gould T. A Summer Plague: Polio and Its Survivors. New Haven, CT: Yale University Press, 1995.
18. Smith JS. Patenting the Sun: Polio and the Salk Vaccine. New York: William Morrow, 1990.
19. De Kruif P. Men against the maiming death. In: De Kruif P. The Fight for Life. New York: Harcourt Brace, 1938,143–220.
20. Berg RH. Polio and Its Problems. Philadelphia: J. B. Lippincott, 1948.

21. Cohn V. Four Billion Dimes. New York: National Foundation for Infantile Paralysis, 1955. Reprint of series in *Minneapolis Tribune*, April 1955.
22. Tomes N. Merchants of health: medicine and consumer culture in the United States, 1900–1940. *Journal of American History* 2001:88:519–48.
23. Burnham JC. How Superstition Won and Science Lost: Popularizing Science and Health in the United States. New Brunswick, NJ: Rutgers University Press, 1987.
24. Blakeslee AL. Polio Can Be Conquered. New York: Public Affairs Committee, 1949, no. 150.
25. Brandt AM, Gardner M. The golden age of medicine? In: Cooter R, Pickstone J (eds.), Medicine in the Twentieth Century. Amsterdam, Netherlands: Harwood Academic, 2000, 21–37.
26. Wilson DJ. A crippling fear: experiencing polio in the era of FDR. *Bull Hist Med* 1998:72:464–495.
27. Fairchild AL. The polio narratives: dialogues with FDR. *Bull Hist Med* 2001:75:488–534.
28. Fishbein M. Morris Fishbein, M.D.: An Autobiography. Garden City, NY: Doubleday, 1969, 342–49.
29. Campion FD. The AMA and U.S. Health Policy since 1940. Chicago: Chicago Review Press, 1984.
30. Engel J. Doctors and Reformers: Discussion and Debate over Health Policy 1925–1950. Charleston, SC: University of South Carolina Press, 2002.
31. Horstmann DM. Problems in epidemiology of poliomyelitis. *Lancet* 1948:251: 273–277. Abstracted, *JAMA* 1948:137:1491.
32. Grimshaw ML. Scientific specialization and the poliovirus controversy in the years before World War II. *Bull Hist Med* 1995:69:44–65.
33. Grey MR. New Deal Medicine: The Rural Health Programs of the Farm Security Administration. Baltimore: Johns Hopkins University Press, 1999.
34. Numbers RL. The fall and rise of the American medical profession. In: Leavitt JW, Numbers RL (eds.), Sickness and Health in America: Readings in the History of Medicine and the Public Health. Madison, WI: University of Wisconsin, 1985, 191–94.
35. Hirschfield DS. The Lost Reform: The Campaign for Compulsory National Health Insurance from 1932 to 1943. Cambridge, MA: Harvard University Press, 1970.
36. Rayak E. Professional Power and American Medicine: The Economics of the American Medical Association. Cleveland, OH: World Publishing Company, 1967.
37. Burrow, JG. AMA: Voice of American Medicine. Baltimore: Johns Hopkins University Press, 1963.
38. Rogers N. Sister Kenny goes to Washington: polio, populism and medical politics in postwar America. In: Johnston RD (ed.), The Politics of Healing: Histories of Alternative Medicine in Twentieth-Century North America. New York: Routledge, 2002:97–116.
39. Burnham JC. American medicine's golden age: what's happened to it? [1982]. In: Leavitt JW, Numbers RL (eds.), Sickness and Health in America: Readings in the History of Medicine and Public Health, 3rd ed. Madison, WI: University of Wisconsin Press, 1997, 284–94.
40. Lederer S, Rogers N. Media. In: Cooter R, Pickstone J (eds.), Medicine in the Twentieth Century. Amsterdam, Netherlands: Harwood Academic, 2000, 487–502.
41. Things You Want to Know about Infantile Paralysis. Educational Health Circular 45. Springfield, IL: Department of Public Health, 1941.
42. Black K. In the Shadow of Polio: A Personal and Social History. Reading, MA: Addison-Wesley, 1966.
43. Daniel TM, Robbins FC (eds.). Polio. Rochester, NY: University of Rochester Press, 1977.

44. Sass EJ, with Gottfried G, Sorem A (eds.). Polio's Legacy: An Oral History. Lanham, MD: University Press of America,1996.
45. Seavey NG, Smith JS, Wagner, P. A Paralyzing Fear: The Triumph over Polio in America. New York: TV Books Inc., 1998.
46. Gallagher HG. FDR's Splendid Deception. New York: Dodd, Mead; 1985.
47. Longmore PK, Umansky L (eds.). The New Disability History: American Perspectives. Albany, NY: New York University Press, 2001.
48. Gritzer G, Arluke A. The Making of Rehabilitation: A Political Economy of Medical Specialization. Berkeley, CA: University of California Press, 1985.
49. Rusk HA. A World to Care For: The Autobiography of Howard A. Rusk, M.D. New York: Random House, 1972.
50. Halpern SA. American Pediatrics: The Social Dynamics of Professionalism 1880–1980. Berkeley, CA: University of California Press, 1988.
51. May ET. Homeward Bound: American Families in the Cold War Era. New York: Basic Books, 1988.
52. Common Childhood Diseases. New York: Metropolitan Life Insurance Company, 1946, foreword.
53. Cohn V. Sister Kenny: The Woman Who Challenged the Doctors. Minneapolis, MN: University of Minnesota Press, 1975.
54. Wilson JR. Through Kenny's Eyes: An Exploration of Sister Elizabeth Kenny's Views about Nursing. Townsville, Queensland, Australia: Royal College of Nursing, 1995.
55. Rogers N. Sister Kenny. Isis 1993:84:772–74.
56. Handbook on Infantile Paralysis: Condensed from an Article in Good Housekeeping as compiled by Maxine Davis [August 1950]. Bloomfield, NJ: Lehn & Fink Products Corporation, 1954.
57. Tomes N. The Gospel of Germs: Men, Women, and the Microbe in American Life. Cambridge, MA: Harvard University Press, 1998.
58. Apple RD. Mothers and Medicine: A Social History of Infant Feeding 1890–1950. Madison, WI: University of Wisconsin Press, 1987.
59. Leavitt JW. Brought to Bed: Childbearing in America 1750–1950. New York: Oxford University Press, 1986.
60. Rosenberg CE. The Care of Strangers: The Rise of America's Hospital System. New York: Basic Books, 1987.
61. Stevens R. In Sickness and In Wealth: America Hospitals in the Twentieth Century. New York: Basic Books, 1989.
62. Wilson DJ. A crippled manhood: infantile paralysis and the constructing of masculinity. Medical Humanities Review 1998:12:9–28.
63. Walker T. Journey Together. New York: David McKay, 1951.
64. Walker T. Rise Up and Walk. New York: E. P. Dutton, 1950.
65. Walker T. Roosevelt and the Fight against Polio New York: A.A. Wyn, 1953.
66. Sterling D, Sterling P. Polio Pioneers: The Story of the Fight Against Polio. Garden City, NY: Doubleday, 1955.
67. Roland J. Ernest Rutherford: Atom Pioneer. London: Werner Laurie, 1955.
68. Rowland J. The Penicillin Man: The Story of Sir Alexander Fleming. New York: Roy Publishers, 1957.
69. Rowland J. The Polio Man: The Story of Dr. Jonas Salk. New York: Roy Publishers, 1960.
70. Altman LK. W.H.O. advises full polio immunization for travelers to Nigeria. New York Times, 1 July 2004.

Suggested Reading

Oshinsky, D.M. Polio: An American Story. New York: Oxford University Press, 2005.

Rogers N. Dirt and Disease: Polio before FDR. New Brunswick, NJ: Rutgers University Press, 1992.

Tomes N. The Gospel of Germs: Men, Women, and the Microbe in American Life. Cambridge, MA: Harvard University Press, 1998

Wilson, D.J. Living with Polio: The Epidemic and Its Survivors. Chicago: Chicago University Press, 2005.

PART III

MATERNAL AND
INFANT HEALTH

6

Safe Mothers, Healthy Babies: Reproductive Health in the Twentieth Century

MILTON KOTELCHUCK

The decline of infant and maternal mortality represents one of the greatest public health achievements of the twentieth century. From 1900 through 2000, infant mortality in the United States declined dramatically from an estimated 10,000–15,000 deaths to 690 deaths per 100,000 births; similarly, maternal mortality declined from an estimated 600–900 deaths to under 10 deaths per 100,000 births. Reductions in both morbidity and mortality have improved the lives of parents and children and have altered expectations for women. Public health action played a central role in the transformation of reproductive health in the twentieth century. This chapter describes decade by decade the evolving concepts and debates about the causes of infant and maternal mortality, the initiatives to ameliorate them, the institutionalization of the major public health advances, and the resulting epidemiologic transformations in the United States.

Infant Mortality Before the Twentieth Century

Before the twentieth century, high rates of infant mortality were considered an unavoidable part of the human experience. In the nineteenth century, infant mortality began to be seen as a social issue that could be amenable to public intervention. The social construct of infant mortality began with the environmental sanitarian movement of the mid-1800s. The early sanitarian reformers believed that poverty and ill health among persons living in growing urban industrial areas were caused by environmental and hygienic factors, not a lack of morals; that children and infants were particularly vulnerable to the population density and lack of sanitation; and that government (i.e., public health) was necessary to reduce the excess morbidity and mortality.[1] In 1860, Edwin Chadwick, a leading sanitarian, argued to use the concept of infant mortality (i.e., infantile death rate) as a measure of a community's sanitary health.[2]

At the end of the nineteenth century, most U.S. births took place in the home and were attended by midwives. Maternal mortality and the birthing experiences of mothers had not yet emerged as distinct public health issues. Obstetrics had just begun its development as a medical specialty. In addition, the biology and pathophysiology of pregnancy and infant mortality were not fully understood, and the "germ" theory of disease was not widely accepted. Epidemiologic and other public health research was limited. No organized national or state efforts to address infant or maternal mortality existed.

1900–1910: Beginnings of the First Public Health Movement to Address Infant Mortality

The epidemiology of infant and maternal mortality at the beginning of the twentieth century was grim. Infant and maternal mortality were the most widespread and visible public health issues. No national data were available regarding infant or maternal mortality rates for the year 1900 because no national data-collection system existed. However, state and city vital statistics registration and census data suggest that mortality rates among infants within the first year of life approached 100–150 deaths per 1000 births; rates in certain urban areas were even higher.[3] Maternal mortality was also exceptionally high during this year; an estimated 600–900 deaths occurred per 100,000 births.[4]

The first decade of the twentieth century was marked by increasing public and professional concern about the high levels of infant mortality in urban areas. The first beginnings of organized government public health action emerged in New York City and other major urban centers, where the nutritional and sanitation interventions were transformed to focus on the education of mothers regarding child hygiene. A reproductive public health movement emerged amid the related Progressive Era struggles for unionization, women's suffrage, immigration reform, child labor protection, and temperance. The ideas that surfaced during this decade, and the increasing trend toward leadership by women, were influential in shaping the early reproductive public health efforts of the twentieth century.

Reducing Infant Mortality through Improving Milk Safety

In the nineteenth century, sanitarians and clinicians had associated mortality among infants living in urban areas with diarrheal disease,[1] which increased substantially during the summer months. Their solutions were environmental in nature (e.g., better garbage collection and improved water supplies) and represented the first public health initiatives to directly address infant mortality. This initial conceptualization of infant mortality led to various efforts in the late nineteenth century and early twentieth century to improve milk products—the perceived cause of infant diarrhea. These efforts included use of infant formulas or percentage feeding (e.g., milk with specific chemical components), purification of the milk supply, and pasteurization.[1] A further public health strategy involved the purchase of "pure" milk from certified farms and then its direct provision to the urban poor. In 1893, Nathan Straus, a philanthropist, established the first milk station to provide free or reduced-priced pasteurized milk in New York City. Milk stations proved very popular and increased in popularity and in number in the early 1900s; by 1910, 15 municipal milk stations had been established in New York City alone.[5] These milk stations were initially a decentralized and charity-oriented initiative, a site-based precursor of today's Special Supplemental Nutrition Program for Women, Infant and Children (WIC) program.

Although popular, studies in the early 1900s suggested that the milk station's provision of pure milk alone had only minimal impact on summertime diarrheal disease; subsequent contamination of milk still occurred in the home.[6] The provision of milk was seen as needing follow-up, in the form of maternal education, to be effective in reducing infant mortality. George Newman's influential book, *Infant Mortality: A Social Problem* (1906), emphasized, "The problem of infant mortality is not one of sanitation alone, or housing, or indeed of poverty as such, but mainly a question of motherhood."[7] Milk stations quickly became sites at which education programs addressing maternal and infant health and hygiene, childcare, and other practical skills could be implemented. They provided a locus for contacting the hard-to-reach urban poor and immigrants. In 1908, the New York City Health Department began to incorporate maternal education and infant examinations in their milk-station activities. Because maternal ignorance, especially among poorer immigrants, was often considered the root of elevated infant mortality in urban areas, the newly emerging social-work profession and progressive urban-settlements movement assumed a critical leadership role in reducing infant mortality.[1]

A series of influential case studies of infant deaths, many from Europe, began to provide evidence that breastfeeding was more hygienic than the use of infant formula and was protective against summertime diarrheal disease and infant mortality.[8,9] Maternal education programs therefore began to encourage breastfeeding as a way to reduce the risk for infant mortality.

Organized Governmental Efforts in Maternal and Child Health

At the start of the twentieth century, governmental efforts directed at maternal and child health (MCH) and welfare in the United States were tentative. The first organized MCH efforts took place in New York City, the major port of entry for immigration at that time and a center for social welfare and progressive political activities. In 1907, after much lobbying, a provisional Bureau of Child Hygiene was established, headed by Dr. Josephine Baker.[1] Because resources were limited, the bureau used school nurses who were not otherwise employed in the summer to visit the homes of the newborns in the districts with the highest infant mortality rates and instruct mothers regarding infant hygiene and breastfeeding. In 1908, partly as a result of the program's use of vital statistics to document its success in reducing infant mortality and its demonstrated financial feasibility, the Bureau of Child Hygiene was made permanent.[1]

By 1910, many of the critical public health programmatic ideas of the twentieth century had been established in New York City, including home visits by nurses, milk supplementation (WIC), breastfeeding and maternal hygienic education, and the use of data to target resources and municipal efforts. Many other large U.S. cities followed suit and established similar children's hygiene bureaus. The word *hygiene* in their name suggests their conceptual orientation. These early governmental efforts, however, remained primarily local initiatives of a few progressive cities—often those dealing with massive immigration.

In response to the increasing calls for a federal role in promoting, if not assuring, the well-being of children, the first White House Conference on Care of Dependent Children was held in 1909 under the auspices of President Theodore Roosevelt. The conference recommendations called for service programs and financial aid to protect the home environment and for the federal government to take responsibility for gathering information regarding problems affecting infant and child health and welfare.[10]

That same year, the American Association for the Study and Prevention of Infant Mortality (AASPIM) was established as the first voluntary national organization dedicated solely to infant mortality. Modeled after its European national committee counterparts (e.g., the Ligue Française contra Mortalité Infantile, founded in 1902), it provided a national forum to coordinate private individuals, voluntary agencies, and urban health departments in addressing infant mortality.[1]

The AASPIM had five goals: (1) to encourage statistical studies of infant mortality to determine the extent and seriousness of the problem; (2) to promote the creation of a network of voluntary philanthropic and health associations devoted to improving maternal ability to carry, bear, and rear healthy infants; (3) to arouse public sentiment and lobby legislatures and government officials to work for the establishment of municipal, state, and federal infant and child health bureaus; (4) to provide a national organizational structure for infant welfare work; and (5) to create a forum and clearinghouse for research into the causes and remedies of infant mortality.[11] AASPIM's agenda was the strategic blueprint for the early twentieth-century public health infant mortality reduction movement.

By the end of 1910, the United States was poised for an aggressive set of local and national activities to address infant mortality problems. Maternal mortality was not yet recognized as a distinct public health problem; efforts to improve reproductive health among women remained secondary to those regarding infant mortality reduction.

1910–1920: Saving Babies—The Campaign to Reduce Infant Mortality

The first national data obtained through the 1915 Birth Registration Act revealed an infant mortality rate (IMR, or the number of deaths within the first year of life per

1000 live births) in that year of 99.9 deaths per 1000 births; and noted 95.7 deaths per 1000 births from 1915 to 1919. Higher infant mortality rates were observed among nonwhite infants (149.7) and in large cities.[12] The neonatal mortality rate (NMR, or the number of deaths within the first 28 days of life per 1000 live births) was 43.4 deaths per 1,000 births in 1915–1919. A subsequent federal study estimated the IMR slightly higher at 111.2 deaths per 1000 births in this period, with 40% of those deaths occurring during the neonatal period.[13] In 1915–1919, the maternal mortality rate was 732.8 deaths per 100,000 births, and was substantially higher (1253.5) for nonwhite women.

Considerable pressure was placed on the federal government by the AASPIM and others to create a children's bureau. In 1912, after years of delay, Congress approved the establishment of this Bureau (P.L. 62–116), that "shall investigate and report to said department upon all matters pertaining to the welfare of children and child life among all classes of our people, and shall especially investigate the questions of infant mortality, the birth rate, orphanage, juvenile courts, desertion, dangerous occupations, accidents and diseases of children, employment, legislation affecting children in the several States and Territories."[14] Julia Lathrop, a social worker, was appointed the Bureau's first director. Although limited by a lack of funding and a narrow mandate, the Children's Bureau provided inspiring leadership in the nation's public health crusade against infant mortality.

Several of the Children's Bureau's initiatives were noteworthy. "Infant Care," published by the bureau in 1914, was the most popular free federal guidebook ever; it provided scientific (rather than traditional) instruction and guidance for mothers. The Children's Bureau also encouraged the development of maternal support groups and motherhood civic activities (e.g., the Little Mother's Leagues and the National Congress of Mothers) and sponsored the first National Baby Week, held in March 1916.

In 1913, the Children's Bureau launched comprehensive investigations of infant mortality in 10 U.S. communities.[13] These birth cohort follow-back studies involved detailed, standardized interviews with all families of infants born in the community during a specified year. Their results shaped the evolving understanding of infant mortality in the United States. They identified a substantially higher overall rate of infant mortality than that previously reported by the Census Bureau or the new Birth Registration Act. They also associated the leading cause of infant deaths with problems of early infancy and maternal conditions of pregnancy (e.g., prematurity, congenital malformations, and birth injuries) rather than gastric and intestinal diseases, supporting the need for improvements in obstetric and prenatal care. Elevated infant mortality was observed most frequently among mothers in the youngest and oldest age groups, twins and triplets, births assisted by instruments, closely spaced births, and artificially fed infants. Family income was inversely related to infant mortality, with an almost fourfold gap in IMR observed between the poorest and the wealthiest families.[13] The economic findings challenged the prevailing view that maternal hygienic education was the principal solution to infant mortality and reinvigorated an enduring debate regarding the role of economic factors in the causation of infant mortality.[1]

By 1918, encouraged by the federal Children's Bureau, four states and 50 large urban cities had established local Children's Bureaus. Funding for these agencies was limited, and smaller and rural municipalities generally lacked the funding to implement similar programs. The first infant mortality reduction program specifically intended for blacks was not developed until 1915 in New York City.[1]

One major barrier for effective public efforts to reduce infant mortality was the absence of reliable birth and death data nationally and in many states and local jurisdictions. In 1915, in response to lobbying by child health advocates, including the AAPSIM and the Children's Bureau, Congress passed the Birth Registration Act— the first national effort to collect standardized national data. This act, the direct predecessor of today's National Center for Health Statistics, began with optional participation and included 10 states and local jurisdictions; other states were gradually added. In 1936, participation was mandated nationally.

Recognizing the Importance of Maternal Health in the Twentieth Century

Prenatal care (PNC) was not a routine part of women's birthing experience at the beginning of the twentieth century. The origins of prenatal care are varied. In the United States, organized PNC was largely introduced by social reformers and nurses, often as a prenatal registration and educational home visit prior to enrollment in outpatient delivery services of a lying-in-hospital.[15] In 1909, the Committee on Infant Social Services of the Boston Women's Municipal League began providing intensive PNC to all obstetric patients at major Boston hospitals. In 1911, AAPSIM's section on Nursing and Social Work passed a resolution urging PNC be made an integral part of infant welfare stations. By 1912, several larger urban municipal Child Hygiene Bureaus established prenatal care subdivisions.[1]

Obstetrics also emerged as a medical specialty in this period, and concurrently, pregnancy came to be perceived as a potentially pathologic state.[16] In 1914, AASPIM President Van Ingen suggested that neonatal mortality was "caused by conditions acting on the child through the mother and must be attacked by methods directed at pregnant women."[17]

In 1915, obstetrician J. Whitridge Williams became the president of AASPIM. He advocated prenatal care to prevent stillbirths and neonatal deaths, and he proposed reforming obstetric delivery practices (including prohibition of midwifery practice), educating mothers to the need for skilled medical attendants, and establishing prenatal and obstetric clinics to educate and supervise pregnant women.[18] This plan elevated obstetric care to a central role in the reduction of infant mortality, and ultimately it fostered more medical and public health attention regarding maternal morbidity and mortality.[1] Other obstetric leaders, such as Joseph DeLee of Chicago, were even more outspoken about the need for medical management and obstetric interventions to enhance the birthing process.[19]

Having determined that prenatal care could reduce infant mortality by 40%, Williams and his colleagues aggressively encouraged PNC (delivered by obstetricians) as part of their infant mortality reduction proposals.[20] This new emphasis on prenatal care readily merged with the educated-mother movement that was then prevalent in the United States. Women began to be advised to receive "skilled professional care" during pregnancy and motherhood.

Williams, DeLee, and other obstetricians also worked to improve hospital-based delivery practices and enhance obstetric education—efforts that diminished the role of midwifery. However, because not enough physicians were available to serve economically disadvantaged women, many public health officials (especially those employed in Child Hygiene Bureaus) advocated instead for improving midwives' skills and increasing their professional scrutiny and regulation.[21]

Maternal Mortality and Public Health

In 1916, the Children's Bureau conducted its first study of maternal mortality.[22] Among women aged 15–44 years, maternal mortality was second only to tuberculosis as a leading cause of death in the United States. Limited availability and underutilization of quality obstetric services were considered the root of the two main killers of pregnant women—puerperal septicemia and eclampsia—both of which are preventable with proper medical and hygienic care.

By 1920, most of the major public health programmatic approaches of the twentieth century to address infant and maternal mortality had become articulated: prenatal care, nutrition intervention, maternal education, home visitation, improved delivery care, sanitary control, and vital statistics usage. The seminal debates about infant and maternal mortality had now been engaged: social welfare versus medical orientation, government versus private responsibilities, and control of the birthing processes.

1920–1930: The Shepard-Towner Act and Maternity Insurance

By the 1920s, infant mortality rates in the United States had begun to decline. The extensive efforts of the prior decade seemed to be having an impact. By 1925, the IMR had dropped to 71.7 deaths per 1000 births, primarily as a result of improvements in postneonatal mortality (PNMR, or number of deaths from 29 days to 1 year of life per 1000 live births); neonatal mortality had declined only slightly to 41.5 deaths per 1000 live births.[21] Most infant deaths now occurred in the neonatal period. Nonwhite IMR declined, but still exceeded 105 deaths per 1000 births. In contrast, only limited progress was being made regarding maternal mortality; the rate of maternal mortality in 1925 was 647.0 deaths per 100,000 births and was substantially higher (1162.0) for nonwhite women.[23]

During the 1920s, Children's Bureau research revealed a strong link between poverty and infant mortality, suggesting that socioeconomic approaches rather than maternal education were needed. These initiatives, broadly labeled "maternity insurance," reflected two central ideas: direct governmental provision of medical services; and economic security for pregnant women (through lost wage compensation/paid leaves, nursing coverage, and domestic assistance),[1] concepts now reflected in the European reproductive public health model. In Europe, pregnancy was viewed as a form of temporary unemployment, and therefore "lost wages" were covered under their employment-based social security insurance systems.

In the late teens and early 1920s, bills mandating maternity insurance as a component of compulsory sickness insurance were unsuccessfully introduced in various state legislatures. Opposition was strong, emanating from concerns over the German and Russian origins of this concept and physician hostility to state regulation of private practice. The rejection of the maternal insurance concept led to a further emphasis on clinical approaches to addressing the problem of infant mortality in the United States and assured private control, rather than any direct state involvement, in the provision of medical services to nonindigent Americans.[1]

Partially in response to the substantial number of young men found to be physically unqualified for military service because of preventable childhood diseases in WWI, the Children's Bureau in 1917 (under the leadership of Julia Lathrop) proposed providing federal matching grants to states to establish infant and maternal health centers and visiting-nurse services, especially in rural areas. This proposal was based on the concept of educated mothers and prevention rather than direct health services or economic support. In 1921, Lathrop's ideas were passed in the form of the Sheppard-Towner Maternity and Infancy Act (P.L. 67–97). The bill galvanized support from virtually all organized women's groups, including suffragettes and motherhood civic associations; fear of women's new votes ensured congressional support.[24]

The Sheppard-Towner Act served as the pioneer national MCH program, the direct predecessor and model for Title V of the Social Security Act. The Children's Bureau assumed administrative responsibility for the program. The Sheppard-Towner Act fostered state children's bureaus, encouraged maternal nutrition and hygiene educational activities, established preventive prenatal and well-baby clinics, and supported visiting nurses for pregnant women and new mothers.

By 1922, a total of 41 states passed enabling legislation. By 1929, a total of 1594 permanent child health and prenatal clinics, administered and staffed largely by women, had been established. They represented a maternal and child public health infrastructure throughout the United States.[10] Many were positioned in rural areas and in areas with large racial or ethnic minority populations. However, many restrictions were also included in the Act, including prohibition of any "maternity insurance," voluntary participation, state control, and a 5-year sunset clause.[1]

During this conservative, pro-business period, the grass-roots popularity of the Sheppard-Towner Act was not matched at the national level.[25] The American Medical Association (AMA) viewed its professional mandate to include preventive as well as curative care; the AMA therefore perceived the Sheppard-Towner Act as direct competition and condemned it as a form of state medicine. Segments of its pediatric section disagreed, leading to the formation of the independent American Academy of Pediatrics in 1930.[26] In 1927, Congress did not renew the Sheppard-Towner Act. In 1929, the Act ceased to function, although 19 states continued the program even without federal funding. Its defeat signified the end of the first sustained period of public health infant mortality reproduction initiatives in the twentieth century. It shifted the provision of preventive services for women and children from public clinics to private offices. The private medical profession's dominance of the infant mortality issue in the United States was manifest, and the involvement of other nonmedical professions waned significantly.[1]

The increased focus on medical approaches to reduce infant and maternal mortality resulted in an expansion of prenatal care during the 1920s. In 1924, the Children's Bureau published "Prenatal Care" as a companion to its popular "Infant Care"; and in 1925, they established professional standards for the content and schedule of PNC visits,[27] standards that are essentially still in use today. The proposed PNC visitation schedule reflected greater attention to maternal rather than infant health, with more PNC visits at the end of the pregnancy to detect the onset of eclampsia, the leading cause of maternal mortality. Clinical prenatal practice became more standardized and widespread, especially among wealthier women.

By the end of this decade, the original five goals of the AAPSIM had mostly been achieved. Infant mortality had begun to decline significantly. The nature of infant mortality-reduction efforts in the United States, however, had been narrowly focused on a medical/clinical care trajectory led by male obstetricians, with an emphasis on preventive prenatal and enhanced delivery care. Infant mortality began to fade as an identifiable social or public health problem.[1]

1930s: The Depression and Title V of the Social Security Act

When the 1930s began, no organized national maternal and infant programmatic efforts were under way, no major infant mortality reduction movement existed, and the United States was in a major economic depression. Progress in reducing mortality rates among both women and infants slowed substantially, especially during the early part of the decade. By 1935, the IMR declined to a rate of 55.7 deaths per 1000 births.[23] Mortality among nonwhite infants (83.2) dropped to rates similar to those that had occurred among white infants more than two decades earlier. IMR improvements continued disproportionately in the post-neonatal period, with neonatal mortality now accounting for 63% of infant deaths. A substantial reduction in maternal mortality began in the second half of the 1930s, most notably in white women, who by 1939 had rates of mortality less than half of those observed among nonwhites (353.3 deaths per 100,000 births versus 762.2).[23]

Upon President Franklin Roosevelt's inauguration, the Children's Bureau (under the leadership of Grace Abbott) proposed three activities to address the consequences of the Depression and improve the health of infants and mothers: aid to dependent children; MCH services, including services for crippled children; and welfare services for children needing special care. These activities were incorporated into the historic Social Security Act of 1935 (P.L. 74–271). Title IV of that Act provided cash payments through the Social Security Board to mothers who had lost paternal support; and Title V, separately administered by the Children's Bureau, provided federal support for state MCH Services. Title V provided the legislative basis for most public health activities regarding maternal and infant mortality for the remainder of the twentieth century.[28] MCH services were a re-establishment of the repealed Sheppard-Towner Maternal and Infancy Act, with expanded matching state grants aimed at strengthening local MCH services, especially in rural areas. It also included new federal funding for Special Projects of Regional and

National Significance (SPRANS), which would serve as the source of many innovative reproductive-health training, research and demonstration programs in future years.

In contrast to the Sheppard-Towner Act, Title V was mandated to focus its services and educational activities more narrowly on economically disadvantaged women, making Title V a poverty-related program and thereby avoiding competition with physicians serving middle-class women.[1] State-level MCH directors were required to be physicians, and state medical societies had the right to approve local state MCH plans. No provisions were made for providing or reimbursing clinical and curative care; referrals were to be made to private physicians, or if the patient were determined to be indigent, to state or charitable agencies. With the legislative split of Title IV and Title V, child welfare was no longer an integral part of public health services for children. States quickly re-established the required state MCH agencies, and once again began to implement publicly supported educational and preventative services.[1]

In 1935, the Vital Registration Act was passed, which mandated that every state establish and maintain a vital registry of all births and deaths. This Act completed the legislative process begun in 1915 and facilitated accurate epidemiologic analyses of maternal and infant morbidity and mortality in the United States. In 1937, the Children's Bureau published "Infant and Maternal Mortality among Negroes" to bring attention to the substantial inequities in their reproductive mortality.[29]

In the 1930s, greater attention was given to maternal mortality. The 1930 White House Conference on Child Health Protection demonstrated a link between poor aseptic practice, excessive operative deliveries, and high maternal mortality.[30] In 1933, a New York Academy of Medicine study on the causes of maternal mortality found that two thirds were preventable; 40% were caused by sepsis (half following delivery and half associated with illegally induced abortions), and the remainder were attributable to poorly managed hemorrhage and toxemia.[31] State maternal mortality committees were established to confidentially examine the medical records of all women who died from maternal causes and ascertain what could have been done to prevent these deaths.[32] These committees were influential in establishing community norms to improve physician behavior and practice. Simultaneously, hospital-based clinical improvements, such as the development of antimicrobial sulfonamides and safer blood transfusions, addressed maternal hemorrhage and infection, two of the leading causes of maternal mortality, and there was a rapid increases in the number of hospital deliveries.[33] The impact was dramatic; within a decade a two-thirds reduction in maternal mortality was observed.

The 1940s: World War II and the Emergency Maternal and Infant Care Program

Despite WWII, the 1940s were a period of substantial improvements in both infant and maternal mortality. The IMR dropped to 38.3 deaths per 1000 deaths in 1945, with improvements among both white (36.9) and nonwhite infants (60.3).[23] The reduction mostly occurred among infants in the post-neonatal period, reflecting the impact of new antibiotics and the growing treatment options for diarrheal diseases, pneumonia, and other infectious disease.

This decade continued the rapid decline in maternal mortality, reaching 207.2 deaths per 100,000 in 1945 and 90.3 by 1949 (more than a 75% decline over the decade). Rates among nonwhites (455.0 in 1945) also improved, but still lagged. Over this decade, hospital births became more common; 56% of births took place at a hospital in 1940, and 88% did 10 years later. Hospital births among nonwhite mothers also dramatically increased (27% to 58%), with an associated marked decline in midwifery deliveries (48% to 26%).[32]

Congress passed the Emergency Maternal and Infant Care (EMIC) program in 1943 in response to the dislocation of soldiers and their families during WWII. Military bases had been overwhelmed by the care demands, and state Title V clinic funding was inadequate. EMIC was a direct revenue-funded program to pay for free prenatal, obstetric, and infant care for the wives of servicemen in the four lowest pay grades. EMIC was administered by the Children's Bureau and operated by state health departments; physicians and hospitals were paid directly for their services. The Children's Bureau stressed the development of licensure and standards for hospital maternity and newborn services to upgrade the quality of reproductive and pediatric care.[34]

The EMIC program represented the only time in the twentieth century that the U.S. government directly provided medical care for large segments of civilian populations. Wartime service needs muted the AMA opposition to this program. EMIC was a very successful and popular; it provided maternity services for 1.5 million births—almost 15% of all U.S. births—and represented a model for a national health service program for mothers and children.[35] The EMIC program, along with many other WWII federal social welfare initiatives, was terminated on June 30, 1949. In 1956, it was resurrected as part of the military's Dependent Medical Care Act, and in 1966 was incorporated into the military's Civilian Health and Medical Program, Uniform Services (CHAMPUS).

Beyond Title V programs, the end of the 1940s was a period of limited federal reproductive public health efforts in the United States, perhaps reflective of the increasingly conservative Cold War period and the dominance of the medical profession in addressing infant mortality. In 1945, the Children's Bureau was moved to the new Federal Security Agency, marking the start of a long period of its decline and influence. There remained opposition to many of the federal MCH programs because they were being run by the Children's Bureau, a non-health-associated agency. By contrast, most European countries, suffering from the aftermath of WWII, implemented comprehensive cradle-to-grave welfare systems, with both government guarantee or provision of health services and maternity insurance benefits (e.g., paid leave, nurse home visits, and maternity and childhood allowances). Two distinct approaches to reducing infant and maternal mortality in the United States and in Europe were now in place.

The 1950s: The Baby Boom

The largest baby boom in U.S. history occurred at the end of WWII, peaking at more than 4 million births per year in 1956. This boom helped spark a demand for high-quality medical and obstetric care. However, this decade also reflected the slowest improvements in infant and neonatal mortality during the twentieth century. The IMR in 1955 was 26.4 deaths per 1000 births (23), declining by only 2.8 deaths over the entire decade, with virtually no improvement in IMR (44.5) or NMR among nonwhite infants. Other countries' IMRs continued to drop in this decade, and as a result, the United States fell from the sixth best IMR in the world to the 13th. Infants with low birth weight (i.e., <2,500 grams) represented 7.6% of all births.[32]

Maternal mortality, by contrast, continued to substantially decline for all women in this decade, reaching 47.0 deaths/100,000 births in 1955, less than 1/10th the rate of 1935. The maternal mortality for nonwhite mothers (110.7), however, remained over three times that for white mothers (32.8).[23]

The 1950s were a very conservative period with few new public health programs and limited public involvement with maternal and infant mortality reduction efforts, possibly the nadir of public health involvement in maternal and infant health in the twentieth century. In 1951, the American College of Obstetricians and Gynecologist (ACOG) was organized to advance the standards of obstetric and gynecologic care of women. With support from the Hill Burton Act of 1946, there was substantial hospital construction (including for obstetric services). A distinctive feature of the decade was the rapid growth in private insurance programs to ensure access, albeit unequal, to the growing private obstetric and pediatric services. Employer-based medical insurance systems with family coverage become firmly established for the middle class, with members of large industrial unions also obtaining such coverage. By 1958, two thirds of Americans had some form of hospital insurance coverage, and 55% of pregnant women had benefits to cover maternity costs.[32] By the end of the 1950s, hospital births were nearly universal for both white (98.8%) and nonwhite (85%) populations.[32] The U.S. maternal and infant care system in the 1950s was characterized as "scientifically advanced, relatively well distributed geographically, and accessible to a majority though not all of American families".[1]

The 1960s: The War on Poverty and Renewal of Federal Interest in Maternal and Infant Health

During the early 1960s, only marginal improvements were made in U.S. IMR, though larger improvements occurred in the second half of the decade. The IMR was 24.7 deaths per 1000 births in 1965;[23] racial disparities narrowed, but remained substantial (21.5 for white infants versus 40.3 for nonwhite infants). More than 75% of infant deaths now occurred during the neonatal period, with over half of the very low birth infants (<1500 grams) dying.[36] In addition, 7.7% of infants were low birth weight in 1965 (6.8% in white infants and 12.8% in nonwhites). By 1969, prenatal care services were widely obtained; 72.4% of white and 42.7% of black mothers initiated PNC during the first trimester.[37] Maternal mortality (31.6 deaths/100,000 births in 1965) slowly declined throughout the decade, with continued marked racial disparities (21.0 white and 83.7 nonwhite MMRs).

In 1962, the Children's Bureau was split; most of its research mandate shifted to the new National Institute for Child Health and Human Development (in the National

Institutes for Health), which eventually supported substantial levels of research into maternal-fetal development and neonatal practice. In its 1963 and 1965 authorizations, Congress gave Title V a new applied MCH research mandate to complement its service orientation;[38] and President John Kennedy, perhaps because of family misfortunes, initiated several small programs in maternal and infant care. The (Mills/ Ribicoff) Maternal and Child Health and Mental Retardation Planning Act of 1963 supported new Title V Maternity and Infant Care (MIC) demonstration projects to provide comprehensive prenatal care (medical care, nutrition, social services, and health education) to high-risk mothers in low-income rural and urban areas. Evaluations of the MIC-enriched PNC programs suggested that they were successful in reducing poor birth outcomes,[39] though only 53 sites were funded by 1969. The MIC model of comprehensive PNC (now supplemented with care-coordination and home visits) has become the standard for publicly supported PNC clinics in the United States.

In 1964, in partial response to the growing civil rights movement, President Lyndon Johnson launched the War on Poverty to address the nation's social and racial inequalities. For the first time in its history, the U.S. government assumed direct responsibility for assuring the well-being of all of its citizens.[40] Three major groups of initiatives emerged from the War on Poverty.[41]

First, in 1965, Congress passed Medicaid—Title XIX of the Social Security Act— to provide health insurance assistance to the poor. Although Medicaid was not a comprehensive maternal and infant health-care program, it directly financed health and hospital services for low-income citizens, many of whom were single mothers and children. Medicaid, however, had at least five limitations.[1] First, state welfare agencies were made responsible for the program because access to health care was considered a poverty issue, not a public health issue. Second, there was substantial variability in eligibility and benefits across Medicaid state programs. Third, with the exception of prenatal care visits, Medicaid paid only for curative health services, not prevention activities. Fourth, Medicaid beneficiaries were vulnerable to changes in categorical eligibility depending on shifting state government budgets and philosophies. And fifth, Medicaid was separated from programs sponsored by Title V. Although Medicaid quickly became the largest provider of funds for MCH-related reproductive health services, Title V programs nationally and locally were not active in setting Medicaid MCH policies. Thus, beginning in 1965 onward, federal maternal and child health services were fragmented among various independent agencies. Despite these limitations, Medicaid was a major step forward in financing the health care during pregnancy for low-income women.

The War on Poverty also addressed the availability of health services for low-income families through a series of categorical initiatives. The Economic Opportunity Act (1965) provided for the construction and financing of neighborhood health centers. These new centers were directly funded to bypass long-standing patterns of racism in state and local health departments; they offered a full range of medical and preventive services and were sites for community development and empowerment. By 1969, more than 150 centers had been established, offering services predominantly to women and children.[42] In 1968, the neighborhood health centers were renamed "community health centers" and their emphasis shifted to more traditional medical care; they were incorporated into the Public Health Services Act (Sections

329 and 330). Other legislation and programs implemented in 1965, including the Health Professions Education Act, Comprehensive Health Planning Assistance, and Regional Medical Programs, further enhanced the availability of maternal and infant health services.

A third set of War on Poverty categorical initiatives focused on specific issues associated with poverty, including Head Start, Community Development Grants, Food Stamps, and Child Nutrition. In 1968, Title X (Family Planning) of the Public Health Services Act was passed to increase availability of family planning services among poor Americans. Because of concerns that family planning would be too narrowly linked to maternity issues, Title X was legislated as a separate program independent of the Title V MCH program. This problematic split has continued into the twenty-first century.

Substantial progress also was made in neonatal medicine. In 1963, RhoGam was introduced to prevent Rh sensitization in women with Rh-negative blood.[15] Progress was also made in managing respiratory problems associated with hyaline membrane disease, the most frequent cause of death among premature infants.[43] Newer clinical advances were, however, still only available in academic medical centers.

In 1968, the U.S. National Birth Certificate was substantially revised, with the collection of additional public health related data (e.g., PNC visits; gestational age; and maternal and paternal age, race, and education). The new certificate provided a much more complete picture of reproductive health in the United States. Its subsequent computerization also made it much more available for local and state analysis. The National Center for Health Statistics (NCHS) initiated a periodic series of national birth cohort follow-back surveys, (e.g., the National Natality Survey) and fertility and family planning surveys (e.g., the National Survey of Family Growth), which allowed for more in-depth studies of reproductive risk and health service utilization.

Out of the political turbulence of the 1960s, a woman's health movement emerged dedicated to the achievement of political and social equality. This movement drew attention to the overmedicalization and male dominance of obstetrical care in the United States, and added a political dimension unseen since the turn of the century to the reproductive health debates of the late 1960s and onward.[44] Substantial grass-roots consumer movements also developed to enhance childbirth.[15] Parent groups, child developmentalists, and pediatricians interested in maternal-infant attachment theory encouraged more "lying in" between hospitalized mothers and their new-borns.[45] These advocates pushed to transform maternity wards to make them more family friendly. In response to the increasing rates of Caesarean deliveries, advocacy groups emerged to encourage women and their families to make informed decisions regarding labor and delivery. Concurrently, the La Leche League encouraged women to breast-feed, a practice that had been long out of favor with many middle-class mothers. Midwifery and natural childbirth (e.g., the Lamaze method) began to reemerge as birthing alternatives that were less medically intrusive.[15]

In the 1960s, through the War on Poverty, the federal government began to address the broader health and social needs of pregnant women that had been ignored since the maternity insurance struggles of the 1920s. A sustained focus directed at maternal or infant mortality reduction, however, had not yet developed. In 1969, the

Children's Bureau was officially abolished, and responsibility for administering the Title V MCH programs shifted to the new Public Health Service in the Department of Health Education and Welfare (DHEW). The dismemberment of the Children's Bureau further diffused federal leadership for mothers and children.[38]

The 1970s: Regionalization and *Roe v. Wade*

The War on Poverty initiatives contributed to the continued decline in infant mortality, which began in 1965 and continued throughout this decade. In 1975, the IMR reached 16.1 deaths per 1000 births, and the racial gap narrowed among white (14.2) and black (26.2) infants.[23] A substantial decline (>40%) in neonatal mortality occurred over the decade to 11.6 deaths per 1000 births, among both white (10.4) and black (18.3) infants. By the end of the 1970s, the United States experienced its lowest post WWII fertility rates and number of annual births. Maternal mortality rates continued to decline to 12.8 deaths per 100,000 births for all populations, but a substantial racial gap remained (9.1 for white and 29.0 for nonwhite mothers). However, by the end of the decade, the MMR began to level off.

By 1975, the number of infants born with low birth weight (7.4%) had declined modestly, although substantial racial disparities (6.3% white and 13.1% black) persisted.[37] The lower infant mortality reflected improved treatment for newborns, not changes in the distribution of birth weights. Initiation of PNC in their first trimester increased to 72.6% in 1975, with more substantial gains among black (55.8%) than white women (75.9%). Caesarian (C-) sections were increasingly performed, representing 10.4% of all hospital-based deliveries in 1975.

Several major new reproductive public health programs and policies began in the 1970s. In 1972, the U.S. Congress authorized the Special Supplemental Nutrition Program for Women, Infants and Children (WIC). Using farm surpluses to provide food for the "special" growth associated with pregnancy, breastfeeding, and early child development, WIC provided nutritional supplementation, nutrition education, and linkages with health-care services for low-income and nutritionally eligible women and infants.[46] After internal federal debate and lack of enthusiasm for the program by DHEW, the U.S. Department of Agriculture (USDA) assumed responsibility for the WIC program, once again further splitting federal maternal and child health programs. WIC was a very popular program that grew rapidly in the 1970s and quickly demonstrated a positive impact on birth outcomes.[47,48] WIC can be viewed as revival of the early era "pure milk" and milk-station movement; nutrition supplementation and advice once again became a major feature of public health prenatal and infant care programs for low-income families in the United States.

In 1973, the Supreme Court ruled in *Roe v. Wade* that states could not restrict access to medical procedures associated with abortion in the first two trimesters of pregnancy. This implicit legalization of abortion provided women with new means to address unwanted pregnancies, control their reproductive rights, and diminish complications associated with illegal abortion—one of the leading causes of maternal death. By the end of the decade, more than 1.5 million legal abortions were obtained annually. Advocacy organizations such as the Guttmacher Institute and

Planned Parenthood, not government agencies, have provided the leadership to ensure available, affordable and safe abortions in the United States. For the first time
in the twentieth century, abortion and family planning had now become substantial
public health issues within the MCH community.[49]

During the 1970s, neonatologists and neonatal intensive care units (NICUs) became more effective at addressing the consequences of prematurity and very low
birth weight, the leading causes of neonatal and infant mortality. To promote increased and equitable access to the nation's 125 NICUs,[50] federal and regional health
planning legislation and organizations, such as the March of Dimes and the Robert
Wood Johnson Foundation,[51,52] supported the creation of regional systems of NICUs.
Under the auspices of state Title V agencies, several states developed comprehensive
programs of regionalized care, including North Carolina and Massachusetts. In
1974, ACOG/AAP established clinical standards for NICUs; a year later, neonatal-
perinatal medicine became a board-certified subspecialty of pediatrics.[53] Regionalization represented a potent combination of improved clinical services and public
health financing and access programs.

In the mid-1970s, the federal MCH Bureau expanded support for selected state
Title V agencies to coordinate comprehensive PNC, regionalize clinical care, and enhance state infrastructure capacity.[54] Premised on state and/or local selection of
needed initiatives, the improved pregnancy outcome (IPO) program served as a model
for several subsequent federal MCH bureau efforts to improve birth outcomes. Infant
mortality reduction, for the first time, had become a separate, and directly funded,
federal public health initiative, beyond its broad inclusion in Title V programs.

Before the 1970s, no overarching federal health policy was in place in the United
States; public health programs (e.g., Title V, Medicaid, and WIC) were each administered independently.[41] The U.S. health policy essentially was the sum of its individual health programs.[40] In the late 1970s, the Carter administration, under the
leadership of Surgeon General Julius Richmond, issued two seminal public health
documents that guided subsequent maternal and child health policy. *Better Health
for Our Children: A National Strategy* included policy recommendations to (1) ensure equitable MCH services, (2) address influences on MCH beyond personal
health services (including nutrition and environmental risks), and (3) build MCH research capacity.[55] The second publication, *Healthy People, 1990*, promulgated a set
of measurable national health objectives for the coming decade.[56] The 1990 goal for
healthy infants was a reduction of infant mortality by 35% to 9 deaths per 1,000
births. Identifying infant mortality reduction as a national health goal provided a
powerful tool to shape and motivate reproductive public health policy and practice.
Over the subsequent decades, federal funds, initiatives, and accountability were increasingly tied to these decade-by-decade numeric national health objectives.

The 1980s: The Second Major Era of Infant Mortality Reduction Efforts in the Twentieth Century

Although the 1980s was a time of conservative politics and government cut-backs,
there was significantly increased attention to infant mortality, racial disparities in

birth outcomes, and enhanced access to comprehensive PNC, ultimately culminating in a major expansion of Medicaid's income eligibility and services for pregnant women and infants. The 1980s can be characterized as the second major national era of public health infant mortality reduction efforts, unparalleled since the 1900–1920s. The 1980s also heralded significant clinical advances, which together with the new public health achievements, set in motion substantial reductions in infant mortality that lasted through the remainder of the century.

Infant mortality rates declined in the 1980s, though more slowly in the early years of the decade. In 1985, the U.S. IMR, now ranked 23rd in the world, dropped to 10.6 deaths per 1000 births, with substantial racial disparity (9.2 for white, 19.0 for black, and 9.9 for Hispanic infants).[23] Rates of low birth weight and premature infants remained essentially constant throughout the decade, at 6.8% and 8.2%, respectively.[37] Little progress was made in enhancing PNC utilization; in 1985, first-trimester initiation rates (76.3%) remained higher for white (79.4%) than black (61.8%) women. The C-section rates continued to rise, reaching 23.8% of births by the end of the decade. Maternal mortality declined only slightly over the prior decade (7.8 deaths/100,000 births), and remained stagnant after 1985, with substantial racial disparities (5.1 for white and 21.3 for black women).

In the early 1980s, economic recession and the adoption of conservative social policy at the federal level under President Ronald Reagan reduced funding for health and social welfare programs and restricted Medicaid enrollment criteria. Title V and six categorical child-health programs were converted into MCH Services Block Grants (P.L. 97–35) with limited federal oversight.[24] The percentage of economically disadvantaged pregnant women covered by Medicaid decreased substantially from 1975. The MCH advocates linked these changes to the reemergence of increased local area IMRs, elevating infant mortality once again as a "social problem."[57]

Improved access to PNC and more comprehensive PNC were proposed as potential solutions to the new infant mortality crisis. Epidemiologic research had documented that increased PNC was associated with better birth outcomes,[58] and that poor and minority women received insufficient PNC.[59] Demonstration projects on case management and home visitation fostered the view that comprehensive PNC was an effective solution to poor birth outcomes and racial health disparities.[60,61] The influential Institute of Medicine (IOM) reports "Preventing Low Birthweight" (1985) and "Prenatal Care: Reaching Mothers, Reaching Babies" (1988) argued that low birth weight could be substantially reduced through improved access to comprehensive PNC and that it was cost-effective, potentially saving $3.38 for each dollar spent.[62,54] Infant mortality began to be viewed again as a social disease with biologic manifestations. Poverty was thought to have both direct (e.g., stress and malnutrition) and indirect (e.g., access to care) effects; racial disparities were thought to reflect underlying socioeconomic differences.[63] European models of enhanced reproductive prevention and social welfare care were reexamined.[64]

The expansion of Medicaid became the driving force to reduce infant mortality, at both the state and national levels. In a series of incremental steps, Congress modified Medicaid's income eligibility using each successive year's Omnibus Budget Reconciliation Act (OBRA).[24] The first step, taken in 1984, was small; pregnant women in two parent families in which both parents were unemployed were made eligible for

Medicaid. In 1985, Medicaid eligibility was expanded to cover all pregnant women in any type of family with income below the state's Aid to Families with Dependent Children (AFDC) welfare eligibility level. In 1986, Medicaid was required to cover pregnant women and infants less than 1 year of age with incomes below 100% of the federal poverty line (FPL), effectively severing the link between receipt of welfare benefits and Medicaid eligibility. Congress continued to gradually expand income eligibility, ultimately allowing Medicaid enrollment up to 185% of the FPL. In addition, states were encouraged to facilitate Medicaid enrollment through outreach by enrollment workers, use of simplified enrollment forms, and presumptive eligibility. The effects on Medicaid enrollment were dramatic; for example, in 20 southern states, Medicaid covered approximately 45% of all births by 1990 compared with only 20% in 1985.[65] The elimination of most financial barriers to medical services for low-income pregnant women was one of the major public health achievements of this decade.

Medicaid reform also expanded to provide a comprehensive, reimbursable package of services for PNC including nutrition, health education, and social services (i.e., the Title V MIC model of PNC services), as well as home visitation and case management. The content of PNC was transformed for low-income women from medical care only to a more "comprehensive" package of prenatal services. In many states, Medicaid programs were transformed from an insurance payer to a purchaser of MCH services. Joint MCH–Medicaid comprehensive PNC projects, such as North Carolina Baby Love program,[66] were touted as successful interagency collaboration and changed perceptions about PNC from clinical care to public health care.[67]

Numerous other national, state, and local initiatives were happening concurrently to promote infant and maternal health. In 1980, the March of Dimes refocused its core efforts from infantile paralysis to improved birth outcomes. The Southern Governors Association and its Southern Regional Task Force on Infant Mortality (1984), which represented the states with the highest infant mortality rates, advocated for Medicaid reform and the creation of state infant mortality commissions. In 1987, Congress established the National Commission to Prevent Infant Mortality, whose subsequent reports proposed a wide range of public health PNC interventions.[68]

Newly established state and local infant mortality commissions organized local efforts and engaged new partners (e.g., politicians, businessmen, and clergy) into infant mortality reduction efforts. The Healthy Mothers, Healthy Baby Coalition galvanized grass-roots efforts. Numerous innovative state programs were developed (e.g., media campaigns, toll-free help lines, PNC incentive coupon books, and payer of last resort programs to insure undocumented immigrants and women not covered by Medicaid). The Healthy Futures/Healthy Generations program (1988–1993), a joint IPO project of the federal MCH Bureau and the Robert Wood Johnson Foundation, attempted to reduce infant mortality in southern states by improving their perinatal health care systems. In 1987, the Center for Disease Control and Prevention (CDC)'s Division of Reproductive Health established the MCH Epidemiology Program and implemented the Pregnancy Risk Assessment Monitoring System (PRAMS) to study birth outcomes and health services at the state level. The Public Health Service Expert Panel Report on the Content of Prenatal Care (1989) recommended that PNC encompass a greater psychosocial focus.[69] Midwifery services reemerged as a solution to the lack of access to providers for low-income women. Fetal and infant mortality review (FIMR) committees, a variant of the earlier era maternal mortality review committees, assessed the underlying social and health system issues involved in local-area infant deaths.[70] The WIC program also continued expanding; by 1989, it served almost 35% of infants born in the United States.[71]

Improved access to medical care and more effective treatment also substantially impacted infant mortality. Despite the repeal of federal planning legislation, regionalization of maternal and neonatal care had become widespread in the 1980s.[41] The number of both neonatologists and NICU beds increased dramatically. Assisted by Medicaid's expanded income eligibility, 700 NICUs were established by 1989, up from only 125 a decade earlier.[43] Surfactant, a lipoprotein that increases the elasticity of immature lungs, provided a new treatment for respiratory distress syndrome, one of the major causes of premature death; its introduction in the mid-1980s may have accounted for up to 20% of the reduction in IMR observed during this decade.[72]

Congress, as part of the OBRA of 1989 (P.L. 101–239), mandated several perinatal system reforms (including a reauthorized and revised Title V MCH Block Grant Program, further Medicaid reform, better coordination among federal programs, enhanced epidemiologic surveillance, and a stronger federal-state partnership) and encouraged many popular programmatic initiatives (e.g., expanded home visiting programs and co-location of prenatal services). These mandates also reestablished public accountability for reproductive health and other MCH-funded programs.[24]

Reproductive public health efforts undertaken toward the end of the decade had a substantial impact. During this time, a widespread movement took place to address the perceived "social problem" of infant mortality, the second such major era in the twentieth century. Public health professionals and political leaders joined forces to implement a wide range of public health activities directed at enhancing access to comprehensive PNC. Comprehensive PNC services provided a framework for the United States to move beyond a narrow focus on medical care and once again address some of the unfinished social welfare and health issues recognized during the 1900–1920s. The long-standing twentieth-century advocacy goal of assuring universal medical services for all pregnant women and their newborns was close to realization via the expansions of Medicaid income eligibility.

The 1990s: The Start-and-Stop Decade for Reproductive Health

The 1990s reflected a politically conflicted decade of new federal public health and welfare initiatives impacting on infant and maternal mortality. The programmatic gains of the late 1980s continued into this decade, but with diminished support for the prior public health consensus on access to comprehensive PNC. Numerous divergent public health and clinical initiatives to further reduce infant and maternal mortality and morbidity characterized the end of the decade.

In the 1990s, infant mortality rates decreased substantially from the prior decade; by 2000 the U.S. rate was 6.9 deaths per 1000 births,[73] exceeding the year 2000 national health objectives for infant mortality of 7.0 deaths per 1000. However, racial disparities in infant mortality rates persisted (6.3 for whites, 15.1 for blacks, and 5.9 for Hispanics). The NMR was 4.9/1000 births, 65% of the IMR. Birth weight–specific mortality rates continued to improve substantially; by the end of the decade, approximately half of babies born weighing 500–750 grams survived,[74] largely because of increased availability of advanced medical care. However, more than 67% of all neonatal deaths occurred among premature, very low birth weight (LBW) infants. By 2000, the number of fetal deaths (non-live birth deaths $\geq$ 20 weeks gestational age) now approximated infant mortality at 6.6 fetal deaths per 1000 live births and fetal deaths. The proportions of low birth weight and premature infants rose gradually during the 1990s (reaching 7.6% and 11.8%, respectively, by 1999).[75] The increased number of multiple births resulting from a wide use of assistive reproductive technologies contributed substantially.[76] Racial disparities continued to disproportionately effect black infants for LBW (6.2% whites; 13.2% blacks; 6.3% Hispanics) and prematurity (9.7% whites; 17.8% blacks; 10.9% Hispanics). The ethnic/racial composition of infants born in the United States shifted reflecting high rates of immigration, especially from Latin America and Asia. Births to unmarried women also increased substantially, to 32.2% in 1995 from 22.0% in 1985.

The efforts to improve access to PNC begun in the 1980s proved effective; there was a steady improvement in PNC utilization throughout the 1990s. In 1995, 81.3% of women (87.1% of white, 70.4% of black, and 70.8% of Hispanic women) initiated PNC in the first trimester, and 28.8% of all women received more than the ACOG-recommended number of PNC visits.[75] The C-section rates dipped slightly mid-decade (20.8%), but rose again by decade's end to 22.8%. Abortion levels declined slightly, but remained at more than 1 million per year.

Maternal mortality rates (MMR; 6.3 deaths/100,000 births in 1995) showed only minimal improvement over this decade, sparking a renewed federal interest in maternal mortality and morbidity. Beginning in 1999, a new, more inclusive classification of maternal deaths was introduced, which better captured nonobstetric causes of deaths related to or aggravated by pregnancy and extended the follow-up time period up to one year post-partum.[77] By 2000, the new maternal mortality rate indicated 9.8 maternal deaths per 100,000 births, with MMRs of 7.5 among white, 22.0 black, and 9.8 Hispanic mothers.

The Healthy Start Initiative

In 1991, the Healthy Start Initiative, the largest dedicated federal infant mortality reduction program in the twentieth century, was implemented. Through the identification and implementation of a broad range of community-based strategies, 16 Healthy Start demonstrations communities, led by local consortia, received substantial funds to develop local services and enhanced systems of care with the goal of reducing their infant mortality rate by 50% over 5 years.[78] Starting in 1997, the Healthy Start Initiative expanded into over 80 replication communities. Healthy Start was made a permanent, authorized program under Title V (Section 514) in the Child Health Act of 2000. The subsequent national evaluation, however, showed that although Healthy Start increased the use of PNC services, it had a limited impact on improving birth outcomes.[79]

Other federal efforts complemented the Healthy Start Initiative. In 1991, an inter-agency Department of Health and Human Service Secretary's Advisory Committee on Infant Mortality (SACIM) was established to guide development of federal infant mortality policy and oversee the Healthy Start Initiative. The CDC implemented a major research initiative "Psychosocial Pathway to Prematurity Prevention in African American Women";[80] NICHD expanded its maternal-fetal and neonatal clinical re-search networks; FIMR projects were institutionalized nationally by ACOG with MCH Bureau funding; and the federal Substance Abuse and Mental Health Services Administration implemented new maternal drug-addiction prevention and treatment programs. In addition, the March of Dimes' initiative, "Towards Improving the Out-come of Pregnancy: the 90's and Beyond," provided policy guidance and encourage-ment for further reproductive public health and clinical activities throughout the decade.[81]

Federal Health and Welfare Policy

In 1992, President William Clinton proposed sweeping legislation—the Health Se-curity Act—to restructure the U.S. health-care system to ensure health care for all Americans. However, lack of support from the medical community, opposition from the health insurance industry, and disorganized advocacy efforts led to the defeat of this act. Despite this defeat, President Clinton supported additional legislation to fur-ther improve infant and maternal health. The Family and Medical Leave Act of 1993 provided for limited, unpaid maternity leave from the workplace—though not paid leave, one of the hallmarks of the European reproductive public health system. In 1997, the State Child Health Insurance Program (S-CHIP), Title XXI of the Social Security Act, addressed the increasing number of uninsured children in the United States, and reflected an incrementalist approach to universal health coverage. Al-though S-CHIP represented the largest expansion of child health services in more than 30 years, its impact on reproductive health is likely to be limited as the Medi-caid program already covers most reproductive health services for similar income eligible women and infants.

The Personal Responsibility and Work Opportunity Reconciliation Act of 1996 transformed the U.S. welfare system. It restricted maternal welfare benefits, which now were time-limited, had a work requirement, and placed a family cap on support for additional children. States also compete for a financial bonus for reducing births to single mothers, and a new abstinence education program was added to Title V (section 510). Although the Act's long-term impact on family welfare and reproduc-tive health remains unclear, it dramatically reduced welfare enrollment.

The Illegal Immigration Reform and Immigrant Responsibility Act of 1996 pro-hibited Medicaid and most other federal health services and welfare benefits for un-documented and many legal immigrants. Analysis of the impact of this reform on access to prenatal care and birth outcomes in immigrant communities has produced conflicted findings.[82,83]

These federal policy decisions reflect competing visions of both increased and de-creased government involvement and responsibility for its citizens' health and wel-fare, perhaps reflective of the political stalemate in this era. Although the Medicaid expansions of the late 1980s remain, the social context for reproductive health services for low-income and immigrant families in the United States has changed.

Clinical Progress in Reproductive Health

Clinical progress continued in the fields of neonatology and maternal-fetal medicine in the 1990s. The number of neonatologists continued to rise, reaching almost 2,500 by 1993.[53] In addition, NICHD's maternal-fetal and neonatal networks fostered cross-institutional research and national clinical trials. Infectious diseases reemerged as a recognized cause of low birth weight, prematurity, and infant mortality; with bacterial vaginosis and fetal fibronectin markers, in particular, identified with prematurity.[84] Efforts to reduce poor birth outcomes through antibiotic treatment protocols for bacterial vaginosis have had mixed results.[85] Pregnant women (and their infants) infected with Human Immunodeficiency Virus (HIV) became a major reproductive clinical and public health challenge in this decade. The utilization of Zidoviudine (AZT) and other anti-retroviral prophylaxis has substantially reduced perinatal transmission.[86]

A Decreased Emphasis on Prenatal Care

In the late 1990s, the prior public health consensus supporting comprehensive PNC as the solution to reduce infant mortality and other poor birth outcomes had broken down.[87,88] Randomized control trials demonstrated that PNC had limited impact on prematurity, low birth weight, or infant mortality. Efforts to establish a direct casual role for social factors in poor birth outcomes have been inconclusive.[89] Moreover, despite the implementation of many new public health programs and continued Medicaid expansions, national rates of prematurity and low birth weight continued to increase. Finally, the emergence of the Latina birth outcome paradox (i.e., good birth outcomes despite elevated poverty rates, lower education levels, and less access to health insurance) undercut the simplistic association between infant mortality and socioeconomic status and race/ethnicity.[90]

Increasing attention is being placed on preconception and interconception health care, rather than prenatal care, to address the reproductive health of both infants and mothers.[91] This orientation perhaps reflects the growth of women's health and longitudinal perspectives in reproductive health care, and responds to the widely cited aphorism, "You can't cure a lifetime of ills in 9 months of a pregnancy."[92] Efforts to convert these concepts into formal intervention services, however, have not yet matured. The CDC has recently focused considerable attention on a Safe Motherhood initiative to address women's health before, during and after pregnancy.[93]

Options for Improving Infant Health in the 1990s

Although no consensus existed in the latter part of the decade regarding the best ways to reduce infant mortality and eliminate racial disparities, many new options were pursued. There was increased attention to preventing infectious diseases in pregnant women (e.g., douching discouragement or antibiotic treatment); better assessing and expanding the social content of prenatal care (e.g., partner violence or maternal depression), and addressing disease-specific contributions to infant mortality (e.g., the AAP's "Back to Sleep" Sudden Infant Death reduction campaign or Smoke Free America's pregnancy smoking cessation campaign). In addition, enhanced MCH epidemiology capacity at state and local levels expanded the availability of data for effective public health action.[94] Addressing birth defects, now associated with over 20% of infant mortality, represented an additional direction for infant mortality prevention efforts. The March of Dimes actively campaigned to increase awareness and consumption of folic acid to prevent neural tube defects. In 1998, the Birth Defects Prevention Act (P.L. 105–168) established a nationwide network of birth defects monitoring and research programs.

Overall, the 1990s were a period of major improvements in infant mortality (and birth-weight specific mortality), but most other markers of infant and maternal health remained stagnant. The efforts to increase PNC utilization appeared successful, but the lack of improvements in low birth weight and prematurity raised questions about its content and efficacy. A host of new federal health and wellness policy initiatives, both progressive and retrogressive, impacted reproductive health in this decade. By the late 1990s, the second major national era of public health efforts to address infant mortality through access to comprehensive PNC would appear to be over, with no overarching reproductive public health policy to replace it. A diverse set of clinical and public health efforts to further reduce maternal and infant mortality are underway.

Conclusions and Challenges for the Twenty-First Century

Over the course of the twentieth century, infant mortality rates declined from upwards of 150 deaths per 1000 births to under 7 deaths per 1000 births—a 95% reduction. Similarly, maternal mortality decreased from 600–900 deaths per 100,000 births to under 10 deaths per 100,000 births—a 97% reduction. Through the implementation of a wide range of public health strategies, infant and maternal mortality have been virtually eliminated as major health scourges in the United States. The twentieth century ended with a broad array of mature and organized public health efforts, backed by extensive clinical knowledge and capacity, to ensure the health and well-being of mothers and infants.

Yet there remains much room for improvement, as the United States ranks but 25th in infant mortality and 21st in maternal mortality in the world.[33] Many unfinished reproductive public health research, practice, and policy challenges still lie ahead. Some of these challenges include:

1. *Preterm birth prevention.* Despite dramatic improvements in infant mortality and neonatal clinical care, the LBW/prematurity rates have steadily increased in the United States for over 20 years and remain much higher than in Europe. While some of the rise is due to ART and multiple births (76), our numerous national prevention initiatives have had seemingly little impact on reversing this trend. The etiology and biologic pathways of very early prematurity (where most infant deaths occur) are still not well understood. Without this critical

knowledge, creating effective public health preventive interventions will remain limited. Additional risk-factor research is still critically needed, especially in the biologic, environmental, and genomic domains. The growing capacity of MCH epidemiology to better assess risk factors and guide public health practice is just becoming evident. To date, little public health attention has been devoted to fetal loss. The recent March of Dimes Prematurity initiative has begun to galvanize national attention on addressing the rising U.S. LBW/prematurity rates.[95]

2. *Racial and social inequities in health and health services.* Perhaps the most enduring reproductive health challenge of the twentieth century has been to understand, address, and ameliorate the ongoing racial and social disparities in reproductive health and health services, especially between black and white infants and mothers. Despite major reproductive gains for all populations, the 2:1 black/white gap for most reproductive outcomes did not diminish throughout the century. As the Latina birth outcome paradox indicates,[90] racial and/or ethnic and socioeconomic disparities are not equivalent. Those factors that influence disparities (such as diffusion of treatment innovation, racism, neighborhood effects) may be distinct from factors that promote better birth outcomes for all, and they need to be independently addressed. One of the two overarching goals of Healthy People 2010 is to "eliminate health disparities,"[96] though that may be difficult to achieve without full etiologic knowledge.

3. *Maternal health and safe motherhood.* The contributions of women's health experiences over their lifetime are increasingly viewed as critical to birth outcomes, yet little is known about what prior history is important or how to measure cumulative experience.[93] Moreover, the sequelae of pregnancy on maternal and women's lifetime health are also poorly appreciated, yet are at the heart of the Safe Motherhood initiative.[94] Research is needed to move beyond maternal mortality to address maternal morbidity.

Transforming women's and maternal longitudinal health concepts into more concrete, efficacious, and equitable reproductive health-service interventions is a challenge for the twenty-first century; many opportunities remain underdeveloped. Preconception care programs to address women's both long-term and immediate pre-pregnancy health needs have not yet become widely institutionalized; they lack funding, have insufficient evidence-based content, and do not address women with unplanned pregnancies. Preconception care must include family planning, as over half of pregnancies in the United States are currently unintended.[97] Yet today, family planning topics (such as birth control, abortion, sex education) are highly politicized and increasingly separated from maternal and child public health efforts (see Chapter 12). Prenatal care—primary care for women during pregnancy—currently has limited impact on prematurity and/or infant mortality. Its efficacy needs to be strengthened; there have been no national consensus conferences to re-evaluate PNC content since 1985.[69] There remains intraprofessional tension over the nature and control of birthing processes. The rising C-section rates in the United States are a clinical and public health challenge. The role of midwives vs. obstetricians in delivering low-risk mothers in the United States continues to simmer as a debate, as does the increasing use of technology in the birthing process. Maternal health in the postnatal period is currently inadequately addressed, primarily by a singular, too often unattended six-week postpartum visit. Many high-risk women receive no further health care until their next pregnancy. The development of a more formal postnatal (or internatal) care program is needed to ensure the delivery of more consistent maternal health care.

4. *Economic and social basis of the infant and maternal mortality*. The key elements of European reproductive/public health model (maternity insurance) do not yet exist in the United States, neither in the provision of universal health services nor the assurance of economic security for pregnant and birthing women. The United States is the only industrial country where health care is not a human right—for children or parents. While Medicaid provides a very broad and important health insurance program for low-income mothers and infants, eligibility, content, and provider availability issues remain. Moreover, the United States lacks any national programs to help cover the direct economic costs associated with parenthood; neither paid maternity leave nor maternity and childhood allowances programs exist. Currently, maternal and child welfare programs remain mostly separated from maternal and infant health programs. The political struggles to address both the economic and clinical basis of poor pregnancy outcomes will continue into the twenty-first century.

5. *New political, social, and historical context of MCH services*. U.S. reproductive health efforts can no longer remain isolated and independent of the reproductive health efforts of the rest of the world. Increasingly, international reproductive health issues (such as HIV/infectious disease transmission, immigrant health, women's status, racism, safe motherhood) affect us. We must begin to rectify the growing gap in reproductive health between rich and poor nations. There is also a need to address the growing militarization of our society. The MCH populations are always the major victims of war, and money spent on the military diminishes revenues for health and social welfare. The reproductive health movement has always been part of the continued struggle for human rights and dignity for women and children. The challenge is to make the United States' reproductive health efforts part of a coordinated global campaign.

Achievements in reproductive health have always involved both professional and political struggles, and this will undoubtedly continue to be so into the twenty-first century. The need for advocacy backed by credible science and practice will be more important than ever. The current debates about the causes and means to ameliorate infant and maternal mortality and morbidity are likely to be revisited in new variations in the years to come. The challenge remains to ensure the equity of reproductive health-care services and ultimately the equity of reproductive health outcomes in the United States and throughout the world.

Public health has dramatically improved the reproductive health of mothers and infants in the twentieth century; it has transformed and enriched all our lives. Our public health predecessors have left a rich professional and political heritage to help realize even further advancements in the twenty-first century.

References

1. Meckel RA. Save the Babies: American Public Health Reform and the Prevention of Infant Mortality, 1850–1929. Baltimore: Johns Hopkins University Press, 1990,15–58; 40–91; 107–11; 119–23; 134–37; 144–48; 172–75; 185–87; 197–99; 211–12; 220–23; 227; 230.
2. Chadwick E. Address on public health. *Trans Natl Assoc Promotion of Social Science* 1860:580.

3. U.S. Census Bureau. Mortality Statistics, 1908, 9th Annual Report. Washington, DC: Government Printing Office, 1909, 242–81.
4. Loudon I. Death in Childbirth: An International Study of Maternal Care and Maternal Mortality, 1800–1950. New York: Oxford University Press, 1992.
5. Barton WH. The work of infant milk stations in relation to infant mortality. *Trans Am Assoc Study and Prevention of Infant Mortality* 1911:2:299–300.
6. Newsholme A. Domestic infection in relation to epidemic diarrhea. *J Hyg* 1906:6:139–48.
7. Newman G. Infant Mortality: A Social Problem. London: Methuen, 1906, 257.
8. Peters OH. Observations upon the natural history of epidemic diarrhea. *J Hyg* 1910: 10:609–11.
9. Davis WH. Prevention of infant mortality by breastfeeding. *Boston Med Surg J* 1912: 166:242–44.
10. Lesser AJ. The origin and development of maternal and child health programs in the United States. *Am J Public Health* 1985:75:590–98.
11. Hendersen CR. Address of the President for 1911. *Trans Am Assoc Study and Prevention of Infant Mortality* 1910:1:17–18.
12. U.S. Census Bureau. Mortality Statistics 1915, 16th Annual Report. Washington, DC: Government Printing Office, 1917, 57.
13. Woodbury RM. Infant Mortality and Its Causes. Baltimore: William and Wilkins, 1926, 23–24, 131.
14. U.S. Children's Bureau. Public Law 62–116. Washington, DC: Department of Labor, 1913.
15. Thompson JE, Walsh LV, Merkatz IR. The history of prenatal care: cultural, social and medical contexts. In: Merkatz IR, Thompson JE, eds. New Perspective on Prenatal Care. New York: Elsevier, 1990, 9–30.
16. Williams JW. Obstetrics: A Textbook for the Use of Students and Practitioners, 3rd ed. New York: Appleton, 1912, 207.
17. Van Ingen. Recent progress in infant welfare work. *Amer J Dis Child* 1914:9:481.
18. Williams JW. The limitations and possibility of prenatal care. *Trans Am Assoc Study and Prevention of Infant Mortality* 1914:5:32–48.
19. DeLee JB. Progress towards ideal obstetrics. *Amer J Obstet Dis Women Child* 1916: 73:407–15.
20. Williams JW. The limitations and possibilities of prenatal care. *JAMA* 1915:44:95–101.
21. Baker, SJ. Schools for midwives. *Trans Am Assoc Study and Prevention of Infant Mortality* 1912:3:232–42.
22. Meigs GL. Maternal mortality from all conditions connected with childbirth in the United States and certain other countries. Children's Bureau publication no. 19. Washington, DC: Government Printing Office, 1917.
23. National Center for Health Statistics. Mortality Statistics, Volume II, Part A, Section 1, Table 1–17 (maternal morbidity), 69; Section 2, Table 2-2 (infant mortality), 3–4. Washington, DC: Government Printing Office, 1993, 3–4.
24. Margolis LH, Cole GP, Kotch JB. Historical foundations of maternal and child health. In: Kotch JR, ed. Maternal and Child Health Programs, Problems and Policy in Public Health. Gaithersburg, MD: Aspen, 1997, 25–26; 35–37.
25. Schmidt W. The development of health services for mothers and children in the United States. *Am J Public Health* 1973:63:419–27.
26. Hughes JG. American Academy of Pediatrics: The First Fifty Years. Elk Grove Village, IL: American Academy of Pediatrics, 1980.
27. Children's Bureau. Standards of Prenatal Care: An Outline for the Use of Physicians. Washington, DC: Government Printing Office, 1925.

28. Hutchins V. Maternal and Child Health Bureau: roots. *Pediatrics* 1994:94:695–99.
29. Tandy E. Infant and maternal mortality among Negroes. Children's Bureau publication no. 243. Washington, DC: Government Printing Office, 1937.
30. Wertz RW, Wertz DC. Lying In: A History of Childbirth in America. New Haven, CT: Yale University Press, 1989.
31. New York Academy of Medicine. Maternal Mortality in New York City. New York: Commonwealth Fund, 1933.
32. Shapiro S, Schleisinger ER, Nesbitt RE. Infant, Perinatal, Maternal and Childhood Mortality in the United States. Cambridge, MA: Harvard University Press, 1968, 115; 145; 146; 225–26; 248; 268.
33. Centers for Disease Control and Prevention. Achievements in public health, 1900–1999: Healthier mothers and babies. *MMWR* 1999:48: 849–58.
34. Sinai N, Anderson OW. EMIC (Emergency Maternity and Infant Care): A Study of Administrative Experience. Bureau of Public Health Economics, Research Series No. 3. Ann Arbor, MI: University of Michigan, 1948. Reprinted New York: Arno, 1974.
35. Klerman LV. Philosophy and History of Maternal and Child Health. Maternal and Child Health Leadership Skills Training Institute, Waltham, MA, 2001.
36. Buehler JW, Kleinman JC, Hogue CJR, et al. Birthweight specific infant mortality, United States, 1960 and 1980. *Public Health Rep* 1987:102:151–61.
37. National Center for Health Statistics. Vital Statistics of the United States 1985, vol. I: natality, table 1–42 (low birthweight), 68; table 1–44 (prenatal care), 70–71. DHHS publication no. (PHS) 88–1113. Public Health Service. Washington, DC: Government Printing Office, 1988.
38. Steiner GY. The Children's Cause. Washington DC: Brookings Institute, 1976, 34–36; 212–14.
39. Sokol R, Woolf R, Rosen M, Weingarden K. Risk, antepartum care and outcome: impact of a maternity and infant care project. *Obstet Gynecol* 1980:56:150–56.
40. Richmond JB, Kotelchuck M. Coordination and development of strategies and policy for public health promotion in the U.S. In: Holland WW, Detels R, Knox G, eds. Oxford Textbook of Public Health, 2nd ed. London: Oxford University Press, 1991, 441–54.
41. Richmond JB, Kotelchuck M. The effect of the political process on the delivery of health services. In: McGuire C, Foley R, Gorr D, Richards R, eds. Handbook of Health Professions Education. San Francisco: Josey-Bass, 1983, 386–404.
42. Schmidt WH, Wallace HM. The development of health services for mothers and children in the U.S. In: Wallace HM, Ryan GM, Oglesby AC, eds. Maternal and Child Health Practices, 3rd ed. Oakland, CA: Third Party Publishing, 1988, 3–38.
43. McCormick MC, Richardson DK. Access to neonatal intensive care. *Future of Children* 1995:5:162–75; 164–167; 169–170.
44. The Boston Women's Health Book Collection. Our Body, Ourselves. Boston: New England Free Press, 1980.
45. Klaus MH, Kennell JH. Parent-Infant Bonding. St. Louis: CV Mosby, 1982.
46. Berkenfield JC, Schwartz JB. Nutrition intervention in the community—the WIC program. *N Engl J Med* 1980:302:579–81.
47. Edozien JC, Switzer BR, Bryan RB. Medical evaluation of the Special Supplemental Food Program for Women, Infants and Children. *Am J Clin Nutr* 1979:32:677–82.
48. Kotelchuck M, Schwartz JB, Anderka MT, Finison KS. WIC participation and pregnancy outcomes: Massachusetts statewide evaluation study. *Am J Public Health* 1984:74:1145–49.
49. Dryfoos JG. Family planning clinics—a story of growth and conflict. *Fam Plann Arch* 1988:20:282–87.

50. Butterfield LJ. Organization of regional perinatal programs. *Semin Perintatol* 1977:1: 217–33.
51. Committee on Perinatal Health. Toward Improving the Outcome of Pregnancy: Recommendations for the Regional Development of Maternal and Perinatal Services. White Plains, NY: March of Dimes National Foundation, 1976.
52. McCormick MC, Shapiro S, Starfield BH. The regionalization of perinatal services: summary of the evaluation of a national demonstration program. *JAMA* 1985:253:799–804.
53. Horbar JD, Lucey JF. Evaluation of neonatal intensive care technologies. *Future of Children* 1995:5:139–61.
54. Institute of Medicine. Low Birthweight. Washington, DC: National Academy Press, 1985, 143; 212–37.
55. Public Health Services. Better health for our children: a national strategy. DHHS publication no. 79-55071. Washington, DC: Government Printing Office, 1981.
56. Public Health Services. Healthy People: the Surgeon's General report on health promotion and disease prevention. DHEW (PHS) publication no. 79-55071. Washington, DC: Government Printing Office, 1979.
57. Sanders A. The Widening Gap: The Incidence of Infant Mortality and Low Birth Weight in the United States, 1978–82. Washington, DC: Food Research and Action Center, 1984.
58. Gortmaker SL. The effects of prenatal care upon the health of the newborn. *Am J Public Health* 1979:69:653–60.
59. Gold RB, Kenny AM, Singh S. Blessed Events and the Bottom Line: Financing Maternity Care in the U.S. New York: Alan Guttmacher Institute, 1987.
60. Korenbrot CC. Risk reduction in pregnancies of low-income women: comprehensive prenatal care through the OB Access Project. *Mobius* 1984:4:34–43.
61. Olds DL, Henderson CR, Tatelbaum R, et al. Improving the delivery of prenatal care and outcomes of pregnancy: a randomized trial of nurse home visitation. *Pediatrics* 1986:77:16–28.
62. Brown SS. Prenatal Care: Reaching Mothers, Reaching Babies. Washington, DC: National Academy Press, 1988.
63. Wise PH, Kotelchuck M, Wilson M, Mills M. Racial and socioeconomic disparities in childhood mortality in Boston. *N Engl J Med* 1985: 313:360–66.
64. Miller CA. Maternal and Infant Survival: Ten European Countries. Washington, DC: National Center for Clinical Infant Program, 1987.
65. Kotelchuck M. Healthy Futures/Healthy Generations evaluation project dissemination conference: final report. University of North Carolina at Chapel Hill, NC, 1995.
66. Buescher PA, Roth MS, Williams D, Goforth CM. An evaluation of the impact of maternity care coordination on Medicaid birth outcomes in North Carolina. *Am J Public Health* 1991:81:625–29.
67. Alexander GR, Kotelchuck M. Assessing the role and effectiveness of prenatal care: history, challenges, and directions for future research. *Public Health Rep* 2001:16:306–16.
68. Chiles L. Death Before Life: The Tragedy of Infant Mortality. Washington DC: National Commission to Prevent Infant Mortality, 1988.
69. Public Health Service Caring for our Future: The Content of Prenatal Care. Washington, DC: Public Health Service, 1989.
70. Wise PH, Wulff LM. A Manual for Fetal and Infant Mortality Review. Washington DC: American College of Obstetricians and Gynecologists, 1991.
71. Henchy J, Weill G, Parker L. WIC in the States: Twenty-five years of Building a Healthier America. Washington, DC: Food Research and Action Center, 1999.
72. Rosenberg KD, Desai RA, Na Y, Kan J, Schwartz L. The effect of surfactant on birthweight-specific neonatal mortality rate, New York City. *Ann Epidemiol* 2001:11: 337–41.

73. Miniño TJ, Arias E, Kochanek MD, Murphy SL, Smith BL. Deaths: final data for 2000. National Center for Health Statistics, Vital Statistics Report 2002:50:100–1 (infant mortality);106 (maternal mortality).
74. MacDorman MF, Menaker F. Infant mortality statistics from the 1999 period linked birth/infant death data set. National Center for Health Statistics, Vital Statistics Report 2002:50:20.
75. Martin JA, Hamilton BE, Ventura SJ, Menacker F, Park MM. Births: final data for 2000. National Center for Healthy Statistics, Vital Statistics Report 2002:50:79 (low birthweight/prematurity); 72 (cesarean deliveries); 12–13 (prenatal care).
76. Russell RB, Petrini JR, Damus K, Mattison DR, Schwarz RH. The changing epidemiology of multiple births in the United States. *Obstet Gynecol* 2003:101:129–35.
77. Callaghan WM, Berg CJ. Maternal mortality surveillance in the United States: moving into the 21st Century. *J Am Med Wom Assoc* 2002:57:1–5.
78. Strobino D, O'Campo B, Schoendorf KC, et al. A strategic framework for infant mortality reduction: implications for Healthy Start. *Milbank* 1995:73:507–33.
79. Devancy B, Howell E, McCormick M, Moreno L. Reducing infant mortality: lessons learned from Healthy Start: final report. Health Services and Resources Administration, USDHHS, July 2000, MPR reference #8166-113.
80. Hogan VK, Ferre CD. The social context of pregnancy for African-American women: implications for the study and prevention of adverse perinatal outcomes. *Matern Child Health J* 2001:5:67–69.
81. March of Dimes. Towards Improving the Outcome of Pregnancy. White Plains, Y: March of Dimes Birth Defects Foundation, 1993.
82. Korenbrot CC, Dudley RA, Greene JD. Change in births to foreign-born women after welfare and immigration policy reforms in California. *Matern Child Health J* 2000: 4:241–50.
83. Ellwood MR, Ku L. Welfare and immigration reform: unintended side effects for Medicaid. *Health Aff* 1998:17:137–51.
84. Goldenberg RL, Iams JD, Mercer BM, Meis PH, et al. Preterm prediction study: the value of new versus standard risk factors in predicting early and all spontaneous preterm births. *Am J Public Health* 1998:88:233–38.
85. Goldenberg RL, Hauth JC, Andres WW. Mechanisms of disease: intrauterine infections and preterm delivery. *N Engl J Med* 2000:342:1500–1507.
86. Sperling RS, Shapiro DE, Coombs RW, et al. Maternal viral load, Zidovudine treatment, and the risk of transmission of human immunodeficiency virus Type I from mother to infant. *N Engl J Med* 1996:335:1621–28.
87. Fiscella K. Does prenatal care improve birth outcomes? A critical review. *Obstet Gynecol* 1995:85:468–79.
88. Goldenberg RL, Rouse DJ. Prevention of premature birth. *New Engl J Med* 1998:339: 313–20.
89. Hughes D, Simpson S. The role of social change in preventing low birth weight. *Future of Children* 1995: 5:87–102.
90. Scribner R. Paradox as paradigm: the health outcomes of Mexican Americans. *Am J Public Health* 1996:86:303–5.
91. Cefalo RC, Moss MK. Preconceptional Health Care: A Practical Guide. St. Louis, MO: Mosby, 1995.
92. Lu MC, Halfon N. Racial and ethnic disparities in birth outcomes: a life course perspective. *Matern Child Health J* 2003:7:13–31.
93. Wilcox LS. Pregnancy and women's lives in the 21st century: the United States Safe Motherhood movement. *Matern Child Health J* 2002:6:215–20

94. Handler A, Gellers S, Kennelly J. Effective MCH epidemiology in state health agencies: lessons from an evaluation of the Maternal and Child Health Epidemiology (MCHEP) program. *Matern Child Health J* 1999:3:217–24.

95. Church-Balin C, Damus K. Preventing prematurity: AWHONN, March of Dimes partner for national campaign. *AWHONN Lifelines* 2003:7:97–101.

96. U.S. Department of Health and Human Services. Healthy People 2010, 2nd ed., 2 vols. Washington, DC: Government Printing Office, November 2000.

97. Henshaw SK. Unintended pregnancy in the United States. *Fam Plann Perspect* 1998: 30:24–29.

Suggested Reading

Meckel RA. Save the Babies: American Public Health Reform and the Prevention of Infant Mortality, 1850–1929. Baltimore, MD: Johns Hopkins University Press, 1990.

Thompson JE, Walsh LV, Merkatz IR. The history of prenatal care: cultural, social and medical contexts. In: Merkatz IR, Thompson JE, eds. New Perspective on Prenatal Care. New York: Elsevier Press, 1990, 9–30.

7

Saving Babies and Mothers: Pioneering Efforts to Decrease Infant and Maternal Mortality

JACQUELINE H. WOLF

When the governor of New York observed that the cholera epidemics striking the United States in 1832, 1833, and 1834 were the work of "an infinitely wise and just God" who "employ[ed] pestilence as one means of scourging the human race for their sins," he was expressing a common view. Most antebellum Americans deemed epidemic disease and premature death the unavoidable fate of the sinful, the ignorant, the poverty-stricken, the immigrant, and the weak.[1] This pervasive attitude reinforced fatalism toward "innocent" death as well. Although Americans considered the high mortality rates of babies and birthing women tragic and undeserved, their deaths seemed as unavoidable as "deserved" death.

This was evident in oft-voiced sentiments of the era. Because infant deaths occurred primarily during the summer when food spoiled quickly, Chicago health officials sheepishly admitted in 1910 that they had previously dismissed those deaths as inescapable. "We calmly accepted the annual harvest of death as if it were as inevitable as the weather; as if indeed a part of the weather. 'Hot weather, babies die,' was our unconscious thought."[2] The attitude toward maternal death and debility was equally defeatist. In 1929, when 15,000 American women died in childbirth, reformers complained that women jeopardizing "life—or at least . . . health—when . . . giv[ing] birth to a child has long been accepted as one of the inexorable laws of nature."[3]

Acceptance of the germ theory of disease eradicated this resignation and preventing all premature death became the overriding goal of public health proponents around the country. Armed with an understanding of infectious disease and its spread, Progressive Era (1890s–1920) reformers prevailed upon municipalities to build and maintain sewage systems, collect garbage, and purify water and food. Coupled with these monumental efforts were educational campaigns to convince the

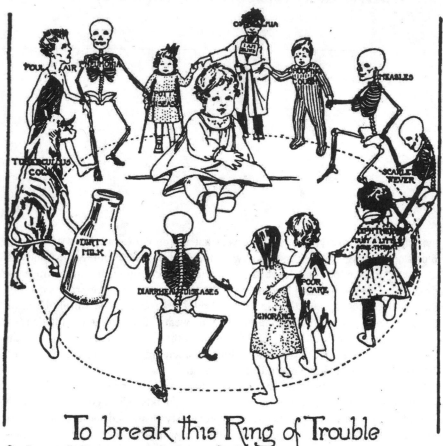

Figure 7.1. The Chicago Department of Health hung this poster in Chicago's neighborhoods as part of the nationwide effort to teach mothers that most infant and child deaths were preventable. Note the three symbols in the lower left portion of the "ring of trouble" representing adulterated cows' milk: the skeleton labeled "diarrheal diseases," the dancing milk bottle labeled "dirty milk," and the emaciated cow labeled "tuberculous cow."

public to change their personal behavior to prevent the spread of disease. Spitting; purchasing, storing, and preparing food; house cleaning; bathing; isolating the sick; and immunizing children each became the subject of public health posters and newspaper and magazine articles (Fig. 7.1). Americans thus came to view epidemic disease as the predictable consequence of unhealthy (but correctable) personal habits, inexcusably callous government, and inadequate public health infrastructure, as opposed to retribution and fate.[4]

This new view of illness and death led not only to public rejection of the state's laissez-faire attitude toward setting and maintaining minimal living standards, it made all premature deaths inexcusable and the deaths of mothers and babies easily the most deplorable. Public health efforts subsequently highlighted the needs of these two vulnerable populations. Newsletters disseminated by public health departments and articles in magazines and newspapers focused on the importance of meticulous infant care, particularly infant feeding, and "scientific" birth practices.

This chapter examines two innovative and influential Progressive Era efforts in Chicago: one to lower infant mortality, the other to lower maternal mortality. Crusades to lower infant mortality focused on regulating the manufacture, shipping, and sale of cows' milk and promoting breastfeeding. Chicago was also the city where physician Joseph DeLee, now dubbed the father of modern obstetrics, standardized obstetric practice as part of his crusade to lower maternal mortality. It is not surprising that these two nationally influential efforts took place in Chicago. The city was a hotbed of Progressive Era activity, home to an array of influential social reformers including Jane Addams, Florence Kelley, Julia Lathrop, Grace Abbott, Sophonisba Breckinridge, and Alice Hamilton—each eventually responsible in innumerable and unique ways for improving the lot of mothers and children around the country.[5]

"Save the Babies"

Initially, campaigns to prevent infant death proliferated in a way that efforts to halt maternal death did not because, by the end of the nineteenth century, the infant death rate had a new and vital meaning. Community leaders now used it to assess societal well-being. As municipalities spent fortunes to build sewer and water filtration systems to end the spread of epidemic disease, governments searched for a yardstick to measure the success of these costly projects. At first municipalities used the overall death rate, but that gauge proved meaningless as it was easily affected by a host of variables unaffected by public works projects, such as old age. Reformers subsequently declared infants the segment of the population most sensitive to environmental threats. Babies thus became canaries-in-the-coalmine for the entire populace.[6] This proved a remarkable blessing for infants because, by the end of the nineteenth century, this use of the infant death rate aroused philanthropic and governmental interest in preventing high infant morbidity and mortality. Spurred by this new incentive, public health officials began paying scrupulous attention to vital statistics and, most significantly for infants, began to correlate cause of death with age at death.

This led to undisputed proof, long known anecdotally to physicians, that diarrhea was the primary cause of infant death in the United States. Infant mortality statistics in Chicago were typical. In 1897, when an estimated 38,764 babies were born in that city, 18% of them died before their first birthday and almost 54% of the dead died of diarrhea.[7] Consequently, early infant welfare efforts highlighted the importance of improving infants' food, the only conceivable source of their gastrointestinal distress. Milk, both bovine and human but especially bovine, became the focus of the most lengthy and visible crusades in early twentieth-century public health reform. "Save the babies" became the justification for a 35-year battle between reformers and the dairy industry as reformers angrily demanded, in a seemingly endless stream of newspaper headlines, pure cows' milk for the nation's infants.

"Give the Bottle-Fed Baby a Chance for Its Life"

The relentless attention paid to cows' milk was justified. The late-nineteenth-century urban milk supply killed tens of thousands of infants each year. Unpasteurized and unrefrigerated as it journeyed from rural dairy farmer to urban consumer for up to 72 hours, cows' milk was commonly spoiled and bacteria-laden. Public health officials dramatically charged that in most U.S. cities, milk contained more bacteria than raw sewage.[8] For years, the Chicago Department of Health kept fanatic track of bacteria in random samples of cows' milk and categorized milk as "clean," "not very clean," and "dirty." The Health Department conspicuously and regularly publicized these findings, warning consumers that even "clean" milk posed a danger to infants and children as "the number of bacteria at the start gives very little indication of the number at the end of twenty-four hours."[9] Officials warned, "Much of the city's milk-supply is better adapted to fertilizing purposes than to feeding purposes. Yet that's the kind of milk so many poor babies get."[10]

Even when infants were able to avoid bacteria-laden milk, milk still proved dangerous. Since milk was a relatively expensive commodity, farmers, shippers, merchants, and consumers often diluted it. One Chicago newspaper decried the babies "gone to a premature grave because . . . [their] cry for milk was unwittingly answered by a supply of a weak . . . mixture of milk and water."[11] The *Chicago Tribune* accused milk dealers of peddling "so-called milk, which is three-fourths water if not something worse" and described the urban milk supply as "worse than fraud, it is murder. The infant mortality in Chicago is very large. How much of it is due to the poisonous germs swallowed in this alleged milk it is hard to determine, but it must play no small part in this colossal crime of infanticide."[12]

Water, however, was probably the least threatening substance added to milk. Since milk was shipped and stored in 8-gallon uncovered vats, wary customers found it easy to sample milk before purchase by plunging a finger into the vat for tasting. Consumers also routinely sampled milk using the dippers intended for ladling milk into a container. Milkmen who delivered their product directly to homes saved money by retrieving an empty, used bottle from one house, ladling milk into it, and delivering it to the next customer on their route. In this way, tuberculosis, diphtheria, typhoid fever, scarlet fever, infant diarrhea, and a host of other illnesses became milk-borne diseases.[13–15]

The open-vat storage system contributed to infants' ill health in additional ways. Not only did dust, dirt, and disease inadvertently enter the milk supply, uncovered vats facilitated the deliberate adulteration of milk. In order to whiten dirty milk, for example, dairy farmers, shippers, and milk dealers customarily added handfuls of chalk dust to milk vats. To make skimmed milk look whole, milk dealers routinely added coloring composed of patent butter, burnt sugar, and aniline dye. Farmers, shippers, and dealers often added a preservative—formaldehyde, salicylic acid, borax, boracic acid, or carbonate of soda—to delay milk spoilage. Consumers likewise contributed to infants' woes. To save money they often mixed two parts "milk expander" (readily available in stores and composed of soda, ammonia, salt, and water) with one part milk. The resulting concoction, noted one sarcastic physician, was "a nice mixture to give a weak infant!"[16-20]

Urban dairy farmers (Chicago's famed Mrs. O'Leary was one of thousands who kept several cows in barns behind their homes) found their own unique ways to save money. To avoid buying the requisite $20-a-ton grain for cow feed, they often purchased a wretched $4-a-ton substitute: the fermented grain (sold at nearby Chicago and Milwaukee breweries) that was a by-product of whiskey manufacture. Feeding distillery waste to cows also guaranteed farmers another bonus: it dramatically increased milk production by overstimulating cows' mammary glands. One angry physician, observing that the resulting inexpensive "swill milk" (as it was known) was a popular baby food, demanded to know: "Would any of us tolerate a sot as a wet nurse for our offspring?"[21-23]

Even contamination of "pure country milk" was largely unavoidable as hygienic dairy practices were virtually nonexistent. Farmers seldom, if ever, washed dairy cattle and the dirt and dung that covered the bodies of these animals invariably fell into the milk pail. One physician complained that the cows he observed at one dairy farm "were so plastered with manure that I could hardly tell their color."[24] Dairy workers seldom washed their hands or changed their clothes before milking, even after spending hours cleaning muck out of the hog pen, the chicken coop, or the horse stable. The interior of dairy barns, with their dirt floors, wooden walls, and improper drainage, were equally filthy.[25]

Infant death was thus a logical consequence of babies' consumption of cows' milk, and by the 1890s, municipal governments, public health departments, physicians, settlement house workers, philanthropists, and newspaper editors decried that fact and demanded reform. In Chicago, the resulting milk crusades lasted more than 30 years. Although Chicago's newspapers first called for pure milk in 1892, dairies in the Chicago milk shed—the vast area spread over seven states that supplied Chicago with milk—did not have to seal milk vats until 1904,[26] did not have to provide milk in bottles until 1912,[27] did not have to pasteurize milk until 1916,[28] did not have to keep milk cold during shipping until 1920,[29] and did not have to test cows for bovine tuberculosis until 1926.[30]

The fight to seal vats was customarily the first of many battles in local milk wars because open vats made adulteration and the spread of bacteria so easy. Like all milk reform efforts, however, the demand proved controversial. Dairies objected not only to the cost of sealing vats, they also argued that it would be "the worst possible contrivance" to ensure milk's purity because "milk, in large cans, more or less exposed to the air . . . improves it."[22]

Pasteurization proved even more contentious than sealing. The mere possibility of pasteurization alarmed members of every conceivable interest group: dairy farmers, dairies, milk dealers, merchants, the medical community, and consumers. The issue was so controversial that the first dairy in New York to pasteurize milk did so secretly, fearing it would hurt business.[31] Objections to the process were many and varied. Dairies insisted that the cost of pasteurization was prohibitive. Physicians argued that nature had not designed milk to be pasteurized and doing so would destroy its nutritive qualities. Public health officials charged that pasteurization would exacerbate the dangerous habits of dairy farmers by masking them. Excuses for avoiding pasteurization abounded: it made milk difficult to digest; prompted scurvy; caused rickets; encouraged the growth of super-toxic bacteria; destroyed flavor.[32–36]

Given the apprehension, the initial emphasis of the clean milk campaigns was on sanitary practice rather than pasteurization. It seemed logical to teach farmers and dairies about hygiene and to enforce basic hygienic standards rather than kill the germs in presumably contaminated milk.[37] One by-product of this sentiment was certified milk—milk produced under the stringent rules and vigilant eyes of a milk commission, usually a group of local doctors working for a municipality or medical charity. Invented in 1892 by Henry L. Coit, a New Jersey physician, certified milk was soon available in every large American city.[38,39] His sick infant son precipitated Coit's design of the certification system. In 1887, "maternal failure" (presumably his wife's inability to breastfeed) prompted Coit's futile search for clean cows' milk for his baby. Twenty years later he told those gathered at the first meeting of the American Association of Medical Milk Commissions, "The vicissitudes through which I passed on the question of pure materials with which to nourish this child, will never be told."[38] His son's death prompted him to form the Essex County Medical Milk Commission to oversee the production of milk in his New Jersey county. Coit had the highest hopes for this "certified milk" and optimistically contended that it would level the playing field for all infants. "The poorest baby in Coomes Alley," he predicted, "will now fare equally well with Thomas Edison's baby in Lewellen Park."[39]

For decades after its introduction, reformers touted certified milk (also called inspected milk in some locales) as the only clean and unadulterated milk to be found in most cities. By the early twentieth century, certified milk stations were familiar fixtures in congested urban neighborhoods, attracting mothers and children in droves. New York businessman Nathan Straus popularized these stations throughout the United States. After opening the first pasteurized milk station in New York City in 1893, he aided medical charities in other cities (including Chicago) in their quest to produce clean milk by providing personnel and equipment for the asking.[40] The pure milk movement—omnipresent for decades in the lives of dairy farmers, dairy workers, shippers, milk dealers, and merchants—was highly visible to the public as well. Because the horrifying specter of shriveled, dying babies was the impetus for milk reform, those bent on improving the urban milk supply did not stop at lobbying the dairy industry. They also publicized the dangers of milk to the public, targeting mothers in particular for their messages. Women learned how to make cows' milk safer for their infants from a barrage of public health messages delivered via posters, pamphlets, and newspaper and magazine articles. Public health nurses made unannounced home visits to discuss infant feeding with the mothers of newborns. Physicians proffered feeding guidance at infant welfare stations scattered throughout congested urban neighborhoods. Typical advice emanated from one Chicago placard headlined "Give the Bottle-Fed Baby a Chance for Its Life!" The sign admonished, "Mothers, Protect Your Babies!" and advised women to buy only fresh milk in bottles, to keep those bottles sealed, to home-pasteurize all milk before serving it to children, and to always keep milk on ice.[41] A pithy slogan summed up the detailed recommendations: "Safe Milk Saves Sickness" (Fig. 7.2). Chicago's Health Department printed these and similar infant welfare placards in eight different languages and posted them on buildings and fences in the city's most vulnerable neighborhoods.[42,43]

During the long years between the first newspaper articles in 1892 decrying spoiled and adulterated milk and the passage of a complete set of state and municipal laws governing milk production 34 years later, the responsibility for preventing infant death due to tainted cows' milk was largely a maternal one. "If the producer and dealer will do their duty," explained one Chicago Health Department newsletter in 1909, "there will be left daily at the consumer's door a bottle of clean, cold, unadulterated milk. It will then be up to the housewife to see that the milk is kept clean and wholesome."[44] Accordingly, articles in women's and infant-care magazines instructed mothers in the meticulous arts of recognizing,[45] pasteurizing,[46–48] refrigerating,[49] and even "humanizing" clean cows' milk.[50–52] The humanization of cows' milk was a laborious process that made the percentages of fat, protein, and sugar in cows' milk akin to those in human milk. As the public came to accept the germ theory of disease, it also became increasingly easy to persuade mothers to take the trouble to pasteurize the milk they purchased (Fig. 7.3). The Chicago Health Department aided this effort by warning ominously, "If you drink . . . milk raw, you take into your body millions of live, disease-producing germs. The only way that you can make . . . milk reasonably safe is to pasteurize it before using."[53,54] Health Departments around the country kept milk and the dangers it posed to infants in the public eye by continuing to churn out posters bearing catchy slogans. One 1914 placard promoting Chicago's efforts to set standards for the dairy industry read, "Bye Baby Bunting Healthman's gone a hunting—To get the dirty milkman's skin and save the baby's life for him."[55]

"Let Us Have More Mother-Fed Babies"

Despite what appeared to be the single-minded rhetoric of the campaigns for pure cows' milk, the medical community was cognizant of their dual responsibility throughout these years. Physicians who watched helplessly as artificially fed infants sickened and died recognized that a dearth of human milk was behind the use of cows' milk as an infant food. Since both babies' lack of access to human milk *and* the dreadful state of the bovine milk supply worked in tandem to generate high infant morbidity and mortality, pediatricians concluded early in the crisis that boosting breastfeeding rates was as vital to infant health as improving the artificial food consumed by babies.

The custom of feeding cows' milk via rags, bottles, cans, and jars to babies rather than putting them to the breast became increasingly common as the last quarter of the nineteenth century progressed. In 1889, one New England physician complained to colleagues in the *New England Medical Monthly* and to mothers in an identical article in *Babyhood* magazine that "the great majority of mothers" were failing to

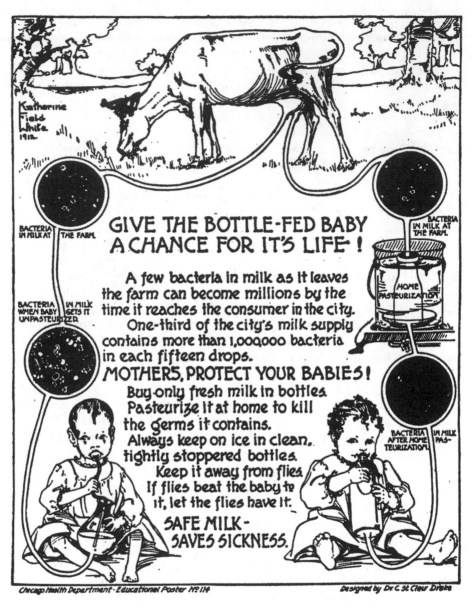

Figure 7.2. This placard, designed by the Chicago Department of Health, instructed the mothers of bottle-fed babies how to select and care for cows' milk in an effort to lower the infant death rate from diarrhea. (*Bulletin. Chicago School of Sanitary Instruction,* 31 August 1912.)

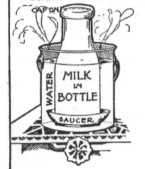

MAKE BABY'S MILK SAFE
PASTEURIZE IT AT HOME
THIS KILLS DISEASE-PRODUCING GERMS in MILK

Directions for Pasteurizing

Use a pail a little shorter than the milk bottle.
Place saucer in bottom of pail and stand the bottle of milk on this saucer. Leave cap on bottle.
Pour hot water into pail until water level is about four inches below top of bottle.
Place on stove and bring water to boiling point.
When water begins to boil immediately remove bottle of milk from pail.
Cool the milk in bottle as rapidly as you can and place it in ice-box as soon as possible.

MILK MUST BE KEPT COLD & TIGHTLY COVERED IN CLEAN BOTTLES TO PREVENT DEVELOPMENT of GERMS IN IT.

Figure 7.3. In Chicago, dairies did not have to pasteurize milk by law until 1916. This 1913 poster instructs mothers how to pasteurize milk at home. (*Bulletin. Chicago School of Sanitary Instruction,* 31 May 1913, 88.)

"fully nurse" their offspring. His emphasis was on "fully."[56] Although the vast majority of mothers did initiate breastfeeding, even breastfed babies received a substantial amount of cows' milk in addition to human milk during their early weeks of life and, increasingly, women weaned babies from the breast by their third month. In 1912, disconcerted physicians complained bitterly that the breastfeeding duration rate had declined steadily since the mid-nineteenth century "and now it is largely a question as to whether the mother will nurse her baby at all."[57] A 1912 survey in Chicago of 55% of the mothers who had given birth that year corroborated the allegation. Sixty-one percent of those women fed their infants at least some cows' milk within weeks of giving birth.[58]

This custom of artificial feeding crossed class lines as upper-, middle-, and working-class women alike—prompted by different social, economic, and cultural pressures—all participated in the practice.[7] Upper-class women relied heavily on servants for infant care and that dependence often precluded breastfeeding. As one wealthy father explained in 1893, servants had cared for all four of his children so his wife "knew nothing about feeding them."[59] New expectations for marriage based on companionship rather than economics shaped middle-class women's infant feeding practices as the bond with their husbands became more important than their relationship with their children.[60] This was reflected in the letter one woman sent to an infant care magazine in 1886 on behalf of her pregnant daughter: "[my daughter] wants to be more of a companion for her husband than she could be if she should nurse Baby; and . . . we wonder if it would not be best for all that the little one be fed [artificially]."[61] Working-class mothers found their infant feeding practices dictated by economics. Women who worked outside the home often had to leave their infants with grade-school daughters and artificial food. The burgeoning number of Little Mothers' Clubs, after-school organizations that trained thousands of young girls to better care for the infant siblings left in their charge, reflected this growing practice. Since these clubs prepared girls not for motherhood, but to care for tiny brothers and sisters, the organizations were particularly adept at drilling girls in the minutiae of artificial feeding.[7,62]

As cows' milk became a staple for all babies (even the breastfed ones as mothers invariably supplemented their breast milk with cows' milk) the medical community launched two campaigns. One, discussed previously, demanded pure cows' milk. The other encouraged all mothers to breastfeed and urged the mothers who did breastfeed to breastfeed longer and to avoid feeding their babies cows' milk while they breastfed. These twin concerns—babies' consumption of too much bad cows' milk and too little good human milk—were exemplified by a poster distributed nationally in 1911. The poster portrayed a long, thin tube attached on one end to a cow's udder and stuck in an emaciated baby's mouth on the other. Between cow and baby, the tube snaked around an unkempt dairy barn, a railroad station, an enclosed railroad car, a horse drawn milk wagon, and a front porch where an uncapped milk bottle surrounded by flies baked in the hot sun. Chicago's version of the poster scolded, "And Yet Some People Wonder Why So Many Babies Die! . . . Let Us Have More Mother-Fed Babies. . . . For Your Baby's Sake—Nurse It!"[63]

The medical community deemed human milk so vital to infants' health that doctors even feared that providing clean cows' milk to babies might be counterproductive since it tended to exacerbate low breastfeeding rates. At a 1910 meeting of the Chicago Milk Commission, a medical charity that provided certified/pasteurized milk at no cost to consumers via dozens of neighborhood milk stations, one doctor complained that the Commission's widely advertised milk made it easy for a mother "to shirk her obligations" and avoid breastfeeding.[64] An exasperated Chicago Medical Society, which managed its own certified milk operation, likewise decried plummeting breastfeeding rates and editorialized in 1909, "We even incline to the opinion that the babies and children would get along very nicely if the entire [cows'] milk supply, whether pasteurized or not, were shut off entirely and permanently."[65]

This debate was not unique to Chicago. New York public health workers grappled with the same observations. In 1911, in response to the accusation that their work harmed babies by discouraging breastfeeding, the four operators of New York's 69 milk stations—Nathan Straus, the New York Milk Committee, the New York City Department of Health, and the Diet Kitchen Association—agreed to require the mothers whose babies received their milk to bring infants in for weekly examinations. If mothers did not produce their infants for these exams, the stations refused to provide them with milk.[66] Yet complaints about the easy provision of cows' milk to mothers did not abate. One angry physician called the American notion of preventive medicine "twisted" because social reformers were devoting their energy to ensuring the ready availability of pure cows' milk for babies while "we have no similarly organized body devoting its attention to the many perplexing problems of the human milk supply."[67]

The sentiment had little effect, however. The only city to dramatically raise breastfeeding rates was Minneapolis, where between 1919 and 1926 the campaign to increase the number of breastfeeding mothers was relentless, going far beyond hanging public health messages on the sides of buildings. Thanks largely to the efforts of one man—Julius Parker Sedgwick, chief of the Department of Pediatrics at the University of Minnesota—workers for the Pediatric Department's Breastfeeding Investigation Bureau followed every woman in Minneapolis for 9 months after the birth of her baby in an effort to keep babies at the breast. Public health nurses visited lactating women ("daily if necessary"), encouraged them frequently via phone calls (if they had telephones), distributed informational brochures on the importance of human milk to human health, and compiled the results of countless infant feeding questionnaires. The labor-intensive effort, a far bigger project than more heavily populated cities like Chicago or New York could muster, paid off. During the first year of the Breastfeeding Bureau's work, infant mortality in Minneapolis declined almost 20%, from 81 deaths per thousand live births in 1918 to 65 in 1919. This decreased mortality was due almost certainly to the work of the bureau because other cities saw similar declines only after they ordered the pasteurization of all cows' milk sold within city limits. As late as 1948 Minneapolis had no such requirement.[68]

Minneapolis's success story appears to have been a lone exception among U.S. cities, however. In other urban areas, infant deaths declined slowly only as each city laboriously cleaned up its cows' milk. In Chicago, infant deaths from diarrhea went from 53.7% of all infant deaths in 1897 to 39.4% in 1912 (after cows' milk was sealed and bottled), to 16.9% in 1924 (after cows' milk was pasteurized), to 1.4% in 1939 (after cows' milk was refrigerated during shipping and tested for bovine tuberculosis). The overall infant mortality rate in Chicago went from 18% in 1897 to 12% in 1912 to 8% in 1924 to 3% 1939.[7]

By the time infant mortality in the United States, and particularly infant death from diarrhea, declined significantly, American mothers had wholly embraced cows' milk as the sanctified product it had become. Given the ubiquitous nature of the milk campaigns, those crusades generated the indelible message that washing cows, scrubbing the walls and floors of dairy barns, and bottling, sealing, refrigerating, and pasteurizing milk nullified the dangers that once seemed inherent in feeding the milk of one species to the offspring of another.

Not until the 1970s, when health reform advocates in the women's movement urged women to learn about and trust their bodies and wrest women's medical care away from "condescending, paternalistic, judgmental and non-informative" physicians,[69] did the United States see an upswing in the number of mothers breastfeeding. Only then did pediatricians, for the first time in almost 50 years, have an opportunity to compare the health of breastfed and bottle-fed babies and to once again link respiratory, ear, and gastrointestinal infections with artificial feeding.[70–79] More recently, researchers have associated some chronic diseases and conditions and higher infant mortality in general to infants' intake of formula and their concomitant inadequate consumption of human milk.[80-96] Thus the purification of cows' milk, while undeniably lowering the infant death rate dramatically, inadvertently contributed to a host of other health problems in subsequent generations by magnifying the importance of cows' milk to health while simultaneously minimizing the importance of human milk.

"Every Case of Labor Should Be Attended By A Good Physician"

Concerted efforts to lower the infant death rate had been ongoing for several decades before reformers focused similar attention on lowering maternal mortality. Spokeswomen for the U.S. Children's Bureau pioneered this latter activity in 1917 when they connected infant and maternal mortality by insisting that infants' welfare depended on their mothers' health. "In the progress of work for the prevention of infant mortality," argued Grace Meigs, director of the Division of Child Hygiene of the Children's Bureau, "it has become ever clearer that all such work is useful only in so far as it helps the mother to care better for her baby. It must be plain, then, to what a degree the sickness and death of the mother lessens the chances of the baby for life and health."[97]

While quality of maternal care is measured today largely in terms of neonatal mortality, health authorities in Grace Meigs's day measured its quality in terms of maternal mortality and, based on that criterion, the U.S. record was abysmal. Among the 20 countries that tracked maternal mortality in the early twentieth century, the United States ranked 19th—ahead of only Chile. The maternal death rate in the United States was twice as high as in Denmark, Italy, Japan, the Netherlands, New Zealand, and Sweden. In 1927, Josephine Baker, chief of the Division of Child Hygiene of the New York Health Department, charged that the United States was "perilously close" to being the least safe country in the world for pregnant women.[98] Indeed, although always much lower than infant mortality, the maternal mortality rate in the United States remained constant, and even increased, long after infant deaths began to decline precipitously. Between 1900 and 1921, deaths from maternity-related causes rose from 13.3 to 16.9 per 100,000 population.[99]

Dorothy Reed Mendenhall, a physician who worked for the U.S. Children's Bureau, blamed antiseptics and anesthesia—"the two things that should make childbirth safer"—for the rise; she charged that the two innovations had made "operative interference [during birth] . . . more possible and more usual."[100] The New York Academy of Medicine agreed. Investigating maternal mortality in New York City, the Academy blamed the rise in maternal death there on the increased use of forceps and the tendency of forceps in unskilled hands to cause postpartum infection. In turn, the Academy study attributed the growing use of forceps to the popularity of obstetric anesthesia and its tendency to diminish "the expulsive powers of the uterine musculature." Investigators concluded, "The mere alleviation or the entire elimination of pain may be achieved at a cost to the mother or infant which should be prohibitive."[101] Despite the studies and concrete allegations, contemporary physicians failed to agree on the cause of increased maternal deaths and so they failed to tackle maternal mortality in a concerted way. Unlike the infant death rate with milk the obvious culprit, individual doctors attributed maternal deaths, not to any carefully culled data, but to their own personal grievances: inadequate prenatal care; "uneducated" midwives; inattention to obstetrics in medical schools; general practitioners ignorant of obstetric technique who nevertheless practiced obstetrics; the low status accorded obstetricians; physicians' "orgy of interference" during birth; and the refusal of hospital administrators to house maternity wards in buildings separate from infectious disease wards.[97,102–8] While vital statistics had pointed unambiguously to infants' food as the primary cause of infant death, triggering unanimity of action among infant welfare reformers, the disparate proposed causes of maternal mortality prompted vitriolic debate among medical professionals rather than solutions.

Despite the bitterness, there were successful, and ultimately influential, efforts to improve the lot of pregnant and laboring women. In 1895, Joseph DeLee, a Chicago obstetrician, opened the Chicago Lying-in Dispensary (also referred to informally as the Maxwell Street Dispensary and in later years as the Chicago Maternity Center) to provide women with prenatal care and physicians to attend their home births, at no charge, and to simultaneously train medical students in the science and art of obstetrics. The Dispensary, which specialized in home births "under adverse conditions with a group of patients physically below par," maintained a maternal mortality rate of .14% of all births even as the United States had a rate more than four times that at .59%.[109]

DeLee, dissatisfied with the obstetric training in medical schools and appalled at women's use of midwives, opened the Chicago Lying-In Dispensary in an immigrant west side neighborhood. There, DeLee and his staff of physicians, nurses, and medical students toiled to standardize aseptic obstetric practice "in the homes of the poor and poorest in Chicago." Their work, an unqualified success from its inception, became the model for similar efforts around the country. In 7000 consecutive cases early in the dispensary's history, only one woman died of postpartum infection. Even European physicians conceded that the Maxwell Street Dispensary sustained "a mortality and morbidity that challenge[d] the work of the best maternities in the world." Sir William J. Sinclair, Professor of Obstetrics and Gynecology at Victorian University in Manchester, England, called DeLee's effort, "the most admirable midwifery work reported in Europe or America in our time."[110]

When DeLee opened the dispensary, the maternal death rate in Chicago was about 57 per 10,000 births.[111,112] Nevertheless, the dispensary elicited no initial enthusiasm among neighborhood women. DeLee tried to attract their attention by posting signs reading Free Prenatal Care and Free Delivery Care in the area surrounding his office, but the immigrant women living in the vicinity of Maxwell Street, accustomed to and comfortable with midwives, ignored the offers. Not easily dissuaded, DeLee knocked on doors to assure pregnant women that their chances for death and debility were markedly less if a physician, rather than a midwife or a neighbor, attended their birth. A handful of women finally accepted his offer for free prenatal care, although even they summoned a midwife after going into labor.[113] Not until DeLee's first delivery more than a month after the dispensary opened did word begin to spread that DeLee could be trusted. Thereafter the dispensary's clientele grew rapidly as former patients, workers at nearby Hull House, and public health nurses from the Chicago Visiting Nurse Association all urged pregnant women to go to the Maxwell Street Dispensary.[111] In the dispensary's third year, physicians provided 5424 prenatal visits, attended the home births of 840 women, and trained 84 medical students in obstetric technique. By 1931, dispensary physicians were attending 2000 home births and training 250 students annually.[114]

In 1895, when DeLee opened the Chicago Lying-in Dispensary, it was the only medical institution in Chicago focusing solely on maternity care. The reason for the paucity of obstetric facilities was obvious—midwife- and general-practitioner-attended home births were the norm. In 1895, when there were 35,000 births in the city, only 800 women gave birth in the hospital.[115] DeLee did not deem this a problem per se; in his entire career (and he worked until his death in 1942) he never considered home birth unsafe or even undesirable. In fact, he vigorously defended home birth, arguing that it was a necessity for most women who could not "go to a maternity" without temporarily dismembering their households at much trouble and expense.[111] Beatrice Tucker, the first woman resident to serve under DeLee, likewise defended home birth, arguing that doctors who attended home births were more highly skilled than other doctors. "When you deliver in homes," she contended, "you develop your ingenuity." She also insisted that the unhygienic surroundings common to the homes of the immigrant women who constituted the vast majority of the dispensary's clientele did not negatively affect birth outcomes. She explained, "Even with the dogs and the cats and the animals swishing about and the flies all around, very rarely were you in trouble with an infection. It just seems as if people in their own homes are probably immune to the kind of bacteria that they're living in, and they don't have pathological bacteria like you have in the hospital, like staphylococcus and strep and this kind of thing."[113]

While DeLee never considered home birth a threat to maternal health, he was gravely concerned about the shortage of medical institutions caring for pregnant and laboring women and the consequent lack of opportunity to formally train physicians in obstetric practice. DeLee thus dreamed of two institutions: a birth dispensary from which to dispatch physicians and nurses to care for women in their homes when they went into labor and a centrally located hospital devoted exclusively to maternity care. He envisioned both institutions addressing his primary concern: training medical students in obstetrics.[115]

DeLee considered physician training the key to lowered maternal mortality. While he deplored the "careless and ignorant midwives" who in 1895 cared for 43% of the women who gave birth in Chicago, he deemed physicians in general practice equally responsible for high maternal morbidity and mortality. Students graduated from medical school, DeLee complained, without ever examining a pregnant woman or attending a birth. Therefore he argued regularly that having a physician at a birth did not necessarily guarantee the presence of a trained specialist.[111]

Thus the Chicago Lying-In Dispensary served two purposes. Its most visible function, at least to the mothers it served directly, was to provide competent physicians to attend home births. Yet the dispensary had a more far-reaching goal as well. Because at least one medical student always accompanied a dispensary physician, the dispensary indirectly served women living well beyond the vicinity of

Maxwell Street.[114,115] As the dispensary board boasted in its first annual report, its free home birthing service provided aid not just to poor, immigrant mothers but also to "the wives of our important citizens [because]. . . . The doctors taught by the dispensary are destined to practice among the affluent as well as the poor and both thus receive the benefits of the institution." The Maxwell Street Dispensary, which relied wholly on donations for its existence, thus quickly became a favorite charity of Chicago's well-to-do, counting among its benefactors members of such prominent Chicago families as the McCormicks, the Loebs, and the Schaffners.[111] Chicagoans were clearly aware that childbirth and its attendant risks threatened all Chicago women.

The dispensary's work was elegant in its simplicity. Early in her pregnancy, a woman desiring services applied for care. Then "from time to time" throughout her pregnancy, she either reported to the dispensary for prenatal care or a physician came to her home. When she went into labor she notified the dispensary, which then dispatched a physician, medical student, and all necessary medical equipment to her home. After giving birth, new mothers and babies continued to receive help. A physician and medical student provided postpartum care daily for 10 days and a visiting nurse arrived each day to change bed linens and bathe the new mother and her baby. The cost to the dispensary for this array of services in 1895 was $6 per case, as opposed to $40–$90 for each hospital birth.[111]

Even as he provided home birth services at no charge to the poor, DeLee fought for a public lying-in hospital for those women whose homes were "entirely too forlorn and unfortunate to be used for confinement" and for particularly complicated cases. He argued that such a hospital would also enhance the training of medical students by enabling them to work under the direct supervision of a hospital medical director and "be drilled in the minutiae of obstetric cleanliness." In 1899, DeLee realized his dream. His charity opened the Chicago Lying-in Hospital in a house containing 15 beds. In 1917, the popular charity abandoned the house and constructed its own hospital building.[114,117] By mid-1919, 24 years after DeLee opened the Maxwell Street Dispensary, physicians working for the Chicago Lying-In Hospital and its associated home birth service had attended a total 33,568 home births and 9301 hospital births and provided obstetric training to 3869 medical students.[118] In subsequent years, dispensary and hospital records reflected the national move of births from the home to the hospital. Between mid-1919 and mid-1930, 40,285 births took place at the Chicago Lying-In Hospital while dispensary physicians attended only 14,591 home births.[119]

DeLee's success was evident not just in Chicago but also nationwide by the 1920s. The need for a rigorously trained doctor at every birth, no matter its location, was now undisputed. As Chicago Health Commissioner Herman Bundesen told the nation's expectant mothers in 1925 via his popular, nationally disseminated infant care booklets, "Every case of labor should be attended by a good physician."[120] This achievement was not unqualified, however. The medical management of obstetrics generated controversy and, by the early 1920s, DeLee was in the eye of that storm.

Despite his ongoing enthusiasm for the aseptic, nonintrusive obstetrics performed so successfully by Maxwell Street Dispensary physicians, DeLee began practicing a host of medical interventions whenever he treated paying patients. This was due in part to the nature of late-nineteenth-century urban society, which was exceedingly class-conscious. Consequently, DeLee's wealthy clients expected special treatment.[121] This type of medical care and its concomitant cost, however, also appear to have been part of DeLee's strategy to make obstetrics a well-respected specialty. After wealthy Chicagoan Ogden McClurg protested DeLee's $1500 fee to attend Mc-Clurg's wife in childbirth in 1922, DeLee implied in a letter to McClurg that twice the charge would not have been unreasonable. He wrote, "This is one of the fundamental reasons for the high mortality in childbirth. The work is hard and burdensome, it restricts one's liberty, robs one of rest at night, requires exceptional skill, and withal, it does not pay. For these reasons there are few obstetric specialists, the bright young physicians seeking more lucrative specialties, and those without the drawbacks mentioned."[122,123]

Even as DeLee and McClurg expressed their mutual annoyance, DeLee's increasingly complex and expensive obstetric treatments were becoming well known to the nation's obstetric community. In an often-quoted article in the premiere issue of the *American Journal of Obstetrics and Gynecology* (*AJOG*) in 1920, DeLee contended that birth is "pathogenic . . . disease producing." He explained dramatically, "So frequent are these bad effects, that I have often wondered whether Nature did not deliberately intend women should be used up in the process of reproduction, in a manner analogous to that of the salmon, which dies after spawning." Among his proposals to subvert the pathology of birth were the administration of morphine (an anesthetic) and scopolamine (an amnesiac) to women during first stage labor, followed by ether during second stage labor to render a woman unconscious so that a doctor could perform an episiotomy and deliver her baby with forceps.[124]

J. Whitridge Williams, a Baltimore obstetrician who taught at Johns Hopkins University and who long was DeLee's philosophical opponent, denounced DeLee's recommendations. "I believe," he told a group of colleagues who had just heard DeLee read the paper that eventually appeared in *AJOG*, "that if his practice were to become general and widely adopted, women would be worse off eventually than had their labors been conducted by midwives. . . . If I have understood Dr. DeLee correctly, it seems to me that he interferes 19 times too often out of 20." Another physician concurred and charged that DeLee's procedures were nothing more than "a hospital 'stunt.' "[125]

Despite colleagues' reservations, DeLee persevered and ultimately triumphed. "The child-bearing woman deserves and must have each and every thing that modern advances in every field of human endeavor can possibly bring her," he wrote in 1930 in *The Chicago Lying-In Hospital and Dispensary Twentieth Annual Report*.[126] Thus, even as DeLee and his dispensary physicians continued to practice much as they had in 1895 while attending home births, at the Chicago Lying-in Hospital these same physicians performed episiotomies on virtually all first-time mothers and routinely injected women with pituitrin to hasten placental delivery. Other hospitals adopted similar techniques and more.[127]

Shortly before his death in 1942, DeLee regretted the dichotomy in obstetric practice that he had fostered and seemed to revert to his philosophical origins. He assured a lay audience that 95% of pregnancies required "only good obstetric treatment" which he defined simply as prenatal care, treatment of complications before they endangered mother or baby, aseptic practice, and the presence of a skilled physician who did not attempt to "streamline" birth. He told listeners: "Mother nature's methods of bringing babies are still the best."[128]

This final assessment by DeLee of appropriate and necessary obstetric practice anticipated the crusade for natural birth, a movement ironically inspired by many of DeLee's methods. An exposé in the *Ladies' Home Journal* in 1958, headlined "Journal Mothers Report on Cruelty in Maternity Wards," was one of the first to voice women's angry demands for reform. As one Indiana woman complained in the article, "So many women, especially first mothers, who are frightened to start out with, receive such brutal inconsiderate treatment that the whole thing is a horrible nightmare. They give you drugs, whether you want them or not, strap you down like an animal. Many times the doctor feels too much time is being taken up and he either forces the baby with forceps or slows things up." Other mothers protested "assembly line techniques" and "not [being] treated as . . . a human being."[129]

The effort to systematize birth, originally championed by DeLee in 1920 and largely institutionalized by the 1950s, continued to elicit bitter reaction. By the 1970s health reform activists in the women's movement were fighting for myriad changes: childbirth classes; "natural" childbirth without medication and equipment; the option to give birth at home; fathers present during labor and delivery; abolition of obstetric routines deemed unnecessary and unpleasant like enemas, shaving pubic hair, and episiotomy; the ability to labor, deliver, and recover in one room; and "rooming-in"—that is, keeping babies with their mothers after birth rather than isolating them in nurseries.[69,130,131]

As demonstrated by the movement for birth reform—described by activists as a crusade to "allow [a woman] the freedom to choose her own way of birth and reclaim the experience as her own"[132]—DeLee's career generated both the greatest accomplishments and the greatest controversies in modern obstetrics. Nor has DeLee's dual legacy ebbed; disagreement among obstetricians about appropriate obstetric practice continues. At the 50th annual meeting of the American College of Obstetricians and Gynecologists in Los Angeles in 2002, organizers extended the time set aside for discussion of elective primary cesarean sections from 15 minutes to an hour "because of the emotions expressed by the audience on this subject."[133] Just as DeLee justified obstetricians' routine use of forceps (in lieu of women pushing) by contending that vaginal birth "retains much morbidity that leaves permanent invalidism,"[124] some contemporary obstetricians similarly defend today's high C-section rate by arguing that vaginal birth causes urinary and fecal incontinence and uterine prolapse.[133,134]

Reminiscent of DeLee in that premiere issue of *AJOG*, one doctor recently likened vaginal delivery to "rolling a bowling ball through the vagina" and argued that up to a third of women who deliver vaginally will have long-term pelvic floor damage.[135] Other obstetricians argue as strenuously that urinary incontinence is just as prevalent in elderly women who have never given birth as in elderly women who have birthed vaginally.[136, 137] These physicians also cite studies that indicate C-sections increase maternal morbidity and mortality and infant morbidity by increasing the risk of hemorrhage and infection in the mother and respiratory problems in infants and children who are deprived of the pulmonary stimulation provided by vaginal birth.[135,138,139] This contentious discussion among contemporary obstetricians is ongoing and mirrors the vitriolic debate between DeLee's and Williams's opposing philosophical camps over the prophylactic use of forceps more than 85 years ago.

Learning from History

As these pioneering efforts to lower infant and maternal mortality in the United States indicate, even the most beneficial work can have unintended, long-term, occasionally detrimental consequences. The United States now enjoys low infant and maternal death rates compared to the years when Henry Coit invented certified milk and Joseph DeLee opened the Maxwell Street Dispensary. When compared with other industrialized countries, however, infant and maternal death rates in the United States are consistently among the highest. One vital lesson to be learned from the histories of maternal and infant mortality rates is that the maintenance of public health and the scrutiny of medical practice are never-ending processes requiring eternal vigilance.

American complacency about the formula feeding of babies, an attitude engendered in part by the widely publicized work done decades ago to purify cows' milk, is a case in point. Although breastfeeding initiation rates in the United States are the highest—at 69.5% in 2001—that they have been since data collection began in 1955,[140] that statistic is not as significant for women's and children's health as breastfeeding exclusivity and duration rates, which are among the lowest in the world. Almost 70% of American mothers initiate breastfeeding, but more than half of American mothers who initiate breastfeeding feed their babies at least some formula within six weeks of giving birth and only 14% exclusively breastfeed their babies for the 6 months recommended by the American Academy of Pediatrics (AAP). Duration rates are equally dismal. Although the AAP advises that babies should be breastfed for at least 12 months, less than 18% of American mothers breastfeed for that minimal year.[141–144] Recent studies suggest that human milk is so vital to long-term human health that low breastfeeding exclusivity and duration rates likely contribute to higher rates of obesity, diabetes, asthma, leukemia, cardiovascular disease, and breast cancer in the general population.[83–96] In the aggregate, new research on the relationship between human milk and human health is so compelling that the American Academy of Pediatrics has called for additional study of the link between formula-feeding in infancy and chronic disease in childhood and adulthood.[141]

Public health officials have also speculated recently that contemporary obstetric practice—specifically the frequent use of assisted reproductive technologies, labor induction, and Cesarean section in high-risk pregnancies—might have contributed to the recent rise in infant mortality in the United States for the first time in more than 40 years. While new technologies have improved the chances of high-risk pregnancies producing a live infant, physicians still find it difficult to keep some premature infants alive beyond their first month.[145–146] In 2002 the infant mortality rate in the United States was 7 per 1000 live births, as compared with 6.8 in 2001.[146,147]

Just as no country can afford to be complacent about infant mortality, maternal mortality continues to garner attention and concern. When compared with other industrialized countries, the United States continues to lag in this arena as well, ranking 12th internationally behind Western Europe, Australia, Canada, and Singapore.

The maternal mortality rate in Switzerland is considerably less than half that in the United States.[148]

As these histories demonstrate, just as infant feeding and birthing practices warranted careful examination and change 100 years ago to mothers' and infants' tremendous gain, ongoing public and professional scrutiny and critique of obstetric and pediatric practice will perpetually benefit mothers and infants.

References

1. Rosenberg CE. The Cholera Years: The United States in 1832, 1849, and 1866. Chicago: University of Chicago Press, 1987.
2. Infant Welfare Service 1909–1910. Report of the Department of Health of the City of Chicago for the Years 1907, 1908, 1909, 1910. Chicago: Department of Health of the City of Chicago, 1911, 177.
3. Bromley DD. What risk motherhood? *Harper's Magazine,* June 1929, 11–22.
4. Tomes N. The Gospel of Germs: Men, Women, and the Microbe in American Life. Cambridge, MA: Harvard University Press, 1998.
5. Schultz RL, Hast A. Women Building Chicago 1790–1990: A Biographical Dictionary. Bloomington and Indianapolis: Indiana University Press, 2001, 6–8, 14–22, 114–16, 345–47, 460–68, 490–92.
6. Meckel RA. Save the Babies: American Public Health Reform and the Prevention of Infant Mortality, 1850–1929. Baltimore: Johns Hopkins University Press, 1990.
7. Wolf JH. Don't Kill Your Baby: Public Health and the Decline of Breastfeeding in the 19th and 20th Centuries. Columbus: Ohio State University Press, 2001.
8. Rosenau MJ. The number of bacteria in milk and the value of bacterial counts. In: Milk and Its Relation to the Public Health. Washington, DC: Government Printing Office, 1908, 421–45.
9. Bacteria in milk. Annual Report of the Department of Health of the City of Chicago for the Year 1906. Chicago: Department of Health of the City of Chicago, 1907, 13–15.
10. Country dairy inspection. Report and Handbook of the Department of Health of the City of Chicago for the Years 1911 to 1918 Inclusive. Chicago: Department of Health of the City of Chicago, 1919, 910–11.
11. Chicago milk. *Chicago Inter Ocean,* 30 September 1892, 4.
12. Stop the bogus milk traffic. *Chicago Tribune,* 23 September 1892, 4.
13. *Bulletin Chicago School of Sanitary Instruction,* 12 October 1907;10;5.
14. *Bulletin. Chicago School of Sanitary Instruction,* 8 July 1911, 223.
15. Trask JW. Milk epidemics, 48–147; Lumdsen L, The milk supply of cities in relation to the epidemiology of typhoid fever, 151–59; and Anderson JF, The frequency of tubercle bacilli in the market milk of the City of Washington, DC, 163–92. In: U.S. Public Health and Marine Hospital Service, Milk and Its Relation to the Public Health. Washington, DC: Government Printing Office, 1908.
16. They water and color the milk. *Chicago Tribune,* 9 August 1894, 7.
17. To secure pure milk what is done in Chicago to prevent adulteration. *Chicago Tribune,* 21 July 1894, 14.
18. Report of the Municipal Laboratory, 1894. Annual Report of the Department of Health of the City of Chicago for the Year Ended December 31, 1894. Chicago: Department of Health of the City of Chicago, 1895, 145–46.
19. Biehn JF. Report of the Health Department Laboratories for 1905. Biennial Report of the Department of Health of the City of Chicago for the Years 1904–1905. Chicago: Department of Health of the City of Chicago, 1906, 7.

20. Scarcely any pure milk. *Chicago Daily News,* 1 September 1892, 2.
21. Pooler HA. The milk supply of large cities, and the improper mode in which it is conducted. *The Medical News* 1886:49:471–72.
22. Kee & Chapell Diary. Facts worth knowing, gathered during twelve years' experience, or points on milk. Chicago: Bowman Dairy Company Papers, Chicago Historical Society, 1885.
23. Edson C. The feeding of cows and its effect on milk. *Babyhood* 1887:3:293–94.
24. Letter from Mahin Advertising Company, 4 September 1913. Health Fraud and Alternative Medicine Collection, American Medical Association Archives, Chicago, IL.
25. Webster EH. Sanitary inspection and its bearing on clean milk. In: U.S. Public Health and Marine Hospital Service, Milk and Its Relation to the Public Health. Washington, DC: Government Printing Office, 1908, 511–14.
26. New milk law in effect. *Chicago Tribune,* 1 May 1904, 7.
27. *Bulletin Chicago School of Sanitary Instruction*, 28 September 1912:15:153.
28. Robertson JD. Foreword. Report and Handbook of the Department of Health of the City of Chicago for the Years 1911–1918 Inclusive. Chicago: Department of Health of the City of Chicago, 1919, xv–xvi.
29. City milk inspection. Report of the Department of Health of the City of Chicago for the Years 1919, 1920, and 1921. Chicago: Department of Health of the City of Chicago, 1922, 324.
30. Lintner JJ. Chicago's pure milk campaign. *Chicago's Health* 1927:21:102–5.
31. Concerning pasteurization. *Bulletin Chicago School of Sanitary Instruction*, 11 June 1921:23:94.
32. State of Chicago's health. *Bulletin Chicago School of Sanitary Instruction*, 26 March 1910:13:2.
33. Freeman RG. Pasteurization of milk. *JAMA* 1910:54:372–73.
34. Moak H. Certified vs. pasteurized milk. Proceedings of the Ninth Annual Conference of the American Association of Medical Milk Commissions, San Francisco, CA, 17–19 June 1915, 138–50.
35. Howe FW. Clean natural vs. pasteurized milk. Proceedings of the Fifteenth Annual Conference of the American Association of Medical Milk Commissions, Boston, MA, 6–7 June 1921, 398–405.
36. Kellogg JH. The supreme importance of clean, uncooked milk for infants and children and the dangers of pasteurized milk. Proceedings of the Fifteenth Annual Conference of the American Association of Medical Milk Commissions, Boston, MA, 6–7 June 1921, 330–61.
37. Important experiments toward maintaining purity of the milk supply. *The Mother's Nursery Guide* 1893:9:315.
38. Coit HL. The origin, general plan, and scope of the Medical Milk Commission. Proceedings of the First Annual Session of the American Association of Medical Milk Commissions, Atlantic City, NJ, 3 June 1907, 10–17.
39. Waserman MJ. Henry L. Coit and the certified milk movement in the development of modern pediatrics. *Bull Hist Med* 1972:46:359–90.
40. Miller J. To stop the slaughter of the babies: Nathan Straus and the drive for pasteurized milk, 1893–1920. *New York History* 1993:74:159–84.
41. *Bulletin Chicago School of Sanitary Instruction*, 31 August 1912:15:140.
42. *Bulletin Chicago School of Sanitary Instruction*, 2 July 1910:13:3.
43. State of Chicago's health. *Bulletin Chicago School of Sanitary Instruction*, 26 March 1910:13:2–5.
44. State of Chicago's health. *Bulletin Chicago School of Sanitary Instruction*, 10 July 1909:12:2.

45. Yale LM. The meaning of clean milk. *Babyhood* 1898:14:183–85.
46. Coit HL. The proper care of milk. *Babyhood* 1894:10:230–32.
47. The preservation of milk. *Babyhood* 1897:3:226–27.
48. How to pasteurize milk. *American Motherhood* 1907:25:55–56.
49. McBride MA. For the children. *New Crusade,* June 1897, 85–86.
50. Rorer ST. Milk: its use and abuse. *Ladies' Home Journal* May 1899, 34.
51. Scovil ER. The truth about baby foods. *Ladies Home Journal,* August 1902, 26.
52. Coolidge EL. The baby from birth to three. *Ladies' Home Journal,* February 1903, 38.
53. *Bulletin Chicago School of Sanitary Instruction,* 26 June 1909:12:2.
54. *Bulletin Chicago School of Sanitary Instruction,* 1 June 1912:15:86.
55. *Bulletin Chicago School of Sanitary Instruction,* 25 April 1914:17.
56. Allen N. The decline of suckling power among American women. *Babyhood* 1889: 5:111–15.
57. The care of infants historical data. *JAMA* 1912:59:542.
58. Infant welfare field work. Report and Handbook of the Department of Health of the City of Chicago for the Years 1911 to 1918 Inclusive. Chicago: Department of Health of the City of Chicago, 1919, 567.
59. Vinton MM. Baby's first month. *Mother's Nursery Guide* 1893:9:69.
60. D'Emilio J, Freedman EB. Intimate Matters: A History of Sexuality in America. Chicago: University of Chicago Press, 1997.
61. Nursery problems. *Babyhood* 1886:2:291.
62. Apple RD. Mothers & Medicine: A Social History of Infant Feeding, 1890–1950. Madison: University of Wisconsin Press, 1987.
63. *Bulletin Chicago School of Sanitary Instruction,* 3 June 1911:14:back cover.
64. Minutes of a meeting of the Milk Commission, 3 May 1910. Chicago Infant Welfare Society Papers, Chicago Historical Society, Chicago, IL.
65. Editorial. *Chicago Medical Recorder* 1909:31:62–63.
66. Summer milk stations in New York. *Arch Pediatrics* (1911):28:561–62.
67. Snyder JR. The breast milk problem. *JAMA* 1908:51:1214.
68. Wolf JH. Let us have more mother-fed babies: early twentieth-century breastfeeding campaigns in Chicago and Minneapolis. *J Hum Lact* 1999:15:101–5.
69. Boston Women's Health Book Collective. Our Bodies, Our Selves: A Book by and for Women. New York: Simon and Schuster, 1976.
70. Uhcard N F. Breast feeding protects against otitis media. *Nutr Rev* 1993:51:275–77.
71. Duncan B. et al. Exclusive breast-feeding for at least 4 months protect against otitis media. *Pediatrics* 1993:91:867–72.
72. Aniansson G. A prospective cohort study on breast-feeding and otitis media in Swedish infants. *Pediatr Infect Dis J* 1994:13:183–87.
73. Goldman AS. Modulation of the gastrointestinal tract of infants by human milk, interfaces and interactions: An evolutionary perspective. *Journal of Nutr* 2000:130:426S–31S.
74. Pickering LK, Morrow AL. Factors in human milk that protect against diarrheal disease. *Infection* 1993:2:355–57.
75. Mitra AK, Rabbani F. The importance of breastfeeding in minimizing mortality and morbidity from diarrhoeal diseases: the Bangladesh perspective. *J Diar Dis Res* 1995:13:1–7.
76. Blaymore BJ, Oliver T, Ferguson A, Vohr BR. Human milk reduces outpatient upper respiratory symptoms in premature infants during their first year of life. *J Perinatology* 2002:22:354–59.
77. Bachrach VR, Schwarz E, Bachrach LR. Breastfeeding and the risk of hospitalization for respiratory disease in infancy: a meta-analysis. *Arch Pediatr Adolesc Med* 2003: 157:237–43.

78. Oddy WH, Sly PD, De Klerk NH. Breast feeding and respiratory morbidity in infancy: a birth cohort study. *Arch Dis Child* 2003:88:224–28.
79. Chantry CJ, Howard CR, Auinger P. Full Breastfeeding Duration and Associated Decrease in Respiratory Tract Infection in US Children. *Pediatrics* 2006:117:425–32.
80. Chen A, Rogan WJ. Breastfeeding and the risk of postneonatal death in the United States. *Pediatrics* 2004:113:e435-e439. Available at: www.pediatrics.org/cgi/content/full/113/5/e435. Accessed 25 April 2006.
81. Forste R, Weiss J, Lippincott E. The decision to breastfeed in the United States: does race matter? *Pediatrics* 2001:108:291–96.
82. Alm B et al. Breast feeding and the sudden infant death syndrome in Scandinavia, 1992–95. *Arch Dis Child* 2002:86:400–2.
83. Von Kries R et al. Breast feeding and obesity: cross sectional study. *Br Med J* 1999: 319:147–50.
84. Gillman MW et al. Risk of overweight among adolescents who were breastfed as infants. *JAMA* 2001:285:2461–67.
85. Armstrong J, Reilly JJ, Child Health Information Team. Breastfeeding and lowering the risk of childhood obesity. *Lancet* 2002:359:2003–4.
86. Bener A, Denic S, Galadari S. Longer breast-feeding and protection against childhood leukaemia and lymphomas. *Eur J Cancer* 2001:37:234–38.
87. Kwan ML, Buffler PA, Abrams B, Kiley VA. Breastfeeding and the risk of childhood leukemia: a meta-analysis. *Public Health Rep* 2004:119:521–35.
88. Chulada PC, Arbes Jr SJ, Dunson D, Zeldin DC. Breast-feeding and the prevalence of asthma and wheeze in children: analyses from the Third National Health and Nutrition Examination Survey, 1988–1994. *J Allergy Clin Immunol* 2003:111:328–36.
89. Oddy W H, Peat JK, DeKlerk NH. Maternal asthma, infant feeding, and the risk of asthma in childhood. *J Allergy Clin Immunol* 2002:110:65–67.
90. Kostraba JN et al. Early exposure to cow's milk and solid foods in infancy, genetic predisposition, and the risk of IDDM. *Diabetes* 1993:42:288–95.
91. Perez-Bravo E, Carrasco E, Guitierrez-Lopez MD, Martinez MT, Lopez G, De los Rios MG. Genetic predisposition and environmental factors leading to the development of insulin-dependent diabetes mellitus in Chilean children. *J Mol Med* 1996: 74:105–9.
92. Martin RM, Ness AR, Gunnell D, Emmett P, Smith GD. Does breast-feeding in infancy lower blood pressure in childhood? *Circulation* 2004:109:1259–66.
93. Owen CG, Whincup PH, Odoki K, Gilg JA, Cook DG. Infant feeding and blood cholesterol: a study in adolescents and a systematic review. *Pediatrics* 2002:110:597–608.
94. Zheng T et al. Lactation reduces breast cancer risk in Shandong Province, China. *Am J Epidemiol* 2000:152:1129–35.
95. Collaborative Group on Hormonal Factors in Breast Cancer. Breast cancer and breast-feeding: collaborative reanalysis of individual data from 47 epidemiological studies in 30 countries, including 50,302 women with breast cancer and 96,973 women without the disease. *Lancet* 2002:360:187–95.
96. Zheng T, Holford TR, Mayne ST, Owens PH, Zhang H, Zhang B, Boyle P, Zahm SH. Lactation and breast cancer risk: a case-control study in Connecticut. *Br J Cancer* 2001:84:1472–76.
97. Meigs GL. Maternal mortality from all conditions connected with childbirth in the United States and certain other countries. U.S. Children's Bureau publication no. 19. Washington, DC: Government Printing Office, 1917.
98. Baker J. Maternal mortality in the United States. *JAMA* 1927:89:2016–17.

99. Woodbury, RM. Infant Mortality and Its Causes with an Appendix on the Trend of Maternal Mortality Rates in the United States. Baltimore: The Williams & Wilkins Company, 1926), 181.
100. Mendenhall, DR. Prenatal and Natal Conditions in Wisconsin. *Wis Med J* 1917:15:363–64.
101. New York Academy of Medicine Committee on Public Health Relations. Maternal Mortality in New York City: A Study of All Puerperal Deaths 1930–1932. New York: The Commonwealth Fund, 1933, 113.
102. DeLee JB. Progress toward ideal obstetrics. *Am J Obstet Dis Wom Child* 1916: 73:407–15.
103. Newman HP. The specialty of obstetrics: present status, possibilities and importance. *Am J Obstet* 1919:80:464–70.
104. Holmes RW. The fads and fancies of obstetrics: a comment on the pseudoscientific trend of modern obstetrics. *Am J Obstet Gynecol* 1921:2:225–37.
105. Williams JW. A criticism of certain tendencies in American obstetrics. *NY State J Med* 1922:22:493–99.
106. Mosher GC. Maternal morbidity and mortality in the United States. *Am J Obstet Gynecol* 1924:7:294–98.
107. Woodbury RM. Maternal mortality: the risk of death in childbirth and from all diseases caused by pregnancy and confinement. U.S. Children's Bureau publication no. 158. Washington, DC: Government Printing Office, 1926.
108. DeLee JB. What are the special needs of the modern maternity? *Mod Hosp* 1927:28:59–69.
109. Tucker BE, Benaron HB. Maternal mortality of the Chicago Maternity Center. *Am J Public Health* 1937:27:33–36.
110. Report of the Board of Directors. Chicago Lying-In Hospital and Dispensary Thirteenth Annual Report 1906–1907, 1907–1908. Northwestern Memorial Hospital Archives, Chicago, IL.
111. The Chicago Lying-In Hospital Dispensary First Annual Report 1895–96. Northwestern Memorial Hospital Archives, Chicago, IL.
112. Deaths and reported causes of deaths: 1895. Biennial Report of the Department of Health of the City of Chicago Being for the Years 1895 and 1896. Chicago: Department of health of the City of Chicago, 1897, 6–33.
113. Berkow I. Maxwell Street: Survival in a Bazaar. New York: Doubleday, 1977.
114. DeLee JB. A Brief History of the Chicago Lying-In Hospital. The Alumni Association of the Chicago Lying-In Hospital and Dispensary 1895–1931 souvenir. Joseph B. DeLee Papers, Northwestern Memorial Hospital Archives, Chicago, IL.
115. The Chicago Lying-In Hospital and Dispensary Fourth Annual Report 1898–99. Northwestern Memorial Hospital Archives, Chicago, IL.
116. The Chicago Lying-In Hospital Dispensary Second Annual Report 1896–97. Northwestern Memorial Hospital Archives, Chicago, IL.
117. The Chicago Lying-In Hospital and Dispensary Fifth Annual Report 1899–1900. Northwestern Memorial Hospital Archives, Chicago, IL.
118. The Chicago Lying-In Hospital and Dispensary Seventeenth Report July 1, 1916 to June 30, 1919. Northwestern Memorial Hospital Archives, Chicago, IL.
119. The Chicago Lying-In Hospital and Dispensary Nineteenth Report July 1, 1926 to June 30, 1930. Northwestern Memorial Hospital Archives, Chicago, IL.
120. Bundesen HN. Before the baby comes. *Chicago Department of Health Weekly Bulletin* 1925:20:330–390.
121. Leavitt JW. Joseph B. DeLee and the practice of preventive obstetrics. *Am J Public Health* 1988:78:1353–60.

122. Letter from OT McClurg to Dr. DeLee, 11 July 1922. Joseph B. DeLee Papers, Northwestern Memorial Hospital Archives, Chicago, IL.

123. Letter from Dr. DeLee to OT McClurg, 8 August 1922. Joseph B. DeLee Papers, Northwestern Memorial Hospital Archives, Chicago, IL.

124. DeLee JB. The prophylactic forceps operation. *Am J Obstet Gynecol* 1920:1:34–44.

125. Discussion. *Am J Obstet Gynecol* 1920:1:77–80.

126. The Chicago Lying-In Hospital and Dispensary Twentieth Report July 1, 1926 to June 30, 1930. Northwestern Memorial Hospital Archives, Chicago, IL.

127. DeLee JB. A message to the alumni. Alumni Bulletin 1927–28 of the Chicago Lying-In Hospital and Dispensary. Northwestern Memorial Hospital Archives, Chicago, IL.

128. DeLee JB. Mother's Day address, May 12, 1940. Joseph B. DeLee Papers, Northwestern Memorial Hospital Archives, Chicago, IL.

129. Shultz GD. Journal mothers report on cruelty in maternity wards. *Ladies Home Journal* 1958:75:44–45;152–55.

130. Mathews JJ, Zadak K. The alternative birth movement in the United States: history and current status. *Women Health* 1991:17:39–56.

131. Morgen S. Into Our Own Hands: The Women's Health Movement in the United States, 1969–1990. New Brunswick, NJ: Rutgers University Press, 2002.

132. Arms S. Immaculate Deception: A New Look at Women and Childbirth in America. New York: Bantam, 1977.

133. Cole D. Highlights in Obstetrics from the 50th Annual Meeting of the American College of Obstetricians and Gynecologists, 4–8 May 2002, Los Angeles, CA. *Medscape Women's Health*. Available at: www.medscape.com/viewarticle/434586_print. Accessed 26 April 2006.

134. Rortveit G, Daltveit AK, Hannestad YS, Hunskaar S. Urinary incontinence after vaginal delivery or cesarean section. *N Engl J Med* 2003:338:900–7.

135. Peck P. Pros and cons of cesarean on demand debated. *Medscape Medical News*. Available at www.medscape.com/viewarticle/453409_print. Accessed 26 April 2006.

136. Buchsbaum GM, Chin M, Glanta C, Guzick D. Prevalence of urinary incontinence and associated risk factors in a cohort of nuns. *Obstet Gynecol* 2002:100:226–29.

137. Buchsbaum GM, Duecy EE, Kerr LA, Huang L-S, Guzick DS. Urinary incontinence in nulliparous women and their parous sisters. *Obstet Gynecol* 2005:106:1253–58.

138. Bernstein PS. Elective cesarean section: an acceptable alternative to vaginal delivery? *Medscape Medical News*. Available at: www.medscape.com/viewarticle/441201_print. Accessed 8 October 2002.

139. Bager P, Melbye M, Rostgaardd K, Benn CS, Westergaard T. Mode of delivery and rise of allergic rhinitis and asthma. *J Allergy Clin Immunol* 2003:111:51–56.

140. Ryan AS, Wenjun Z, Acosta A. Breastfeeding continues to increase into the new millennium. *Pediatrics* 2002:110:1103–09.

141. American Academy of Pediatrics. Breastfeeding and the use of human milk. *Pediatrics* 2005:115:496–506.

142. Ruowei L, Ogden C, Ballew C, Gillespie C, Grummer-Strawn L. Prevalence of exclusive breastfeeding among U.S. infants: the Third National Health and Nutrition Examination Survey (Phase II, 1991–1994). *Am J Public Health* 2002:92:1107–10.

143. Centers for Disease Control. Breastfeeding practices: results from the 2003 National Immunization Survey. Available at: http://www.cdc.gov/breastfeeding/NIS_data/. Accessed 22 September 2004.

144. Jones G, Steketee RW, Black RE, Bhutta ZA, Morris SS, and Bellagio Child Survival Study. How many child deaths can we prevent this year? *Lancet* 2003:362:65–71.

145. O'Connor A. U.S. infant mortality rises slightly. *New York Times,* 12 February 2004, 30.
146. MacDorman MF, Martin JA, Mathews TJ, Hoyert DL, Ventura SJ. Explaining the 2001–02 infant mortality increase: data from the linked birth/infant death data set. National Vital Statistics Reports, January 24, 2005:53.
147. Kochanek KD, Smith BL. Deaths: preliminary data for 2002. National Vital Statistics Reports, February 11, 2004:52.
148. State of the world's mothers 2003. (Save the Children, 2003). Available at www.savethe children.org/publications/SOWMPDFfulldocument.pdf. Accessed 25 April 2006.

Suggested Reading

Infant Health History

Apple RD. Mothers & Medicine: A Social History of Infant Feeding 1890–1950. Madison: University of Wisconsin Press, 1987.

Baker JP. The Machine in the Nursery: Incubator Technology and the Origins of Newborn Intensive Care. Baltimore: Johns Hopkins University Press, 1996.

Brosco JP. The early history of the infant mortality rate in America: a reflection upon the past and a prophecy of the future. *Pediatrics* 1999:103:478–85.

Cheney RA. Seasonal aspects of infant and childhood mortality: Philadelphia, 1865–1920. *Journal of Interdisciplinary History* 1984:14:561–85.

Curry L. Modern Mothers in the Heartland: Gender, Health, and Progress in Illinois 1900–1930. Columbus: Ohio State University Press, 1999.

Klaus A. Every Child a Lion: The Origins of Maternal and Infant Health Policy in the United States and France, 1890–1920. Ithaca: Cornell University Press, 1993.

Ladd-Taylor M. Mother-Work: Women, Child Welfare, and the State, 1890–1930. Urbana: University of Illinois Press, 1994.

Ladd-Taylor M. My work came out of agony and grief: mothers and the making of the Sheppard-Towner Act. In: Koven S, Michel S, eds. Mothers of a New World: Maternalist Politics and the Origins of Welfare States. New York: Routledge, 1993, 321–42.

Lindenmeyer K. A Right to Childhood: The U.S. Children's Bureau and Child Welfare, 1912–46. Urbana: University of Illinois Press, 1997.

Meckel RA. Save the Babies: American Public Health Reform and the Prevention of Infant Mortality, 1850–1929. Baltimore: Johns Hopkins University Press, 1990.

Melvin PM. Milk to motherhood: the New York Milk Committee and the beginning of well-child programs. *Mid-America* 1983:65:111–31.

Miller J. To stop the slaughter of the babies: Nathan Straus and the drive for pasteurized milk, 1893–1920. *New York History* 1993:74:159–84.

Preston SH, Haines MR. Fatal Years: Child Mortality in Late Nineteenth-Century America. Princeton, NJ: Princeton University Press, 1991.

Stern AM, Markel H, eds., Formative Years: Children's Health in the United States, 1880–2000. Ann Arbor: University of Michigan Press, 2004.

Strong TH. Expecting Trouble: The Myth of Prenatal Care in America. New York: New York University Press, 2000.

Waserman MJ. Henry L. Coit and the certified milk movement in the development of modern pediatrics. *Bull Hist Med* 1972:46:359–90.

Wolf JH. Don't Kill Your Baby: Public Health and the Decline of Breastfeeding in the 19th and 20th Centuries. Columbus: Ohio State University Press, 2001.

Wolf JH. Low breastfeeding rates and public health in the United States. *Am J Pub Health* December 2003:93:2000–10.

Maternal Health History

Antler J, Fox DM. Movement toward a safe maternity: physician accountability in New York City, 1915–1940. *Bull Hist Med* 1976:50:569–95.

Borst CG. Catching Babies: The Professionalization of Childbirth, 1870–1920. Cambridge: Harvard University Press, 1995.

Devitt N. The transition from home to hospital birth in the United States 1930–1960. *Birth and the Family Journal* Summer 1977:4:47–58.

Dye NS. Mary Breckinridge, the frontier nursing service and the introduction of nurse-midwifery in the United States. *Bull Hist Med* 1983:57:485–507.

Edwards M, Waldorf M. Reclaiming Birth: History and Heroines of American Childbirth Reform. Trumansburg, NY: The Crossing Press, 1984.

Ettinger LE. Nurse-Midwifery: The Birth of a New American Profession. Columbus: Ohio State University Press, 2006.

Hoffert SD. Private Matters: American Attitudes toward Childbearing and Infant Nurture in the Urban North, 1800–1860. Urbana: University of Illinois Press, 1989.

Kass AM. Midwifery and Medicine in Boston: Walter Channing, M.D. 1786–1876. Boston: Northeastern University Press, 2002.

King CR. The New York Maternal Mortality Study: A conflict of professionalization. *Bull Hist Med* 1991:65:476–502.

Leavitt JW. Brought to Bed: Childbearing in America, 1750–1950. New York: Oxford University Press, 1986.

Leavitt JW. Joseph B. DeLee and the practice of preventive obstetrics. *Am J Pub Health* 1988:78:1353–61.

Leavitt JW. Strange young women on errands: obstetric nursing between two worlds. *Nursing History Review* 1998:6:3–24.

Lesser AJ. The Origin and development of maternal and child health programs in the United States. *Am J Pub Health* June 1985:75:590–98.

Loudon I. Death in Childbirth: An International Study of Maternal Care and Maternal Mortality, 1800–1950. Oxford: Oxford University Press, 1992.

Loudon I. The Tragedy of Childbirth Fever. Oxford: Oxford University Press, 2000.

Mathews JJ, Zadak K. The alternative birth movement in the United States: history and current status. *Women & Health* 1991:17:39–56.

McMillen S. Motherhood in the Old South: Pregnancy, Childbirth, and Infant Rearing. Baton Rouge: Louisiana State University Press, 1990.

Mitchinson W. Giving Birth in Canada 1900–1950. Toronto: University of Toronto Press, 2002.

Reagan LJ. When Abortion Was a Crime: Women, Medicine, and Law in the United States, 1867–1973. Berkeley: University of California Press, 1997.

Scholten CM. On the importance of the obstetrick art: changing customs of childbirth in America, 1760–1825. *William and Mary Quarterly* 1977:34:426–45.

Ulrich LT. A Midwife's Tale: The Life of Martha Ballard, Based on Her Diary, 1785–1812. New York: Vintage Books, 1990.

Wertz RW, Wertz DC. Lying-In: A History of Childbirth in America. New Haven: Yale University Press, 1989.

PART IV

NUTRITION

8

The Impact of Improved
Nutrition on Disease Prevention

RICHARD D. SEMBA

In the twentieth century, major achievements in nutrition and public health in the United States led to the decline in nutritional disorders such as rickets, pellagra, iodine deficiency disorders, infantile scurvy, and iron deficiency due to hookworm infection. There was a tremendous growth in knowledge about nutrition that helped shape food policy, regulations, and education. The overall nutritional status of the U.S. population improved over the last century, but these gains have been clouded by the emergence of obesity. Many nutritional deficiency disorders were addressed through public health strategies such as fortification, promotion of nutrition education, home gardening, and school lunch programs.

In *The Modern Rise of Population* (1976), Thomas McKeown (1912–1988) proposed that improved nutrition, clean water, and better hygiene were the main factors that reduced morbidity and mortality from infectious diseases in developed countries since the eighteenth century.[1] Improved nutritional status gave stronger immunity against infectious diseases.[2] Mortality rates from infectious diseases were falling prior to the growth of hospitals or technological advances in medicine such as new vaccines and development of antibiotics. In *The Role of Medicine: Dream, Mirage, or Nemesis?* (1979), McKeown further reinforced his argument.[3] The McKeown hypothesis, as it later became known, has become widely accepted, orthodox, and a powerful argument for public health efforts in nutrition.

Trends in height show that nutrition has improved since the late nineteenth century in Europe and the United States.[4-10] The average height of college students,[11-16] prison inmates,[17] and military personnel[18] increased. Americans have continued to show a secular increase in height, as shown by the Fels Institute growth study[19] and the U.S. Army Anthropometric Survey.[20] Improved nutrition played an important role in the reduction of morbidity and mortality in the United States, and many major nutritional deficiency disorders largely disappeared during the twentieth century. These diseases are highlighted in this chapter and include rickets, pellagra, iodine deficiency disorders, infantile scurvy, iron deficiency and hookworm, vitamin A deficiency, and folate deficiency.

Rickets

Vitamin D deficiency results in rickets, the disordered growth and mineralization of the long bones with stunted growth and a bow-legged appearance. Rickets generally occurs between 6 months and 3 years of age.[21] Vitamin D, which consists of a group of fat soluble seco-sterols such as ergocalciferol (vitamin D_2) and cholecalciferol (vitamin D_3), is synthesized in the skin upon exposure to ultraviolet B in sunlight and is also available in a few foods such as fatty fish, fish liver oils, eggs, and in vitamin D-fortified foods such as milk and breakfast cereals. In the early twentieth century, rickets was a major public health problem in some cities and regions of the United States,[22] Great Britain,[23] and central Europe.[24] In the Northern Hemisphere, the incidence of rickets was higher in the winter and peaked in March and April.[25]

In the early 1920s, Edward Mellanby (1884–1955) showed that experimental rickets in puppies could be cured by cod-liver oil.[26,27] The substance in cod-liver oil that was originally thought to prevent rickets was vitamin A. Further studies in 1922 showed that after bubbling air through heated cod-liver oil (which destroyed the vitamin A), there was still a factor in the cod-liver oil that promoted calcium deposition in bones.[28] This substance was isolated in the sterol fraction of cod-liver oil[29] and was termed vitamin D in 1925.[30] Later, ultraviolet radiation was shown to induce vitamin D activity in foods.[31,32] In 1932, Adolf Windaus (1876–1959)[33] and Frederic A. Askew[34] independently isolated vitamin D_2.

Prevalence of Rickets in the United States

Around the turn of the century, a high prevalence of rickets occurred in many northern U.S. cities.[35–40] The prevalence of rickets among infants in the Columbus Hill district of New York City, an impoverished black community, was an estimated 90% in 1917.[35] A large hospital-based survey showed that 80% of infants and young children had rickets in Boston.[37,38] Rickets was found among 49.8% of white and 87.6% of blacks in Memphis.[41] Large autopsy series in Baltimore showed a prevalence of rickets among children of about 45–75%,[42,43] and rickets was highly prevalent in Denver.[44]

Infants and children with rickets were generally from a low socioeconomic level.[35] Blacks[45] and some immigrants were considered at high risk.[46,47] The Columbus Hill neighborhood of New York City had both a high prevalence of rickets and the highest infant mortality rate in New York City (314 per 1000 live births)[35] compared to overall rates in New York City (96 per 1000 for whites and 202 per 1000 for blacks).[35] The susceptibility of darker skinned persons to rickets was not understood[48] until studies showed that increased skin pigment reduces the capacity of the skin to synthesize vitamin D.[49,50]

Prophylactic and Therapeutic Measures Against Rickets

Cod-liver oil was long used as an empirical remedy for rickets,[35,45,51,52] and more systematic investigation of cod-liver oil as a treatment for rickets was conducted in the early twentieth century. The pediatrician Alfred Hess (1875–1933) and others showed that cod-liver oil could be used to treat rickets,[35,52,53] and it became the accepted treatment and prophylaxis for rickets.[54–56] Hess showed that rickets was related to sunlight exposure[57,58] and direct sunlight exposure, or heliotherapy, for one half hour to several hours was an effective treatment.[59,60] Direct outdoor sunlight exposure was necessary because ordinary window glass blocked the action of sunlight against rickets.[61–63] In 1923, cod-liver oil and regular sunlight exposure led to a marked reduction of rickets in a poor neighborhood in New Haven, Connecticut.[64]

By the 1930s, academic and popular publications on nutrition emphasized the importance of cod-liver oil and sunlight as prophylaxis against rickets.[65–71] Cod-liver oil became a daily morning ritual for millions of infants and young children. In 1929 the consumption of cod-liver oil in the United States totaled 4.9 million pounds[72] compared to a population of children under five years of about 11.4 million.[73] Irradiated ergosterol was a potent treatment for rickets,[74,75] and in 1934, the direct irradiation of evaporated milk was undertaken on a commercial basis for preventing rickets[76,77] but appeared to be less effective for premature infants.[78] In 1934, the Committee on Foods of the American Medical Association approved vitamin D-fortified pasteurized milk.[79] Adequate vitamin D intake was deemed necessary for optimal growth in children.[80]

By 1940, commercial vitamin D milk began to appear in many U.S. cities, and the three main forms of vitamin D milk were metabolized milk from cows that were fed irradiated yeast, milk that was irradiated with ultraviolet light, and milk that was fortified with vitamin D.[81] By the late 1950s, rickets occurred in one of 2791 pediatric admissions.[82] Although rickets has been considered to be largely vanquished from the United States, there has been a recent increase in reports of rickets, perhaps due to a combination of factors such as less outdoor activity time for children and substitution of nonfortified juices instead of vitamin D-fortified milk.[83]

Pellagra

Pellagra is a deficiency disease due to the lack of niacin, a water-soluble vitamin that is essential for oxidation and reduction reactions of both catabolic pathways of carbohydrates, lipids, and proteins, and of anabolic pathways of fatty acid and cholesterol synthesis. Tryptophan, an essential amino acid, can also be metabolized to niacin, thus, foods containing either niacin or tryptophan can be used to treat pellagra. Rich dietary sources of niacin include red meat, liver, fish, poultry, legumes, eggs, oil seeds, cereal grains, and yeast. In the early twentieth century, pellagra was endemic in the American South, and was known by the mnemonic 4 Ds: dermatitis, diarrhea, dementia, and death.[84] Pellagra has protean clinical manifestations that include erythema and exfoliative dermatitis on exposed areas of the skin such as the neck, back of the hands, and ankles, stomatitis and diarrhea, mental status changes including depression, loss of memory, paranoia, and dementia, vertigo, peripheral muscle weakness with burning sensation in the extremities, cachexia, and death. Pellagra was already recognized in Italy, France,[85] and Spain, where it was widely believed to be caused by toxins in corn.[86]

The Appearance of Pellagra in the American South

In 1907, George Searcy described an outbreak of pellagra among the inmates of the Mount Vernon Insane Hospital in Alabama that resulted in 88 cases of pellagra with 57 deaths.[87] Searcy noted: "No nurses had the disease. They handled the patients, slept in the halls near them, and the chief difference in their way of living was in the diet. They ate little corn bread . . . they had a little more variety of diet." Searcy prevented pellagra among the inmates by modifying the diet, but his observations were largely overlooked. New outbreaks of pellagra occurred in mental institutions and orphanages elsewhere in the South.[84]

Toxins and infections were considered the most plausible causes of pellagra at the National Pellagra Conferences held in South Carolina in 1909[88] and 1912.[89] A diet high in corn was also suspected to cause pellagra but could not be linked to pellagra in experiments among hospital inmates.[90] Pellagra continued to increase across the southern United States, and from 1907 to 1911 there were 15,870 cases (excluding those in insane asylums) reported from eight states[91] (see Fig. 8.1). The associated

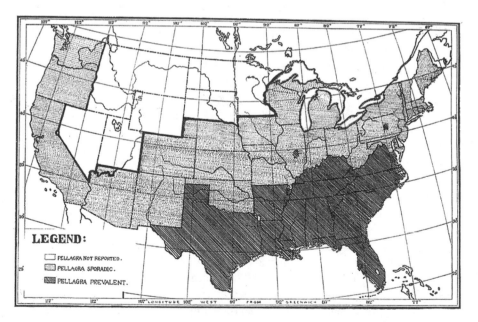

Figure 8.1. Distribution of pellagra in the United States. (From Lavinder CH. The prevalence and geographic distribution of pellagra in the United States. *Public Health Rep* 1912: 27:2076–88.)

mortality rate was an alarming 39.1%. Two wealthy philanthropists, Colonel Robert Thompson of New York City and J. H. McFadden of Philadelphia funded a research expedition for the investigation of pellagra. The Thompson-McFadden Pellagra Commission centered many of their investigations in Spartanburg County, South Carolina. This county had many cotton mills, and the prevalence rate of pellagra in these mill villages was about 104 cases per 10,000 population.[92]

The cotton mill villages in the American South were part of the larger cotton economy spread across the Cotton Belt extending through the southern states from eastern North Carolina through western Texas.[93,94] In this one-crop system, the incomes of workers and tenant farmers were intricately tied to the fluctuations in the price of cotton.[95] The predominant diet among tenant farmers was the "three M diet" of meat, meal, and molasses, where the "meat" was actually salt fat pork and "meal" was corn bread. Few had vegetable gardens.[93] Since 1880, the number of tenant farmers grew steadily in the United States, especially in the South.[96] New cotton mill villages arose in many counties in the Piedmont, especially in the Carolinas,[94] and the mill villages of the South were plagued by pellagra.[97] The Thompson-McFadden Pellagra Commission pursued the hypothesis that pellagra was an infection spread person to person by unknown means.[98,99] When the commission used a crude food frequency questionnaire in their investigations, no association was found between food and pellagra.[100] Pellagra cases were found to occur in some neighborhoods and were considered to have spread from preexisting index cases.[100]

The Epidemiologic Studies of Pellagra by Joseph Goldberger

In 1914, Joseph Goldberger (1874–1929) was asked by the Surgeon General to investigate pellagra in the United States. Goldberger was an infectious disease specialist who had previous experience working with yellow fever, typhoid fever, dengue, typhus, and diphtheria. A great deal of public anxiety and concern had been raised about this new epidemic, and out of a total budget of $200,000 for public health in the United States, the Public Health Service devoted $45,000, or nearly a quarter of the entire budget, for pellagra in 1913. When Goldberger was appointed to the investigation in 1914, the budget for pellagra was almost doubled to $80,000.[84]

In his initial investigation of pellagra, conducted at an orphanage in Mississippi, Goldberger noted that the employees of the institution never contracted pellagra, which was inconsistent with an infectious disease.[101] Instead, Goldberger called attention to the differences in diet between the employees and the children. In two orphanages in Jackson, Mississippi, where pellagra was highly prevalent, Goldberger radically changed the diet by providing eggs, fresh milk, fresh meat, beans and peas, and oatmeal instead of corn grits. No changes were made in the hygienic and sanitary conditions of the orphanages. In the first orphanage that previously had 79 cases of pellagra, there were no further cases of disease, and in the second orphanage that previously had 130 cases, there was one case of pellagra.[102] Goldberger also prevented pellagra by similar dietary changes at the Georgia State Sanitarium.[102,103] He and his colleagues recommended ownership of a milk cow, an increase in home milk consumption, poultry and egg raising for home consumption, stock raising, and diversification of home food crops, including an adequate pea patch, to safeguard against crop failure.

After the Thompson-McFadden Pellagra Commission published their study of six cotton mill villages,[100] Goldberger undertook his own investigation of diet and pellagra in seven cotton mill villages, including some that were involved in the Thompson-McFadden investigation.[104,105] Goldberger and his colleagues were careful to define criteria for active cases of pellagra, to characterize the incidence of pellagra by house-to-house visits every two weeks, to assign cases of pellagra to households, and to record the relationship between season, diet, and cases of pellagra. Instead of asking members of the household about the relative frequency of consumption of certain types of foods, Goldberger obtained records of household food supply for 15-day sample periods before or coincident with the seasonal rise of the incidence of pellagra and matched the records with the mill store records of food purchases of the mill workers and members of their households. Goldberger and his colleagues concluded that households with more lean meat, milk, butter, cheese, and eggs had a lower risk of pellagra.[104,105]

Goldberger and colleagues later showed that pellagra was more common among middle-aged women, and that there was a sharp rise in the incidence during April and May, with a well-defined peak in June.[106] A thorough investigation involving R. E. Tarbett, a sanitary engineer in the U.S. Public Health Service, showed no relationship between sanitation and pellagra.[107] Goldberger and his colleagues also noted: "In general, pellagra incidence was found to vary inversely according to family income."[108] When analyses were controlled for household income, there was less risk of pellagra in the households that had food supplies from sources such as home-owned cows, poultry, and home vegetable gardens.

In the spring of 1914, Goldberger and his associate George Wheeler began a study to produce experimental pellagra in previously healthy men by "feeding a one-sided, monotonous, principally cereal diet of the type found in previous studies to be associated with a high incidence of pellagra."[109] The study population consisted of white male convicts at Rankin Prison Farm of the Mississippi State Penitentiary. Twelve subjects volunteered for the experiment in exchange for consideration of a pardon by Governor Earl Brewer of Mississippi. The other 108 convicts on the farm served as controls. Goldberger described the prison farm in detail in order to show that the sanitation and hygiene situation was similar for intervention and control groups.[109]

The experimental diet consisted of white wheat flour, corn meal, hominy grits, corn starch, white rice, granulated cane sugar, cane syrup, molasses, sweet potatoes, cabbage, collards, turnips, turnip greens, pork fat, coffee, baking powder for biscuits and corn bread—the typical diet of the southern sharecropper. The control diet consisted of considerably more meat and dairy products than the experimental diet. The convicts who volunteered for the experiment were known as the "pellagra squad." Initially, 12 volunteers were observed for about 4 months. During the period of observation, one convict escaped, but he was soon recaptured and reassigned to the control group. After approximately 6 months, six of the members of the "pellagra squad" developed pellagra. No pellagra was observed among the control convicts. Goldberger and Wheeler concluded: "In relation to the production of pellagra, this study suggests that the dietary factors to be considered as possibly essential are

(1) an amino acid deficiency, (2) a deficient or faulty constitution of the mineral supply, possibly, but doubtfully, (3) a deficiency in the fat soluble vitamin intake, and perhaps (4) an as yet unknown (vitamin?) factor."[109]

To show that pellagra was not a contagious disease, Goldberger and other volunteers, including his wife, inoculated themselves with the blood, nasopharyngeal secretions, epidermis from pellagrous skin lesions, urine, and feces, via intramuscular injection, subcutaneous injection, application to nasopharyngeal mucosa, and oral cavity.[110] None of the volunteers developed pellagra.[110] Goldberger and Wheeler also produced experimental pellagra in dogs, a condition known as blacktongue, by feeding with a diet similar to that which produced pellagra in humans.[111,112]

Flood and Drought in the Mississippi River Valley, 1927–1931

The death rates from pellagra continued to climb in 13 Southern states, and it peaked in 1928 after a devastating flood of the Mississippi River in the spring of 1927. Goldberger and the statistician Edgar Sydenstricker (1881–1936) visited parts of the flood area, where local health officials estimated that pellagra was increasing in the overflow area of the Mississippi from Illinois to Louisiana.[113] Goldberger and Sydenstricker recommended yeast distribution as an immediate measure and the cultivation of vegetable gardens and an increase in dairy activities as long-term solutions.[113] In response, the American Red Cross distributed nearly 12,000 pounds of powdered brewers yeast.[114]

Drought followed in 1929 and 1930, and in the most extensive peacetime relief operation in the United States to that time, the Red Cross distributed more than 600,000 four-pound seed packages and promoted home gardening.[115] For the treatment of pellagra victims, an additional 30 tons of powdered yeast were distributed.[115] The home gardening effort reinforced the value of crop diversification, as "many farmers were surprised to find the improvement in health of all members of the family, with a corresponding gain in energy and ambition."[115]

The vitamin deficiency that caused pellagra had not been completely elucidated by the early 1930s, but there was sufficient empirical knowledge to combat pellagra by homestead food production and administration of yeast. The approach taken was somewhat similar to that advocated by Théophile Roussel (1816–1903) to eradicate pellagra from rural France in the nineteenth century.[85] Although Casimir Funk (1884–1967) first isolated nicotinic acid in 1911,[117] the relationship to pellagra was not clear until nicotinic acid and nicotinic acid amide were found to be effective in curing blacktongue in dogs[118] and pellagra in humans.[119] Corn is rich in niacin, but the niacin is biologically unavailable unless there is prolonged exposure to extreme Ph,[120] and corn was not prepared in this manner in the typical Southern diet.

The Role of Food Fortification in the Elimination of Pellagra

In 1938, the joint committee of the Council on Foods and Nutrition and the Council Pharmacy and Chemistry of the American Medical Association recommended the fortification of certain staple foods, including flour.[121] Thiamin and niacin, contained in wheat bran, was largely removed in the mechanized milling that produced white flour. Standards were developed to fortify flour with thiamin, niacin, and riboflavin. This enriched flour, as proposed by the recently organized Food and Nutrition Board, was adopted by the National Nutrition Conference for Defense in Washington, D.C., in May 1941. By the end of 1942, 75%–80% of all family flour and baker's white bread was enriched, and the Army, Navy, and all federal institutions used enriched flour. Between 1938 and 1939 when most bread was not enriched and 1942–1943 when 75% of the bread was enriched, a large decrease in beriberi and pellagra was reported at Bellevue Hospital in New York.[121] By 1942, the number of deaths from pellagra was already declining, having peaked in 1929, followed by an overall decrease in the following three decades.[122] An analysis of federal regulations and state laws suggests that food fortification contributed to the decline of pellagra in the South.[123]

Iodine Deficiency Disorders

The iodine deficiency disorders include mental retardation, impaired physical development, increased perinatal and infant mortality, hypothyroidism, cretinism, and goiter. Goiter is defined as an enlargement of the thyroid gland, and cretinism represents a severe form of iodine deficiency characterized by severe mental retardation. The effects of iodine deficiency on brain development are most pronounced during periods of rapid growth—that is, in the fetus, neonate, infant, and young children. The iodine deficiency disorders were once a significant problem in the United States.

By the beginning of the twentieth century, studies in Europe had shown that iodine was a cure for goiter[124] and lack of iodine in drinking water was implicated as a cause of goiter and cretinism.[125] In the nineteenth century, iodized salt and tablets were used as prophylaxis on a limited scale in France.[126,127] Jean-Baptiste Boussingault (1802–1887), an agricultural chemist, observed in Colombia, South America, that the local people used salt from nearby salt deposits for treating goiter; analysis of the salt showed that it contained high concentrations of iodine.[128,129]

Widespread Recognition of Goiter in the United States

During World War I, goiter was widespread among men drafted into the service.[130,131] In 1928, a survey of schoolchildren in 43 states showed rates greater than 50% in some localities, including New York, Pennsylvania, Ohio, Indiana, Michigan, Illinois, Wisconsin, Minnesota, Montana, and Washington.[132,133] The goiter rates in the United States correlated closely with the iodine concentrations in the water supply.[131] The number of simple goiters per 1000 men drafted in the United States during World War I appeared to represent a "goiter belt" across the northern United States (see Fig. 8.2).[132]

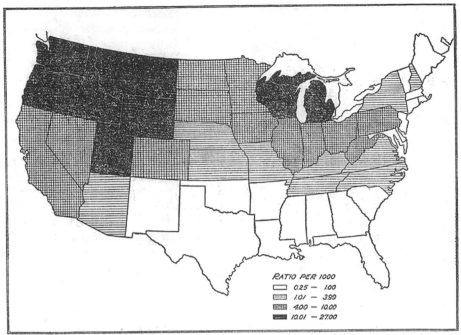

Map showing ratio of simple goiter per 1,000 men examined for military service in each State of the United States during the
World War. The rates are based on a total of 2,510,701 examinations

Figure 8.2. Number of persons with goiter per 1000 men drafted in the United States during
World War I. (From Olesen R. Distribution of endemic goiter in the Untied States as shown by
thyroid surveys. *Public Health Rep* 1929:44:1463–87.)

Work of David Marine and Oliver P. Kimball

Early pioneering work by the pathologist David Marine (1880–1976) and Oliver P.
Kimball led the way for eventual iodine prophylaxis in the United States.[134] Marine's
investigation of goiter among brook trout led to human studies. Between 1916 and
1920, Marine and Kimball studied goiter among school girls in Akron, Uhio, and
found that sodium iodide was effective in treatment and prevention of goiter.[136–140] In
1922, Kimball noted that when people in West Virginia changed from using local
brownish salt that contained 0.01% of iodine to using out-of-state, white, refined salt
that contained no iodine, there was an dramatic increase in the prevalence of goiter.[140] Kimball's observations on the use of naturally iodized salt in West Virginia
were reminiscent of Jean-Baptiste Boussingault's previous description of the use of
naturally iodized salt in Colombia.[128,129]

Largely through the advocacy of David Murray Cowie (1872–1940), the nation's
first iodized salt goiter prevention program was initiated in Michigan in 1924.[141] The
program required the cooperation of the salt producers, grocers, and the State Department of Health. No advertisement or comment by the salt producers was allowed, but the U.S. Department of Agriculture originally insisted that the salt cartons

be labeled with a skull and crossbones because iodine was considered a poison.[140] Eventually over 90% of homes were using iodized salt, and subsequent observations showed that endemic goiter practically disappeared in the state.[142]

The use of iodized salt was not without its critics, as some adults with goiter experienced iodine-induced hyperthyroidism (Jod-Basedow reaction)[143-145] Marine attributed this small peak of hyperthyroidism to the enthusiasm for iodine medication in the 1920s that came in the form of iodine in candies, tablets, and chewing gum.[146] The use of iodized salt became more widespread in the United States, and by 1955, three-quarters of households were using iodized salt.[147] Other sources of iodine have contributed to a rise in iodine consumption in the United States, including the use of iodate by the baking industry and the use of iodophors in the milk industry.[148] In the 1970s, thyroid examinations of nearly 36,000 persons in the Ten-State Nutrition Survey showed that goiter and iodine deficiency were rare.[149] The Third National Nutrition and Health Examination Survey (NHANES III), 1988–1994, showed that iodine intake was adequate but that was a decline in iodine intake in the United States over the past 20 years.[150] By the late 1990s, the total consumption of iodized salt accounted for 50%–60% of salt consumed in the United States.[150]

Infantile Scurvy

Vitamin C is a generic term for ascorbic acid, dehydroascorbic acid, and all compounds that have the biological activity of ascorbic acid. Vitamin C is essential for the biosynthesis of collagen, carnitine, and catecholamines. Lack of vitamin C results in infantile scurvy, a syndrome characterized by subperiosteal and intramuscular hemorrhages and red, swollen gums that are prone to bleeding. Although adult scurvy was well known through the centuries, infantile scurvy was not recognized until the late nineteenth century. William Cheadle (1836–1910)[151] and Thomas Barlow (1845–1945) made early descriptions of infantile scurvy, the latter of which earned the eponym of Barlow disease for infantile scurvy.[152]

In 1898, the American Pediatric Society investigated infantile scurvy and found that it occurred mostly among infants who received commercial infant formula or condensed milk, and "in general the cases reported seem to indicate that the farther a food is removed in character from the natural food of a child the more likely its use is to be followed by the development of scurvy.[153] In 1907, Axel Holst (1861–1931) and Theodor Frölich produced experimental scurvy in the guinea pig, a step that facilitated the eventual characterization of vitamin C.[154] Elmer McCollum (1879–1967) argued that scurvy was caused by excessive constipation and toxins of bacterial origin in the gastrointestinal tract,[155] but Alfred Hess noted that scurvy was often observed when orange juice was removed from the diet of young infants and disappeared with the return of orange juice to the diet.[156-158] Scurvy was also more likely to occur among infants who were fed milk that had been pasteurized at 165° F compared to 145° F.[156] Thus, excessive heating of milk to reduce bacterial contamination also contributed to loss of its vitamin C content.

By the 1920s, most infants received orange juice or tomato juice, and infantile scurvy became rare.[159-161] Popular manuals in child nutrition emphasized the need to provide anti-scorbutics such as orange juice to prevent scurvy in young infants, especially if they were being fed formula foods.[162–165] In 1932, Albert Szent-Györgyi (1893–1986)[166] and Charles Glen King (1896–1988)[167] isolated the anti-scorbutic factor. The following year, Norman Haworth (1883–1950) and Edmund Langley Hirst (1898–1975) described the structure of ascorbic acid and its synthesis.[168] Infantile scurvy declined in the United States and accounted for only one in 3300 pediatric admissions by the late 1950s.[82]

Iron Deficiency and Hookworm

Hookworm infection was once a major cause of iron deficiency, leading to anemia and mortality in the South.[169] Two species of hookworm, *Ancyclostoma duodenale* and *Necator americanus*, account for morbidity and mortality in humans, with the latter accounting for most infections in the United States.[170] Hookworm is usually spread from person-to-person through contamination of soil and vegetation with feces that contain hookworm eggs. In the soil, the eggs develop into larvae that can penetrate human skin on contact. The infective larvae may leave a pruritic, papulovesicular eruption on the skin, so-called ground itch. The hookworm larvae migrate through the skin, through the alveoli of the lungs, where they may be coughed up and ingested. The hookworms attach to the intestinal mucosa and cause chronic blood loss and depletion of iron stores.[171]

In 1843, *A. duodenale* was described[172] and implicated as a cause of profound anemia.[173] In 1902 *N. americanus* (*Uncinaria americana*) was described by the parasitologist Charles Wardell Stiles (1867–1941).[174] A former student of Stiles, Bailey K. Ashford (1873–1934), showed that the widespread tropical anemia in Puerto Rico was due to hookworm.[175,176] Early survey work by Stiles suggested that hookworm infection was widespread in the South, especially among poor whites.[177] The discovery of widespread hookworm infection became an explanation for some stereotypes of the South, including the proverbial laziness of poor white farmers.[177]

The surgeon-general, Walter Wyman (1848–1911), requested Stiles to initiate a campaign against hookworm disease based on "20 per cent. thymol and epsom salts [treatment] combined with 80 per cent. sanitation [prevention]."[178] Thymol and oil of chenopodium were early treatments used for hookworm.[179] Stiles noted that most rural schools and churches did not have a privy, and as a result the soil became contaminated with hookworm eggs and larvae.[178] Many poor children and adults went barefoot, exposing them to new hookworm infection. The U.S. Public Health Service distributed pamphlets regarding the construction of sanitary privies. Stiles continued to lecture widely in the South about the importance of sanitary privies, earning him the nickname of "Privy Councillor."[178]

In 1909, the Rockefeller Sanitary Commission for the Eradication of Hookworm Disease was established, and the commission had three goals: to determine the geographical distribution of the disease and degree of infection, to cure those who were infected, and to take measures to stop soil pollution in order to remove the source of infection.[180] In 1914, a survey of at least 200 rural schoolchildren, aged 6 to 18 in every county, was undertaken in 11 Southern states.[181] Of 548,992 children examined,

216,828 (39%) were infected with hookworm. Hookworm infection was found in almost every county except those in the western three-fourths of Texas.[181]

From 1911 through 1914, the Rockefeller Sanitary Commission sponsored a dispensary campaign, examining and providing treatment for over a million persons.[181] The county hookworm dispensary resembled an old Southern tent revival, with lectures on how hookworm was stunting the children and leaving them mentally incapable, testimonials from those who had been treated, exhibits containing bottles full of worms collected from those who had been treated, and then free diagnosis and treatment for those in the audience.[182] The commission also educated local physicians about hookworm. Bulletins on hookworm disease were published and distributed to local schools, and new laws required the construction and use of sanitary privies.[181] In 1915, the Rockefeller Sanitary Commission went out of existence.[178,182]

Studies of Hookworm Infection and Child Health in the United States

In 1926, the physician Wilson G. Smillie (1886–1971) showed that deworming of heavily infected schoolchildren improved hemoglobin concentrations and increased growth.[183,184] Hookworm infection was associated with poor mental development.[185,186] Edward K. Strong (1884–1963) of the Rockefeller Sanitary Commission, found that infected children who were treated for hookworm had better performance on mental development tests than infected children who were not treated.[187] School-based deworming programs were undertaken in heavily affected areas of the South such as Covington County, Alabama.[188] The rural school was considered the unit of control, and installation of sanitary toilets was combined with mass treatment with anthelminthics.[188]

A second survey conducted in 1920–1923 was compared with the original infection rates reported by the Rockefeller Sanitary Commission in 1910–1915.[189] Although the prevalence of hookworm was less than in the original survey, the overall prevalence of infection was still 27.8%.[189] The prevalence of hookworm infection continued to drop in the United States, perhaps due to improvements in hygiene and sanitation. Hookworm infection has largely been eradicated in the United States, but it was still prevalent in some areas of the South in the 1970s.[190–193]

Other Dietary Deficiencies

Vitamin A Deficiency

Vitamin A, or all-trans retinol, is essential for normal growth, immunity, hematopoiesis, and vision. Vitamin A is available as preformed vitamin A in foods such as butter, cheese, cod-liver oil, and eggs, or as pro-vitamin A carotenoids in foods such as dark green leafy vegetables and carrots. The vitamin A deficiency disorders are characterized by a spectrum of abnormalities that include impaired immunity, increased morbidity and mortality from some infectious diseases, impaired growth, and xerophthalmia.[194] Vitamin A was characterized through a long process that took nearly 60 years from

demonstrations that there was a substance in milk or egg yolk that supported the survival of animals,[195–198] extraction of this fat-soluble substance from milk,[199,200] eggs,[201]
or butter-fat,[201,202] naming the substance "fat-soluble A,"[203] distinguishing vitamin A
from vitamin D,[28] and description of the chemical structure,[20,205] to crystallization of
vitamin A in 1937.[206] Carotene was described as a precursor to vitamin A in 1929.[207]

Vitamin A was originally termed the "anti-infective" vitamin because vitamin
A-deficient animals were found to be more susceptible to infections.[208,209] It was well
known that children with clinical vitamin A deficiency had high morbidity and mortality from infectious diseases. The pediatrician Kenneth D. Blackfan (1883–1941)
and pathologist Simeon Burt Wolbach (1880–1954) showed that widespread pathological alterations occurred in the respiratory, gastrointestinal, and genitourinary
tracts of vitamin A-deficient infants.[210] From 1920 through 1940, vitamin A underwent considerable evaluation in at least 30 therapeutic trials to determine whether
vitamin A supplementation could reduce morbidity and mortality from infectious
diseases.[211] The studies were conducted during a period when there was an increased
awareness of the problem of infant and child mortality in Europe and the United
States. Among these trials, Joseph Ellison discovered that vitamin A supplementation reduced mortality in children with measles,[212,213] and Edward Mellanby and colleagues found that vitamin A reduced the morbidity of puerperal sepsis.[214]

Clinical vitamin A deficiency, as characterized by xerophthalmia (night blindness, Bitot spots, corneal ulceration, or keratomalacia), appeared only in occasional
case reports in the United States in the early twentieth century.[211,215] Erik Widmark
(1889–1945) recognized that subclinical vitamin A deficiency was likely associated
with increased infectious disease morbidity,[216] and a state of subclinical vitamin A
deficiency was acknowledged as "the borderline between health and disease" where
a child would appear healthy but was more susceptible to poor outcomes in face of
an infection.[217] In the 1930s and 1940s, subclinical vitamin A deficiency appeared to
be prevalent in the United States, as reflected by low plasma or serum vitamin A concentrations[218–220] and impaired dark adaptation.[221,222] Cod-liver oil, a rich source of
vitamins A and D, was marketed in the United States not only as prophylaxis against
rickets but also as a means of increasing the resistance of children to infectious
diseases.[211,217]

In 1939, the Council on Foods and Nutrition of the American Medical Association recommended that margarine be fortified with vitamin A.[223] In the early 1950s,
skimmed milk, which lacked vitamin A, was fortified with 2000 International Units
(IU) of vitamin A per quart, and in 1961, the Food and Nutrition Board of the U.S.
National Nutrition Council and the Council on Foods and Nutrition of the American
Medical Association reaffirmed their endorsement that margarine, fluid skim milk,
and dry nonfat milk should be fortified with vitamin A.[224] Federal assistance for providing milk for school children began in 1940 in Chicago and New York. The Special
Milk Program was authorized in 1954 and was implemented in order to encourage
fluid milk consumption by serving milk at the lowest possible price or at no cost for
eligible students. The Special Milk Program became part of the Child Nutrition Act
of 1966. Milk consumption in the schools increased over 10-fold in the period between 1946–47 and 1969–70, from 228 million cups of milk served to 2.7 billion
cups served under the Special Milk Program of the Child Nutrition Act.[225]

In the United States, there now appears to be sufficient vitamin A intake to prevent clinical manifestations such as night blindness.[226] Serum retinol distributions from the third National Health and Nutrition Examination Survey, 1988–1994, show that the vitamin A status of the U.S. population is generally good, but that the vitamin A status of minority children could be improved.[227] Some lower income groups are at risk of subclinical vitamin A deficiency in the United States.[228,229]

Folate Deficiency

Folate is a generic term used to describe a family of compounds with the biological activity of folic acid (pteroylglutamic acid). Folate plays an important role as coenzymes in the synthesis of nucleic acids and amino acids, thus, cells that undergo more rapid synthesis such as hematopoietic cells and epithelial cells are affected earlier in folate deficiency. In the 1930s, Lucy Wills (1888–1964) described megaloblastic anemia among pregnant women in India which responded to yeast taken orally.[230] This unknown hematopoietic factor became known as Wills' factor. In 1941, a growth factor in spinach was termed folic acid.[231] The factor that cured megaloblastic anemia was isolated from liver and yeast, and pteroylglutamic acid was purified in 1943[232,233] and synthesized in 1945.[234]

Folate deficiency is associated with an increased risk of neural tube defects. In the U.S. population, the risk of neural tube defects is about 1 per 1000 pregnancies.[235] Clinical trials show that improving maternal folate status around the periconceptual period will reduce the risk of neural tube defects.[236] The U.S. Food and Drug Administration mandated that all enriched cereal products be fortified with folate after January 1, 1998,[237] and fortification appears to have had an impact on overall improvement of folate status among adults in the United States.[238–240] From 1991 to 2001, there was a 23% decline in neural tube defects, a decrease attributed largely to folic acid fortification.[241]

Nutrition Education and Feeding Programs

Knowledge about nutrition grew rapidly in the first half of the twentieth century with the characterization of vitamins and trace elements and their role in human health. Large changes took place in the diet of Americans, and nutrition education, fortification, marketing, and advances in agriculture and food technology were among the factors that contributed to these changes.[242] With the discovery of the vitamins, a new ideology of scientific motherhood emerged—women were in charge of the care and raising of children but needed the assistance of scientists in order to have the knowledge about vitamins to keep their children healthy.[243]

The U.S. Food Administration

During World War I, the U.S. Food Administration took a major role in disseminating information about proper nutrition and home gardening. Allied populations in parts of Europe were facing serious food shortages and famine, and government intervention was needed to conserve food supplies, stabilize domestic markets, and allow for foreign food aid. In 1917, the U.S. Food Administration was created under the Food Control Act, and Herbert Hoover (1874–1964) was appointed administrator.[244] Hoover recognized that "famine does not occur according to popular ideas. . . . The poor get weak, and weaker, and die—of something else than famine. They die of tuberculosis; they die of epidemic disease; they die of whatever it is that finds fertile soil for its fatal growth among a people weakened by mal-nutrition or under-nutrition."[245] Patriotism and food became linked as part of the war effort.[245]

The U.S. Food Administration emphasized that certain foods could be conserved for exportation abroad without sacrificing the nutritional needs of people in the United States.[246,247] In order to maintain good nutrition at home, nutrition education was aimed at both college students and school children. Among the strategies for conservation of foods was an effort to increase the domestic supply of fruits and vegetables through gardening, including school gardens.[246,247] The U.S. Department of Agriculture facilitated home gardening with pamphlets.[248,249] Vegetable gardens were planted in school yards, empty lots, and backyards, and colorful posters were used to educate the public (see Fig. 8.3). The U.S. Food Administration reported that in 1917, an estimated 3 million gardens were planted, not including the acreage planted by farmers.[247] Another organization, the National War Garden Commission,[250] promoted "war gardens" to increase the national food supply, and instructions were provided for planting, fertilizing, controlling pests, harvesting, and storing fruits and vegetables.[251]

With the accumulation of food surpluses after the close of World War I, the home gardening efforts declined.[252] At the same time, horse manure became less available as fertilizer because of increased use of automobiles.[252] Home gardening increased again with the outbreak of war in Europe in 1939, despite initial restraint by the U.S. Department of Agriculture.[252] The actual public health impact of the U.S. Food Administration and home gardening efforts on the nutrition and health of Americans is difficult to assess precisely, but such efforts undoubtedly helped to educate the general public about the newer knowledge of nutrition. Previous ideas about nutrition, which basically held that the essential foods consisted of protein, carbohydrates, and fats, were overturned by the discovery of the vitamins, and there was the revelation that green leafy vegetables, once held in lesser esteem, were of great importance owing to their vitamin content.[242] The per capita consumption of fruits and vegetables increased by nearly 45% from 1911 to 1945.[253] Consumers continued to receive strong messages about the benefits of an adequate diet, and nutrition became established "not only as a branch of preventive medicine but as a major instrument of social policy."[242]

School Lunch Programs

In the beginning of the twentieth century, the problem of child malnutrition was raised by Robert Hunter (1874–1942) in *Poverty* (1904)[254] and John Spargo (1876–1966) in *The Bitter Cry of the Children* (1906).[255] Child malnutrition was a cause célèbre that incited public interest in school feeding.[256] Hunter suggested that there were 60,000 to 70,000 children in New York City alone who arrived at school hungry and unfit to learn,[254] and Spargo estimated that not less than 2 million school children nationwide were suffering from poverty and inadequate nourishment.[255]

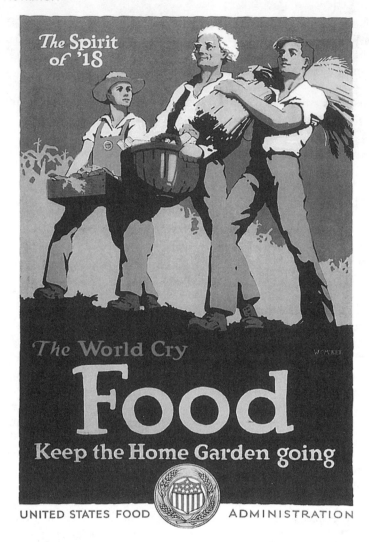

Figure 8.3. "The Spirit of '18" poster of the U.S. Food Administration, 1918, emphasizing home gardening. (Collection of the author.)

Various attempts were made to provide school lunches in the schools of large cities.[257] The educator William R. P. Emerson (1869–1951) estimated that 20–40% of children graduating from elementary schools were not well nourished, and he established nutrition clinics in the schools.[258,259] With the cooperation of the child, physician, teacher, and parent, the malnourished children were put in a separate class where the curriculum included nutrition education, dietary assessment, and monitoring of weight and height.[260] A Bureau of School Lunches was established by the Department of Education in New York City in 1918.[257]

In 1935, the Federal Surplus Commodities Corporation engaged in school feeding with surplus food from U.S. farmers. By 1938, 45 states and the District of Columbia were participating in school lunch programs.[242] The National School Lunch Act provided permanent status to school lunch programs in 1946 and was further strengthened by the Child Nutrition Act in 1966. By 1974, the National School Lunch Program was feeding nearly 25 million American school children each day. In 2001, the National School Lunch Program served more than 27 million lunches in over 97,700 schools across the United States.[261]

Conclusions

In the twentieth century, major progress was made in the near elimination of many nutritional deficiencies disorders in the United States, such as rickets, pellagra, iodine deficiency, infantile scurvy, iron deficiency due to hookworm, and subclinical levels of vitamin A deficiency and folate deficiency. Milestones in this process are summarized in Table 8.1. The vitamins and their roles in human health were characterized, and dietary requirements were established. The fortification of foodstuffs, nutrition education, home gardening, and federally supported feeding programs all were aimed at improving the nutrition of the U.S. population. In many cases, there was existing empirical knowledge to take measures against specific nutritional deficiency disorders even though the nutritional factors involved had not been fully elucidated. When specific vitamins were finally characterized and synthesized, the knowledge was often translated quickly into public health measures such as food fortification. The American diet also evolved in light of the newer knowledge of nutrition, with increased consumption of fruits and vegetables. Despite the tremendous advances in the twentieth century, not all nutritional problems have been addressed.

Challenges for the Twenty-First Century

The progress that has been made in the reduction of nutritional deficiency disorders has been offset by an epidemic of obesity that has occurred mostly over the last two to three decades. Obesity has now become the most common nutritional disease in the United States.[262] From 1991 to 1999, there was a substantial increase in the proportion of adults who were overweight (body mass index 25 kg/m^2) and obese (body mass index 30 kg/m^2).[263] In 2000, the prevalence of adults who were overweight was 56% and obese was 19.8%.[263] The consequences of this epidemic of obesity include increased morbidity and mortality, diabetes mellitus, hypertension, and cardiovascular disease.[262] Overweight and obesity have also become a problem among children in the United States, with 8% of children 4 to 5 years of age being overweight.[264] The risk of overweight and obesity in adulthood is especially high for those who are overweight during childhood.[264] Little progress has been made to reduce iron deficiency among women of childbearing age in the United States. Vitamin D deficiency is still common among older adults. These challenges remain for nutrition and public health efforts in the twenty-first century.

Table 8.1. Some notable milestones in nutrition in the 20th century.

1903	High prevalence of hookworm found in the South by Charles Wardell Stiles.[177]
1904	Child hunger highlighted in Robert Hunter's *Poverty*.[254]
1906	John Spargo describes child malnutrition in *The Bitter Cry of the Children*.[255]
1907	George Searcy describes pellagra in an "insane asylum" in the South.[87]
1907	Axel Holst and Theodor Frölich produce experimental scurvy in guinea pigs.[154]
1909	First National Pellagra Conference held in Columbia, South Carolina.[88]
1909	Rockefeller Sanitary Commission for the Eradication of Hookworm Disease established.
1911	Casimir Funk isolates nicotinic acid (niacin).[117]
1911–1914	Rockefeller Sanitary Commission conducts mass hookworm campaigns in the South.
1911	Wilhelm Stepp extracts fat-soluble substance in milk that supports growth.[199]
1911	Pellagra Commission of Illinois shows that an excessive corn diet does not cause pellagra (90).
1912	Second National Pellagra Conference held in Columbia, South Carolina.[89]
1912	Frederick Hopkins demonstrates the presence of a substance in milk that supports growth.[198]
1913	U.S. Public Health Service devotes nearly one quarter of total budget for pellagra.
1913	Elmer McCollum extracts fat-soluble substance from butter or egg that supports growth.[201]
1913	Thomas Osborne and Lafayette Mendel extract fat-soluble substance from butter that supports growth.[202]
1914–1915	Joseph Goldberger investigates pellagra in orphanages in the South.[101,102]
1914–1918	Infantile scurvy prevented by addition of orange juice to diet.[157,158]
1916	Edward Strong shows that deworming improves mental development in children.[187]
1916–1920	David Marine and Oliver Kimball conduct iodine prophylaxis studies of goiter.[136–139]
1917	Food Control Act creates the U.S. Food Administration.
1917–1918	Major public health and nutrition efforts to promote vegetable gardens.
1918–1920	Joseph Goldberger investigates pellagra in Southern mill villages.[104–108]
1920	Experimental pellagra produced in inmates on the Rankin Prison Farm, Mississippi.[109]
1920	High prevalence of goiter found among draftees in World War I; "goiter belt" described.
1921	Edward Mellanby produces experimental rickets in dogs.[26]
1922	Elmer McCollum separates anti-rachitic substance from vitamin A in cod-liver oil.[28]
1922	Theodore Zucker isolates anti-rachitic substance in sterol fraction of cod-liver oil.[29]
1924	Iodized salt program started in Michigan.[142]
1926	Hookworm associated with growth retardation.[183]
1926	Deworming reduces anemia and improves growth in children.[184]
1927	Lydia Roberts focuses on nutrition education in *Nutrition Work with Children*.[258]
1928	High goiter rates found in school children, especially in northern United States.[133]
1928	Vitamin A termed the "anti-infective" vitamin.[208]
1928	Experimental blacktongue produced in dogs by feeding them a typical sharecropper's diet.[111,112]
1928–1941	Clinical trials of vitamin A as prophylaxis or treatment for various infections.[211]
1929	Peak of total deaths from pellagra in the United States.
1929–1931	Promotion of homestead food production and distribution of yeast to combat pellagra in Mississippi after flood of 1927 and drought of 1929–1930; pellagra deaths decline.
1931	Paul Karrer describes the chemical structure of vitamin A.[204,205]
1932	Adolf Windhaus and Frederic Askew independently isolate vitamin D_2.[33,34]
1932	Albert Szent-Györgyi and Charles King independently isolate vitamin C.[166,167]
1932	Joseph Bramhall Ellison discovers that vitamin A supplementation reduces mortality in children with vitamin A deficiency and measles.[212]
1933	Kenneth Blackfan and S. Burt Wolbach describe pathology of vitamin A-deficient infants.[210]
1933	Structure of vitamin C determined by Norman Haworth.[168]

Table 8.1. (*continued*)

1934	American Medical Association approves fortification of milk with vitamin D.[79]
1937	Holmes and Corbet crystallize vitamin A.[206]
1937	Nicotinic acid (niacin) cures blacktongue in dogs.[118]
1938	Joint Commitee of the Council on Foods and Nutrition and Council on Pharmacy and Chemistry, American Medical Association, recommend fortification of certain staples foods such as flour with thiamin, niacin, and riboflavin.[121]
1939	Council on Foods, American Medical Association, recommends fortification of margarine with vitamin A.[223]
1939	Nicotinic acid (niacin) cures pellagra in humans.[119]
1940	Milk producers begin to fortify skim milk with vitamin A.
1942	75–80% of all family flour and baker's white bread in United States is enriched.
1946	National School Lunch Program is begun.
1954	Special Milk Program is established.
1966	Child Nutrition Act strengthens school lunch programs and Special Milk Program.
1975	Ten-state Nutrition Survey shows that goiter is rare.[149]
1998	U.S. Food and Drug Administration mandates folate fortification of all enriched cereal products.[237]

References

1. McKeown T. The Modern Rise of Population. New York: Academic Press, 1976.
2. Scrimshaw NS, Taylor CE, Gordon JE. Interactions of Nutrition and Infection. World Health Organization Monograph Series no. 57. Geneva, World Health Organization, 1968.
3. McKeown T. The Role of Medicine: Dream, Mirage, or Nemesis? Princeton: Princeton University Press, 1979.
4. Floud R, Wachter K, Gregory A. Height, Health and History: Nutritional Status in the United Kingdom, 1750–1980. Cambridge Studies in Population, Economy and Society in Past Time no. 9. Cambridge, UK: Cambridge University Press, 1990.
5. Cone TE Jr. Secular acceleration of height and biologic maturation in children during the past century. *J Pediatr* 1961: 59:736–40.
6. Boas F. Age changes and secular changes in anthropometric measurements. *Am J Phys Anthropol* 1940: 26:63–68.
7. Lloyd-Jones O. California tall children. *Am J Dis Child* 1940:60:11–21.
8. Tanner JM. Growth at Adolescence, 2nd ed. Oxford: Blackwell Scientific Publications, 1962.
9. Michelson N. Investigations in the physical development of Negroes. I. Stature. *Am J Phys Anthropol* 1943:1 ns:191–213.
10. Meredith HV. Change in the stature and body weight of North American boys during the last 80 years. *Adv Child Dev Behav* 1963:1:69–114.
11. Blunt K, Cowan R. Ultraviolet Light and Vitamin D in Nutrition. Chicago: University of Chicago Press, 1930.
12. MacKinnon DC, Jackson CM. Changes in physical measurements of the male students at the University of Minnesota during the last thirty years. *Am J Anat* 1931: 47:405–23.
13. Bowles GT. New Types of Old Americans at Harvard and at Eastern Women's Colleges. Cambridge, MA: Harvard University Press, 1932.
14. Hunt EE Jr. Human growth and body form in recent generations. *Am Anthropol* 1958: 60:118–31.
15. Chenoweth LB. Increase in height and weight and decrease in age of college freshmen over a period of twenty years. *JAMA* 1937:108:354–56.

16. Deegan WA. A fifty-nine year survey at Yale reveals freshmen are becoming younger, heavier and taller. *Res Quart* 1941:12:707–11.

17. Karlan SC. Increase in height and weight among the underprivileged. *NY State J Med* 1941: 41:2425–2426.

18. Trotter M, Gleser GC. Trends in stature of American whites and Negroes born between 1840 and 1924. *Am J Phys Anthropol* 1951:9:427–40.

19. Bock RD, Sykes RC. Evidence for continuing secular increase in height within families in the United States. *Am J Hum Biol* 1989:1:143–48.

20. Greiner TM, Gordon CC. Secular trends of 22 body dimensions in four racial/cultural groups of American males. *Am J Hum Biol* 1992:4:235–46.

21. Cokenower JW. Rickets in its early stages and best treatment to prevent deformities. *JAMA* 1911:57:1506–7.

22. Hess AF. Rickets Including Osteomalacia and Tetany. Philadelphia: Lea & Febiger, 1929.

23. Ferguson MF. A Study of Social and Economic Factors in the Causation of Rickets. Medical Research Committee Special Report Series No. 20. London, Medical Research Committee, 1917.

24. Chick H, Dalyell EJ, Hume EM, Mackay HMM, Smith HH. Studies of Rickets in Vienna 1919–1922. Medical Research Council Special Report no. 77, London, His Majesty's Stationery Office, 1923.

25. Hess AF, Unger LJ. Infantile rickets: the significance of clinical, radiographic and chemical examinations in its diagnosis and incidence. *Am J Dis Child* 1922:24:327–38.

26. Mellanby E. Experimental Rickets. Medical Research Council Special Report Series no. 61. London, His Majesty's Stationery Office, 1921.

27. Mellanby E. Experimental Rickets. The Effect of Cereals and Their Interaction with Other Factors of Diet and Environment in Producing Rickets. Medical Research Council Special Report Series no. 93. London, His Majesty's Stationery Office, 1925.

28. McCollum EV, Simmonds N, Becker JE, Shipley PG. Studies on experimental rickets. XXI. An experimental demonstration of the existence of a vitamin which promotes calcium deposition. *J Biol Chem* 1922:53:293–312.

29. Zucker TF, Pappenheimer AM, Barnett M. Observations on cod-liver oil and rickets. *Proc Soc Exp Biol Med* 1922:19:167–69.

30. McCollum EV, Simmonds N, Becker JE, Shipley PG. Studies on experimental rickets. XXVI. A diet composed principally of purified foodstuffs for use with the "line test" for vitamin D studies. *J Biol Chem* 1925:65:97–100.

31. Steenbock H. The induction of growth promoting and calcifying properties in a ration by exposure to light. *Science* 1924:60:224–25.

32. Hess AF, Weinstock M. Antirachitic properties imparted to inert fluids and to green vegetables by ultra-violet irradiation. *J Biol Chem* 1924:62:301–13.

33. Windaus A, Linsert O, Lüttringhaus A, Weidlich G. Über das krystallistierte Vitamin D$_2$. *Justus Liebigs Ann Chem* 1932:492:226.

34. Askew FA, Bourdillon RB, Bruce HM, Callow RK, Philpot J St L, Webster TA. Crystalline vitamin D. *Proc Roy Soc London Ser B* 1932:109:488–506.

35. Hess AF, Unger LJ. Prophylactic therapy for rickets in a Negro community. *JAMA* 1917:69:1583–86.

36. Blau AI. Rickets among children in New York City. *Month Bull Dept Health City New York* 1919:9:144–53.

37. Morse JL. The frequency of rickets in infancy in Boston and vicinity. *Boston Med Surg J* 1899:140:163–65.

38. Morse JL. The frequency of rickets in infancy in Boston and vicinity. *JAMA* 1900: 34:724–26.

39. Parry JS. Observations of the frequency and symptoms of rachitis, with the results of the author's clinical experience. *Am J Med Sci* 1872:63:17–52.
40. Thomas JJ, Furrer AF. A review of one hundred cases of rachitis. *Cleveland Med J* 1907: 6:491–95.
41. Mitchell FT. Incidence of rickets in the South. *South Med J* 1930:23:228–35.
42. Follis RH Jr, Jackson D, Eliot MM, Park EA. Prevalence of rickets in children between two and fourteen years of age. *Am J Dis Child* 1943:60:1–11.
43. Follis RH Jr, Park EA, Jackson D. The prevalence of rickets at autopsy during the first two years of age. *Johns Hopkins Hosp Bull* 1952:91:480–97.
44. Forbes RP, Green B, Stephenson FB. Rickets in Colorado. *Arch Pediatr* 1926: 43:131–37.
45. Acker GN. Rickets in Negroes. *Arch Pediatr* 1894:11:893–98.
46. Snow IM. An explanation of the great frequency of rickets among Neapolitan children in American cities. *Arch Pediatr* 1895:12:18–34.
47. Southworth TS. The importance of the early recognition and treatment of rachitis. *JAMA* 190850:89–93.
48. Hess AF, Unger LJ. The diet of the Negro mother in New York City. *JAMA* 1918: 70:900–2.
49. Hess AF. Newer aspects of the rickets problem. *JAMA* 1922:78:1177–83.
50. Clemens TL, Adams JS, Henderson SL, Holick MF. Increased skin pigment reduces the capacity of skin to synthesize vitamin D_3. *Lancet* 1982:1:74–76.
51. De Jongh LJ. The Three Kinds of Cod Liver Oil; Comparatively Considered with Reference to Their Chemical and Therapeutic Properties. Philadelphia: Lea & Blanchard, 1849.
52. Park EA, Howland J. The radiographic evidence of the influence of cod-liver oil in rickets. *Bull Johns Hopkins Hosp* 1921:32:341–44.
53. Asserson MA. Study of the effect of cod liver oil to prevent rickets in Negro children. *Month Bull Dept Health City New York* 1918:8:198–204.
54. Garland J. The importance of cod liver oil as an anti-rachitic agent. *Boston Med Surg J* 1924:191:347–49.
55. Barnes D. Clinical effectiveness of a cod liver oil concentrate. *Am J Dis Child* 1933: 46:250–61.
56. Morse JL. Progress in pediatrics: a summary of the literature of the last few years on rickets. *Boston Med Surg J* 1922:186:507–13.
57. Hess AF. The influence of light in prevention and cure of rickets. *Lancet* 1922:2:367–69.
58. Hess AF. The prevention and cure of rickets by sunlight. *Am J Pub Health* 1922:12: 104–7.
59. Hess AF, Unger LJ. An interpretation of the seasonal variation of rickets. *Am J Dis Child* 1921:22:186–92.
60. Hess AF, Gutman MB. The cure of infantile rickets by sunlight accompanied by an increase in the inorganic phosphate of the blood. *JAMA* 1922:78:29–31.
61. Shipley PG, Park EA, Powers GF, McCollum EV, Simmonds N. The prevention of the development of rickets in rats by sunlight. *Proc Soc Exp Biol Med* 1921:19:43–47.
62. Hess AF, Unger LJ, Pappenheimer AM. Experimental rickets in rats. III. The prevention of rickets by exposure to sunlight. *J Biol Chem* 1922:50:77–82.
63. Hess AF, Unger LJ, Pappenheimer AM. A further report on the prevention of rickets in rats by light rays. *Proc Soc Exp Biol Med* 1922:19:238–39.
64. Eliot MM. The control of rickets: preliminary discussion of the demonstration in New Haven. *JAMA* 1925:85:656–63.
65. Plimmer RHA, Plimmer VG. Food, Health, Vitamins, 5th ed. London: Longmans, Green, 1932.

66. Chenoweth LB, Morrison WR. Community Hygiene. New York: F. S. Crofts, 1934.

67. Thoma KM. Food in Health and Disease. Preparation, Physiological Action and Therapeutic Value. Philadelphia: F. A. Davis Company, 1936.

68. Funk C, Dubin HE. Vitamin and Mineral Therapy. New York: U. S. Vitamin Corporation, 1936.

69. Gauger ME. Vitamins and Your Health. New York: Robert M. McBride, 1936.

70. Bacharach AL. Science and Nutrition. London: Watts & Co., 1938.

71. Kenyon JH. Healthy Babies Are Happy Babies. A Complete Handbook for Modern Mothers. Boston: Little, Brown, 1940.

72. Prescott SC, Proctor BE. Food Technology. New York: McGraw-Hill, 1937.

73. U.S. Bureau of the Census. Historical Statistics of the United States. Colonial Times to 1957. Washington, D.C.: Government Printing Office, 1960.

74. Hess AF, Lewis JM. Clinical experience with irradiated ergosterol. *JAMA* 1928:91:783–88.

75. May EW. The prevention of rickets in premature infants by the use of Viosterol 100 D. *JAMA* 1931:96:1376–80.

76. Jeans PC, Stearns G. Effectiveness of vitamin D in infancy in relation to the vitamin source. *Proc Soc Exp Biol Med* 1934:31:1159–61.

77. Rapoport M, Stokes J Jr, Whipple DV. The antirachitic value of irradiated evaporated milk in infants. *J Pediatr* 1935:6:799–808.

78. Davidson LT, Merritt KK, Chapman SS. Prophylaxis of rickets in infants with irradiated evaporated milk. *Am J Dis Child* 1937:53:1–21.

79. Committee on Foods. American Medical Association. Vitamin D fortified pasteurized milk. *JAMA* 1934:103:1069.

80. Jeans PC. Vitamin D milk. The relative value of different varieties of vitamin D milk for infants: a critical interpretative review. *JAMA* 1936:106:2066–69, 2150–59.

81. Roadhouse CL, Henderson JL. The Market-Milk Industry. New York and London: McGraw-Hill, 1941.

82. Committee on Nutrition. American Academy of Pediatrics. Infantile scurvy and nutritional rickets in the United States. *Pediatrics* 1962:29:646–47.

83. Abrams SA. Nutritional rickets: an old disease returns. *Nutr Rev* 2002:60:111–15.

84. Etheridge EW. The Butterfly Caste: A Social History of Pellagra in the South. Westport, CT: Greenwood Press, 1972.

85. Semba RD. Théophile Roussel and the elimination of pellagra from 19th century France. *Nutrition* 2000:16:231–33.

86. Roe DA. A Plague of Corn: The Social History of Pellagra. Ithaca: Cornell University Press, 1973.

87. Searcy GH. An epidemic of acute pellagra. *JAMA* 1907:49:37–38.

88. National Association for the Study of Pellagra. Transactions of National Conference on Pellagra held under auspices of South Carolina State Board of Health at State Hospital for the Insane, Columbia, SC, 3–4 November 1909. Columbia, SC: The State Company Printers, 1910.

89. National Association for the Study of Pellagra. Transactions of the National Association for the Study of Pellagra. Second Triennial Meeting at Columbia, SC, 3–4 October 1912. Columbia, SC: T. L. Bryan Company, 1914.

90. Pellagra Commission. Report of the Pellagra Commission of the State of Illinois. Springfield, IL: Illinois State Journal Company State Printers, 1911.

91. Lavinder CH. The prevalence and geographic distribution of pellagra in the United States. *Public Health Rep* 1912:27:2076–88.

92. Siler JF, Garrison PE, MacNeal WJ. Pellagra. A summary of the first progress report of the Thompson-McFadden Pellagra Commission. *JAMA* 1914:62:8–12.

93. Vance RB. Human Factors in Cotton Culture: A Study in the Social Geography of the American South. Chapel Hill, NC: University of North Carolina Press, 1929.

94. Vance RB. Human Geography of the South: A Study in Regional Resources and Human Adequacy. Chapel Hill, NC: University of North Carolina Press, 1932.

95. Wheeler GA, Sebrell WH. The control of pellagra. *JAMA* 1932:99:95–98.

96. Public Affairs Committee. Farmers Without Land. New York: Public Affairs Committee, 1937.

97. Beardsley EH. A History of Neglect: Health Care for Blacks and Mill Workers in the Twentieth-Century South. Knoxville: University of Tennessee Press, 1987.

98. Siler JF, Garrison PE, MacNeal WJ. The relation of methods of disposal of sewage to the spread of pellagra. *Arch Intern Med* 1914:14:453–74.

99. Siler JF, Garrison PE, MacNeal WJ. Further studies of the Thompson-McFadden Pellagra Commission. A summary of the second progress report. *JAMA* 1914: 63: 1090–93.

100. Siler JF, Garrison PE, MacNeal WJ. A statistical study of the relation of pellagra to use of certain foods and to location of domicile in six selected industrial communities. *Arch Intern Med* 1914:14:292–373.

101. Goldberger J. The etiology of pellagra. The significance of certain epidemiological observations with respect thereto. *Public Health Rep* 1914:29:1683–86.

102. Goldberger J, Waring CH, Willets DG. The prevention of pellagra. A test of diet among institutional inmates. *Public Health Rep* 1915:30:3117–31.

103. Goldberger J, Waring CH, Tanner WF. Pellagra prevention by diet among institutional inmates. *Public Health Rep* 1923:38:2361–68.

104. Goldberger J, Sydenstricker E. A study of the diet of nonpellagrous and of pellagrous households in textile mill communities in South Carolina in 1916. 1918:71:944–49.

105. Goldberger J, Wheeler GA, Sydenstricker E. A study of the relation of diet to pellagra incidence in seven textile-mill communities of South Carolina in 1916. *Public Health Rep* 1920:35:648–713.

106. Goldberger J, Wheeler GA, Sydenstricker E. Pellagra incidence in relation to sex, age, season, occupation, and "disabling sickness" in seven cotton-mill villages of South Carolina during 1916. *Public Health Rep* 1920:35:1650–64.

107. Goldberger J, Wheeler GA, Sydenstricker E, Tarbett RE. A study of the relation of factors of a sanitary character to pellagra incidence in seven cotton-mill villages of South Carolina in 1916. *Public Health Rep* 1920:35:1701–14.

108. Goldberger J, Wheeler GA, Sydenstricker E. A study of the relation of family income and other economic factors to pellagra incidence in seven cotton-mill villages of South Carolina in 1916. *Public Health Rep* 1920:35:2673–714.

109. Goldberger J, Wheeler GA. The experimental production of pellagra in human subjects by means of diet. *Hygienic Lab Bull* 1920:120:7–116.

110. Goldberger J. The transmissibility of pellagra. Experimental attempts at transmission to the human subject. *Pub Health Rep* 1916:31:3159–73.

111. Goldberger J, Wheeler GA. Experimental black tongue of dogs and its relation to pellagra. *Public Health Rep* 1928:43:172–217.

112. Goldberger J, Wheeler GA, Lillie RD, Rogers LM. A further study of experimental blacktongue with special reference to the blacktongue preventive in yeast. *Public Health Rep* 1928:43:657–94.

113. Goldberger J, Sydenstricker E. Report of an inquiry relating to the prevalence of pellagra in the area affected by the overflow of the Mississippi and its tributaries in Tennessee, Arkansas, Mississippi, and Louisiana in the spring of 1927. *Public Health Rep* 1927:42:2706–25.

114. American Red Cross. The Mississippi Valley Flood Disaster of 1927: Official Report of the Relief Operations. Washington, DC: American National Red Cross, 1927.

115. American Red Cross. Relief Work in the Drought of 1930–31: Official Report of the American National Red Cross. Washington, DC: American National Red Cross, 1931.

116. True AC. A History of Agricultural Extension Work in the United States, 1785–1923. United States Department of Agriculture Misc. Publication No. 15. Washington, DC: Government Printing Office, 1928.

117. Funk C. On the chemical nature of the substance which cures polyneuritis in birds induced by a diet of polished rice. *J Physiol* 1911:43:395–400.

118. Elvehjem CA, Madden RJ, Strong FM, Woolley DW. Relation of nicotinic acid and nicotinic acid amide to canine black tongue. *Am Chem Soc J* 1937:59:1767–68.

119. Spies TD, Bean WB, Ashe WF. Recent advances in the treatment of pellagra and associated deficiencies. *Ann Intern Med* 1939:12:1830–44.

120. Laguna J, Carpenter KJ. Raw versus processed corn in niacin-deficient diets. *J Nutr* 1951:45:21–28.

121. Wilder RM, Williams RR. Enrichment of Flour and Bread: A History of the Movement. Bulletin of National Research Council no. 110. Washington, DC: National Research Council, National Academy of Sciences, 1944.

122. Miller DF. Pellagra deaths in the United States. *Am J Clin Nutr* 1978:31:558–59.

123. Park YK, Sempos CT, Barton CN, Vanderveen JE, Yetley EA. The effectiveness of food fortification in the United States: the case of pellagra. *Am J Publ Health* 2000:90:727–38.

124. Coindet JF. Découverte d'un nouveau remède contre le goître. *Bibliotheque Universelle* 1820:14:190–98.

125. Chatin A. Existence de l'iode dans l'air, les eaux, le sol et les produits alimentaires. *Annales Société Météorol France* 1859:7:50–107.

126. Goitre in Savoy. *Lancet* 1869:2:518.

127. Merke F. History and Iconography of Endemic Goitre and Cretinism. Berne: Hans Huber, 1984.

128. Boussingault [JB]. Mémoire sur les salines iodifères des Andes. *Ann Chim Phys* 1833:54:163–77.

129. Boussingault [JB]. Viajes científicos a los Andes ecuatoriales ó coleccion de memorias sobre física, química é historia natural de la Nueva Granada, Ecuador y Venezuela, presentadas à la Academia de Ciencias de Francia. Paris: Libreria Castellana, 1849.

130. U.S. Army Surgeon General's Office War Department. Defects Found in Drafted Men. Statistical information compiled from the draft records showing the physical condition of the men registered and examined in pursuance of the requirements of the Selective-Service Act. Washington, DC: War Department, 1920.

131. McClendon JF, Williams A. Simple goiter as a result of iodine deficiency. *JAMA* 1923:80:600–1.

132. Olesen R. Distribution of endemic goiter in the United States as shown by thyroid surveys. *Public Health Rep* 1926:41:2691–703.

133. Olesen R. Distribution of endemic goiter in the United States as shown by thyroid surveys. *Public Health Rep* 1929:44:1463–87.

134. Harvey AM. David Marine: America's pioneer thyroidologist. *Am J Med* 1981:70: 483–85.

135. Marine D, Lenhart CH. Observations and experiments on the so-called thyroid carcinoma of brook trout (Salvalinus fontinalis) and its relation to ordinary goitre. *J Exp Med* 1910:12: 311–37.

136. Marine D, Kimball OP. The prevention of simple goiter in man. A survey of the incidence and types of thyroid enlargement in the schoolgirls of Akron (Ohio), from the 5th to the 12th grades, inclusive—the plan of prevention proposed. *J Lab Clin Med* 1917:3:40–48.

137. Kimball OP, Marine D. Prevention of goiter in man. Second paper. *Arch Intern Med* 1918:22:41–44.

138. Kimball OP, Rogott JM, Marine D. The prevention of simple goiter in man. Third paper. *JAMA* 1919:73:1873–74.

139. Marine D, Kimball OP. Prevention of simple goiter in man. Fourth paper. *Arch Intern Med* 1920:25:661–72.

140. Kimball OP. History of the prevention of endemic goitre. *Bull World Health Organ* 1953:9:241–48.

141. Markel H. "When it rains it pours": endemic goiter, iodized salt, and David Murray Cowie, M.D. *Am J Pub Health* 1987:77:219–29.

142. Altland JK, Brush BE. Goiter prevention in Michigan: results of thirty years' voluntary use of iodized salt. *J Mich State Med Soc* 1952:51:985–89.

143. Hartsock CL. Abuse of iodine, especially of iodized salt, in the prevention of goiter. *Ann Intern Med* 1927–1928:1:24–27.

144. Hartsock CL. Iodized salt in the prevention of goiter. Is it a safe measure for general use? *JAMA* 1926:86:1334–38.

145. Kohn LA. The midwestern American "epidemic" of iodine-induced hyperthyroidism in the 1920s. *Bull NY Acad Med* 1976:52:770–81.

146. Marine D. Endemic goiter: a problem in preventive medicine. *Ann Intern Med* 1954: 41:875–86.

147. U.S. Department of Agriculture. Household Food Consumption Survey, 1955: Dietary Levels of Households in the United States. Report no. 6:19. Washington, DC: Government Printing Office, 1957.

148. Matovinovic J, Trowbridge FL. North America. In: Stanbury JB, Hetzel BS, eds. Endemic Goiter and Endemic Cretinism: Iodine Nutrition in Health and Disease. New York: John Wiley and Sons, 1980.

149. Trowbridge FL, Hand KE, Nichaman MZ. Findings relating to goiter and iodine in the Ten-State Nutrition Survey. *Am J Clin Nutr* 1975:28:712–16.

150. Hollowell JG, Staehling NW, Hannon WH, Flanders DW, Gunter EW, Maberly GF, Braverman LE, Pino S, Miller DT, Garbe PL, DeLozier DM, Jackson RJ. Iodine nutrition in the United States. Trends and public health implications: iodine excretion data from National Health and Nutrition Examination Surveys I and III (1971–1974 and 1988–1994). *J Clin Endocrinol Metab* 1998:83:3401–08.

151. Cheadle WB. Clinical lecture on three cases of scurvy supervening on rickets in young children. *Lancet* 1878:2:685–87

152. Barlow T. On cases described as "acute rickets" which are probably a combination of scurvy and rickets, the scurvy being an essential, and the rickets a variable, element. *Med Chir Trans* 1883:66:159–220.

153. American Pediatric Society. The American Pediatric Society's collective investigation on infantile scurvy in North America. *Arch Pediatr* 1898:15:481–508.

154. Holst A, Frölich T. Experimental studies relating to ship beri-beri and scurvy. II. On the etiology of scurvy. *J Hygiene* 1907:7:634–71.

155. McCollum EV, Pitz W. The "vitamine" hypothesis and deficiency diseases. A study of experimental scurvy. *J Biol Chem* 1917:31:229–53.

156. Hess AF. The pathogenesis of infantile scurvy. *Trans Assoc Am Phys* 1918:33:367–86.

157. Hess AF, Fish M. Infantile scurvy: the blood, the blood-vessels and the diet. *Am J Dis Child* 1914:8:385–405.
158. Hess AF. Infantile scurvy. II. A new aspect of the symptomatology, pathology and diet. *JAMA* 1915:65:1003–6.
159. Hess AF. Recent advances in knowledge of scurvy and the anti-scorbutic vitamin. *JAMA* 1932:98:1429–33.
160. Aikman J. Infantile scurvy. *Arch Pediatr* 1921:38:41–51.
161. Faber HK. Infantile scurvy following the use of raw certified milk. *Am J Dis Child* 1921:21:401–5.
162. McCollum EV, Simmonds N. The American Home Diet: An Answer to the Ever Present Question What Shall We Have for Dinner. Detroit: Frederick C. Mathews Company, 1920.
163. Holt LE. Food, Health and Growth. A Discussion of the Nutrition of Children. New York: Macmillan Company, 1922.
164. Bell AJ. Feeding, Diet and the General Care of Children. A Book for Mothers and Trained Nurses, 2nd ed. Philadelphia: F.A. Davis Company, 1927.
165. Callow AB. Food & Health: An Introduction to the Study of Diet. London: Oxford University Press, 1928.
166. Svirbely JL, Szent-Györgyi A. The chemical nature of vitamin C. *Biochem J* 1932:26:865–70.
167. King CG, Waugh WA. Isolation and identification of vitamin C. *J Biol Chem* 1932:97:325–31.
168. Haworth WN, Hirst EL. Synthesis of ascorbic acid. *Chemistry and Industry* 1933:52:645–56.
169. Deaderick WH, Thompson L. The Endemic Diseases of the Southern States. Philadelphia: WB Saunders Company, 1916.
170. Stiles CW. Hookworm Disease (or ground-itch anemia): Its Nature, Treatment and Prevention. Treasury Department, Public Health and Marine-Hospital Service of the United States, Public Health Bulletin no. 32. Washington, DC: Government Printing Office, 1910.
171. Pawlowski ZS, Schad GA, Stott GJ. Hookworm Infection and Anemia: Approaches to Prevention and Control. Geneva: World Health Organization, 1991.
172. Dubini A. Nuovo verme intestinale umano (Agchylostoma duodenale), costituente un sesto genere dei Nematoidei proprii dell'uomo. *Ann Univ Med* (Milano) 1843:106:5–51.
173. Perroncito E. Osservazioni elmintologiche relative alla malattia sviluppatasi endemica negli operai del Gottardo. *Atti della R. Accademia dei Lincei* 1879–80 (3 ser.):7:381–433.
174. Stiles CW. A new species of hookworm (Uncinaria americana) parasitic in man. *Amer Med* 1902:3:777–78.
175. Porto Rico Anemia Commission. Report of the Permanent Commission for the Suppression of Uncinariasis in Porto Rico, 1906–1907. San Juan, PR: Bureau of Printing and Supplies, 1907.
176. Ashford BK, Gutiérrez Igaravidez P. Uncinariasis (hookworm disease) in Porto Rico: A Medical and Economic Problem. San Juan, Porto Rico, August 5, 1910. U.S. 61st Congress, 3d. Session, Senate Doc, 808. Washington, DC: Government Printing Office, 1911.
177. Stiles CW. Report Upon the Prevalence and Geographic Distribution of Hookworm Disease (Uncinariasis or Anchylostomiasis) in the United States. Hygienic Laboratory Bulletin no. 10. Washington, DC: Government Printing Office, 1903.
178. Stiles CW. Early history, in part esoteric, of the hookworm (uncinariasis) campaign in our southern United States. *J Parasitol* 1939:25:283–308.

179. Chandler AC. Hookworm Disease: Its Distribution, Biology, Epidemiology, Parasitology, Diagnosis, Treatment and Control. New York: Macmillan, 1929.
180. Rockefeller Sanitary Commission for the Eradication of Hookworm Disease. Organization, activities, and results up to December 31, 1910. Washington, DC: Offices of the Commission, 1910.
181. Rockefeller Sanitary Commission for the Eradication of Hookworm Disease. Fifth Annual Report for the year 1914. Washington, DC: Offices of the Commission, 1915.
182. Ettling J. The Germ of Laziness: Rockefeller Philanthropy and Public Health in the New South. Cambridge, MA: Harvard University Press, 1981.
183. Smillie WG, Augustine DL. Hookworm infestation. The effect of varying intensities on the physical condition of school children. Am J Dis Child 1926:31:151–68.
184. Smillie WG, Augustine DL. The effect of varying intensities of hookworm infestation upon the development of school children. South Med J 1926:19:19–28.
185. Smillie WG, Spencer CR. Mental retardation in school children infested with hookworms. J Educ Psychol 1926:17:314–21.
186. Waite JH, Neilson IL. Effects of hookworm infection on mental development of North Queensland schoolchildren. JAMA 1919:73:1877–79.
187. Strong EK. Effects of Hookworm Disease on the Mental and Physical Development of Children. Rockefeller Foundation. International Health Commission Publication no. 3. New York: Rockefeller Foundation, 1916.
188. Smillie WG. Control of hookworm disease in south Alabama. South Med J 1924:17: 494–99.
189. Jacocks WP. Hookworm infection rates in eleven southern states as revealed by resurveys in 1920–1923. JAMA 1924:82:1601–2.
190. Gloor RF, Breyley ER, Martinez IG. Hookworm infection in a rural Kentucky county. Am J Trop Med 1970:19:1007–9.
191. Sargent RG, Dudley BW, Fox AS, Lease EJ. Intestinal helminths in children in coastal South Carolina: a problem in southeastern United States. South Med J 1972:65:294–98.
192. Martin LK. Hookworm in Georgia. I. Survey of intestinal helminth infections and anemia in rural school children. Am J Trop Med Hyg 1972:21:919–29.
193. Martin LK. Hookworm in Georgia. II. Survey of intestinal helminth infections in members of rural households of southeastern Georgia. Am J Trop Med Hyg 1972:21:930–43.
194. McLaren DS, Frigg M. Sight and Life Manual on Vitamin A Deficiency Disorders (VADD), 2nd ed. Basel: Task Force Sight and Life, 2001.
195. Lunin N. Über die Bedeutung der anorganischen Salze für die Ernährung des Thieres. Zeitschr Physiol Chem 1881:5:31–39.
196. Socin CA. In welcher Form wird das Eisen resorbirt? Zeitschr physiol Chem 1891:15: 93–139.
197. Pekelharing CA. Over onze kennis van de waarde der voedingsmiddelen uit chemische fabrieken. Nederl Tijdschr Geneesk 1905:41:111–24.
198. Hopkins FG. Feeding experiments illustrating the importance of accessory factors in normal dietaries. J Physiol 1912:44:425–60.
199. Stepp W. Experimentelle Untersuchungen über die Bedeutung der Lipoide für die Ernährung. Zeitschr Biol 1911:57:136–70.
200. Wolf G, Carpenter KJ. Early research into the vitamins: the work of Wilhelm Stepp. J Nutr 1997:127:1255–59.
201. McCollum EV, Davis M. The necessity of certain lipins in the diet during growth. J Biol Chem 1913:15:167–75.
202. Osborne TB, Mendel LB. The relationship of growth to the chemical constituents of the diet. J Biol Chem 1913:15:311–26.

203. McCollum EV, Kennedy C. The dietary factors operating in the production of polyneuritis. *J Biol Chem* 1916:24:491–502.
204. Karrer P, Morf R, Schöpp K. Zur Kenntnis des Vitamins-A aus Fischtranen. *Helv Chim Acta* 1931:14:1036–40.
205. Karrer P, Morf R, Schöpp K. Zur Kenntnis des Vitamins-A aus Fischtranen II. *Helv Chim Acta* 1931:14:1431–36.
206. Holmes HN, Corbet RE. The isolation of crystalline vitamin A. *J Am Chem Soc* 1937:59:2042–47.
207. Moore T. The relation of carotin to vitamin A. *Lancet* 1929:2:380–81.
208. Green HN, Mellanby E. Vitamin A as an anti-infective agent. *Brit Med J* 1928:2:691–96.
209. Green HN, Pindar D, Davis G, Mellanby E: Diet as a prophylactic agent against puerperal sepsis. *Brit Med J* 1931:2:595–98.
210. Blackfan KD, Wolbach SB. Vitamin A deficiency in infants. A clinical and pathological study. *J Pediatr* 1933:3:679–706.
211. Semba RD. Vitamin A as "anti-infective" therapy, 1920–1940. *J Nutr* 1999:129:783–91.
212. Ellison JB. Intensive vitamin therapy in measles. *Brit Med J* 1932:2:708–11.
213. Semba RD. On Joseph Bramhall Ellison's discovery that vitamin A reduces measles mortality. *Nutrition* 2003:19:390–94.
214. Green HN, Pindar D, Davis G, Mellanby E. Diet as a prophylactic agent against puerperal sepsis. *Brit Med J* 1931:2:595–98.
215. Hess AF, Kirby DB. The incidence of xerophthalmia and night-blindness in the United States — a gauge of vitamin A deficiency. *Am J Publ Health* 1933:23:935–38.
216. Widmark E. Vitamin-A deficiency in Denmark and its results. *Lancet* 1924:1:1206–9.
217. Semba RD. The vitamin A and mortality paradigm: past, present, and future. *Scand J Nutr* 2001:45:46–50.
218. May CD, Blackfan KE, McCreary JF, Allen FH. Clinical studies of vitamin A in infants and in children. *Am J Dis Child* 1940:59:1167–84.
219. Lewis JM, Bodansky O, Haig C. Level of vitamin A in the blood as an index of vitamin A deficiency in infants and in children. *Am J Dis Child* 1941:62:1129–48.
220. Robinson A, Lesher M, Harrison AP, Moyer EZ, Gresock MC, Saunders C. Nutritional status of children. VI. Blood serum vitamin A and carotenoids. *J Am Diet Assoc* 1948:24:410–16.
221. Jeans PC, Zentmire Z. The prevalence of vitamin A deficiency among Iowa children. *JAMA* 1936:106:996–97.
222. Rapaport HG, Greenberg D. Avitaminosis A: incidence in a group of one hundred hospitalized children as measured by the biophotometer. *NY State J Med* 1941:879–80.
223. Council on Foods and Nutrition, American Medical Association. Fortification of foods with vitamins and minerals. *JAMA* 1939:113:681.
224. Bauernfeind JC, Arroyave G. Control of vitamin A deficiency by the nutrification of food approach. In: Bauernfeind JC, ed. Vitamin A Deficiency and Its Control. New York: Academic Press, 1986, 359–88.
225. Gunderson GW. National School Lunch Program Background and Development. Food and Nutrition Service publication no. 63. Washington, DC: Food and Nutrition Service, U.S. Department of Agriculture, 1971.
226. Food and Nutrition Board. Dietary Reference Intakes for Vitamin A, Vitamin K, Arsenic, Boron, Chromium, Copper, Iodine, Iron, Manganese, Molybdenum, Nickel, Silicon, Vanadium, and Zinc. Washington, DC: National Academy Press, 2001.
227. Ballew C, Bowman BA, Sowell AL, Gillespie C. Serum retinol distributions in residents of the United States: third National Health and Nutrition Examination Survey, 1988–1994. *Am J Clin Nutr* 2001:73:586–93.

228. Duitsman PK, Tanumihardjo SA, Cook L, Olson JA. Vitamin A status of low-income pregnant women in Iowa as assessed by the modified relative dose-response. *Ann N Y Acad Sci* 1993:678:344–45.

229. Spannaus-Martin DJ, Cook LR, Tanumihardjo SA, Duitsman PK, Olson JA. Vitamin A and vitamin E statuses of preschool children of socioeconomically disadvantaged families living in the midwestern United States. *Eur J Clin Nutr* 1997:51:864–69.

230. Wills L. Treatment of "pernicious anaemia of pregnancy" and "tropical anaemia" with special reference to yeast extract as a curative agent. *Brit Med J* 1931:1:1059–64.

231. Mitchell HK, Snell EE, Williams RJ. The concentration of "folic acid" [letter]. *J Am Chem Soc* 1941:63:2284–90.

232. Stokstad ELR. Some properties of growth factors for Lactobacillus casei. *J Biol Chem* 1943:149:573–74.

233. Stokstad ELR. Historical perspective on key advances in the biochemistry and physiology of folates. In: Picciano MF, Stokstad LR, Gregory JF III, eds. Folic Acid Metabolism in Health and Disease. New York: Wiley-Liss, 1990, 1–21.

234. Angier RB, Boothe JH, Hutchings BL, et al. Synthesis of a compound identical with the L. casei factor isolated from liver. *Science* 1945:102:227–28.

235. Food and Nutrition Board, Institute of Medicine. Dietary Reference Intakes for Thiamin, Riboflavin, Niacin, Vitamin B_6, Folate, Vitamin B_{12}, Pantothenic Acid, Biotin, and Choline. A report of the Standing Committee on the Scientific Evaluation of Dietary Reference Intakes and its Panel on Folate, Other B Vitamins, and Choline, and Subcommittee on Upper Reference Levels of Nutrients. Washington, DC: National Academy Press, 1998.

236. Czeizel AE. Folic acid-containing multivitamins and primary prevention of birth defects. In: Bendich A, Deckelbaum RJ, eds. Preventive Nutrition: The Comprehensive Guide for Health Professionals, 2nd ed. Totowa, NJ: Humana Press, 2001, 349–71.

237. Food and Drug Administration. Food standards: amendment of standards of identity for enriched grain products to require addition of folic acid. *Federal Register* 1996:61: 8781–97.

238. Jacques PF, Selhub J, Bostom AG, Wilson PWF, Rosenberg IH. The effect of folic acid fortification on plasma folate and total homocysteine concentrations. *N Engl J Med* 1999:340:1449–54.

239. Lawrence JM, Petitti DB, Watkins M, Umekubo MA. Trends in serum folate after food fortification. *Lancet* 1999:354:915–16.

240. Centers for Disease Control. Folate status in women of childbearing age — United States, 1999. *MMWR* 2000:49:962–65.

241. Mathews TJ, Honein MA, Erickson JD. Spina bifida and anencephaly prevalence — United States, 1991–2001. *MMWR* 2002:51 (RR13):9–11.

242. Cummings RO. The American and His Food. A History of Food Habits in the United States. Chicago: University of Chicago Press, 1941.

243. Apple RD. Vitamania: Vitamins in American Culture. New Brunswick, NJ: Rutgers University Press, 1996.

244. Surface FM, Bland RL. American Food in the World War and Reconstruction Period. Stanford, CA: Stanford University Press, 1931.

245. Kellogg V, Taylor AE. The Food Problem. New York: Macmillan, 1917.

246. U.S. Food Administration. Food and the War: A Textbook for College Classes. Boston: Houghton Mifflin, 1918.

247. U.S. Food Administration. Food Saving and Sharing: Telling How the Older Children of America May Help Save from Famine Their Comrades in Allied Lands Across the Sea. Garden City, NY: Doubleday, Page, 1918.

248. Beattie JH. The Farm Garden in the North. Farmers' Bulletin no. 937. Washington, DC: U.S. Department of Agriculture, 1918.

249. Thompson HC. Home Gardening in the South. Farmers' Bulletin no. 934. Washington, DC: U.S. Department of Agriculture, 1918.

250. Pack CL. The War Garden Victorious. Philadelphia: J. B. Lippincott, 1919.

251. National War Garden Commission. War Vegetable Gardening and the Home Storage of Vegetables. Washington, DC: National War Garden Commission, 1918.

252. Tucker D. Kitchen Gardening in America: A History. Ames: Iowa State University Press, 1993.

253. Black JD, Kiefer ME. Future Food and Agricultural Policy: A Program for the Next Ten Years. New York: McGraw-Hill, 1948.

254. Hunter R. Poverty. New York: Macmillan, 1904.

255. Spargo J. The Bitter Cry of the Children. New York: Macmillan, 1906.

256. Bryant LS. School Feeding. Its History and Practice at Home and Abroad. Philadelphia: J. B. Lippincott, 1913.

257. Duffy J. A History of Public Health in New York City, 1866–1966. New York: Russell Sage Foundation, 1974.

258. Roberts LJ. Nutrition Work with Children. Chicago: University of Chicago Press, 1927.

259. Emerson WRP. The malnourished child in the public school. *Boston Med Surg J* 1920: 182:655–58.

260. Emerson WRP. Nutrition clinics and classes: their organization and conduct. *Boston Med Surg J* 1919:181:139–41.

261. U.S. Senate Select Committee on Nutrition and Human Needs. Compilation of the National School Lunch Act and the Child Nutrition Act of 1966 with related provisions of law and authorities for commodities distribution. Washington, DC: Select Committee on Nutrition and Human Needs, 1974.

262. Pi-Sunyer FX, Laferrère B, Aronne LJ, Bray GA. Obesity — a modern-day epidemic. *J Clin Endocrinol Metab* 1999:84:3–7.

263. Mokdad AH, Bowman BA, Ford ES, Vinicor F, Marks JS, Koplan JP. The continuing epidemics of obesity and diabetes in the United States. *JAMA* 2001:286:1195–200.

264. Deckelbaum RJ, Williams CL. Childhood obesity: the health issue. *Obesity Res* 2001:9 (suppl 4):239S–243S.

Suggested Reading

Apple RD. Vitamania: Vitamins in American Culture. New Brunswick, NJ: Rutgers University Press, 1996.

Etheridge EW. The Butterfly Caste: A Social History of Pellagra in the South. Westport, CT: Greenwood Press, 1972.

Ettling J. The Germ of Laziness: Rockefeller Philanthropy and Public Health in the New South. Cambridge, MA: Harvard University Press, 1981.

McKeown T. The Role of Medicine: Dream, Mirage, or Nemesis? Princeton, NJ: Princeton University Press, 1979.

9

The More Things Change: A Historical Perspective on the Debate over Vitamin Advertising in the United States

RIMA D. APPLE

Vitamins are mystical and magical. Their popularity has been evident from the time the micronutrients were discovered, named, and championed in the scientific literature and the popular press in the early twentieth century. The dramatic growth in vitamin sales demonstrates unequivocally the public's confidence in micronutrients to restore and maintain health. Vitamin sales amounted to slightly more than $12 million in 1931; by 1939 this figure had increased more than sixfold to over $82.7 million. Its meteoritic rise continued. By 1942 sales topped $130 million.[1] In the early 1990s, we spent more than $4 billion on vitamin supplements. Today vitamins represent a more than $17.7 billion industry.[2,3]

To some, the growth of the vitamin industry was a threat to the general population's health and well-being. Public health leaders, including officials at the Food and Drug Administration (FDA) and officers of the American Medical Association (AMA), denounced vitamin promotions as offering false hopes. They warned that little evidence existed to document the power of vitamins, except in clear cases of vitamin deficiency. They also claimed that vitamins were a waste of the consumer's money. With no conclusive scientific data demonstrating the effectiveness of vitamin supplementation, these products were at least useless and at worst harmful, they argued. Opponents of vitamin supplementation believed they were protecting the consumer's health and the consumer's wallet.[1]

Despite vehement arguments from physicians and other public health officers, the popularity of vitamin supplementation has grown steadily over the years. At the same time, within the industry, the focus has shifted from one micronutrient to another over the years as health conditions and social issues have changed. In the 1930s, there was particular concern about vitamin D intake. Rickets was spreading throughout war-ravaged Europe, children needed to be protected from this vitamin-deficiency condition. Consequently, manufacturers rushed to advertise that their products were vitamin D enriched (Fig. 9.1). In the early 1940s, promotions turned to vitamin B_1, which promised to enhance the health and well-being of patriotic Americans. As with

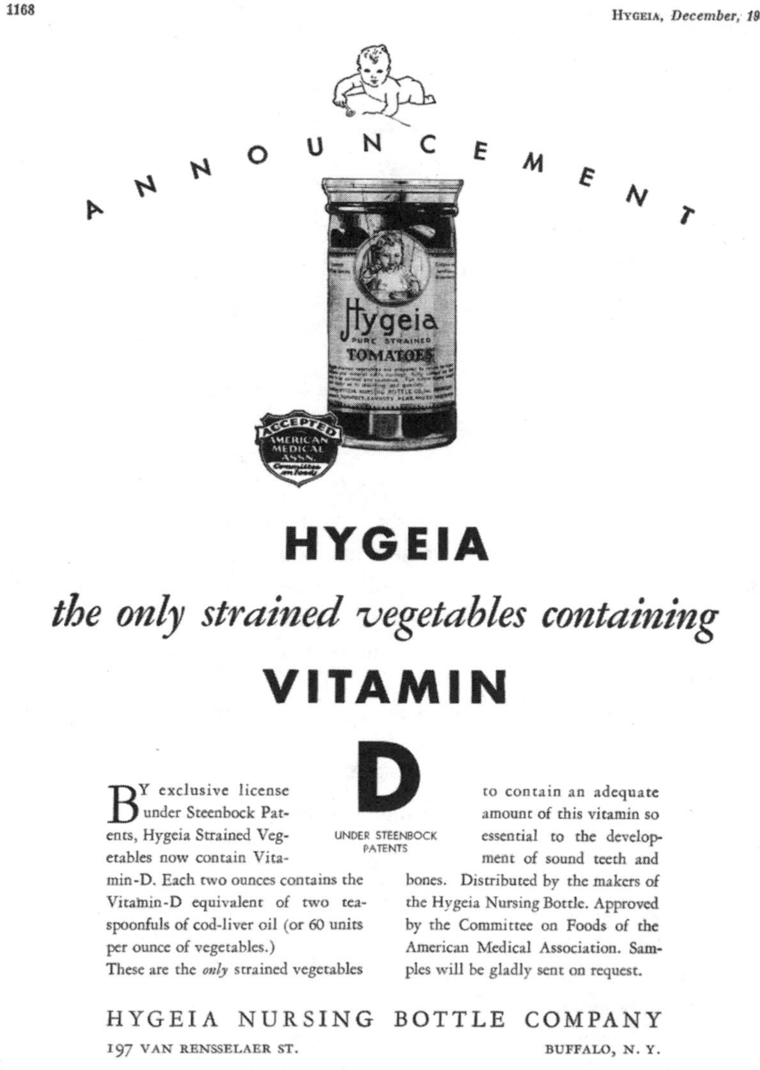

Figure 9.1. Hygeia advertisement, 1931.

vitamin D, concern for the B$_1$ content of the American diet stimulated practical efforts to mitigate potential problems, and food enrichment programs in the United States expanded significantly as an important adjunct to public health. In later decades other micronutrients came center stage. In the late 1960s and 1970s much attention was paid to Linus Pauling and his promotion of the power of vitamin C;[1,4] today the spotlight is on the vaunted power of antioxidants.[5]

Though the focus of concern changed over the decades, several overarching themes have remained constant in the history of vitamin supplementation in the United States. Two in particular keep reappearing: insurance and beauty. Vitamins were, and are, vitally important to maintaining health, but how to be certain one's diet contains sufficient quantities of these critical micronutrients? Supplementation was the ready answer, according to the popular news media and advertisements, despite the disclaimers of public health officials and medical practitioners. Press and advertising campaigns reminded consumers that beauty depended on good health and assured them that they could secure a healthy, lovely, fresh appearance through the use of vitamin supplementation. Emerging in the interwar period, the themes of beauty and insurance were reinterpreted and reinforced through successive eras, reverberating in the contemporary promotion of the cancer fighting potential and beautifying effects of antioxidants.

It is an often-stated maxim that the basis of beauty is good health. Enterprising pharmacists often have employed this idea to promote the general sale of vitamin supplements. Rationalizing that "women buy vitamins for beauty as well as for health because they regard the two things as inseparable," a pharmacist in Lincoln, Nebraska, used an aggressive vitamin campaign to increase store traffic in 1940.[6] In another successful promotion a few years later, a druggist in Missouri placed vitamins on the cosmetic counter and boosted cosmetic sales and vitamin sales with a war theme that "Beauty is your duty."[7] In addition to general good health, other vitamin products promised more specific "beautifying" effects.

In the 1930s, when the print media were filled with alerts about the need for vitamin D in the American diet, much of this discussion centered on children. However, the question of the vitamin D requirements for adults received significant attention as well.[8] Advertisers were not oblivious to the potential markets this created. Soon products such as "Vita-Ray: Vitamin all purpose cream" were widely publicized in the national press (see Fig. 9.2), with claims that the work of physicians and scientists had demonstrated the beneficial effects of vitamin D enriched face cream:

> If you use just one jar of Vita-Ray Cream feeding the wonderful sunshine Vitamin D right through to the tiny capillaries which carry the blood that nourishes the skin, your skin will look noticeably younger. Lines and wrinkles will begin to grow dim and become smoothed out.[9]

The belief that vitamin D contributed to healthy skin, and thus beauty, was not limited to advertisers of vitamin-enriched creams and soaps. In the June 1938 issue of the popular women's magazine *Good Housekeeping*, the bold headline "Now You Can Feed Your Skin" announced an article by Walter H. Eddy, director of the Good Housekeeping Bureau. Eddy was a familiar source of information for readers, producing a monthly column that frequently employed highly dramatic language to announce

BECAUSE <u>SHE</u> RISKED AN UGLY BURN . .

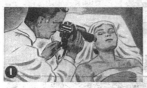

HER DOCTOR knew that too intense x-ray . . . like age . . . often "dries out" *cholesterin*—the element that supplies Vitamin D to the capillaries which nourish the skin. But how to *replace* Vitamin D?

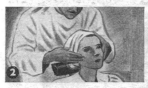

THE DOCTOR HAD AN IDEA. "Suppose," he reasoned, "we combine Vitamin D with *cholesterin*, which skin *can* absorb. Perhaps this life-giving Vitamin D will be *absorbed with it* to revitalize tissues."

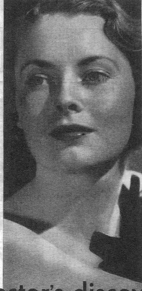

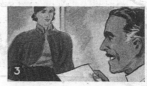

HIS REASONING WAS SOUND. Harmful effects of x-ray were reduced! But something else happened! The skin, *wherever vitamin cream was applied*, became younger — freer from dryness and lines.

GOOD HOUSEKEEPING TESTED VITA-RAY. University doctors confirmed amazing records. Typical microphotos, as above, show change in 28 days. Read below how Vita-Ray can *noticeably* beautify your skin.

Her Boston doctor's discovery can make

your skin more beautiful

AT LAST A WAY HAS BEEN FOUND to feed Vitamin D direct through the pores . . . with Vita-Ray Cream. And results have astonished doctors who tested this vitamin cream on "normal skins," "dry" skins — skins of every type.

From the first day complexions took on a new delicacy. Pores were restored to normal size. Skin lost its dryness. Even the exacting tests of microphotographs revealed an amazing change. *The skin was actually growing young again.*

Praised by Beauty Editors

Beauty editors of leading publications, invited to view these experiments, commented upon the amazing record. Good Housekeeping tested and approved Vita-Ray Cream, authorized the use of its seal.

Invited to Hall of Science . . .

Then, a crowning triumph! Vita-Ray, because of its vitamin research, was invited to sponsor the vitamin exhibit in the Hall of Science at A Century of Progress. And this scientific discovery has already become the most popular cream sold in many outstanding stores.

To the eye, Vita-Ray is just a delightful white cream. The great difference is that Vita-Ray, *and Vita-Ray alone*, contains 750 A. D. M. A. Vitamin D units . . . to make your skin grow fresher, younger, lovelier.

If you use just one jar of Vita-Ray Cream . . . your skin will look *noticeably younger.* It will feed the wonderful sunshine Vitamin D through to the tiny capillaries—the sole source of nourishment for the skin.

Soon, any enlarged pores you have will become smaller. Your complexion will take on a new softness. If your skin has a tendency to dryness it will become firmer and fresher and younger again. Lines and wrinkles will begin to grow dim and become smoothed out. What Vita-Ray *has done* for others it *can* for you.

Vita-Ray also contains special cleansing ingredients and it is used just as you would any other cream. After your pores are thoroughly cleansed apply another thin film and leave it on as a powder base. Thousands of women have found that Vita-Ray is the one *all-purpose* cream for day and night. And it is *one* cream scientifically tested to make the skin grow younger again.

Seeing is Believing, Try Vita-Ray Under this Inviting Offer!

Only the most outstanding stores have been appointed to sell Vita-Ray. If your favorite store hasn't yet been selected — mail coupon with $1.00 for a 30-day supply. Unless you begin immediately to find the freshness and beauty which Vita-Ray gives, we will refund your money without question or delay.

Vita-Ray
vitamin ALL PURPOSE CREAM

March 1935 Good Housekeeping

Figure 9.2. Vita-Ray advertisement, 1935.

the latest discoveries in nutritional science. Eddy's article cited several studies that described how vitamins, through the medium of cod-liver oil, "can enter the body via the skin in quantities sufficient to produce their health-giving benefits."[10] Not limiting his praise to cod-liver oil, Eddy declared that the Good Housekeeping Bureau determined that vitamin-enriched face creams, too, were potent and affected skin health.

There were, however, those who disagreed with this prescription of vitamin D for the skin. Federal agencies such as the Federal Trade Commission (FTC) and the Food and Drug Administration, as well as publications such as *Hygeia*, the health journal produced by the American Medical Association for nonprofessionals, attacked these advertisements as baseless and even forced some of the companies to modify their claims.[11–13] In addition, though the Good Housekeeping Bureau portrayed itself as an impartial, scientific investigative agency, consumer activists and other critics frequently challenged this representation.[14,15] So, on the one hand, a widely read author in a popular women's magazine affirmed the beautifying effects of vitamin face cream; on the other hand, government officials and medical authorities denounced these products as shams, a situation guaranteed to spread the controversy through the popular media.

The controversy over vitamin D enriched cream was an indication of how public the debate was. No minor skirmish between the industry and public health officials; the debate permeated the popular media and popular culture, influencing how people thought about the health claims of vitamin producers. The dispute was so well known that movie writers employed it as a shorthand to define their characters and capitalism in the RKO film *Beauty for the Asking*. The 1939 movie stars Lucille Ball as Jean Russell, a hard-working entrepreneur. Russell develops her own face cream in the kitchen of her New York apartment. She hires a Madison Avenue advertising executive to help her market the product. Together they devise a marketing plan that involves changing Ball's name to Jeanne de la Varelle, designing a whole line of cosmetics and establishing a "salon de beauté" to promote the line. Some of Russell's customers resist the new products and want what is familiar. One woman insists the salon use "turtle oil cream." As she tells Russell, "turtle oil must be good. It is the most expensive cream on the market." Russell's simple retort is a telling reflection of the cosmetic industry's hype: "Well, it's not as expensive as ours." From this, it is clear that Ball's character, the screenwriters, and the audience understand how the cosmetic industry works. As this and other scenes show, she certainly is not above extravagant promotion.

But later in the film a discussion over vitamin-enriched face creams shows the viewers that she does draw the line at false advertising. Russell is a shrewd business woman, but she has moral stature, unlike her partner, Denny Williams (played by Patrick Knowles), who is interested only in money. He is willing to utilize any claim, no matter how empty, to encourage sales. During a marketing meeting, Williams informs Russell that he has just heard about a new product—"vitaminized cream." He suggests that they add vitamins to their products as well. But this is where Russell draws the line: "No, it's all right to charge women eight times what we should; they won't buy if we don't," she concedes. "But that's as far as I'll go." She considers vitamin claims with face creams to be cheating. To Williams the solution is simple: add vitamins to the cream, then their claims will be truthful. But Russell will not agree, patiently explaining that "only vitamin D can be absorbed by the skin. We can't get enough of that into the cream to do any good." Because of their approach to the issue of vitamins in face cream, we know that Russell is a sharp, but "ethical" entrepreneur, while Williams is sleazy. The fact that the screenwriters employed a current controversy to describe their characters with just a few lines suggests that the film's viewers were quite familiar with the debate over "beautifying" vitamins. The idea of vitamins for beauty, though not accepted by all, was current in American culture.

This connection between vitamins and beauty appeared time and time again in promotions for various products. For instance, Walter Eddy also supported the use of vitamin-enriched soaps. The AMA's *Hygeia* rejected this claim as well. The Federal Trade Commission evidently concurred. In May 1938 it issued a complaint against some manufacturers of vitamin-fortified soaps; in September 1941, it ordered manufacturers to cease and desist claims of the "beneficial value upon the skin by reason of [the soap's] vitamin content."[12]

Vitamins Plus, another, and apparently more successful commercial venture that coupled vitamin supplementation and beauty, was promoted as a treatment for "avitaminosis" (see Fig. 9.3). Introduced late in 1937, this combination of vitamins, liver extract, and iron was sold as a beauty aid through department stores.[1] The target audience for these vitamins, as for so many other vitamin products, was women. In its first 6 months alone, Vitamins Plus spent $150,000 in magazine advertising and $30,000 in newspaper promotions matched by $30,000 of department store funds.

This product's primary advertising claims centered on its role as a beauty aid, though the company also proudly announced that Vitamins Plus had been purchased by the Byrd Antarctic Expedition.[16] The promise of Vitamins Plus was both more extensive than those for vitamin D creams and soaps, and more specific. Advertisements emphasized the positive benefits of the product and enjoined women to "Wake up and enjoy life . . . be happily healthy the year 'round . . . With Vitamins Plus, the complete vitamin routine."[17]

In order to attract consumers with the income to purchase Vitamins Plus, the company consciously sought to dissociate "avitaminosis" from malnutrition and poverty. Its brochure, "Beauty Building from A to G,"[18] maintains that the condition was not restricted to "poor people" and demonstrates this point with a testimonial about a woman whose circumstances led her doctor to diagnose avitaminosis.

> People would meet her on the street and say "You just don't look a bit well." And it was true. Her make-up wouldn't stay put. Her hair came all out of curl ten minutes after it was set. No use to put on nail polish . . . it just chipped right off again.[18]

The solution in this sad situation was, of course, Vitamins Plus, available at the cosmetic counters of department stores throughout the United States at $2.75 for 1 month's supply.

Though the concept of "beautifying" vitamins appeared in magazines, advertisements, and even Hollywood films, it was not universally accepted. The FTC put a halt to vitamin-enriched soaps. In the case of Vitamins Plus, this supposedly miraculous product raised questions in the minds of some consumers, who asked the Food and Drug Administration if the product was "good and worth the $2.75." According to the FDA, many of the claims for the product "have no adequate scientific basis" and "are not supported by the consensus of reliable medical opinion."[19] The agency felt, though,

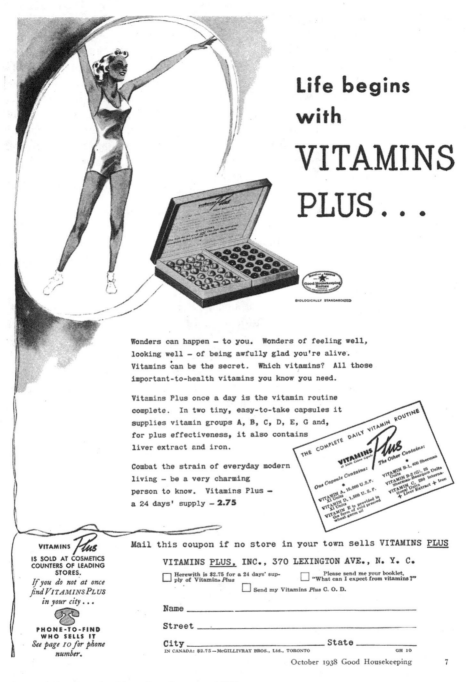

Figure 9.3. Vitamins Plus advertisement, 1938.

that given the extent of its regulatory powers in the 1930s, it did "not have a satisfactory basis for legal action."[20]

Other queries came to the FDA from the Federal Trade Commission, the agency charged with regulating advertising in the United States. At the request of the FTC, the FDA commented on many of the Vitamins Plus claims, stating unequivocally, for instance: "We are familiar with no scientific evidence which indicates that deficiency of vitamins has any bearing of whether make-up will stay put, curls remain in the hair, or nail polish adheres to the finger nails."[21,22] Soon after, Vitamins Plus, under a stipulation with the FTC, agreed to halt promotions informing consumers that cloudy, lusterless eyes were due to a vitamin A deficiency, that vitamin in-take determined the staying power of cosmetics, and that vitamin B removed lactic acid from the blood stream and consequently eliminated fatigue.[23,24] Despite this setback, Vitamins Plus enjoyed a long life. Sales statistics are unavailable, but popular culture attests to its prominence. By late 1938 in Manhattan, a prestigious hotel, the Waldorf-Astoria, had placed the pills on its breakfast menu, and a popular nightclub, the Stork Club, stocked Vitamins Plus along with cigarettes and cigars, a situation recorded in a *New Yorker* cartoon.[25-27] Moreover, the product appeared on store shelves until at least 1960.[28]

The marketing of other vitamin products—Retin-A being a recent example—produced similar accounts in the historical record. And, today, of course, the media are filled with stories and advertisements promoting the importance and "beautifying" effects of antioxidants, particularly in skin care. We are bombarded with headlines like "Forever Young?", "Face Food," and "Stop Aging Now"; with articles detailing the devastating effects of free radicals and extolling the miraculous virtues of vitamin A, vitamin C, vitamin E, beta-carotene, and the like; and with grand promises—for example, that antioxidants will enable us to develop suntans healthfully. We are urged to eat foods rich in antioxidants, supplement our diets with vitamin pills, and slather our faces with antioxidant-rich creams and moisturizers. The connection between beauty and vitamins continues to be a dominant theme in the history of vitamin supplementation.[5,29-32]

Another significant theme explicitly woven into the history of vitamins in American culture is the promise of optimal health through supplementation. Since at least the 1930s, vitamin supplementation has been promoted as a form of health insurance. The history of vitamin supplementation developed from the initial discovery of vitamins, through announcements about the curative and preventative value of emerging micronutrients, through the development of methods of extraction and synthesis. During these years, the question most commonly asked by researchers, clinicians, and the public was: How will I know that I am getting enough of each vitamin? From the earliest years, the response was "eat a well-balanced diet." But at the same time, the media were filled with stories that many, if not most, Americans were not eating a well-balanced diet. Worse yet, newspapers and magazines reported, the foods we ate were deficient in necessary vitamins and minerals because of modern modes of food production and food processing that stripped out critical micronutrients before the food arrived at our tables. The earliest vitamin products were promoted in the 1920s and 1930s as crucial adjuncts to the depleted American diet. Critically, this was not only an advertising ploy. Nutrition writers too debated this point and, though not as committed as manufacturers to supplementation, they did acknowledge the possible benefits of vitamin products.

By 1939, Walter Eddy of *Good Housekeeping*, used the metaphor of automobile insurance to promote the use of vitamin supplementation.[33] Explaining that researchers have developed minimum standards for daily vitamin intake, standards sufficient to "prevent active, physical manifestations of disease," he cautioned that what we don't know is how much is needed for "optimal or buoyant health." Furthermore, he noted that most people do not eat the recommended amounts of fruits, vegetables, and dairy products; therefore, he claimed, "vitamin deficiency is fairly common" in the United States. He had a solution to this conundrum of how to ensure sufficient vitamin intake: "There is one way of being on the safe side, however—that is to add a sufficiently large factor of safety to the average minimum vitamin requirement to cover possible contingencies. That's the insurance method, and it's being widely practiced in dietetics today." By analogy, Eddy asserted, though $10,000 to $20,000 of liability auto insurance may be all you need, still $100,000 to $300,000 is safer. "Therefore," he concluded, "take your vitamin concentrates, increase your vitamin-rich foods, if you will. You are following a perfectly safe dietary insurance program."[33]

Beginning in the 1940s, the insurance concept attained even greater currency through the well-publicized advertising campaigns of Miles Laboratory for its popular product line of One-A-Day Brand vitamin pills (Fig. 9.4). The focus of One-A-Day's promotional campaigns was the vitamin tablet's role as health "insurance." The company sought to use its labels and its advertising to create an earnest image of thoughtful health guidance: "Don't tuck the bottle away in your medicine cabinet. Don't take the tablets at irregular intervals or only when you are feeling ill. One-A-Day brand Vitamin A and D tablets are food supplements, and should be taken one a day—every day—preferably with a meal. You will not get the greatest benefits from ONE-A-DAY tablets unless you take them regularly."

Intending to avoid a repetition of the protracted dispute Miles had had with the Food and Drug Administration over earlier products,[34] the company discussed the creation of One-A-Day labels with the agency even before the product was on the market shelves. FDA officials objected to the label,[35] claiming that it "implie[d] that it is necessary in order to fully protect the user from vitamin A and D deficiencies that the product be taken every day. This does not appear to be in accord with generally accepted scientific opinions."[36] In other words, the Miles presentation suggested that consumers risked vitamin deficiencies unless they took One-A-Day every day. The FDA officials found this counsel unacceptable and false. They consistently maintained that the general American diet contained sufficient sources of all the vitamins needed for a healthful diet. They balked at any suggestion that vitamin supplementation was necessary and that the American diet was insufficient without daily vitamin supplementation. They insisted that Americans could and should get vitamins from food and not waste their money on vitamin supplements.

Yet the idea that the American diet was not necessarily sufficient and that therefore the consumer needed the assurance of a daily vitamin tablet was the very rationale for vitamin supplementation. Even more significant, it was the hallmark of Miles's One-A-Day campaign. Consequently, Miles faced the problem of recommending

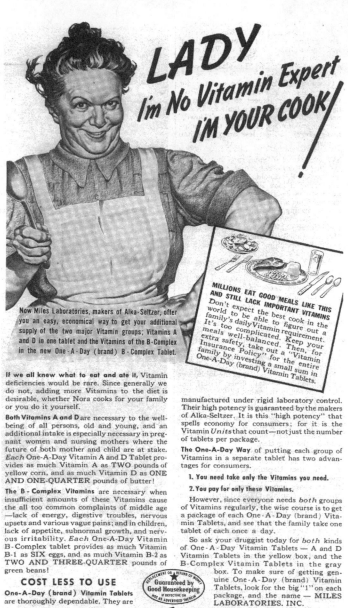
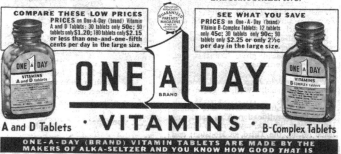

Figure 9.4. Miles One-A-Day advertisement, 1941.

202

daily vitamin tablets in a way that the Food and Drug Administration, a group adamantly opposed to vitamin supplementation, would find acceptable. This it did by skillful indirection: rather than instructing consumers to take the pills regularly, the labels gently urged them to remember their daily One-A-Day. The new inserts read: "One-A-Day (brand) Vitamins A and D Tablets furnish an easy, inexpensive way to insure that you get enough of these essential Vitamins. Why not put the bottle on the breakfast table as a pleasant reminder to make taking a tablet every day a part of your daily routine?"[37]

In booklets and in advertisements, over the decades, Miles consistently drove home the message "Now we know how essential Vitamins are in our everyday life." With One-A-Day, consumers need not "risk the diseases caused by [vitamin] deficiency."[38,39] (See Fig. 9.4.)

This became a common refrain in the promotional material of the vitamin industry.[40,1] And it was reflected to some extent by the consuming public. Typical was one Pittsburgh woman who wrote the FDA, defending her use of vitamins. "Yes, we have vitamin bottles on our breakfast table," she wrote, "But just as some days my family does not eat their 'standard American diet,' so too on many days I forget to pass out the vitamins. I think it evens itself out in the long run."[41] She did not see vitamins as always necessary, but rather as insurance for times when family members might not be eating well.

Despite the longevity of the "insurance" motif among manufacturers and consumers, groups and agencies such as the American Medical Association and the Food and Drug Administration through the decades steadily insisted that the American diet was sufficient and that Americans did not need megadoses, or even multivitamins, to maintain their health. They claimed that there was no evidence to document the need for vitamin supplements. Those who did promote supplementation were frequently labeled as "health nuts," or misguided citizens, or more interested in monetary gain than public health.[1]

In the new century, the vitamin debates continue and the idea of vitamin supplementation as insurance finds new proponents: researchers and clinicians. Most significantly, contemporary proponents of vitamin supplements, especially supplementation with antioxidants, typically do not claim scientific certainty. Contemporary advocates are more likely to appraise today's research and concur with Jeffrey Blumberg's assessment,[42] that there is "enough evidence already on which to base a judgment that the potential benefits of supplements will outweigh by a large degree the potential risks."[43–46]

Articles in the popular press of the late twentieth century further reinforced the belief in the power, even the necessity, of vitamin supplementation for optimal health. Earlier advocates of vitamin pills had confidently asserted that we needed these dietary adjuncts to ward off disease and secure optimal health, and some contemporary writers are equally confident. Asks one bold headline in the popular women's magazine *Glamour*: "Do you need to take supplements?" The reply is unambiguous: "The smart answer is yes." The author's rationale is not unique to the late twentieth century: "It's theoretically possible to get all the nutrients you need from food. But the fact is most women don't. In other words, vitamin supplementation is 'nutritional insurance.' "[47]

More common in the popular press of the 1990s are authors who equivocate, but ultimately prescribe vitamin supplements. Headlined queries such as "Can these pills make you live longer?" are answered with a cautious "Maybe" and careful conclusions that "many physicians, believing that the potential benefits [of vitamin supplementation] outweigh the possible risks, say go ahead and take them."[48]

In the popular press of the twenty-first century, there is less ambiguity. Physicians, nutritionists, and others committed to improving the health of the American public continue to point out the difficulties in interpreting contemporary research about the need for and the effects of vitamin supplementation. They emphasize the dangers in generalizing from limited studies. Yet, the popular press shows little such equivocation in articles that describe conditions that can be prevented with the conscientious use of vitamin supplements. Commonly, popular health writers insist: "Most of us don't get enough of the vitamins we need. . . . Some general guidelines: Take a multivitamin . . . every day with meals."[49–51] They admit that the "proof of the benefits of multivitamins is still far from certain" and that more research is needed to rigorously evaluate the effects of vitamin supplementation. And yet, they typically conclude: "At some point, while researchers work on figuring out where the truth lies, it just makes sense to say that potential benefit [of vitamin supplementation] outweighs the cost.[52] Now, even the Food and Drug Administration has modified its long-standing opposition to vitamin supplementation, titling a 2002 article in its popular magazine *FDA Consumer* "Tips for the Savvy Supplement User" and informing readers that "the choice to use a dietary supplement can be a wise decision that provides health benefits."[53]

Though the focus may change over the decades—from vitamin D, to vitamin B_1, to vitamin C, to antioxidants—significant themes keep recurring in the history of nutrition. Are vitamin supplements efficacious? Are they necessary? So far, definitive answers to these questions consistently elude us. But lack of certainty does little to dim the claims and counter-claims that flood the public media and advertising campaigns. It is both instructive and sobering to realize that these contemporary nutritional and public health concerns are not unique to our era. These historical patterns alert us to scientific and emotional factors—the concern for the adequacy of the American diet, the quest for physical health and beauty—that shape public debates over vitamin supplementation today, and in all likelihood, will continue to in the future.

References

1. Apple RD. Vitamania: Vitamins in American Culture. News Brunswick, NJ: Rutgers University Press, 1996.
2. Gorman C. Vitamin overload? *Time*, 10 November 1997, 84.
3. Vitamins, minerals, and supplements: North American Retail Market Review (Theta Reports). Available at: url: http://www.marketresearch.com/map/prod/932761.html. Accessed 9 February 2004.
4. Richards E. Vitamin C and Cancer: Medicine or Politics? New York: St. Martin's Press, 1991.
5. Forever young? *Mademoiselle*, October 1994, 56.
6. Cosmetics, vitamins, hosiery double women traffic in year. *Drug Topics*, 3 June 1940, 35.
7. Vitamins on cosmetic bar link good looks to health. *Drug Topics*, 1 May 1944, 47.
8. Eddy WH. Milk plus: that is what you get when you buy milk with vitamin D added to it. *Good Housekeeping*, May 1934, 98, 136.

9. Vita-Ray advertisement. *Good Housekeeping,* February 1935, 232.

10. Eddy WH. Now you can feed your skin. *Good Housekeeping*, June 1938, 80.

11. Vitamin ads under fire. *Business Week*, 27 November 1937, 49–50.

12. Fishbein M. Modern medical charlatans, II: Vitamin follies. *Hygeia,* 16 February 1938, 115.

13. Miller LM. The vitamin follies. *Hygeia*, 16 November 1938, 1004–5.

14. Lamb RD. American Chamber of Horrors. New York: Farrar & Rinehart, 1936.

15. Kallet A, Schlink FJ. 100,000,000 Guinea Pigs: Dangers in Everyday Foods, Drugs, and Cosmetics. New York: Grosset & Dunlap, 1933.

16. Vitamin Plus advertisement. *Drug Topics*, 22 January 1940, 9.

17. Vitamins Plus file. Food and Drug Administration Archives, RG88 Acc# 63A292, box 480.

18. Beauty building from A to G. Vitamins Plus file. Food and Drug Administration Archives, RG88 Acc# 63A292, box 480.

19. WRH to Durrett JJ, 1938 January 8. Vitamins Plus file. Food and Drug Administration Archives, RG88 Acc# 63A292, box 480.

20. Memo from FDA Drug Division to Chief, Easter Division, 19 August 1938. Vitamins Plus file. Food and Drug Administration Archives, RG88 Acc# 63A292, box 480.

21. Dunbar PB. Memo to the Federal Trade Commission, 11 January 1939. Vitamins Plus file. Food and Drug Administration Archives, RG88 Acc# 63A292, box 480.

22. Davidson WF to Dunbar PB, 10 December 1938. Vitamins Plus file. Food and Drug Administration Archives, RG88 Acc# 63A292, box 480.

23. Trade Commission cases. *New York Times*, 24 October 1940.

24. Stipulation (02652). Vitamins Plus file. Food and Drug Administration Archives, RG88 Acc# 63A292, box 480.

25. Vitamin vistas. *Tide* 1938:12:22–23.

26. Vitamins. *Tide* 1938:12:9–11.

27. Again, vitamins. *Tide* 1938:12:11–12.

28. R.E.D. to FDA 4 February 1960. Vitamins Plus file. Food and Drug Administration Archives, RG88 Acc# 63A292, box 480.

29. Astley A. Face food. *Vogue,* January 1996,140–41.

30. Carper J. Stop aging now. *Ladies' Home Journal*, September 1995, 154–57.

31. Gilbert S, Is it possible to get a safe suntan? *New York Times,* 17 July 1997, C.2.

32. Tannen M. Hope springs nocturnal. *New York Times Magazine*, 5 November 1995, 62–63.

33. Eddy WH. How many vitamins a day do we need? *Good Housekeeping*, January 1939, 55.

34. Cray WC. Miles, 1884–1984: A Centennial History. Englewood Cliffs, NJ: Prentice-Hall, 1984, 40–46.

35. Memorandum. 4 June 1941. FDA Archives, Acc# 63A292, AF 13007.

36. Larrick to Clissold. 5 December 1940. FDA Archives, Acc# 63A292.

37. Attachment to letter from MR Stephens, Chief, St. Louis Station, FDA, to Chief, Central District," 4 February 1942. FDA Archives, Acc# 63A292, AF13007.

38. Miles One-A-Day advertisement. *Parents' Magazine*, December 1941, 80.

39. Year 'round: One-A-Day vitamins for your whole family. Elkhart, IN: Miles Laboratories, [1945]. Miles Laboratories Archive.

40. Vitamin Information Bureau. Vitamins and your health. New York, 1970. Files concerning Nutrition research and FDA controversy, 1961–1970. Miles Laboratories Archives Acc# 8446a.

41. N ["Mrs. WA"] to FDA. 15 October 1972. FDA Archives, Acc# 88-78-19, o51.18.

42. Brody JE. Personal health. *New York Times*, 22 May 1996, C.11.

43. New AR. Vitamins: health or hype? *Better Homes and Gardens*, March 1995, 56.

44. Packer L, Sullivan JL. The promise of antioxidants. *Saturday Evening Post*, January/February 1995, 50.
45. Chartrand S. With winter a whisper away, the question is how much vitamin C should a person take each day? *New York Times*, 7 October 1996, D.2.
46. Brody JE. Vitamin E may enhance immunity, study finds. *New York Times*, 7 May 1997, A.16.
47. Howkins MA. The big vitamin debate: Do supplements help or hurt? *Glamour*, August 1994, 204–7.
48. Murray M. Can these pills make you live longer? *Reader's Digest* September 1994,19.
49. Take your vitamins. *Parade Magazine*, 22 September 2002, 23.
50. Will a vitamin a day keep the doctor away? *Health Letter* (Public Citizen Health Research Group) 2002: 18:3–4.
51. Folate and arteries. *Nutrition Action* 2004:31:12.
52. The great multivitamin debate. *Time*, 31 December 2001/7 January 2002, 150.
53. Tips for the savvy supplement user. *FDA Consumer* 2002:36:17–21.

Suggested Reading

Apple RD. Vitamania: Vitamins in American Culture. New Brunswick, NJ: Rutgers University Press, 1996.

Hilts PJ. Protecting America's Health: The FDA, Business, and One Hundred Years of Regulation. New York: Alfred A. Knopf, 2003.

Levenstein H. Paradox of Plenty: A Social History of Eating in Modern America. New York: Oxford University Press, 1993.

Nestle M. Food Politics: How the Food Industry Influences Nutrition and Health. Berkeley: University of California Press, 2002.

PART V

OCCUPATIONAL HEALTH

10

Safer, Healthier Workers: Advances in Occupational Disease and Injury Prevention

ANTHONY ROBBINS

PHILIP J. LANDRIGAN

This chapter will examine the epidemiology of occupational disease and injury in the United States during the twentieth century. We shall present data on changing rates and patterns of work-related illness and offer explanations for the successes that were achieved in occupational health as well as for failures in prevention. We shall introduce heroes whose work substantially advanced the science of occupational medicine and who contributed to major reductions in incidence of work-related illness.

Worker Health and Safety in the Twentieth Century

During the twentieth century, the American workforce faced many types of job-related injuries and illnesses, ranging from exposures to hazardous chemical agents to extreme emotional stress and trauma. Such exposures and experiences can have numerous negative health outcomes that can manifest immediately or after varying periods of time.

The Nature and Costs of Occupational Disease

In the United States, an estimated 6500 job-related deaths from injuries, 13.2 million nonfatal injuries, 60,300 deaths from disease, and 862,200 illnesses occur annually.[1] The range of illnesses caused by work is broad and can involve every organ system. Diseases linked classically to occupation include lung cancer and malignant

209

mesothelioma in workers exposed to asbestos; cancer of the bladder in aniline dye workers; pneumoconiosis in coal miners; leukemia and lymphoma in chemical and rubber workers exposed to benzene; skin cancer in farmers and sailors chronically exposed to the sun; and chronic bronchitis in workers exposed to dust particles. Additional conditions have been more recently associated with occupation and include dementia in persons exposed to solvents, sterility in men and women exposed to certain pesticides, asthma in workers exposed to latex and toluene diisocyanate, and carpal tunnel syndrome in workers engaged in repetitive, stressful wrist motion. These conditions can be either acute or chronic. They may be manifested through symptoms that are easily identified or through the emergence of subtle dysfunction that can be discerned only through careful medical testing.

Recent calculations put the direct costs (i.e., the amount of money spent on medical care, property damage, and services related to injury or illness) of work-related injuries and illnesses at $65 billion annually.[1,2] When an estimated $106 billion of indirect costs (i.e., those associated with lost work days or reduced productivity) are added, the total cost to society reaches $171 billion annually. Of this amount, $145 billion is spent for work-related injuries and $26 billion on occupationally acquired illness.[1,2]

In March 2000, the National Institute of Occupational Safety and Health (NIOSH) compared the costs of occupational disease and injury in the United States with the costs of cancer, circulatory disease, Alzheimer's disease, and human immunodeficiency virus (HIV)/acquired immune deficiency syndrome (AIDS). Costs (both direct and indirect) for circulatory diseases and for cancer were comparable to those associated with occupational injuries and illness. Work-related injuries and disease cost the nation more than twice as much as Alzheimer's disease and more than four times as much as HIV/AIDS.

Workplace-related injuries and diseases are distinctly different from most other problems in public health in that deaths, diseases, and disabilities acquired in the workplace are all products of economic activity undertaken within our society. They are therefore, in theory, preventable.

Changing Patterns of Employment

The health and safety of workers is affected by (1) the industries in which they are employed, (2) the technologies and materials used in those industries, and (3) the duration and intensity of workers' exposures to technologies and materials. Level of production also is critical to determining how rapidly exposure accumulates. Changing patterns of employment can result in profound shifts in the incidence and distribution of work-related morbidity and mortality.

There were major changes in industry and employment in the United States during the twentieth century. Agriculture, mining, and basic manufacturing employ a much smaller faction of the workforce today than they did 100 years ago. Workers now are increasingly exposed to new synthetic chemicals, and they face communications technologies, forms of transportation, and machines that were unimagined 100 years ago. Service-producing industry jobs now outnumber goods-producing industry jobs, creating new types of work-related health issues.[3] Eighty-five million Americans (70% of the workforce) now work in service-oriented industries, and the number of Americans who function in executive, administrative, and management positions continues to grow.[4]

The relationship between changing patterns of employment and workplace injury and illness is reflected in morbidity and mortality data. The National Safety Council (NSC) has estimated that in 1912, a total of 18,000–21,000 U.S. workers died as a consequence of work-related injury; similarly, the Bureau of Labor Statistics reported the number of industrial-associated deaths for 1913 to be 23,000, or 5.9 deaths per 100,000 workers. The U.S. workforce at that time was 38 million.[5] By 1997, with fewer people employed in manufacturing, mining, and agriculture, the death rate had dropped to 5100, or 3.9 per 100,000, in a workforce of 130 million. The NSC also has collected data on work-related morbidity: the rate of unintentional work-related injuries for 1997 was 4 per 100,000 workers—substantially lower than the rate of 37 per 100,000 observed in 1933.

Additionally, NIOSH has identified the industries with the highest rates of occupation-related fatalities for 1980–1995. Despite a more than 10-fold reduction in fatality rate since the early 1900s, mining remains the industry that poses the highest risk for workplace mortality (30.3 deaths per 100,000 workers). Other industries that place workers at high risk include agriculture/forestry/fishing (20.1 deaths per 100,000 workers), construction (15.2 deaths per 100,000 workers), and transportation/communications/public utilities (13.4 deaths per 100,000 workers; see Fig. 10.1). At the start of the twentieth century, machine-related injuries were the most common

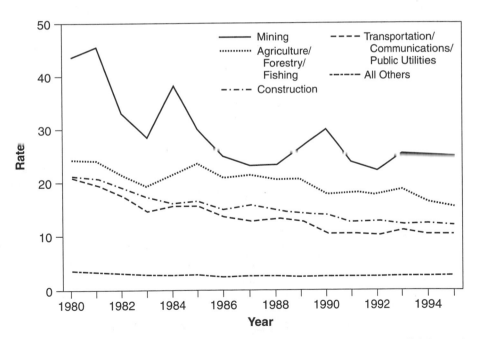

Figure 10.1. Occupational injury death rates (per 100,000 workers), by industry division and year—United States, 1980–1995. All others include public administration, manufacturing, wholesale trade, retail trade, services, and finance/insurance/real estate.

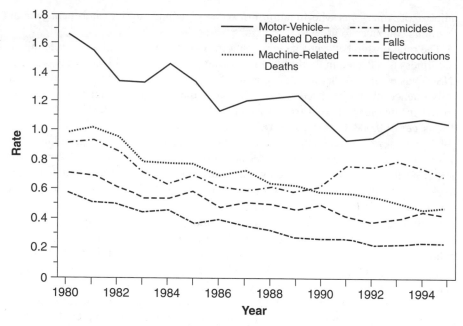

Figure 10.2. Rates (per 100,000 workers) for leading causes of occupational injury deaths, by cause and year—United States, 1980–1995.

direct cause of death. By century's end, motor vehicle-related injuries and workplace homicides had become the two leading causes of acute, traumatic work-related deaths[5] (see Fig. 10.2).

The Science of Occupational Health and the Pioneers in the Field

Diseases that are caused by work are underdiagnosed. Many illnesses of occupational origin are incorrectly ascribed to other causes because most work-related illnesses are not clinically distinct from diseases resulting from other causes. Diagnosis of occupational disease is complicated further by the long latency period that frequently must elapse between a toxic exposure and the appearance of signs and symptoms of disease. A further impediment to the correct diagnosis and effective prevention of occupational disease is that influential persons and organizations with vested interests frequently argue that no connection exists between a particular exposure and disease. This pattern of opposition has been observed repeatedly when substances (e.g., asbestos, arsenic, benzene, lead, and beryllium) are identified as posing a health threat to persons who work with them.[6]

    Researchers, practitioners, and advocates of workplace health and safety who have been willing to confront vested interests for the sake of worker health have been critical to building the field of occupational medicine. These heroes of occupational health have advanced the science even during periods when scientific progress was not accompanied by improved protection of workers. Early heroes, including Bernardino Ramazzini in the early 1700s, Charles Turner Thackrah in the nineteenth century, and Sir Thomas Legge, and Alice Hamilton in the first half of the twentieth century laid the foundations for the practice of occupational health. They publicized the problem of work-related illness and injury by describing the harsh working conditions that they observed in factories and mines, and they helped to establish the tradition of clinical recognition of occupational disease.

In the late twentieth century, Irving Selikoff and other researchers employed epidemiology to characterize the causes of occupational disease in working populations. Through this work the concept of latency (i.e., the delay between exposure and development of disease) was formulated, alerting health professionals to the potential for disease manifestation years or even decades after workplace exposures. David Rall and other modern toxicologists contributed further to the understanding of workplace safety and health, moving the field of toxicology from a descriptive understanding of dose-response relationships to the prediction of human effects based on studies in microorganisms and laboratory animals.

Investigation of Lead Exposure

Investigation of health hazards posed by exposure to lead in the workplace exemplifies the critical role that heroes in occupational health have played in advancing science and prevention. Occupational lead poisoning was clearly described by Nikander, a Greek poet and physician of the second century BC Nikander, in his poem *Theriaca and Alexipharmaca*, detailed the adverse consequences of exposure to cerussa (lead carbonate) and specifically noted the occurrence of colic, paralysis, visual disturbance, and encephalopathy.[8]

Nearly 2000 years later, Bernardino Ramazzini, the father of occupational medicine, in his *de Morbis Artificum Diatriba* (1713),[9] described lead poisoning in potters and in portrait painters:

> In almost all cities there are other workers who habitually incur serious maladies from the deadly fumes of metals. Among these are the *potters*. . . . When they need roasted or calcined lead for glazing their pots, they grind the lead in marble vessels. . . . During his process, their mouths, nostrils, and the whole body take in the lead poison. . . . First their hands become palsied, then they become paralytic, splenetic, lethargic, and toothless.
>
> I have observed that nearly all the *painters* whom I know, both in this and other cities, are sickly. . . . For their liability to disease, there is an immediate cause. I mean the materials of the colors that they handle and smell constantly, such as red lead, mercury and white lead.[9]

In Great Britain, Charles Turner Thackrah (1832) described chronic occupational lead poisoning in plumbers, white lead manufacturers, house-painters, paper-stainers, and potters.[10] A major figure in the history of occupational lead poisoning in Great Britain was Sir Thomas Legge, who in 1897 was appointed first Medical Inspector of Factories. Legge stressed that industrial lead poisoning was "due almost entirely to lead dust or fume," and he proposed the following four axioms for the control of occupational lead poisoning:[10]

- Unless and until the employer has done everything—and everything means a good deal—the workman can do next to nothing to protect himself, although he is naturally willing enough to do his share.
- If you can bring an influence to bear external to the workman (i.e., one over which he can exercise no control) you will be successful; and if you cannot or do not, you will never be wholly successful.
- Practically all industrial lead poisoning is due to the inhalation of dust and fumes; and if you stop their inhalation you will stop the poisoning.
- All workmen should be told something of the danger of the material with which they come into contact and not be left to find it out for themselves—sometimes at the cost of their lives.

Under Legge's influence (and despite considerable opposition from the lead industry), lead poisoning was made a nationally notifiable disease in Britain in 1899. With ensuing surveillance and control, the number of reported cases in Britain fell from 1058 in 1900 to 505 in 1910[7] and to 59 in 1973,[11], despite considerable increases in lead consumption.

In the United States, cases of lead poisoning were noted during the seventeenth and eighteenth centuries in the pottery, pewter-making, shot-dropping, and lead smelting industries. A substantial increase in incidence occurred in the latter half of the nineteenth century following the discovery of lead deposits in the Rocky Mountain States. An estimated 30,000 cases of lead poisoning may have occurred during 1870–1900 in Utah, the state in which the largest number of workers were affected. An interesting feature of the Utah epidemic was the abundance of cerussite (lead carbonate) ore, which is more soluble and thus more readily absorbed than the more common ore, galena (lead sulfide).

Only minimal systematic attention was given to the prevention and control of lead poisoning in the United States until Dr. Alice Hamilton, late Assistant Professor Emeritus of Industrial Medicine at Harvard, began her surveys of lead exposure in 1910. Hamilton observed that:

> Only a few years ago, we were most of us under the impression that our country was practically free from occupational poisoning . . . that our lead works were so much better built and managed, our lead workers so much better paid, and therefore better fed, than the European, that lead poisoning was not a problem here as it is in all other countries. . . . As a matter of fact, the supposed advantages . . . obtained only in a few of the lead trades . . . [and] that far from being superior to Europe in the matter of industrial plumbism, we have a higher rate in many of our lead industries than have England or Germany.[12]

Hamilton and her colleagues investigated lead exposure in various industries, among them storage-battery manufacture. Among 915 men employed in five battery manufacturing plants, as well as among workers who engaged in type founding, smelting, enameling of sanitary ware, and pigment production, 164 (18%) cases of lead poisoning were reported. Hamilton faced considerable opposition from both employers and members of her own profession when these findings were publicized; nevertheless, she persisted heroically, and her work improved conditions of exposure in the North American lead industries.[13]

In recent years, lead poisoning has continued to occur with disturbing frequency in the United States. Episodes of lead poisoning have been reported in a range of industries from battery manufacture to brass casting, bridge construction, demolition, missile silo construction, chemical manufacture, shipbuilding and ship-scrapping, and police work. Particularly high blood lead levels have occurred among workers at scrap smelters.

Asbestos Exposure

Dr. Irving J. Selikoff of the Mount Sinai School of Medicine in New York City is another hero of occupational medicine. A preeminent physician and researcher, Dr. Selikoff made numerous landmark contributions to medicine, saving the lives of millions. In the 1960s, Selikoff noted an unusually high occurrence of lung disease among workers at the United Asbestos and Rubber Company in Paterson, New Jersey. His detailed examination of these patients constituted the first recognition of the occupational dangers of exposure to asbestos.[14] Recognizing asbestos as the cause of lung cancers and mesotheliomas that occur two decades or more after exposure, he conducted epidemiologic studies necessary to persuade physicians and lawmakers of a causal relationship. This work laid the foundation for the establishment of strict asbestos-exposure limits and generated concern over the potential hazards of other occupational materials.

Selikoff also demonstrated the existence of a synergistic interaction between asbestos and cigarette smoking in the causation of lung cancer. He is credited with development of a bank of scientific information implicating asbestos exposure as a major public health hazard, providing the basis for effective disease prevention and control.

In identifying the life-threatening effects of asbestos exposure, Dr. Selikoff gave the then new science of occupational medicine the champion it needed, proving the association between the workplace and negative health outcomes. Dr. Selikoff expanded his work beyond asbestos to examine the risks present in a diversity of occupational environments. From shipyard workers to firefighters, Dr. Selikoff endowed workers from diverse industries with a new right, that of a safe working environment.

Formation of the National Toxicology Program

Another hero of occupational health was Dr. David P. Rall, director of the National Institute of Environmental Health Sciences (NIEHS) from 1971 to 1990. Although Rall is renowned for his role in the NIEHS's evolution from a small nucleus of people with large ideas to a preeminent center for environmental health science research, perhaps his most remarkable legacy is his development of the National Toxicology Program (NTP). Established in 1978, the NTP is a cooperative effort to coordinate toxicologic testing programs within the Department of Health and Human Services. The major objectives of the NTP are to (1) increase the depth of knowledge about the toxicology of chemicals, (2) evaluate the full range of toxic effects of chemicals, (3) develop and validate more effective assays for toxicity, and (4) disseminate toxicologic information resulting from its studies.

In 1978, NIEHS was designated the focal point for establishment of the NTP, and Rall was appointed its director. The NTP became the only comprehensive toxicology testing program in the world, providing researchers with a body of toxicologic data that is essential to bettering public health. In addition, the NTP set a course of research for animal testing that will extend into the twenty-first century. In describing the work of NTP, Rall stated, in 1988: "It is our job as scientists to attempt, as best we can, to look into the future, see the changes ahead, and anticipate the side effects of these changes. But we know from the past experiences that there are few important and useful discoveries that do not have some unanticipated, undesirable side effects. It is our responsibility to alert leaders in public policy and suggest to them how we might prevent or minimize any negative health consequences."[15]

The Defining Features of Occupational Health

A unique feature of occupational health is that the population exposed to workplace hazards is usually easy to define. Because employment is a regularized feature of society and involves keeping records, obtaining information about who has worked at a job, in what capacity, and for how long is a relatively straightforward process; therefore, identifying who is potentially exposed and who needs to be protected also is rarely problematic. By contrast, for most non-workplace environmental exposures, boundaries are less precise, and populations at risk become more difficult to define.

Researchers learn about the exposures of workers by studying the relatively closed environment of the workplace. Physical hazards (e.g., temperature, radiation, noise, vibration, and pressure) and exposures through the skin, respiratory, and digestive systems can be characterized and quantified. The level and time period of exposure also can be obtained accurately. When an injury or disease can be enumerated (e.g., through a case definition), epidemiology permits the quantification of the association between exposure and disease occurrence. Dose-response relationships can be defined. When these associations are causal, they are also by definition preventable.

Another unique feature of occupational health is that every workplace exposure occurs because an employer has created the work environment and the worker has chosen (not always without coercion) to work in that environment. What a society chooses to produce and how it chooses to produce them are thus the underlying causes of occupational disease and injury. Although these societal decisions have presented American consumers with opportunities, these decisions limit public health professionals in protecting workers from injury and disease.

Primary Prevention of Occupational Disease

Primary prevention is defined as etiologic prevention (i.e., as prevention directed against the source of disease). A classic example from the field of infectious disease epidemiology is vaccination against poliomyelitis. Primary prevention differs from later (i.e., secondary and tertiary) forms of prevention, as these involve, respectively, the early detection of disease and the treatment of disease to prevent death. Examples of secondary prevention include medical screening of exposed persons to detect early disease, and behavioral modification. A classic example of tertiary prevention from infectious disease epidemiology is the use of the iron lung to prevent death in persons already infected with the poliomyelitis virus. Primary prevention is inherently more efficient and effective than either secondary or tertiary prevention.

Premarket Toxicologic Screening

Evaluation of the toxicology of new chemical compounds prior to their commercial introduction constitutes an effective means for preventing toxicity. Such assessment can include review of structure-activity relations, the application of short-term tests, and the conduct of long-term animal bio-assays. Such tests must be universally and systematically applied, and resulting data must be made publicly available.

Epidemiologic Surveillance

Another approach to the primary prevention of occupational disease involves epidemiologic surveillance. Although epidemiologic studies require by definition that disease or death must have already occurred in a population, the detection by epidemiologic means of occupationally induced disease provides a powerful basis for the prevention of future cases. A particular advantage of this approach is its potential to detect disease resulting from interactions among multiple factors. For example, the interaction between cigarette smoke and asbestos in the etiology of lung cancer likely would have gone undetected if epidemiologic study of workers had not been undertaken.

Application of Biological Markers

Biologic markers are anticipated to provide a new mechanism for the primary prevention of occupational disease in the twenty-first century.[16] Markers are the biological, cytogenetic, physiologic, or functional changes that result from exposure to a toxin and that appear to presage the development of disease. The application of markers to the early detection of disease produces the following gains: (1) earlier detection of environmentally induced illnesses, (2) detection of a larger percentage of affected persons, (3) detection of early preclinical change at low levels of exposure, and (4) possibility of early treatment or early interruption of exposure before irreversible cellular transformation has occurred. Additionally, the use of newly developed markers of chemical exposure permits more precise assessment of past exposures, clearer delineation of exposure-effect relations, and better delineation of disease mechanisms, particularly at low-dose levels. The application of such techniques in epidemiologic studies of populations exposed to occupational toxins is expected to lead to substantial increases in the understanding of the etiology of occupational illness.

Disease Prevention in the Workplace

A unique feature of occupational health and safety is the existence of a well-described hierarchy of strategies for protecting workers. The most effective are those approaches most closely tied to the production process; the least effective are those that depend on workers to protect themselves.

At the top of the protection hierarchy is the design or redesign of the production process. The production of polyvinyl chloride illustrates the role of production design in protecting workers. When BF Goodrich first manufactured vinyl chloride polymer from vinyl chloride monomer, the work was performed in largely open reactor vessels. Workers in the vicinity of the reactors were exposed to vapor containing vinyl chloride monomer. Only after a physician working for Goodrich associated this exposure with four cases of an extremely rare cancer—angiosarcoma of the liver—was action taken by the plastics industry to redesign the production process. The redesign occurred only after the industry lost in its effort in a court of law to defeat a government regulation limiting workplace exposure to vinyl chloride monomer. The industry had claimed that the ultimately successful solution to the problem of worker exposure to vinyl chloride monomer—a closed reactor vessel—would be prohibitively expensive and put the industry out of business. However, when it was finally enclosed, the polymerization process proved to be more efficient than in the open vessel because the monomer vapor to which workers had previously been exposed was now contained and incorporated into product. Expensive waste was eliminated, and workers' exposure to vinyl chloride monomer minimized.[17]

The concept of substitution also is high in the protection hierarchy. Because different chemicals pose unique hazards, using less hazardous agents to perform the same function can protect workers. For example, various chemicals can be used effectively to remove dirt and lubricants from machine parts and electrical circuits. Traditionally, petroleum-based solvents have been employed for such cleaning and degreasing; however, these solvents often are toxic to the liver and nervous system. Increasingly, soap and water have been found to be effective substitutes for the solvents, posing far less hazard for workers. In situations where water and detergents cannot be used, better information on the toxicity of solvents permits the selection of the least dangerous, yet effective, chemical.

When neither process design nor chemical/material substitution can make the workplace safer, engineering controls—principally ventilation and enclosure—constitute the next best intervention on the prevention hierarchy. The goal of this type of intervention is to separate the worker from the toxic fumes or dust by removing the hazard. Typically, fresh-air flow or an enclosed workstation with supplied air provide the worker with a safer environment. Hoods and fans remove dust generated by machinery (e.g., drills). Wetting down dust can also control exposures. Spray booths can protect workers from vapors when paint and other materials are applied and are particularly effective for protecting workers who remain in one location. An advantage to this strategy is that exposures are rarely singular, and ventilation protects workers from all contaminants in the air they breathe.

Finally, when the design of safe workplaces is not feasible, workers must be protected by the least preferred strategy, personal protective equipment (PPE), including respirators, hard hats, hard-toe shoes, safety glasses, gloves, and body suits. None of this equipment is fully effective or reliable; its effectiveness is dependent on the way in which a worker uses it (e.g., when the mask is removed because it is uncomfortable or does not supply air easily enough to perform heavy work). Protection may be incomplete when a mask leaks or when gloves protect the hands from solvents for only a limited time.

The Role of Legislation and Regulation

Government laws and programs constitute another defining feature of the worker health and safety environment. Worker compensation, mine regulation, and workplace regulation were all introduced in the twentieth century, along with government programs to study workplace hazards.

Workers Compensation

State worker-compensation acts were introduced in 1910, when New York passed a law requiring compensation for industrial accidents. Mississippi passed the last of these laws in 1948. Gradually, all states amended workers compensation programs to provide compensation for specific occupational diseases that were officially listed in state laws. They offered no coverage for diseases of the workplace that were not included on these official lists. More recently, workers compensation programs in most states have expanded to cover all occupational injuries and diseases. These programs not only shield employers from lawsuits by making payments to harmed workers but also create an incentive for employers (whose insurance premiums pay for the compensation) to make their workplaces safer. Like other insurance programs, premiums create a fund to pay in the future for "rare events" resulting in injuries and diseases. However, because these premiums level the contribution of all employers in an industry and can be considered a cost of doing business that offers no competitive advantage, minimal incentive to protect workers devolves from the program.[18]

Mine Regulation

For centuries, mining has been recognized as the most dangerous industry. In the twentieth century, coal miners have had short working lives; many died or ended their working years prematurely as a result of complications of silicosis (e.g., tuberculosis) and disaster-related injury. The Bureau of Mines was created in 1910 in response to a series of mine disasters. In 1907, 11 incidents caused 869 of the 2534 deaths reported in bituminous coal mines that year. Methane gas and coal dust explosions caused most of coal mine disasters, but collapsing roofs and walls and haulage-related incidents resulted in the greatest number of deaths. The Bureau helped the industry improve mining technology, both to increase production and to improve safety, but the industry remained the country's most dangerous. In 1969, Congress enacted the Coal Mine Health and Safety Act to focus on the safety and health of coal miners. In addition, the role of the Department of Labor was expanded to protect all miners with the creation of the Mine Safety and Health Administration (MSHA) in 1977.

Workplace Regulation

The Occupational Safety and Health Act of 1970 (the OSHA act) created a nation-wide regime of workplace inspections to enforce federal worker-protection laws and regulations in the United States. The OSHA act affected every industry, covering many more workers than MSHA. Although MSHA has established a long-standing tradition of regulating mines, the rules and inspections set forth in the OSHA act introduced a new aspect of labor law to most employers and workers. The focus of the government moved beyond child labor, wages, and hours; attention was instead given to the most intimate details of how work is organized and the way in which these details affect workers. Inspectors were authorized to enter any workplace without notice and respond to complaints from workers or labor unions.

The Occupational Safety and Health Act charged the Department of Labor's Occupational Safety and Health Administration (OSHA) with promulgation of standards that would assure safe and healthy workplaces. The law also created the National Institute for Occupational Safety and Health (NIOSH) to study workplace hazards and to make recommendations to OSHA and MSHA regarding best practices for protecting workers and miners. For the first time, Congress had created a separate research agency to enhance scientific contributions to rules and regulation. Government took responsibility for the research needed to establish a scientific basis for regulation. Organizationally, Congress placed NIOSH in the government's health agency (the Department of Health, Education and Welfare, now Health and Human Services), thus separate from the standard-setting and enforcement functions in the Department of Labor. Like OSHA, NIOSH was granted the right of entry into any workplace to learn whether new or altered rules were needed to protect workers. These research visits could be triggered by a request from a worker or union or from an employer concerned about a workplace hazard.

Labor Unions

Organized worker groups (i.e., labor unions) constitute another distinctive feature of occupational safety and health. Unions have long been involved in the struggle for occupational health and safety on many issues, usually at the state and local level. During the Progressive Era (1890–1910), unions advocated state factory-inspection laws, workers compensation, child labor protection, safer work for women, and the eight-hour work day (see Chapter 11). During the twentieth century, American unions were involved in occupational safety and health, although this role was less formal than in other industrial countries. In Europe, particularly in the Nordic countries, society recognizes labor unions as one of the labor market parties, along with employers and government officials, who collectively, through negotiations, determine conditions of work. Unlike the United States, where fewer than 15% of workers belong to unions, most European workers belong to unions and most large workplaces have union/management health and safety committees responsible for worker protection. Europe thus relies less on government inspection and enforcement, and more on consensus among the involved parties.

In the United States, the relationships have evolved in a more adversarial manner, with unions using strikes and political pressure and claiming fewer formal roles. Government health and safety agencies have been slower to rely on labor/management cooperation to agree on national standards or to set safe conditions of work. However, the research, standard setting, inspection, and enforcement programs of NIOSH, OSHA, and MSHA still accord to workers and their representatives the privilege of participating in inspections and "exit conferences," as well as the opportunity to request research, new regulations, and inspections.

In the United States, the value of labor/management cooperation to study or solve occupational health problems has been demonstrated in many industries within the last century. In the 1960s, The United Rubber Workers and the tire industry collaborated to fund academic occupational health researchers to study exposures and their consequences in the industry. Beginning in the 1980s, the United Automobile Workers and auto industry adopted a similar joint health and safety program; in addition, the aluminum industry and the United Steelworkers joined with NIOSH to create a tripartite program to study pot rooms and other dangerous jobs. Labor unions remain weak in the United States. Employer groups and conservative state and federal governments have deliberately thwarted union organizing and attempted to restrain the power of organized workers. An ideological commitment to the market and free enterprise has made Americans reluctant to adopt practices from other industrial democracies where unions have been encouraged as a way to stabilize labor management relations. One consequence of the U.S. policy is for both labor and management to move worker health and safety issues into the broader labor/management struggle.

Impediments to Prevention

Despite the many available prevention strategies, generic impediments to prevention exist. These impediments fall into three categories: economic, cultural and psychological, scientific and regulatory.

Economic Obstacles

Economic obstacles to prevention generally involve costs.[19,20] When investment to prevent disease and injuries occurs as part of building a new plant or completely reconstructing a process and equipment, such an investment is often acceptable to the investor or employer. Within new investment for plant and equipment, the marginal cost of greater safety is minimal. However, because the U.S. regulatory system is not focused on new plants and equipment, but rather on ongoing compliance with exposure standards, most investments to achieve better protection of workers are made for that purpose alone and involve retrofitting an existing plant or process; such investments can be daunting to employers, who therefore resist government and union pressure to retrofit for the sake of worker protection alone. Virtually every new rule promulgated by OSHA has been greeted by industry claims that the regulation will put one or more establishments or even entire industries out of business.

Changes in manufacturing, particularly substitutions, intended to protect workers also have economic consequences for employers. The cost of raw materials, the disposal or sale of by-products, and the management of wastes may be affected by such changes. The cost of protecting workers intersects also with the broader economy. Ventilation is more expensive in very cold or hot climates and increases energy costs. Environmental rules may increase costs of waste management. Shortages and gluts can change the economics of purchasing raw materials and supplies and selling by-products. These uncertainties become impediments to investments in worker protection.

Cultural and Psychological Obstacles

The American culture attributes special value to persons who serve as the decision makers in the workplace, an attitude that may be a holdover from the rugged frontier

---

Box 10.1. The Precautionary Principle.

The question of whether to regulate and at what level of certainty is perennial in occupational health.[21] Advocates of aggressive regulatory intervention point to John Snow's triumph in halting the London cholera epidemic by removing the handle of the Broad Street pump more than three decades before discovery of the *Vibrio cholerae*. Proponents of a more cautious approach cite scientific exactitude, the risk of provoking unnecessary anxiety, costs, and the undoubted benefits to modern life of the chemical revolution as bases for their anti-regulatory position.

These issues embody profoundly differing views of the nature of science. Not surprisingly, therefore, regulators and members of the judiciary, particularly the large majorities of those bodies not formally trained in science, approach them with trepidation.

Unfortunately, regulatory delay, as much or more than regulation itself, may be costly. Regulators and the courts should be wary of the argument that a chemical is innocent until proven guilty. Also, they must come to appreciate the difference between a "negative" study, which truly exonerates a chemical from suspicion of hazard, and an inconclusive study. The proper verdict in the latter instance is "not proven," rather than "innocent."

In the case of benzene, data generated by NIOSH indicate that the risk of death from leukemia is elevated approximately 150 times above background in workers exposed for a 40-year working lifetime at the previous legally enforceable standard of 10 parts per million (ppm). The risk of leukemia from lifetime exposure at 5 ppm is approximately 12 times above background. At 1 ppm, the standard proposed by OSHA in 1977, but overturned by the Supreme Court and not reinstated until 10 years later, a 10% increase in risk is evident. In the decade following the Supreme Court decision on benzene, many thousands of workers in the United States were exposed to benzene at levels of 1–10 ppm. For several hundred of these men and women, the cost of regulatory delay is death.[22]

of the nineteenth century. Psychologically, these persons maintain a sense of being in control. Thus, efforts to inspect, criticize, or change the workplace often are perceived to be challenges to authority or sovereignty, even in circumstances where the consequences may be good for the company as well as for workers.

Scientific and Regulatory Obstacles

The import of traditions from scientific research into the regulatory process has in some instances become an impediment to prevention.[19] Conflict frequently exists between the cautious and conservative standards needed for scientific proof and the deliberately precautionary standards that are needed to assure that workers are protected. In laboratory and epidemiologic science, researchers typically require that findings be validated statistically to ensure a less than 5% chance that the results can be attributed to "chance." This approach requires great certainty before a scientist can declare proof. By contrast, in the arena of public health protection when reasonable data provide strong, though less than definitive evidence that a particular chemical may cause a serious disease in humans, policy makers and researchers should err in the direction of caution to reduce the likelihood of injury even while they await final proof of a cause-and-effect relation. Recently, the precautionary principle (Box 10.1) has been invoked as an unifying principle that may balance between the often conflicting needs of protecting health and establishing scientific proof.[21]

Prevention: Successes and Failures

Successes

Success, in terms of prevention of workplace injury and illness, reflects a combination of changing employment patterns and direct efforts by government to protect workers. The importance of these two factors varies by industrial sector. In mining, an industry with a heavy regulatory presence, close correlations can be made between governmental action and changing rates of injury and illness. By contrast, in general industry, where coverage by OSHA inspectors is much more sparse, changes in patterns of employment are the principal cause of changing rates of illness and injury, although a marginal contribution is made by the intervention of governmental agencies.

The overall decline in incidence rates of workplace injuries and disease in the twentieth century can be attributed principally to the declining share of the American workforce employed in manufacturing, mining, and agriculture—the industries providing the most dangerous jobs. The occupations that expanded most rapidly in the twentieth century, primarily those that are office-based or service-producing, pose fewer physical threats to workers than jobs in agriculture and heavy manufacturing.

Some of the most dangerous work environments have been modified to protect workers. In many cases, however, disaster or tragedy precipitated public attention to these problems. For example, in the 1930s, more than 700 deaths, mostly from acute silicosis, occurred among persons working to dig the Gauley Junction water tunnel, a four-mile-long tunnel through a mountain of quartz in West Virginia[23] Another example of tragedy surrounds asbestos, the cause of the largest number of occupational cancers, which remained unrecognized as an occupational hazard until pictures of former workers suffering from asbestosis and dying of lung cancer were publicized.[14]

The MSHA and OSHA regulations have had a prominent political component. For instance, miners and foundry workers were unionized, and the United Mine Workers and the Steelworkers pressed MSHA and OSHA to adopt protective standards. Similarly, unions for chemical workers advocated for the benzene standard, and textile unions pushed for the cotton-dust standard. By contrast, in agriculture, where much of the workforce is migrant labor, only limited regulatory action has been taken to protect farm workers from poor sanitation, pesticides, and dangerous equipment.

Failures

Failure to apply scientifically valid technologies in the workplace to protect the health of workers against known and strongly suspected hazards constituted the greatest safety and health failure of occupational health in the twentieth century. Perhaps the strongest indication of this failure is the lack of formal education of engineers (the professionals responsible for designing plants, equipment, and production processes) in the science of safety and health. The following are examples of failures that occurred in the prevention of workplace illness and injury in the twentieth century.

Pre-Market Testing of Chemicals

According to the precautionary principle, any new exposure should be studied before workers are subjected to it. Makers of new drugs and pesticides are required by law to study the toxicology of their products so that appropriate precautions can be taken. For chemical exposures in the workplaces, regulatory precautions derive from the Toxic Substance Control Act (ToSCA) of 1977, administered by the Environmental Protection Agency (EPA). Under ToSCA, EPA requires toxicity testing of chemicals before they enter commerce; however, despite this Act, this testing was conducted infrequently.

The National Toxicology Program was created, in part, to strengthen EPA's ability to require testing and to assure that new chemicals are tested. A National Academy of Sciences study of chemical use in commerce demonstrated that only 43% of commonly sold chemicals have ever been tested for health effects.[24] Even for new compounds, testing requirements have not yet been standardized. Responsibility for deciding whether to assess toxicity, as well as that for deciding which tests to perform, is left principally with the chemical manufacturers.[25]

Thus, despite a gain in knowledge of how to prevent worker exposure, U.S. employers remain inadequately informed regarding the hazards of chemicals they use (see Box 10.2). Often workers are informed about the hazards associated with the use of certain chemicals solely via materials safety data sheets (MSDS), which contain information that can be largely inadequate.[26]

Box 10.2. The Lucel-7 Outbreak. An Example of Regulatory Failure.[27]

In 1979, NIOSH investigated an outbreak of encephalopathy and neuropathy in work-ers in a plant in Texas making fiberglass bathtubs.[1] The workers developed vision problems, and peripheral neuropathy. The affected workers had all been previously healthy, but developed central and peripheral neurologic dysfunction shortly after the introduction to the plant of a new catalyst, 2-t-butylazo-2-hydroxy-5-methylhexane (BHMH), trade name Lucel-7.

The first case of disease occurred shortly after introduction of BHMH; symptoms were most severe in persons most heavily exposed. The outbreak ended abruptly after use of the chemical was discontinued. BHMH was the only new chemical in use in the process. Three other plants operated by the same manufacturer used the same materi-als as the Texas plant, except that they used methyl ethyl ketone peroxide (MEKP) in-stead of BHMH; workers in none of those other plants developed neurological disease.

Experimental animal studies conducted after this outbreak demonstrated unequivo-cally the neurotoxic potential of BHMH. Pathological findings in exposed animals included: (1) loss of nerve fibers in the peripheral nerves and spinal cord; (2) degener-ation of nerve fibers in the optic tracts; and (3) development of lenticular cataracts. These findings provide a rational explanation for the pattern of neurological dysfunc-tion observed in the affected workers.

The tragic lesson of this epidemic is that it could have been entirely prevented by adequate premarket evaluation of BHMH. Premarket testing is the most effective means of assessing the toxicity of new chemicals compounds.[24,25]

Psychological and Physical Stress

In circumstances in which workers are subjected to stress and strain as part of their interaction with machines, only a limited set of rules exists to guide employer be-havior. For example, noise standards limit worker exposure to excessive sound lev-els; however, as is illustrated by the design of most commonly used workstations, minimal attention has been given to worker comfort or to ergonomics.

The controversy over an ergonomics standard intended to protect workers from repetitive strain trauma has been hard fought. Because most work environments have been designed without attention to protecting workers, ergonomics problems have come to outnumber all other forms of injury in the American workforce. In 2000, after many years of debate, OSHA adopted an ergonomics standard to protect workers from repet-itive strain and trauma. This standard generated much employer opposition. In February 2001, the Bush administration withdrew the ergonomics standard in the first month af-ter President Bush's inauguration.

Radiation Hazards

Ironically, radiation, one of the exposures that was monitored carefully throughout the 20th Century, was never adequately prevented. Because early studies showed that exposure to ionizing radiation was deadly (either acutely in large doses or latently because of the cancer it caused), the practice of regular dosimetry was adopted to monitor most exposed workers. However, because of the need for tight national security and defense during the Cold War, the U.S. government chose to override evidence of the dangers associated with radioactive materials and continue to allow workers to be exposed. In the military and the massive atomic weapons industry, workers were routinely exposed to dangerous levels of ionizing radiation, as evidenced by dosimetry readings. The U.S. government discounted the dangers by publicly comparing these workers' exposures to patient exposure to medical X-rays.[28] However, whereas X-rays subject the body to radiation for milliseconds, radioactive dusts accumulate in the lungs. In addition, radioactive isotopes (e.g., iodine and strontium) can accumulate in particular organs of the human body, remaining there for many years.

In the uranium mines that operated to meet the needs of the nuclear weapons program and the nuclear power industry, employers monitored ambient radiation. As required by MSHA rules, employers also kept airborne radon levels below the regulatory standard, which had been established on the basis of studies of radiation exposure. As NIOSH studied uranium miners in the late 1970s and 1980s, one of us (Robbins) commented frequently that NIOSH was finding a greater number of cancers than had been anticipated during the nuclear weapons build-up. He noted that the prevalence of these cancers indicated that either the mining industry had deliberately under-measured or under-reported environmental surveillance data to remain in compliance with MSHA regulations or this radiation was more carcinogenic than previously believed. In either case, MSHA is considering new rules for environmental monitoring and permissible exposure levels.

International Export of Hazards

American corporations are increasingly exporting hazardous materials to developing nations largely because occupational and environmental protections and rules often are weak in these countries. When U.S. plants move abroad, employers can operate under less stringent environmental and worker health and safety rules. Sometimes the result of lenient regulations is disaster, as in Bhopal, India, where an explosion that released methyl isocyanate from Union Carbide's pesticide plant resulted in the deaths of thousands of persons living in the vicinity.[29]

Similarly, although certain pesticides (e.g., DDT) that pose a threat to the health of both makers and applicators have disappeared from the developed world, production and use have moved overseas. Whether the free trade regimes of the North American Free Trade Agreement and World Trade Organization will encourage exportation of hazards or expose American workers to weaker standards of our trading partners remains unknown.

Attacks on Worker Protection

Alarming new efforts are underway to weaken worker protections. These efforts can be evidenced by the withdrawal of the OSHA ergonomics standard noted above and the decrease of the OSHA inspection budget despite evidence that inspections are too infrequent to constitute an adequate incentive for employers to provide a safe and healthful workplace.

Conclusions

The United States experienced great reductions in rates of workplace deaths, injuries, and diseases during the twentieth century. Most of this improvement can be attributed to changes in patterns of employment, although direct intervention by governmental agencies has also made a difference, particularly in mining, the most closely regulated industry. The most dangerous jobs—mining, farming, and timbering, and manufacturing—declined in number, while safer service industry employment increased to dominate the economy. Advances in technology and employer safety programs also helped to make the most dangerous jobs safer.

Advances in science and technology contributed to safer workplaces in the twentieth century. Better toxicology to predict the dangers of chemical agents, better surveillance to detect environmental hazards and their human effects, and most recently biomarkers that can detect very small exposures and pre-clinical states of disease in exposed workers have enhanced safety programs. The strategies for protecting workers represent a hierarchy of approaches: the most efficient and effective are safe process design and change to safer production processes, including substituting safer for more dangerous agents. The next most effective strategy is use of technologies (e.g., ventilation and enclosure) to control exposures; the least effective and efficient is reliance on personal protective equipment.

Government regulation, particularly the enactment of OSHA and MSHA, contributed greatly to increased awareness of workplace hazards. However, U.S. employers often have viewed government efforts to protect workers as an undesirable intrusion on employer sovereignty. The United States, with fewer unionized workers than almost any other industrially developed nation, has relied on workers and their unions far less than other industrial countries to help set workplace conditions to protect worker health. Workers have instead applied political pressure on government. Consequently, the greatest advances in workplace regulation have occurred in unionized industry.

Worker safety and health in the United States in the twentieth century can be viewed either as impressive progress (as evidenced by statistics) or as inadequate and incomplete given the great gap that exists between current knowledge of workplace hazards and continuing failure to apply that knowledge to protect human health against many of the hazards of the workplace.

Challenges for the Twenty-First Century

It is not possible to be clairvoyant, thus the safest way to predict the future is to envision a continuation of the past. Many trends we see in the United States today paint a bleak future for worker safety and health at home and abroad. We mention only a few:

1. While a continuing shift of jobs away from manufacturing to the service sector will reduce toxic exposures and trauma, and thus injuries and work related death rates may decline in the United States, the resulting outsourcing and globalization will move dangerous jobs to parts of the world that do far less to protect workers and we can expect the global consequences to be a greater number of toxic exposures, injuries, and deaths.
2. The 2004 reelection of President Bush may represent an endorsement of his policies, and some of these might have serious consequences for worker health:

   • Rejection of science-based policy making, evident in the withdrawal of the ergonomics and diesel particulates rules.
   • Tort reform that would eliminate many lawsuits that could protect workers from hazardous products.
   • Extension of the Data Quality Act, which slows all science-based regulation.
   • Diminished enforcement of worker protection rules.
   • Tax cuts that leave less money for government programs.
   • Increased secrecy, including facts about hazardous industries, in the name of homeland security.

3. Further decline in trade union membership.
4. Public health attention drawn away from worker safety and health to other problems.

The raw statistics on worker injury and disease may continue to decline owing largely to a change in jobs, but globally and compared to what might be possible, we predict a picture of worker safety that our heroes would have spoken out against.

References

1. Leigh JP, Markowitz SB, Fahs M, Shin C, Landrigan PJ. Occupational injury and illness in the United States: estimates of costs, morbidity, and mortality. *Arch Intern Med* 1997, 157:1557–1568.
2. Leigh JP, Markowitz S, Fahs M, Landrigan P. Costs of Occupational Injuries and Illnesses. Ann Arbor, MI: University of Michigan Press, 2000.
3. Kuhn S, Wooding J. The changing structure of work in the United States: part 1—the impact of income and benefits. In: Levenstein C, Wooding J, eds. The Political Economy of Occupational Disease, in Work, Health, and Environment: Old Problems, New Solutions . . . New York: Guildford Press, 1997, 22.
4. Levenstein C, Tuminaro D. The cost effectiveness of occupational health interventions. In: Levenstein C, Wooding J, eds. The Political Economy of Occupational Disease, in Work, Health, and Environment: Old Problems, New Solutions. New York: Guilford Press, 1997, 4.
5. Centers for Disease Control and Prevention. Improvements in workplace safety—United States, 1900–1999. *MMWR* 1999:48:461.
6. Ozonoff D: Failed warnings: asbestos-related disease and industrial medicine. In: Bayer R. The Health and Safety of Workers: Case Studies in the Politics of Professional Responsibility. New York and Oxford: Oxford University Press, 1988, 139–218.
7. Oliver T. Lead Poisoning from the Industrial, Medical and Social Points of View. London: H.K. Lewis, 1914.

8. Major RH. Classic Descriptions of Disease with Biographical Sketches of the Authors, 2nd ed. Baltimore, MD and Springfield IL: Charles C. Thomas, 1939.
9. Ramazzini B. de Morbis Artificum Diatriba. Wright, WC, trans. Chicago: University of Chicago Press, 1973.
10. Hunter D. The Disease of Occupations, 4th ed. Boston: Little, Brown, 1969.
11. H.M. Chief Inspector of Factories Annual Report. London: Her Majesty's Stationery Office, 1973.
12. Hamilton A. Lead poisoning in the United States. *Am J Public Health* 1914:4:477.
13. Hamilton A. Lead poisoning in American industry. *J Ind Hyg* 1919:1:8.
14. Selikoff IJ, Churg J, Hammon EC. Asbestos exposure and neoplasia. *JAMA* 1964:188: 22–26.
15. In Memoriam. David P. Rall, 1926–1999. *Environ Health Perspect* 1999:107:A538–A539.
16. Goldstein B, Gibson J, Henderson R, et al. Biological markers in environmental health research. *Environ Health Perspect* 1987:74:3–9.
17. Markowitz G, Rosner D. Deceit and Denial: The Deadly Politics of Industrial Pollution. Berkeley: University of California Press & Milbank Memorial Fund, 2002.
18. Geoffrey C, Beckwith J. The myth of injury prevention incentives in workers' compensation insurance. In: Levenstein C, Wooding J, eds. The Political Economy of Occupational Disease, in Work, Health, and Environment: Old Problems, New Solutions. New York: Guildford Press, 1997, 93–127.
19. Robbins A, Freeman, P. Congress looks at the evidence. *J Public Health Policy* 1985:6: 335–39.
20. Page T, Robbins A. Cost-benefit analysis in occupational health. In: McDonald C, ed. Advances in Occupational Health. London: Churchill and Livingstone, 1981, 22–37.
21. Kriebel D, Tickner J, Epstein P, et al. The precautionary principle in environmental science. *Environ Health Perspect* 2001:109:871–76.
22. Nicholson WJ, Landrigan PJ. Quantitative assessment of lives lost due to delay in regulation of occupational exposure to benzene. *Environ Health Perspect* 1989:82:185–88.
23. Cherniack MG. The Hawk's Nest Incident: America's Worst Industrial Disaster. New Haven: Yale University Press, 1986.
24. Toxicity Testing: Needs and Priorities. Washington, DC: National Academy of Sciences, 1984.
25. Baseline of Hazard Information that Is Readily Available to the Public: Chemical Hazard Data Availability Study—What do we really know about the safety of high production volume chemicals? Washington, DC: Office of Pollution Prevention and Toxics, Environmental Protection Agency, 1998.
26. Karstadt M, Bobal R. Access to data on chemical composition of products used in auto repair and body shops. *Am J Ind Med* 1984:6:359–72.
27. Horan JM, Kurt T, Landrigan PJ, Melius JM, Singal M. Neurologic dysfunction from exposure to 2-t-butylazo-2-hydroxy-5-methylhexane (BHMH): a new occupational neuropathy. *Am J Public Health* 1985:75:513–17.
28. Brugge D, Goble R, The history of uranium mining and the Navajo people. 1: *Am J Public Health* 2002:92:1410–19.

Suggested Reading

Levenstein C, Wooding J, eds. The Political Economy of Occupational Disease in Work, Health, and Environment: Old Problems, New Solutions. New York: Guildford Press, 1997.

11

A Prejudice Which May Cloud the Mentality: The Making of Objectivity in Early Twentieth-Century Occupational Health

CHRISTOPHER SELLERS

Today, when health and environmental professionals want to assess the seriousness of some hazard either in the workplace or the outside air, they gather a sample of the suspicious air to analyze and measure. They read safety, or danger, in the resulting numbers. At least since World War II, when the first official list of Threshold Limit Values (TLVs) was endorsed by a group of professional industrial hygienists, the notion that there are "maximum safe concentration levels" has served as a central tenet of American efforts to control pollutants within the factory and without.[1] Upon the federal government's deepening involvement in both occupational and environment health after 1970, quantitative atmospheric controls have been written into nationwide law, to be enforced by the Environmental Protection Agency (EPA) and the Occupational Safety and Health Administration (OSHA). Many other countries as well have followed these American examples.[2-5] Atmospheric chemical analysis is so fundamental to the way modern occupational and environmental health expertise works that it has become difficult to imagine how industrial disease or air pollution could be controlled without it.

Yet prior to American adoption of these quantitative tools correlating atmospheric chemical levels and disease, industrial health practices were neither unimaginably primitive nor unscientific. Earlier methods, as practiced by early industrial hygiene pioneers like Alice Hamilton, not only had their own logic but also their virtues. During this time, medical and scientific compilers of this knowledge wrote at once for

230

physicians or hygienists and for those without scientific training, aspiring to reports that would remain comprehensible and persuasive for all these groups. Unshielded by a veil of pre-calculated numbers, successful practitioners like Hamilton had to cultivate their own communicative and persuasive skills with lay audiences. Their knowledge itself remained closely tied either to preventive interventions through factory inspection or to curative ones through the clinic, though these realms remained largely separate from one another.

A quantitative chemical approach to occupational disease and a thorough synthesis of workplace and clinical information began with Europe's relatively longstanding national systems for monitoring and controlling occupational disease.[6-8] Only following World War I, when such a system was taking shape in the United States, did Americans fully embrace this kind of laboratory investigation and its products. The new epistemological emphasis arrived in this country hand in hand with the advent of a new community of experts, centered in the public health schools, in company medical clinics, and in state divisions of industrial hygiene. Yet the fervor with which America's industrial hygienists turned to the laboratory and quantification reflected their dissatisfaction with both the imprecision of existing methods and the social politics with which those methods had become enmeshed.

By the mid-1920s, debate swirled especially around a crucial element in the emerging American system of workplace health regulation: the company physician. Recognizing the unavoidable contentiousness of company doctors' claims to be scientific, as well as those of the fewer doctors allied with labor unions, postwar researchers in the new public health schools and government study initiatives seized upon the integrated and laboratory-oriented methods pioneered by the Europeans. They also began to address their work increasingly to each other and to a specialized audience of physicians and hygienists, rather than to laypersons. Alice Hamilton herself became instrumental in introducing a new "objectivity" talk about the new methods, which located them on the scientific side of a newly discovered boundary between science and policy. The impartiality they claimed for this new knowledge, in contrast to the ideologically manipulable knowledge they saw as belonging to an earlier era, actually laid the groundwork for a new form of policy prescription. Exemplified by their estimates of safe concentration levels, forerunners of what the American Conference of Government Industrial Hygienists would enshrine as "TLVs," it relied more on the authority of a community of experts than the art of persuasion.

Control of Occupational Disease During the Late Progressive Era

American texts on the diseases associated with particular vocations long predate the Progressive Era (1890s–1920), appearing sporadically throughout the nineteenth century.[9-11] Late nineteenth-century sanitarians in New York City and elsewhere published reports on their investigations of factories, giving rise to the first state factory inspection bureaus in New Jersey (1885) and in New York and Massachusetts (1886).[12-14] Factory inspectors, though they concentrated on protecting child and women laborers, also enforced laws regulating dust and ventilation. Private companies in the mining and railroad industries also began hiring their own physicians to treat employees long before the turn of the century, though mostly out of concern for industrial accidents rather than disease.[15,16]

In the Progressive Era, especially from 1910 onward, the research, writing, and intervention on industrial health multiplied dramatically. Some historians have portrayed the Progressive Era as a time of overwhelming belief in "science," when claims to scientific practice came to dominate the rhetoric of professions like medicine, forestry, and management, and became a familiar cry in the political arena.[17–20] Others have remarked on the moral fervor that pervaded the era, from the settlement houses to Theodore Roosevelt's Progressive political crusade of 1912.[21–23] Though these two features of the era may seem somewhat incongruous, their coexistence becomes more understandable in the light of the contemporary norms for knowledge about occupational disease. This knowledge, comprehensible to laymen yet fully scientific in its time, had to serve at once as fact and as prod to the economic or humanitarian aspirations of its audience. A summary of the arenas in which knowledge about occupational disease came to be collected and applied around 1914 in this country, and the types of interventions available within each, sheds light on the distinctive social apparatus that emerged early on to deal with industrial health hazards. Both government and industry adopted strategies for monitoring occupational maladies and their causes in which observations and conclusions had to remain easily accessible to laypeople and closely linked either to cure or to prevention.

By 1914, some 33 of the more industrial states had established factory inspection bureaus.[24] Though not all of these agencies had clear legal authority to act against chemical causes of occupational diseases, 22 had laws against injurious dusts and 15 against poisonous gases, fumes, and vapors.[24] Some of the laws required the presence of specific devices to remove dust or fumes in industries. Others relied upon the judgment of inspectors as to whether the dust in a particular factory was "excessive" or the preventive methods already in use were "suitable."[25] Invariably, inspectors could carry out the laws by simple visual observation and purely qualitative determinations. Neither laboratories nor expert personnel for measuring atmospheric dust or chemical concentrations seemed practical or necessary. But most early inspectors also made little effort to enforce laws against fumes and dust.[26,27]

Some of the more active factory inspection units had begun to experiment with quantitative chemical analyses. In particular, C. T. Graham Rogers, the medical inspector of factories for the state of New York, acquired access to a chemical laboratory in 1910 and undertook numerous atmospheric measurements. Though such efforts seemed to resemble the later forms of regulation, the measurements almost invariably served the essentially qualitative, prevention-focused regulatory system of the time. In his reports, for instance, Rogers used quantitative measurements as arguments for expanding the regulatory power of the state Department of Labor in dangerous workplaces. In arguing for the regulation of a factory process involving arsenic, Rogers found it sufficient to mention that a room contained 0.093 grams per cubic meter, without providing any other number for comparison. Simply the measured presence of a poison was argument enough.[28] When Rogers called for "standards" for the arsenic-laden workroom, or for a "specific method" to deal with gases such as carbon monoxide, he was asking not for rules similar to Threshold

Limit Values, but for standards of preventive practice, for a clarified sense of when vents or hoods or masks would be required.[28]

Rogers was one of only a handful of physicians employed in state factory inspection prior to World War I. By 1915, only Illinois, Massachusetts, New York, and Pennsylvania had medical factory inspectors.[29] Rogers's training allowed him to make occasional use of another investigative technique that soon became a much more integral part of occupational disease control than quantitative measurements: the physical examination. In his capacity as a government factory inspector, Rogers usually examined either children, to determine their fitness or age, or the victims of occupational disease.[30]

Whether involving preventive mechanisms or exams, the laws those such as Rogers enforced became part of a growing governmental mechanism to monitor illnesses due to working conditions. Between 1911 and 1914, some 15 states passed laws requiring all physicians to report any cases of occupational disease to the state labor or health department.[31] This attempt to enlist the aid of private practitioners and company and academic physicians in a government-based program of surveillance had only limited success. Though the reports that did arrive in state agencies sometimes produced leads for factory or medical inspectors, private physicians by and large rarely asked about their patients' places of work, and made few occupational diagnoses.[32-34] Their apathy partly reflected the dearth of instruction about this kind of malady in the medical schools, but also the difficulty of distinguishing between occupational and other causes of disease.

Better to catch what familiarity with the voluminous European literature had led them to suspect were vast numbers of undiagnosed industrial maladies, some academic physicians took it upon themselves to devise and encourage a medicine more geared to diagnosis and treatment of job-related disease. In a few medical schools, professors sponsored clinics devoted solely to occupational disease. W. Gilman Thompson started the first one at the Columbia College of Physicians and Surgeons in 1910, but the largest opened at Harvard a few years later under the guidance of David Edsall.[35-37] Some unions, as well, including New York's Cloak and Skirt Makers' Union, began to sponsor their own clinics.[38]

Efforts against occupational disease by the employers themselves probably had the most widespread impact on the health of the working population in this period. The earliest attempts of companies to supervise the health of their employees emerged as an important facet of "welfare work," those paternalistic efforts to care for the workers' broader needs that, often, also aimed to fend off trade unions.[39-41] For public health advocates as well, company physical exams seemed a potent and effective weapon in anti-tuberculosis campaigns.[42] From the start, however, many workers viewed these initiatives with mistrust and suspicion.[43] The advent of workmen's compensation further propelled the spread of physical examinations in industry. In 1909, Montana passed the first state workmen's compensation law; by 1914, a total of 24 states had enacted similar laws.[44,45] In the wake of these laws, company officials found the physical exam a useful way to collect evidence about employees that could later combat any false compensation claims. Early compensation law only covered accidents, and a diagnosis of occupational disease generally served to invalidate a claim, which meant further incentive for companies to put their own doctors on the job.[46] The new laws provided further inducements for firms to hire their own physicians and set up their own factory clinics. An American Association of Industrial Physicians and Surgeons, founded in 1916, heralded the arrival of a "new specialty" called "industrial medicine."[47,48] Expanding ranks of industrial physicians probably devoted greater attention to job-related illness than the average private practitioner, but often not so much to the satisfaction of their worker patients.

Between the turn of the century and 1914, the social mechanism both to detect and prevent or treat work-related illness came to encompass a expanding array of government agencies and some key new groups of physicians outside the companies themselves. Physical examinations and visual inspection of workplaces, occasionally along with laboratory analysis of air, dust, or other material, provided the main modes of information gathering. But for the most part, the information from physical examinations about workers' bodies remained in the clinics among physicians, while the information on factory environments, from observation and analysis, remained within the inspection bureaus. Even C. T. Graham Rogers performed physical exams and sampled factory air at mutually exclusive times and places, and he never systematically correlated the two kinds of information.

During the Progressive Era, clinical and environmental knowledge did come together in the numerous studies of working environments unassociated with any regulatory or medical treatment functions. A diverse group of reformers, muckraker journalists, social scientists, lawyers, and physicians, employing what they termed social surveys, often included workplaces in their purview.[49] Publishing articles in popular magazines such as *Harpers'* and *The Survey* or in social science journals, they paired attention to conditions and diseases of the factory with scrutiny of workers' home environments, and usually emphasized industrial accidents over poisonings.[50-52] Only rarely did these studies closely examine the connection between the dust or fume exposure they reported and actual cases of disease. As for investigations that concentrated exclusively on occupational disease and its environmental causes, these usually depended on government sponsorship. Between 1909 and 1914, the national Bureau of Labor Statistics supported both John Andrews's investigation of the phosphorus match industry and Alice Hamilton's of the lead industries.[53-55] Unlike investigators in the twenties, however, the early Hamilton as well as Andrews only aimed to establish the significant presence of lead or phosphorus poisoning in the industries they studied, not to map in any extensive or quantifiable way the relations between increasing exposure and disease. Their qualitative goal meant that their reports on the factory environment and their clinical case histories could remain spatially and conceptually separate within their reports, except for common references to particular tasks within the factory. In contrast to C. T. Graham-Rogers, neither Hamilton nor Andrews found laboratory measurements or physical examinations to be necessary to their purpose. They relied largely on interviews, hospital records, and direct observation.

The assumed audience for these industrial disease studies further inclined their authors to this qualitative approach. Hamilton and Andrews wrote their reports for the scattered and diverse assortment of laymen and technically trained experts who then had some power over the factories and the inspection laws: company managers, factory inspectors, and the politicians and the public, as well as physicians and hygienists. They did not clearly discern any expert community in a position to appreciate a more quantitative or interventionist approach, or to interpret it effectively. Three or 4 years later, the authors of the earliest American textbooks on occupational disease also stressed forms of knowledge that would remain comprehensible for a lay audience.

W. Gilman Thompson's *The Occupational Diseases: Their Causation, Symptoms, Treatment and Prevention*, which appeared in 1914, constituted the first textbook on the subject in the United States. Within a couple of years, two additional textbooks joined his volume, one by George Price, and another by George Kober and William Hanson.[56,57] Not surprisingly, given the training of the authors and the growing role of physicians within the existing system for controlling occupational disease, these textbooks primarily addressed physicians, whether in the public health or mainstream medical communities. At the same time, each claimed in their preface or foreword to speak as well to a diverse crowd that included most of those groups engaged in efforts to control job-related illnesses in the Progressive Era. Thompson, Price, Kober, and Hanson all expressed the hope that those without technical backgrounds, such as employers, social workers, and labor leaders or employees, would consult their texts. These textbooks also recognized a certain lack of integration between the two major means for intervening against occupational diseases at the time: through the clinic and through state factory inspection. Thompson, who concentrated on characterizing occupational illness in clinical terms, still included sections on the nonchemically defined hazards covered by the factory laws—"impure air" and general "dust" and "fumes"—alongside his accounts of the clinical appearance of poisonings from specific chemicals. Kober and Hanson evinced a more equal balance between clinical and factory inspection approaches, categorizing diseases by specific causes and by industry, and paying greater attention to prophylaxis within the factory itself, though less to clinical diagnosis and cure. Their differing emphases reflected contrasting backgrounds: Kober in military medicine, Hanson in public health, and Thompson in a medical school.[58,59] Like C. T. Graham-Rogers, all these authors leaned almost entirely on qualitative observations. They cited chemical analyses only to show a poison's presence, made little of clinical laboratory results, and when mentioning Europeans' estimates of safety levels, noted how, for instance, "the point of toxicity will vary in individuals."

In the arenas of both traditional medicine and public health, these textbook writers faced an uphill struggle for recognition of their subject matter. Within medicine, even the eighth edition in 1915 of the most famous medical textbook of the era, William Osler's *The Principles and Practices of Medicine*, devoted only seven of 1225 total pages to industrial chemical disease.[60] Physicians in academic medicine or private practice remained hesitant or ignorant about industrial maladies, in part because of fears about the potentially controversial or even "socialistic" implications of occupational diagnoses. Those in companies had little interest in publicizing any such diseases they discovered.[61] As for public health officials, their enthusiasm for bacteriology led many of them to overlook or de-emphasize the most typical occupational maladies, which had chemical causes. In 1913, Hibbert W. Hill proclaimed a "New Public Health" that stressed individual measures like immunization and personal hygiene over environmental tactics such as factory sanitation.[62] J. Scott Mac-Nutt's *A Manual for Health Officers* published in 1915, devoted only four of some 600 pages to industrial hygiene.[63]

Yet whether the target was a public who could press for new laws or the manufacturers themselves, both Andrews and Thompson expressed similar notions about the proper nature of knowledge about occupational disease. It consisted of "facts" or "data" that met only minimal formal requirements. They could be collected, disseminated, and used without any necessary special training. Most important, however, they had to be, in Thompson's words, "effective" and "reliable." The requirement of effectiveness meant that they were not simply what we would call objective knowledge. They had to activate a moral compulsion or imperative, that would lead their recipient toward a particular line of action. Essentially, this knowledge had to harbor an ethical content for its intended audience, or at least to speak to its audience's values in an imperative manner. Thompson put it this way: "The employer, when presented with such data, may be convinced of the extent and seriousness of the disease hazards as they concern his industry; and if practical and reasonable suggestions for betterment are simultaneously issued, he is almost certain to be convinced, at least, of the economic value of the suggestions, and may put them into effect for greater efficiency if not for humanitarian reasons." Though avowedly scientific, this knowledge had to remain comprehensible to physicians and laymen alike. It was to stir them not just to greater awareness but to social betterment.

This understanding of scientific knowledge about occupational disease accorded well with contemporary institutions and practices. The means for gathering information about job-related illnesses remained closely linked to responsibilities for treatment or regulation. Even those who undertook government studies without any official ameliorative duties often made personal efforts to see that the prescriptions necessitated by their facts were translated into action. Following his study of the phosphorus match industry, John Andrews successfully lobbied for legislation placing a prohibitive tax on that industry's product. Alice Hamilton personally presented the results of her studies, along with her recommendations for improvement, to company managers or owners.[64] Practically nowhere in the United States were the problems of industrial chemical disease studied without a view toward effecting immediate changes, either in particular factories or in cases of disease. For those involved in this era's system for recognizing and combating occupational disease, facts, to make sense, took shape from values. The "is" remained explicitly inseparable from the "ought."

The Growth of a Community of Experts

In the 10 years between 1915 and 1925, several new institutions arose for the study and control of work-related disease. World War I stimulated increased federal interest in research into occupational disease, as well as a new organizational structure for government research efforts. Before the war, responsibility for federal research in industrial disease had been divided between the Bureau of Labor Statistics and the field studies office within the Public Health Service. The wartime surge of government interest in this research, partly a response to new American munitions and chemical industries, culminated in the centralization of these efforts within the Public Health Service.[65] At the Bureau of Mines, investigations of ways of countering chemical weaponry gave way during the postwar years to research into industrial chemical effects, often in cooperation with the PHS's new Office of Industrial Hygiene and Sanitation.

Another important institutional development started in 1918, when Harvard established the nation's first Department of Industrial Hygiene, with Alice Hamilton as its first professorial appointment. By the early twenties, a few medical schools joined the new public health schools in creating university niches for laboratory and clinical research into occupational disease. Harvard, with an entire department devoted to industrial subjects, became the academic center for the new forms of science and ways of thinking that developed in the twenties. Other schools sponsored more limited but similar research, often within different departmental divisions. The Johns Hopkins School of Public Health included significant research on industrial disease in its Department of Physiological Hygiene. The medical school at Yale created a similar division, though the University of Pennsylvania's School of Hygiene followed Harvard and Hopkins's public health model more closely.[66] These same departments also began to offer formal instruction on industrial health topics.

Coupled with the emergence of these new research efforts, new audiences for the research also coalesced. Within the medical profession, physician groups created local forums where the new specialists could present their work. In 1917, the College of Physicians of Philadelphia established a Section on Industrial Medicine and Public Health that invited experts to give lectures to its members and any other interested public.[67] The New York State Society of Industrial Medicine, formed in 1921, not only sponsored lectures but in 1923 began its own journal.[68] State and local medical societies welcomed discussions of industrial topics at their general meetings. Texts of many of these lectures found their way into society *Proceedings* or *Transactions*.[69–71] In 1919, two new journals also appeared devoted partly or solely to industrial topics: *Modern Medicine* (soon to become *The Nation's Health*) and the *Journal of Industrial Hygiene*, published out of the Harvard Division. The American Medical Association in 1922 even went so far as to add "industrial medicine" to the title of its section devoted to "public health."[72] As for public health professionals themselves, they joined the physicians in establishing new outlets for discussion of industrial health during this period. The supranational Conference of State and Provincial Health Authorities of North America created a Committee on Industrial Hygiene in 1919 to promote activities on job-related illness within health departments.[73] In consultation with the Public Health Service's Office of Industrial Hygiene, it also undertook periodic surveys of state and local activities regarding industrial health.

Changes in the compensation system also began to demand further attention to occupational disease, among both company physicians and many private practitioners. Though in 1919, only Massachusetts provided workmen's compensation for such diseases, 4 years later, some seven other states had passed legislation granting coverage, particularly for work-related chemical disease.[74,75] Sociologist Anthony Bale has found that this wave of legislation arose as an attempt to stave off the efforts of the American Association for Labor Legislation and others to enact plans providing workers with a system of general health insurance. In its wake, medical involvement in compensation decisions became more of a necessity. Unlike accidental injuries, whose extent and effects on an employee were often obvious, diseases were often more subtle entities, requiring the diagnostic skills of a physician. Almost all state compensation boards could appoint physicians to carry out official physical exams, and an increasing number of states hired permanent medical directors or advisors. Long-term physician appointments helped to ensure that claim decisions would reflect consistent diagnostic criteria. Yet with the growing numbers of claims, the requirements of the compensation boards for an efficient and uniformly even-handed appraisal of cases helped convince many that explicit standardized principles of diagnosis were necessary as well for the major industrial chemical diseases.[76–78] The compensation system thus began to exert pressure on the form that medical knowledge should take.

Only after World War I did the first studies reveal the extent to which companies had begun to hire their own physicians, as the widening coverage of the compensation acts probably led even more companies to hire their own physicians and thereby broadened the audience for new occupational disease research. In 1927, a study of the Philadelphia area revealed that of 873 firms employing more than 25 people, 473 reported some form of medical service.[79] If a 1926 study by the National Industrial Conference Board was representative, then around half of these firms with medical service, or a quarter of all larger firms, gave physical examinations to prospective and actual employees.[80]

The growth in the numbers of company physicians and the increasing resort to the physical examination met with considerable resistance in some quarters. Many labor leaders believed the technique to be an invasive and all-too-manipulatable evil. When John Andrews wrote some 20 labor leaders in 1915 to ask them where they stood on the issue, "without exception a vigorous protest against medical examination came with every reply." More than anything, labor worried that management might unjustly exploit the exam to deny them jobs. The abolition of physical exams became a major union demand in the labor-management struggles of the late 1910s.[81,82] The shadow of this conflict extended into the programmatic statements of company physicians during the twenties, and also came to haunt those occupying the new academic posts in industrial hygiene.[83–85]

New Modes of Research and Self-Justification

Around the time that new research positions began to open up in industrial hygiene and new forums and audiences appeared, along with worker resistance, the researchers themselves began to alter their ways of gathering knowledge about industrial chemical disease. New textbooks began to appear in the mid-twenties reappraising both the kind of knowledge considered scientific and the social role of that knowledge. No textbook more fully embodied the changes than Alice Hamilton's first book, *Industrial Poisoning in the United States*, published in 1925.[86]

Hamilton's role as advocate of the new approach might at first seem surprising. After all, she had been one of the major architects of the earlier form of knowledge. Yet the trajectory of her career symbolized as well as anything else the institutional changes that made a new kind of science possible. In 1919, receiving the Harvard appointment as the nation's first professor of industrial medicine, she thenceforth left field studies of the looser, qualitative, earlier sort almost entirely behind. Within her new academic abode, she joined with Cecil and Philip Drinker, David Edsall, and other Harvard colleagues during the ensuing years in their attempts to convert "industrial hygiene" into a more coherent and prestigious scientific pursuit. Her *Industrial Poisons in the United States* was the first book-length compendium to emerge from the nation's only academic department devoted strictly to research and teaching in occupational health.

In a striking departure from the pre-1920 textbooks, Hamilton included no direct mention of the audience she intended. With the arrival of organized forums and recipients for knowledge about chemical disease within medicine and public health, she could now assume who her readers would be. She alluded to the new situation by noting an "enormous increase in the interest of the medical world in industrial toxicology of late years."[86] In contrast to earlier, when she had also aimed for her reports to reach and convince factory managers, she now wrote scientific texts almost exclusively for physicians and other technically trained professionals. Hamilton would continue to compose articles on her work for popular magazines throughout her long career, but these would be of a very different character. Her 1925 textbook gave clear witness that the science of industrial disease native to the Progressive Era, with its potential audience of both laymen and physicians, had now quietly met its demise.

The topography she offered for her subject matter bore only modest resemblance to those in the earlier American textbooks. Rather than attempting to encompass all diseases thought to have some causal relation to particular occupations, she restricted herself to "industrial poisons"—the chemical diseases. Her maneuver reflected a growing sensitivity about disciplinary boundaries of her field. As the public health schools like Harvard had begun to undertake research and teaching on industrial health, they partitioned the subject into tentative specialty areas whose full content they left to the discretion of the new faculty. At Harvard, Hamilton called her particular pursuit industrial toxicology. She handed over the dust diseases to Philip Drinker with his interest in "ventilation and illumination," while Cecil Drinker and others in applied physiology took responsibility for investigating fatigue and other nonchemical industrial complaints. Hamilton hoped by her textbook to definitively establish the boundaries of her specialty and to further consolidate it as a discipline. Not only did she confine herself to chemical health effects, she also asserted from the beginning that she would stress "chronic, not acute" forms of poisoning.[86] This last objective did not result in much practical difference between the pre-1920 texts and her own, but it did mark a programmatic shift.

Hamilton's attempt to carve out a coherent area of specialty also involved a newly explicit address of the proper form of scientific investigation of industrial chemical disease. "There are already some studies of poisonous trades in the United States which for thoroughness leave nothing to be desired," she could now write.[86] She had in mind a particular study of manganese poisoning conducted by some of her Harvard colleagues, David Edsall and Cecil Drinker, in 1919.[87] The "thoroughness" of their work, investigating mysterious ailments at a New Jersey factory, inhered mainly in the several types of information which they were able to collect and assemble into a single integrated understanding of industrial manganese poisoning. They brought together data on: "the incidence in a large group of workmen, the conditions under which poisoning occurred, the mode of entrance, and the clinical manifestations, of early stages of poisoning as well as of later stages."[86]

Hamilton used her praise of "thoroughness" to designate a new exemplar for research in occupational disease. Its standards were integrative, more closely and coherently combining techniques that for the most part had remained in separate realms before World War I. Quantitative studies of working environments would have to be combined with clinical laboratory data and the results of physical exams. Preferably, large numbers of subjects and both short and extended terms of exposure would be involved. The new scientific exemplar, with its more extensive correlations of data from the clinic and factory environment and its more comprehensive and interventionist scrutiny of the relation between exposure and poisoning, promised greater certainty in scientific judgments about the chemical causes of disease.[88]

As she promoted these new scientific practices, the concept of safe concentration levels gained greater prominence in her textbook than in earlier ones. The new methodological standard duplicated the combinations of knowledge by which European authors had derived the earliest such figures. Not only did American researchers now undertake similar calculations, but an independent estimate of the safety limit became an obligatory task for Hamilton as textbook author, when the appropriate data on a chemical were available. She offered figures for carbon monoxide, lead, mercury, ammonia, and benzene, among others.[88]

Alongside the new notions about the best scientific methods for studying chemical disease, Hamilton expressed a new self-consciousness about her own role as a scientist in the field. Her solidifying sense of professionalism now incorporated a critical stance toward the partisanship that often accompanied medical testimony about occupational diseases. "Mental reservations may have to be made," she averred; "one must always remember in a study of this kind the existence of a prejudice which may cloud the mentality of some first-class men." And, "Apparently it is impossible for some physicians to treat industrial diseases with the detachment and impartiality with which they approach those diseases which are not confined to the working classes." The example she then cited, from a government bulletin, made it clear that she was talking about the occluded vision of doctors who served unions as well as the company hires. While "the physician retained by the men shows so strong a sympathy for them as to quite dull his critical sense, . . . the physicians for the companies accept evidence which is on the face of it one-sided. . . ."[87]

For the first time in an American textbook about occupational disease came a plea for a more objective attitude toward the study of workers' health. Enabling this appeal was not just her long experience but new methodological benchmarks that seemed to be emerging, which Hamilton hoped might better ensure the same results under any social circumstance. Her own example also points up how this need for a more exacting and objective standard of practice originated at least partly in social crisis. Only after controversies over knowledge had arisen within the existing system for controlling industrial disease, in the context of on-going struggles between labor and management, did the purveyors of medical knowledge such as Hamilton seek to construct a more self-consciously objective science. Here, objectivity had a meaning specific to Hamilton's own time and place: the evaluation of industrial diagnoses only on the basis of agreed upon scientific standards, without regard for the economic ideology of the particular physician who reported it or the social or economic position of his patients.

Hamilton's call to a more objective professional ideal applied not only to researchers such as herself; it had a special meaning for the physician hired to treat patients in the factory: "let him be careful never to sacrifice his own intellectual integrity nor adopt the standards of the non-medical man to whom the proper working of the plant is of first importance. His task is to safeguard the health of the patients who are entrusted to him. . . ."[88]

The physician's "intellectual integrity" did not necessarily involve sympathy for the working class, even though it might lead him or her into conflict with the plant managers apparently on the workers' behalf. Rather, Hamilton meant steadfastness to the standards of diagnosis, judgment, and treatment that he or she had acquired through professional training. Presumably, researchers such as Hamilton were responsible for these standards. In conceiving of the pursuit of worker health as an objective undertaking, Hamilton asserted the role of her own kind in developing the standards upon which the research community could agree. She also assumed that the main responsibility for intervening on behalf of worker health should rest with those who followed these standards, which assured the disinterestedness of their actions—namely, properly trained physicians. Her plea for an objective approach toward industrial health constituted an argument for the centrality of expertise in the study, prevention and treatment of occupational disease.

The new self-consciousness which Hamilton expressed about the necessity for objective standards for research and practice in occupational medicine did not by itself guarantee that the field would become less subject to economic interests. The subsequent history of industrial hygiene research and practice is full of examples of how similar claims to objectivity have continued to serve as a new disguise especially for pro-management agendas.[89,90] Still, Hamilton became the earliest American researcher to articulate this kind of ideal by which her colleagues' and successors' work could be judged. Her new self-justificatory strategy provided a vital prop to the new system of knowledge and regulation as it widened in scope and influence.

The Widening New System and Its Consequences

Hamilton's textbook captured many of the newer currents in the contemporary system of knowledge about industrial chemical disease, which were to become even more pronounced as the 1920s progressed. Shortly after her work appeared, in 1926, the PHS's Office of Industrial Hygiene established an even more elaborate and synthetic exemplar for research with its tetraethyl study.[91] The office included significantly more workers in its investigation than the manganese study involved. By including physical scientists on its research team, the office was also able to undertake more extensive quantitative studies of the working environment. In subsequent field studies, office researchers followed the methods they had established in the tetraethyl lead study, and they began to calculate safe concentration levels as well.[92-94] They also helped to extend the same research practices into the area of dust diseases.[95]

Compensation law may well have had an impact on the move to more standardized scientific practices, but the precise form these standards took most likely had some influence on legal thinking as well. When workers in New Jersey filed a total of 110 different claims for compensation for benzene poisoning in 1927 and 1928, the state compensation commission used a set of three postulates as a "standard and guide" for decision making on claims: "1. The claimant must demonstrate an exposure to benzol poisoning. 2. The claimant must present symptoms of benzol poisoning. 3. The claimant must demonstrate a change in his blood picture."[96] These three kinds of information, which were all necessary for a "positive diagnosis" and full compensation under the law, paralleled the array of knowledge in the manganese study. Law followed science in asserting the need to know about chemical exposure and absorption as well as disease. The compensation system thus evolved its own hybrid system of medicolegal logic.

Finally, the new scientific standards of both method and attitude helped drive and guide the making of new forms of government intervention in the workplace. New or expanded divisions and bureaus of "industrial hygiene" emerged within state departments of labor and health. New York increased the postgraduate trained personnel in its Division of Industrial Hygiene from one doctor in 1922 to four doctors and two engineers in 1924.[97,98] Connecticut began a Division of Occupational Diseases in 1928, which included both a physician and an industrial hygienist on its staff by 1930.[99] In that year, Connecticut and New York conducted the most extensive industrial hygiene activities in the country, but 12 other states reported special groups devoted to industrial hygiene work, evenly distributed between departments of health and labor.[100] A clear division of responsibilities arose between researchers in the public health schools and federal agencies and these new state officials in the field of industrial hygiene.

The state industrial hygienists investigated problems of occupational disease in specific factories, usually at the request of employers but also at the invitation of the regular factory inspectors.[101,121,122] The industrial hygiene organizations in both Connecticut and New York preferred to offer recommendations to factory owners or managers, though they could legally order preventive measures in collaboration with their respective inspection bureaus.[102] With engineers as well as doctors on their staffs, they could carry out physical examinations, atmospheric chemical analyses, and clinical laboratory work. Though their capabilities reproduced the range of information in the investigational exemplars of the time, they became increasingly reliant upon the conclusions of the researchers about maximum safe atmospheric concentrations and the proper diagnostic use of laboratory tests or X-rays. More and more, they turned away from drawing conclusions based on the naked eye, whether in the workplace or the clinic. Instead, environmental and clinical laboratory tests moved to center stages as the final arbitrators of the safety of working environments.[103,104] Connecticut's Bureau of Preventable Diseases performed some physical examinations in the mid-twenties to follow up official reports of occupational disease.[105] After 1928, however, the reports of the new Division of Occupational Diseases rarely mentioned physical examinations, though they included extensive quantitative environmental analyses.[106]

To see how this new complex of experts, knowledge, and rhetorical defenses operated, we need only consider why safe concentration estimates proved so central to it. They preserved the combination of fact with imperative in the knowledge of Gilman Thompson, but now in a technical form suitable to a professional audience of state and company industrial hygienists and physicians. For their expert audience they addressed an unsentimental professional obligation to promote safety, and for much of this audience and the public they seemed to belong to the realm of objective science. The standardized methods which some researchers such as those at the PHS developed to calculate these estimates reinforced such perceptions, along with the political and cultural authority of the new research community. The PHS investigators regularly determined their estimates of what was "safe" from the least atmospheric concentrations at which their field studies uncovered no full-blown clinical cases of poisoning.[107–109] This decision itself involved numerous other determinations that at least since 1970, our laws have reserved instead for policy makers, from whether or not to include a safety margin to whether cases of asymptomatic chemical absorption should be ignored or avoided.[110,111] Despite pretenses otherwise, when these researchers distinguished between what was appropriate for scientific experts to decide and what was not, the lines they drew actually served to disguise and protect what we now see as a highly value-laden process.

The state industrial hygiene divisions became the final leg in the circuit of specialized study and intervention that constituted a new system of knowledge about industrial disease. By 1940, some 31 states sponsored industrial hygiene work.[112,113] By this time, as well, the American Conference of Government Industrial Hygienists (ACGIH) had formed, out of a seminar sponsored by the PHS's Division of Industrial Hygiene that brought together industry hygienists as well as state and local public health officials. By 1946, it had begun work on establishing the first set of what were to become the Threshold Limit Values—essentially safe concentration levels on which the ACGIH's Threshold Committee could reach agreement. Not only did the ACGIH make use of Hamiltonian appeals to objectivity, its estimates largely duplicated those set by a committee of Hamilton and her colleagues some 6 years before, following their recommendations to the letter in 28 of 38 cases. Of the rest, six ACGIH estimates were lower and only 4 were higher.[114,115] The apparently consensual and numerically precise nature of the TLVs reinforced their proponents' claims to objectivity and expertise, on which the prescriptive power of the estimates now almost entirely depended. While the history of the TLV's application makes for another story, the formulation of an entire, official list of them brought the system of knowledge from the twenties to full fruition. In the American science of industrial hazards, the same patterns of investigations, attitudes and practices dominated the field of industrial health for another quarter of a century.

Patterns set in the mid-twentieth century have persisted: warring sides in modern controversies over occupational risks still attempt to draw boundaries between the parts of their arguments that are science and those that are policy, and thus subject to interest group pressures.[116] In the field of occupational and environmental health, this strategy, which is not just a rhetorical ploy but a gesture closely tied to one's professional identity, had its origins in the sweeping changes of the twenties. It began with the emergence of a new system for the production and usage of knowledge in the field of occupational disease. As research institutions grew separate from regulatory ones, and as groups of trained experts emerged within the regulatory agencies,

a new type of knowledge and a new stance toward knowledge evolved, in close relation. As objectivity came to seem opposed to the "cloud" of economic interest, the
invocation of science developed a different and more characteristically modern
meaning.

For the progressives, the science of occupational disease had been a democratic
knowledge, which would rally public support and the commitment of factory owners
to improve the factory environment. From the twenties onward, claims to science
served increasingly as defenses of expertise, and arguments for closing particular
decisions and rationales to lay scrutiny and debate. The new system did better assure
the reliability of what was known about occupational diseases, and chemical diseases
in particular. Their toxicological approach proved more difficult to apply to the dust
diseases, but even there, the more elaborate standards for knowledge may have better
guaranteed that the prescriptions of its bearers would be heeded. What also seems
clear in retrospect is that the new requirements helped ensure that this knowledge
would remain accessible to a limited audience only. Except for occasional flurries of
unavoidable public attention, such as that surrounding the silicosis deaths at Gauley
Bridge, knowledge about industrial diseases came up against new barriers in circulating to a lay public, and remained largely sealed within the same community of experts until the challenges of the 1960s.[117]

In the early twenty-first century, the basic scientific methods, disciplinary boundaries, and institutions from the 1920s persist, and appeals to a more scientific or
objective knowledge remain a cornerstone of debate on occupational and environmental health issues.[118] In more recent times, the conventional notion of scientific
objectivity has come under assault from across the political spectrum. From the
1980s, scholars wielding the perspectives of sociology of science and feminism,
many of them left-leaning, have attacked the kinds of intellectual and institutional
partitions that arose in the 1920s in the field of industrial chemical disease. Sylvia
Tesh, after analyzing the attempts of scientists to assess the toxicity of Agent Orange, concluded that Hamiltonian objectivity about such socially embedded issues
is impossible: "science, because it does not exist without scientists, necessarily
requires value-filled human decisions at every step."[119,120] On the other hand, as
American unions have lost much of their ability to serve as a countervailing influence, the government funding that supported a surge of new research in occupational
and environmental health from the 1960s onward has plateaued, and remains politically vulnerable to erosion. Corporations and conservative foundations have meanwhile ever more brazenly turned to supporting researchers who will come up with
the "right" questions: whether about the disease effects of tobacco or the human impact and reality of global warming.

Specialists in occupational and environmental health still need the ideal of objectivity. They need it every bit as much as when, back in the 1920s, Hamilton first
enunciated what was at stake. Yet after nearly a century of experience with Hamilton's version of this ideal, it has become difficult to follow Hamilton in believing that
objectivity can become, for an entire group of scientific professionals, a fully accomplished reality. It now seems unlikely that scientific standards will completely
suppress pressures and influences external to the expert community. Indeed, interests, even warring ones within a scientific profession, are precisely what makes it

tick. Scientists and physicians in the field of occupational and environmental health need to find new ways of acknowledging up-front how their scientific judgments can be influenced by the standards of the research community, and by their own interests and inclinations, personal and political as well as professional. The historical making of Hamiltonian objectivity stands as an inspiring example, dated as its terms and circumstances may be. In a field so contested as industrial hygiene was by the 1920s, it is not surprising that such a strong insistence on scientific impartiality would emerge. Yet the ever-present vulnerability of science to partisanship makes an explicit and balanced appraisal of its status all the more necessary, not just in Hamilton's time but in our own.

Note

A revised version of this article originally published in *Toxic Circles; Environmental Hazards from the Workplace into the Community*, edited by Helen Sheehan and Richard Wedeen (New Brunswick: Rutgers University Press, 1993), 231–63.

References

1. Paull JM. The origin and basis of Threshold Limit Values. *Am J Ind Med* 1984:5:231.
2. Ashford N. Crisis in the Workplace: Occupational Disease and Injury. Cambridge, MA: MIT Press, 1976.
3. Salter L. Mandated Science; Science and Scientists in the Making of Standards. Dordrecht, Holland: Kluwer Academic Publishers, 1988, 53–54.
4. Vigliani E et al. Methods Used in Western European Countries for Establishing Maximum Permissible Levels of Harmful Agents in the Working Environment. Milan: Fondazione Carlo Erba, 1977.
5. Noweir MH. Occupational health in developing countries with special reference to Egypt. *Am J Ind Med* 1986:9:134.
6. Teleky L. History of Factory and Mine Hygiene. New York: Columbia University, 1948.
7. Kober GM. History of industrial hygiene and its effect on public health. In: Mazyck Ravenel, ed. A Half Century of Public Health. New York: American Public Health Association, 1921, 361–411.
8. Rosen G. A History of Public Health. New York: MD Publications, 1958, 264–75, 419–39.
9. McCready B. On the Influence of Trades, Professions and Occupations in the United States, in the Production of Disease. New York: Arno Press, 1972 [originally published in 1837].
10. Rohe GH. The hygiene of occupations. *Public Health Pap Rep* 1885:10165–73.
11. McCord CP. Occupational health publications in the United States prior to 1900. *Ind Med Surg* 1955:24:363–68.
12. Rosen G. Urbanization, occupation and disease in the United States, 1870–1920: the case of New York City. *J Hist Med Allied Sci* 1988:4:391–425.
13. Galishoff S. Safeguarding the Public Health, Newark 1895–1918. Westport, CT and London: Greenwood Press, 1975, 135–38.
14. Price GM. Factory inspection and factory inspectors. *J Ind Hyg* 1919:1:165–66.
15. Hazlett TL, Hummel W. Industrial Medicine in Western Pennsylvania, 1850–1950. Pittsburgh: University of Pittsburgh Press, 1957, 31–47.
16. Derickson A. Workers' Health: Workers' Democracy; the Western Miners' Struggle, 1891–1925. Ithaca and London: Cornell University Press, 1988.

17. Vogel M, Rosenberg C, eds. The Therapeutic Revolution: Essays in the Social History of Medicine. Philadelphia: University of Pennsylvania Press, 1979, 3–108.
18. Rosenberg C. The Care of Strangers: The Rise of America's Hospital System. New York: Basic Books, 1987.
19. Hays S. Conservation and the Gospel of Efficiency: The Progressive Conservation Movement, 1890–1920. New York: Atheneum, 1969.
20. Nelson D. Frederick Taylor and the Rise of Scientific Management. Madison: University of Wisconsin Press, 1980.
21. Davis A. Spearheads for Reform: The Social Settlements and the Progressive Movement, 1890–1914. New York: Oxford University Press, 1967.
22. Andrews W, ed. The Autobiography of Theodore Roosevelt. New York: Charles Scribner's Sons, 1958, 340–45.
23. Blum JM. The Republican Roosevelt. Cambridge, MA: Harvard University Press, 1967, 149–50.
24. Thompson WG. Occupational Diseases: Their Causation, Symptoms, Treatment and Prevention. New York: D. Appleton and Co., 1914, 136, 140.
25. Andrews J. Scientific Standards in Labor Legislation. *American Labor Legislation Review* 1911:1(June):123–34.
26. Report of Massachusetts Commission to Investigate the Inspection of Factories, Workshops, Mercantile Establishments and Other Buildings. Boston: Wright and Potter Printing Co., 1911, 14.
27. Hamilton A. Exploring the Dangerous Trades: The Autobiography of Alice Hamilton, M.D. Boston: Northeastern University Press, 1985, 132.
28. Report of Bureau of Factory Inspection. In: Annual Reports of Department Bureaus for the Twelve Months Ended September 30, 1911. Albany: State Department of Labor, 1913, 36, 37.
29. Price G. Medical supervision in dangerous trades. *J Sociol Med* 1915:16:96.
30. Twelfth annual report of the commissioner of labor for the twelve months ended September 30, 1912. In: Albany: State Department of Labor, 1913, 74–74, 82.
31. Committee on Occupational Hygiene. Occupational hygiene. *American Labor Legislation Review* 1914:6:525.
32. Annual report of the industrial commissioner for the twelve months ended June 30, 1921. Albany: State Department of Labor, 1922, 108, 152.
33. Thirtieth report of the Bureau of Labor for the period ending June 30, 1922. Hartford, CT: Connecticut Department of Health,1922, 12.
34. Stenographer's notes of public hearing before the Joint Standing Committee on Public Health and Safety, January Session, 1923. Connecticut State Law Library, Hartford, 1923.
35. Kober GM. History of industrial hygiene and its effects on public health. In: Mazyck Ravenel, ed. A Half Century of Public Health. New York: American Public Health Association, 1921, 393–94.
36. Curran JA. Founders of the Harvard School of Public Health, with biographical notes, 1909–1946. New York: Josiah Macy, Jr. Foundation, 1970, 154–55, 159.
37. Aub J. Pioneer in Modern Medicine: David Linn Edsall of Harvard. Boston: Harvard Medical Alumni Association, 1970, 182–93.
38. Garment Workers' Union tackling tuberculosis. *Survey* 1913:31:313.
39. Andrews J. Physical examination of employees. *Am J Public Health* 1916:6:825.
40. Nugent A. Fit for work: the introduction of physical examination in industry. *Bull His Med* 1983:57:579–81.
41. Nelson D. Managers and Workers: Origins of the New Factory System in the United States, 1880–1920. Madison, WI: University of Wisconsin Press, 1975, 101–21.

42. Teller ME. The Tuberculosis Movement: A Public Health Campaign in the Progressive Era. New York: Greenwood Press, 1988, 88–92.
43. Transactions of the Tenth Annual Meeting of the National Association for the Study and Prevention of Tuberculosis, Washington, DC, 7–8 May 1914. Philadelphia: William F. Fell, 1914, 54–58.
44. National Industrial Conference Board. Workmen's Compensation Acts in the United States: The Legal Phase. Boston: National Industrial Conference Board, 1917, 5.
45. American Association for Labor Legislation. Standards for workmen's compensation laws. *American Labor Legislation Review* 1914:4:585.
46. Bale A. Compensation crisis: the value and meaning of work-related injuries and illnesses in the United States, 1842–1932. Ph.D. dissertation, Brandeis University, 1986, 444–521.
47. Mock HE. Industrial medicine and surgery: a résumé of its development and scope. *J Ind Hyg* 1919:1:1, 3–5.
48. Selleck H, Whittaker A. Occupational Health in America. Detroit: Wayne State University Press, 1962, 57–69.
49. Rosner D, Markowitz G. The early movement for occupational safety and health, 1900–1917. In: Leavitt JW, Numbers R, eds. Sickness and Health in America: Readings in the History of Medicine and Public Health. Madison: University of Wisconsin Press, 1985, 507–24.
50. McFarlane AE. Fire and the skyscraper: the problem of protecting the workers in New York's tower factories. *McClure's Magazine* 1911:37:467–82.
51. Sanville FL. A woman in the Pennsylvania silk-mills. *Harper's Monthly* 1910:120:615–62.
52. Butler EB. Pittsburgh women in the metal trades. *Charities* 1908–9:21:34–47.
53. Andrews J. Phosphorus poisoning in the match industry in the United States. *Bulletin of the U.S. Bureau of Labor* 1910:86.
54. Hamilton A. Lead poisoning in potteries, tile works, and porcelain enameled sanitary ware factories. *Bulletin of the U.S. Bureau of Labor* 1912:104
55. Hamilton A. Hygiene of the painters' trade. *Bulletin of the U.S. Bureau of Labor Statistics* 1913:120:42–43.
56. Price G. The Modern Factory: Safety, Sanitation, and Welfare. New York: John Wiley and Sons, 1914.
57. Kober GM, Hanson WC. Diseases of Occupation and Vocational Hygiene. Philadelphia: Blakiston's Son & Co., 1916.
58. Rosen GM. From frontier surgeon to industrial hygienist: the strange career of George Martin Kober. *Am J Public Health* 1975:65: 638–43.
59. Hanson WC. The Hygiene of Occupation and Its Administrative Control. Transactions of the Fifteenth International Congress on Hygiene and Demography, Washington, DC, 23–28 September 1912. Washington, DC: Government Printing Office, 1912, vol. II, part II, 899–900.
60. Osler W, McCrae T. The Principles and Practice of Medicine. New York and London: D. Appleton and Company, 1915, 393–95, 402–7.
61. Edsall D. Some of the relations of occupations to medicine. *JAMA* 1909:53:1873–74.
62. Hill HW. The New Public Health. Minneapolis: Press of the Journal-Lancet, 1913.
63. MacNutt JS. A Manual for Health Officers. New York: John Wiley and Sons, 1915, 434–37.
64. Sellers C. Hazards of the Job: From Industrial Disease to Environmental Health Science. Chapel Hill: University of North Carolina Press, 1997, chap. 3.
65. Young AN. Interpreting the dangerous trades: workers' health in America and the career of Alice Hamilton, 1910–35. Ph.D. dissertation, Brown University, June 1982, 68–106.

66. Fee E. Disease and Discovery: A History of the Johns Hopkins School of Hygiene and Public Health. Baltimore and London: Johns Hopkins University Press, 1987, 124–26, 172–76.
67. Meeting of the College, Wednesday, May 2, 1917. Record of the College of Physicians of Philadelphia, archives of the College of Physicians of Philadelphia, 86.
68. Our first number. *The Industrial Doctor* 1923:1:13–14.
69. Ziegler SL. The peril of wood alcohol toxemia and the remedy. *Pa Med J* 1921:25:177–81.
70. Utley FB. Anthrax. *Pa Med J* 1922:25:831.
71. Programs of county meetings. Proceedings of Connecticut State Medical Society, Hartford, CT, 1921, 207.
72. Clark WI. Industrial medicine and public health. *N Engl J Med* 1930:202:1188.
73. Proceedings of the Conference of State and Provincial Health Authorities of North America, Washington, D.C. St. Paul: Conference of State and Provincial Health Authorities, 24–25 May 1920, 122.
74. Mock H. Industrial Medicine and Surgery. Philadelphia and London: W.B. Saunders, 1919, 678.
75. National Industrial Conference Board, Workmen's Compensation Acts in the United States: The Medical Aspect. New York: National Industrial Conference Board, 1923.
76. Controversy obscures facts in compensation decisions. *Nation's Health* 1922:4:25.
77. Hatch LW. Industrial medicine in its relation to workmen's compensation. *The Industrial Doctor* 1923:1:209.
78. Sayer H. Report of the Committee on Medical Questions. *The Industrial Doctor* 1923:1:13.
79. Proceedings of the Conference of State and Provincial Health Authorities of North America, Washington, D.D. St. Paul: Conference of State and Provincial Health Authorities, 14, 16 May 1927, 188.
80. National Industrial Conference Board. Medical Care of Industrial Workers. New York: National Industrial Conference Board, 1926, 25.
81. Derickson A. Workers' Health, Workers' Democracy. Ithaca and London: Cornell University Press, 1988, 205–9.
82. Brody D. Labor in Crisis: The Steel Strike of 1919. Philadelphia: J.B. Lippincott, 1965, 101.
83. Kerr JW, McCurdy SM, Geier O. The scope of industrial hygiene. *JAMA* 1916:77:1822.
84. Selby CD. Modern industrial medicine. *Modern Medicine* 1919:1:35.
85. Mock H. Industrial medicine and surgery: the new specialty. *JAMA* 1917:63:3.
86. Hamilton A. Industrial Poisons in the United States. New York: Macmillan Company, 1925.
87. Edsall D, Wilbur FP, Drinker C. The occurence, cause, and prevention of chronic manganese poisoning. *J Ind Hyg* 1919–20:1:183–94.
88. Sellers C. The PHS's Division of Industrial Hygiene and the transformation of industrial medicine. *Bull His Med* 1991:65:42–73, 234, 319, 380–81, 480–81.
89. Markowitz G, Rosner D. The street of walking death: silicosis, health and labor in the tri-state region, 1900–1950. *Journal of American History* 1990:77:540.
90. Rosner D, Markowitz G. Research or advocacy: federal occupational safety and health policies during the New Deal. In Rosner D and Markowitz G eds. Dying for Work: Workers' Safety and Health in Twentieth-Century America. Bloomington and Indianapolis: Indiana University Press, 1989, 83–102.
91. Leake J, Kolb L, et al. The use of tetraethyl lead gasoline in its relation to public health. *Public Health Bull* 1926:163.
92. Bloomfield JJ, Blum W. Health hazards of chromium plating. *Public Health Rep* 1928: 43:2330–47.

93. Greenberg L. Benzol poisoning as an industrial hazard. *Public Health Rep* 1926: 41: 1356–65, 1410–31,1516–35.

94. Neal P, Jones R, Bloofield JJ, Dallavalle M, Edwards T. A study of chronic mercurialism in the hatters; fur-cutting industry. *Public Health Bull* 1937:234.

95. Sayers RR et al. Anthraco-silicosis among hard coal miners. *Public Health Bull* 1935:221.

96. Kessler HH. Some medicolegal aspects of occupational disease. *Arch Intern Med* 1929: 43:875.

97. New York State Department of Labor. Annual Report of the Industrial Commissioner for the Twelve Months Ended June 30, 1922.. Albany: J.B. Lyon Company, 1923, 40.

98. New York State Department of Labor. Annual Report of the Industrial Commissioner for the Twelve Months Ended June 30, 1924. Albany: J.B. Lyon Company, 1925, 110.

99. Annual Report of the Connecticut State Department of Health, 1930. Hartford, CT: Connecticut Department of Health, 1931, 241.

100. Proceedings of the Conference of State and Provincial Health Authorities of North America, Washington, DC, 18–20 June 1930. St. Paul: Conference of State and Provincial Health Authorities, 106.

101. Annual Report of the Department of Health of the State of Connecticut, 1928. Hartford, CT: Connecticut Department of Health, 1928, 207.

102. Communication. Tone J, Commissioner of the Department of Labor and Factory Inspection, to Stanley Osborne, Commissioner of the Department of Health, 18 February 1937. In Folder 943, Box 69, Series III, C.E.A., Winslow Papers, Sterling Library Manuscripts and Archives, Yale University, New Haven, CT. For New York, see note 101.

103. New York State Department of Labor. Annual Report of the Industrial Commissioner for the Twelve Months Ended June 30, 1921. Albany: State Department of Labor, 1922, 110.

104. New York State Department of Labor. Annual Report of the Industrial Commissioner for the Twelve Months Ended December 31, 1931. Albany: J.B. Lyon Company, 1932, 123.

105. Annual Report of the Department of Health for the State of Connecticut, 1925; Hartford, 1925, 93.

106. Annual Report of the Department of Health of the State of Connecticut, 1931; Hartford, 1931, 427–433.

107. Russell A, Jones R, Bloomfield JJ, Britten R, Thompson L. Lead poisoning in a storage battery plant. *Public Health Bull* 1933:205:32, 55.

108. Dreessen W, Edwards T, Reinhart W et al. The control of the lead hazard in the storage battery industry. *Public Health Bull* 1941:262:58–59.

109. Bloomfield JJ, Blum W. Health hazards in chromium plating. *Public Health Rep* 1928:43:2345.

110. Henderson Y, Haggard H, Teague M, Prince A, Wunderlich R. Physiological effects of automobile exhaust gas and standards of ventilation for brief exposures. *J Ind Hyg* 1921:3: 92.

111. Dreessen W, Edwards T, Reinhart W et al. The control of the lead hazard in the storage battery industry. *Public Health Bull* 1941:262:58–59.

112. Proceedings of the Conference of State and Provincial Health Authorities of North America, Washington, DC, 8, 10–11 May 1940. St. Paul: Conference of State and Provincial Health Authorites, 1940, 86.

113. Proceedings of the Conference of State and Provincial Health Authorities of North America, Washington, DC, 18–20 June 1930. St. Paul: Conference of State and Provincial Health Authorities, 1930, 106.

114. Bowditch M, Drinker CK, Drinker P, Haggard HH, Hamilton A. Code for safe concentrations of certain common toxic substances used in industry. *J Ind Hyg* 1940:22:251.

115. Report of the Sub-Committee on Threshold Limits. Proceedings of the Eighth Annual

Meeting of the American Conference of Governmental Industrial Hygienists, 7–13 April 1946, Chicago. St. Paul: Conference of State and Provincial Health Authorities, 54–55.

116. Jasanoff S. Contested boundaries in policy-relevant science. *Social Studies of Science* 1987:17:195–230.

117. Cherniak M. The Hawk's Nest Incident; America's Worst Industrial Disaster. New Haven and London: Yale University Press, 1986.

118. Castleman B, Ziem G. Corporate influence on Threshold Limit Values. *Am J Ind Med* 1988:13:531–59.

119. Tesh S. Hidden Arguments: Political Ideology and Disease Prevention Policy. New Brunswick and London: Rutgers University Press, 1988, 5.

120. Salter L. Mandated Science: Science and Scientists in the Making of Standards. Dordrecht, Holland: Kluwer Academic Publishers, 1988.

121. McBurney R. Industrial hygiene practice: typical case illustrating aid rendered to manufacturers. *Ind Hyg Bull* 1927:3:41–44.

122. Flexner J. The work of an industrial hygiene division in a state department of labor. *U.S. Department of Labor Bulletin* 1939:31:9–10, 19–22.

Suggested Reading

Hamilton A. Exploring the Dangerous Trades; The Autobiography of Alice Hamilton, M.D. Boston: Northeastern University Press, 1985.

Kober GM. History of industrial hygiene and its effect on public health. In: Mazyck Ravenel, ed. A Half Century of Public Health. New York: American Public Health Association, 1921, 361–411.

Rosner D, Markowitz G. The early movement for occupational safety and health, 1900–1917. In: Leavitt JW, Numbers R, eds. Sickness and Health in America: Readings in the History of Medicine and Public Health. Madison: University of Wisconsin Press, 1985, 507–24.

Sellers, C. Hazards of the Job: From Industrial Disease to Environmental Health Science. Chapel Hill, N.C.: University of North Carolina Press, 1997.

Warren, C. Brush With Death: A Social History of Lead Poisoning. Baltimore, MD: Johns Hopkins University Press, 2000.

PART VI

FAMILY PLANNING

12

Family Planning: A Century of Change

JACQUELINE E. DARROCH

During the twentieth century, technologic changes in family-planning methods available to American women and men increased couples' ability to successfully control the number and timing of children, increased women's control over fertility, separated contraceptive behavior from intercourse, and gave rise to alternative medical provider networks for women's reproductive-health care. This chapter summarizes key changes in family planning over the last century and provides an overview of changes in contraceptive technology and in the provision of reproductive health and contraceptive services.

Background

As the twentieth century dawned, American women typically became biologically capable of conceiving children at age 15, were married at age 22, and had their first babies at age 24.[1] They had an average of 3.6 children during their reproductive lives,[2] but only 2.9 of these children would live to reach their fifth birthdays. The risk of dying from childbirth for these women was almost 1 in 100.[3] By the end of the century, these reproductive-health statistics had shifted substantially.[4] Women born during the last third of the 1900s experienced menarche 2 years earlier, at 13 years of age, and first engaged in sexual intercourse at age 17; however, women typically were married later, at age 25, and had their first babies at 26. They would have an average of 2.1 children over their lifetimes,[5] and their children had a 99% likelihood of living until age 5 years.[6] The risk of dying from childbirth among these women was 1 in 10,000.[7] Most American women and their sexual partners living during both of these time periods took measures to control the number and timing of their children. Without use of contraceptive measures, most women are capable of having as many as 18 children before menopause.[8] The average number of births per woman has varied over time. The number among white women (the only group for which the statistic is available for early years) declined steadily from the 1800s through the early 1900s, from about 7.0 in 1800, to 3.6 in 1900, and to 2.1 in the mid-1930s.[9] Average number of births rose sharply during the post-World War II baby boom to 3.8 in 1957, reflecting an average number of 3.6 among white and 4.8 among black and other women.[10] The average number fell to 1.7 in 1976 (1.7 among whites and 2.2 among black women), and then rose again to 2.1 among both white and black women in 1999.[11]

Fertility Control in the First Half of the 1900s: Withdrawal, Douche, and Condom

Throughout the twentieth century, most U.S. couples used contraceptive methods or practices. This occurred in spite of informal and formal prohibitions against contraceptive use. In 1873, the federal Comstock Act, "An Act for the Suppression of Trade in, and Circulation of, Obscene Literature and Articles of Immoral Use," defined contraceptives as obscene and illicit and made it a federal offense to disseminate methods through the mail or across state lines.[12] Ultimately, 30 states had laws on the books prohibiting or restricting the sale and advertisement of contraceptives, though they were seldom enforced. Connecticut law prohibited use of contraception. When Margaret Sanger opened the first birth control clinic in the United States in 1916 in Brooklyn, New York, in 1916, it was closed after 10 days by the New York City "vice squad."[13] Although she was jailed for a month, the case, *People v. Sanger*, resolved in 1918 with a court decision allowing women in New York to use birth control for therapeutic purposes. In 1936, a federal appeals court ruled in *United States v. One Package*, that doctors could distribute contraceptives and information across state lines. Nationwide legal recognition of rights of couples to practice contraception occurred through Supreme Court decisions late in the century—for married couples in 1965 (*Griswold v. Connecticut*) and in 1972 for the unmarried (*Eisenstadt v. Baird*).[4]

The types of measures people used, however, changed dramatically from the beginning to the end of the 1900s. Measuring national patterns of sexual and fertility-control behavior of women began only in the mid-1900s, starting with the Growth of American Families studies in 1955 and 1960,[14] followed by the National Fertility Studies in 1965, 1970, and 1975,[15–17] and the National Survey of Family Growth in 1973, 1976, 1982, 1988, 1995, and 2002.[18]

Despite the lack of national data during the first half of the century, direct evidence of fertility-control patterns is available from studies of women visiting birth-control clinics and from women hospitalized for childbirth. Several studies collected and analyzed by sociologist Norman Himes indicated widespread contraceptive knowledge and use in the early part of the century.[19] Himes compiled a wide-ranging history of fertility-control practices from preliterate to modern times. He presented data on fertility-control practices ascertained through large-scale surveys of women and men during the 1920s that collected data regarding marital life and sexuality. He also summarized pioneering research conducted in the 1920s to measure effectiveness of birth control practices, including studies carried out by Marie Kopp at the New York City Birth Control Bureau; Hannah Stone at the Newark New Jersey Maternal Health Center; and by Raymond Pearl, who used data from surveys of women hospitalized in multiple cities around the United States.

In the early 1930s, Raymond Pearl determined the effectiveness of fertility-control practices by measuring the ratio of pregnancies among users of a particular method to exposures measured in women-years of method use. This measure proved easy to compute and continues to be widely used, despite the potential for inconsistent outcomes resulting from variations in the duration of exposure used.[20] Information from these researchers provided the first scientific data regarding the effectiveness of available methods of contraception and variations in contraceptive success among users by sociodemographic characteristics, by childbearing intentions, and by the regularity of contraceptive use.

The multi-city study of 4945 women hospitalized for childbirth conducted by Pearl revealed that 37% of first-time mothers and approximately 50% of women giving birth a subsequent time had used contraceptives before pregnancy.[19] (These levels might have been underestimates because of overrepresentation of Roman Catholic women in some of the cities studied.) Use was highest among "well-to-do and rich" whites (78%), moderate among whites of "moderate circumstances" (51%), and low among blacks and low-income whites (21%–39%). Other studies of women visiting birth-control clinics from the late 1910s to the early 1930s demonstrated that 59%–93% had already used some form of contraceptive, with four of the seven studies indicating that ≥90% had already used one or more methods.

In 1978, a nationally representative, retrospective survey was conducted involving 1049 white women born during 1901–1910 who had been married at some time during their lifetimes and who had reached their prime reproductive ages in the 1920s and 1930s. This study found that 749 (71%) of these women had used a contraceptive during their lifetimes and that another 169 (16%) had used a douche for feminine hygiene.[20] These data are consistent with Himes's estimate that the most commonly used methods (accounting for 80% of methods used) in the first part of the twentieth century were withdrawal, douche, and condom in almost equal proportions. Other methods cited by women included suppositories and jellies, diaphragms, sponges, intrauterine devices (IUDs), lactation, and periodic abstinence.[19]

A 1934 report by Kopp of 9250 contraceptive clinic clients demonstrated that more than half of women who had used withdrawal or douche as contraceptive methods and almost half of those who had used the condom prior to attending the clinic believed they had become pregnant while using these methods.[22] Pregnancy rates among women attending health clinics who had been using contraceptive methods were only one fourth those of women using no method. According to a 1933 report by Stone, of 1987 women surveyed at the Newark Maternal Health Center in Newark, New Jersey, 92% had already used contraceptives and 80% had tried more than one method. Women visited the center not because they wanted to learn something about birth control, but because they wanted to obtain accurate and scientific information.[23]

The Mid-1900s: Condom, Diaphragm, and Periodic Abstinence

In 1955, a study called the Growth of American Families (GAF) was undertaken to examine factors affecting control of fertility to shed light on why postwar birthrates were so much higher than those before the war and to help improve birth forecasts in the United States. The GAF was the first study of fertility regulation in the United States that was nationally representative, using area probability sampling techniques. Because the focus of this study was on women's expectations of the number of children they would have over the next 5 years, it was limited to married women, and it included only the white population. It was followed in 1960 by a similar survey aimed at determining how well the 1955 reports of future births predicted aggregate levels of births over the next 5 years. (The 1960 survey collected information on both white and nonwhite women, but published comparisons with 1955 include only those who were white.)

The 1955 nationally representative survey of 2713 married white women aged 18–39 years found that 70% had used a contraceptive during their lifetime, and 34% had used a method before their first pregnancy. The most commonly used methods had changed, however. Among women who had used contraceptives, the most recently used method was the condom (27%), the diaphragm (26%), and periodic abstinence (21%); 6% used contraceptive sterilization and 20% used other methods (see Fig. 12.1).[14,15,24–28]

The shift in types of contraception being used by the mid-1900s reflected several technological developments. Condoms have been traced to use of animal membranes as "penis protectors" in ancient Egypt, and over the centuries men have used cloth sheaths both for protection against syphilis and for contraception. Rubber condoms were first marketed in 1850, shortly after the vulcanization of rubber in 1844; the development of latex and modern manufacturing methods in the twentieth century made them both more durable and inexpensive.[19] Building on earlier informal use of lemon halves for contraception, the vaginal diaphragm was developed in the early 1800s in Europe, as was first described in published accounts in the 1880s. Diaphragms were smuggled into the United States in the early 1920s by Margaret Sanger because U.S. law banned importation of contraceptives. U.S. manufacture began in 1925 by a company formed by Sanger's husband and other associates.[29,30] Parallel with the development of new methods, an understanding of the biology of reproduction advanced with establishment of the timing of ovulation in 1928.

The development of reproductive-health delivery services to distribute these new technologies contributed to changes in the methods used by U.S. couples. In 1937, 1 year after the federal court ruling, in *United States v. One Package,* that doctors could legally distribute contraceptive information and supplies across state lines, the American Medical Association officially endorsed birth control, and North Carolina became the first state to include birth control in a public health program. (See Chapter 13.) During 1937–1957, six additional southeastern states (i.e., Alabama, Florida, Georgia, Mississippi, South Carolina, and Virginia) initiated family-planning services.[31] Many such clinics offered vaginal foam and condoms with no medical supervision, organized patient recruitment, follow-up, or evaluation. In 1942, the

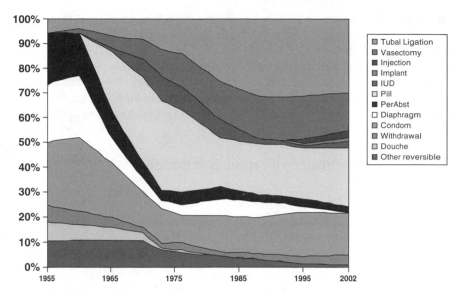

Figure 12.1. Methods used by currently-married contraceptive users, 1955–2002. 1955: white married women ages 18–39 years; other years: all married women ages 15–44 years. (From Whelpton PK, Campbell AA, Patterson JE. Fertility and Family Planning in the United States. Princeton: Princeton University Press,1966; Ryder NB, Westoff CF. Reproduction in the United States. Princeton: Princeton University Press,1971; Westoff CF. The modernization of U.S. contraceptive practice. *Fam Plann Perspect* 1972:4:9–12; Bachrach CA. Contraceptive practice among American women, 1973–1982. *Fam Plann Perspect* 1984:16:253–59; 1988 NSFG, 1995 NSFG; Mosher WD, et al. Use of contraception and use of family planning services in the United States: 1982–2002. *Adv Data* 2004:350.)

Planned Parenthood Federation of America was established and began to coordinate the operation of affiliated birth-control clinics around the country, offering diaphragms, spermicidal foam, and condoms under physician supervision.[3] These clinic programs sought to provide economically disadvantaged women and other women who had difficulty accessing private physicians with contraceptive-associated information and supplies.

During 1955–1960, contraceptive use further increased.[14] The 1960 National Growth of American Families survey found that 81% of the 2414 married white women aged 18–39 years who were survey respondents had used some type of contraceptive method. Another 7% expected to use contraceptives in the future and 10% were subfecund. The proportions of women who had used condoms increased, as did the proportion who had undergone sterilization and used spermicidal jelly independent of the diaphragm; use of douche for contraceptive purposes declined. Compared to other women, contraceptive use was highest among college-educated women, those whose husbands' incomes were higher, and Protestant (vs. Roman Catholic) women. Married, nonwhite women aged 18–39 years were less likely to have used a contraceptive method than their white counterparts (59% vs. 81%), though the differences were narrow in the Northeast and among college-educated women.

Nonwhite wives were most likely to have used the condom, douche, and diaphragm, whereas the top three methods among whites were the condom, diaphragm, and the practice of periodic abstinence.[15] However, wide differences in method occurred by religious affiliation. Among Protestant and Jewish wives who had used contraceptives, 69% had most recently used the condom or diaphragm, and only 7% had practiced periodic abstinence. In contrast, 53% of Catholic wives who had used contraceptives most recently used periodic abstinence, and 33% relied on the condom or the diaphragm.

1960–2000: Pill, Sterilization, and Condom

Technologic Innovation

Before 1960, when oral contraceptives were approved by the Food and Drug Administration (FDA), and the intrauterine device (IUD) began to be marketed, almost all available contraceptives short of surgical sterilization were used around the time of intercourse (e.g., condom, diaphragm, withdrawal, and douche) or were linked to the timing of coitus (e.g., periodic abstinence). All such methods worked by preventing the sperm from meeting the egg. Some of them required male participation, whereas the others involved his knowledge, if not approval. In addition, all of these methods had high failure rates (See below: Contraceptive Use—Effectiveness). In 1960, the advent of the oral contraceptive, and to a lesser extent the IUD, offered the prospect of a highly effective contraceptive that women could use regardless of knowledge or approval from their male partner. In addition, these new options for birth control could be used independently from the act of sexual intercourse. They worked by blocking release of an egg (oral contraceptives) or by disrupting sperm transport through women's reproductive tracts (IUD), with backup mechanisms of blocking implantation.

Over time, changes were made to these methods to improve safety and effectiveness. Estrogen and progestin levels in oral contraceptives were reduced, and IUDs changed in shape and size, were made with new materials (i.e., copper), and were redesigned to release progestins. Other method innovations followed. In the 1970s, new procedures for tubal sterilization that could be performed under local anesthesia on an outpatient basis became widely available. In 1983, the FDA approved the contraceptive sponge. In 1990, progestin-releasing subdermal implants active for 5 years became available, followed in 1992 by a 3-month injectable progestin. In 1993, a polyurethane female condom was approved by the FDA, and in 1997, emergency use of oral contraceptive pills for postcoital application was approved. At the end of 2000, the FDA approved a long-acting progestin-releasing IUD.

Increased Contraceptive Use and Changing Method-Use Patterns

The advent of these additional contraceptive technologies to block fertilization, and the social changes that accompanied them resulted in increased use of contraceptives. After the peak of the baby boom in 1957, the annual number of births in the United States began to recede; women increasingly were receiving higher education and becoming employed, spurred in part by the assurance that they could control their fertility. The women's liberation movement took root in the frustrations of 1950s housewives and captured the hopes of young women freed from the fear of pregnancy. In addition, the movement coincided with the 1960s' antiwar and free-love movements that inspired young people to question past patterns of marriage and family-building.[32]

In 1965, a new series of national surveys began monitoring contraceptive use among U.S. women. These National Fertility Surveys followed in earlier traditions: personal interviews of women in U.S. households who were randomly selected to be representative of all women of reproductive age living in households. The samples became larger and included over-samples of nonwhite women; they also broadened to include not only currently married women but also those who had been married at some time in their lives. In the 1965 survey of 5617 currently married women aged less than 54 years, 89% of couples at risk for unintended pregnancy (i.e., those consisting of a woman aged 15–44 years who, along with her husband, would be physically able to become pregnant if they were not using a contraceptive method, but not trying to become pregnant) were using a contraceptive method.[24]

The National Fertility Surveys were succeeded by the National Survey of Family Growth, which was conducted five times from 1973 through 1995 and again during 2002. It expanded from surveying women aged 15–44 years who had ever been married or had a child living with them in 1973 and 1976 to all women aged 15–44 years in 1982,[25] 1988,[26,33] and 1995;[27,34] the survey was modified to include men aged 15–44 years in 2002.[28] By 1995, the level of contraceptive use had increased to 95% of currently married and 93% of all women at risk for unintended pregnancy. Subgroup differences in contraceptive-use levels narrowed; by 1995, contraceptive-use levels by family poverty status, by religious affiliation, and by race and Hispanic ethnicity varied by ≤3 percentage points.[27]

Within 5 years of entering the U.S. market, the pill had become the most popular single method. By 1965, 33% of white married women aged 18–39 years had used oral contraceptives. During this year, the contraceptives used most frequently were the pill (23%), condom (15%), and periodic abstinence (11%); the diaphragm and sterilization had been used most recently by 8% of these women, and 19% had used other methods.[16]

Survey data allow these trends to be tracked to the end of the twentieth century, with data available for all currently married women in 1965, all women who were ever married from 1973 forward, and all women aged 15–44 years from 1982 onward. Although data for unmarried women are less complete than for currently married women, patterns of change in method use are similar for never-married and formerly married women, despite differences in levels of use of specific methods (see Fig. 12.2).[25–28]

Oral Contraceptives

Use of the pill peaked in 1973, when 36% of all currently married women who used contraceptives relied on this method of birth control.[18] By 1982, the level of pill use dropped to 19%, primarily because of reports in the mid-1970s that linked pill use with cardiovascular disease.[36–40] As a result of this association, studies were initiated to identify the levels of this and other side effects of oral-contraceptive use, and to tease out the independent contributions of pill use and other co-factors.

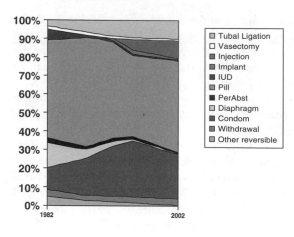

Figure 12.2. Methods used by never-married contraceptive users, 1982–2002. (From Bachrach CA. Contraceptive practice among American women, 1973–1982. *Fam Plann Perspect* 1984:16:253–59; 1988 NSFG, 1995 NSFG; Mosher WD, et al. Use of contraception and use of family planning in the United States: 1982–2002. *Adv Data* 2004; 350.)

By 1988, a slight rise in pill use occurred, although for married women, the level of use remained below that of 1965. Many factors contributed to this slow increase, including (1) changes in pill formulations to lower dosages that produced fewer health and "nuisance" side effects (e.g., nausea), (2) greater recognition of health benefits of oral contraceptive use (e.g., prevention of ovarian and endometrial cancer; reduced menstrual bleeding, cramps, and pain; reduced risk for benign breast disease; prevention of ectopic pregnancy; and improvement of acne),[41] and (3) an overall delay in childbearing.

In 2002, a total of 11.6 million women aged 15–44 years used oral contraceptives, accounting for 31% of all method use.[28] Pill use increased slightly during 1988–2002 among currently married women, but use decreased for women who had never married. Lower use among unmarried women coincided with increased awareness of human immunodeficiency virus (HIV) and other sexually transmitted diseases (STDs), diseases that could be prevented by use of condoms.

IUD

Use of IUDs also increased steadily following their introduction in the early 1960s. In 1973, IUD use peaked when 10% of currently married women using contraceptives relied on this method, and then decreased to only 2% in 1988. The rise reflected the demand for female-controlled, effective, coitus-independent contraceptives and the expectation that the IUD would fulfill these needs without recourse to hormones. The drop in use reflects fear of this method that resulted from the Dalkon Shield disaster.[42] The Dalkon Shield IUD, marketed nationwide during 1971–1974, was linked to spontaneous, septic abortions and pelvic inflammatory disease. These complications resulted from its unique materials and design. Intense media coverage of Dalkon Shield litigation extending into the mid-1980s, combined with a general crisis in the United States in liability and liability insurance, gave rise to widespread concern that all IUDs could increase women's risk for upper-genital-tract infection. In this climate, all but one IUD manufacturer (a progesterone-releasing device that had been used by a small number of women) left the U.S. market.[43] Research eventually demonstrated that IUDs other than the Dalkon Shield were not independent risk factors for these complications although they do not protect against STDs and offer no protection against the development of upper-genital-tract infection and subsequent tubal infertility.[44] However, levels of use remained low because these devices.[45] Despite the introduction of a new copper-containing IUD in 1988 and a long-term progestin-releasing IUD in 2001, by 2002 only 775,000 women were using IUDs, representing 2% of all contraceptive users.[35]

Contraceptive Sterilization

In contrast to the fluctuations in pill and IUD use during the twentieth century, contraceptive sterilization rose steadily from 12% of all currently married women who practiced birth control in 1965 to 48% in 1995. The level dropped slightly to 45% in 2002 as some couples opted instead for long-acting hormonal methods and the IUD. In 2002, female sterilization was the second most commonly used contraceptive method in the United States. In total, 10.3 million women had been sterilized for contraceptive reasons, and an additional 3.5 million of their partners had had vasectomies.

Until the mid-1970s, female and male procedures contributed about equally to contraceptive sterilization. However, tubal ligation became much more common than vasectomy during the last third of the century because of several factors, including (1) changes in relative cost and safety in tubal sterilization as an outpatient procedure was developed and became widely available, and (2) concerns (later shown to be unfounded) regarding long-term health risks associated with vasectomy (e.g., heart disease).[8,44] With improved surgical procedures, including development of laparoscopic techniques for tubal ligation and increased use of local anesthesia with light sedation, both tubal ligation and vasectomy became ambulatory procedures. Many tubal ligations also began to be performed immediately postpartum (i.e., within 48 hours of delivery) because of greater convenience, lower costs, ease of surgery, and more efficient use of health resources. During the 1990s, a no-scalpel vasectomy procedure, developed in 1974 in China, was adopted by many vasectomy providers in the United States.[41] Sterilization procedures also became more financially feasible. By the end of the century, contraceptive sterilization was covered by the Medicaid program for eligible women, and according to a 1993 survey, most private employment-based health insurance plans covered tubal ligation and vasectomy.[46]

In 1995, 63% of women using contraception who intended to have no more children reported contraceptive sterilization of themselves or their partner,[34] and in 2002, 59% were relying on female or male sterilization.[28] In 1995, the typical U.S. woman was aged 30.9 years when she had all the children she intended to have.[4] One fourth of women obtaining tubal ligations in the mid-1990s were less than 25 years of age and half were less than 29 years.[47]

Condom

Condom use decreased among married couples during the 1960s and early 1970s, from 22% of currently married contraceptive users in 1965 to 11% in 1976. (Women reporting concurrent or alternative use of condoms and another nonsystemic method were coded as condom users, but those reporting use of condoms as well as sterilization, implant, injectable, pill, or IUD were not coded as relying on those systemic methods.) During the 1980s and early 1990s, however, condom use increased steadily. By 1995, 17% of married contraceptive users were relying on condoms. Condom use among unmarried users also increased steeply during the 1980s and early 1990s, from 2% and 12% of formerly married and never-married users, respectively, in 1982 to 15% and 30%, respectively, in 1995. Increased use of condoms by unmarried couples undoubtedly reflected growing awareness of and concern about the risks of HIV and other STDs.

Condom use decreased between 1995 and 2002 among unmarried contraceptive users, to 12% of noncohabiting formerly married couples and 24% of unmarried couples in 2002. These drops may reflect (1) lowered concerns about HIV and other STDs, (2) campaigns by some nongovernmental groups and the federal government stressing abstinence as the appropriate option for unmarried couples and calling into question the effectiveness of condoms for disease and pregnancy prevention, and (3) formal and informal restrictions on teaching young people about how to use condoms effectively.[48–50]

In 2002, 6.9 million women were relying on their partners' use of condoms as their most effective birth-control method, accounting for 18% of all methods used. In addition, another 1.6 million women who were using oral contraceptives also were using condoms. Such dual-method use was most common among younger, unmarried persons, the group most likely to be seeking to prevent both STDs and pregnancy.[28]

Private and Public Contraceptive Service Providers in the Twentieth Century

With the advent of oral contraceptives and IUDs in the 1960s, the most commonly used methods required that women visit a health-care provider for a prescription or IUD insertion and, eventually, for injection or implant insertion. Heavy use of these methods, coupled with the growing uptake in surgical sterilization and small numbers of women continuing to use the diaphragm and cervical cap, forged a strong link between contraception and medical providers. However, by the late 1960s, it had become clear that many low-income and minority women were unable to obtain modern contraceptives because they could not afford physician visit fees or contraceptive supply costs. While women of all income levels wanted about the same number of children, the lower their income, the more children they had.[4] For example, studies in Louisiana in 1964–1965 (when disseminating family-planning information was a felony in the state) demonstrated that only 28% of economically disadvantaged women of reproductive age in New Orleans used contraception, compared with 85% of middle- and upper-income women.[51] Although 60% of economically disadvantaged women wanted no more than three children, on average, these women had had nearly five children before age 26 years, and three fourths did not want to become pregnant again. In 1967, such information led to reinterpretation of the criminal code and initiation of postpartum family-planning services in Louisiana.

Services were first offered to postpartum women, and efforts soon expanded to include training outreach workers and providing postpartum, well-child, and family-planning services.

The growing awareness of the difficulties encountered by economically disadvantaged women when trying to obtain prescription methods of contraception coincided with rising public attention to the general problems of poverty and the commitment of the Great Society to alleviate them. In 1964, the first federal grant for family-planning services was made by the Office of Economic Opportunity (OEO) to Corpus Christi, Texas; by 1967, 63 family-planning projects had been established in the United States. By 1969, that number had grown to 230 OEO-funded projects in 42 states and Puerto Rico, and the Department of Health and Welfare (DHEW) Children's Bureau was funding family-planning projects in 79 cities. In addition, some federal funding was provided by DHEW Maternity and Infant Care projects, the Indian Health Service, the Model City programs, and the Department of Defense; federal research efforts to improve contraceptive methods also were expanding.[52] In the federal fiscal year 1968, of the 3072 counties in the United States, 1200 had some type of subsidized family-planning services available, although most served only small numbers of clients.[53] Family-planning clinic providers served only 773,000 women, but an estimated 5,367,000 low-income women of childbearing age were sexually active, nonsterile, and seeking to avoid pregnancy and therefore likely to need subsidized care. Of the women served, 41% received family-planning services from health-department clinics, 27% from hospitals, 27% from Planned Parenthood clinics, and 5% from other agencies. In contrast, only small numbers roughly estimated at 45,000–55,000 of women covered by the Medicaid program begun in 1965 were receiving medical family-planning services from private physicians.[54]

The growing provision of family-planning services within the public sector was supported by public health officials, private physicians, and volunteer service organizations (e.g., the Planned Parenthood Federation of America). Provision of these services was also spurred by research and advocacy from the non-profit Center for Family Planning Program Development, founded in 1968 to help support the development of a nationwide family-planning service delivery network and a new field of family planning and reproductive health. Working with providers, academic researchers, legal experts, and policy makers, the center developed estimates of the need for subsidized services and monitored the gap between need and available care.

In 1968, the President's Committee on Population and Family Planning recommended that family-planning services be made available by 1973 to all U.S. women who wanted but could not afford them.[55] In 1969, President Richard Nixon asked for consolidation of existing family-planning services into a separate unit within DHEW and for increased funding to provide expanded services. Bills introduced in the Senate by Joseph D. Tydings (D-MD) and Ralph Yarborough (D-TX) and in the House by James H. Scheuer (D-NY) and George Bush (R-TX) led to the 1970 enactment of Title X of the Public Health Service Act. This act provided federal grants for family-planning services, funds for training of family-planning service personnel, guidelines for service-delivery standards, and funding of contraceptive research and development. Providers receiving Title X public funding were required to offer contraceptive services for free or low-cost to poor and low-income persons. Contraceptive service funding also became integrated into Medicaid (with a beneficial federal matching rate), into federal-state block grants, and into state budgets.[4] The Center, which was named The Alan Guttmacher Institute in 1974, in honor of the obstetrician-gynecologist who was one of the country's greatest supporters of making reproductive health information and services available to all U.S. women, provided technical assistance to organizations around the country to help them initiate services. The network of publicly funded clinics grew rapidly to the mid-1970s, but growth leveled off due to (1) plateaus in dedicated funding, (2) political opposition to government provision of family planning care to young, unmarried women, and (3) opposition by groups opposed to abortion against public funding of contraceptive services provided by organizations that independently also provided abortion.[56] In 2004, a total of 2953 separate agencies provided publicly funded contraceptive services at 7683 clinic sites.[57]

In 1995, 21.4 million women (36% of all women aged 15–44 years) visited a health-care provider for contraceptive services.[58] Of these, 15.0 million (70%) visited a private or health maintenance organization physician, 5.1 (24%) went to a publicly supported family-planning clinic, and 1.3 million (6%) went to a hospital or other type of medical provider that was likely also to have received public funding. Of the 6.5 million women who visited publicly funded family-planning clinics in 1997, 35% visited state or local health departments, 29% went to Planned Parenthood clinics, 12% to community health clinics, 12% to hospital-based family-planning clinics, and 12% to other independent providers.[4] Most of the women using publicly funded family-planning clinics either had family incomes under the federal poverty level or had incomes at 100%–249% of the poverty level. Agencies providing publicly funded contraceptive services also provide clients with access to a range of other services (e.g., immunizations and prenatal care).

About two thirds (69%) of the family-planning visits women made to private physicians regarding contraceptive care were to obstetrician-gynecologists; 21% of women visited general/family practitioners, and 10% of women sought care from other types of physicians.[59] Of all men making contraceptive-related health-care visits, 43% went to urologists. The provision of contraceptive care in the private health-care setting was often in the context of other services; 81% of women and 64% of men who received contraceptive-associated services reported having had another reason for the visit (e.g., general medical care, a gynecologic exam, a Pap test, and a prenatal or postpartum exam). Private insurance or managed care was the expected source of payment for 60% of all visits; 12% were covered by Medicaid or other government programs, 22% were paid by the patient (who may later have been reimbursed by insurance), and 6% by other sources.

During the latter part of the century, persons visiting publicly funded family-planning clinics instead of private providers for medical contraceptive services were more likely to have a low household income, lack private insurance, and be covered by Medicaid. Such persons also were more likely to be less than 30 years of age, unmarried, black or Hispanic, and not to have attended college.[58] Although some of these persons had private insurance, many insurance policies did not cover all contraceptive supplies or services. In 1995, 71% of women aged 15–44 years at risk for unintended pregnancy had some type of private insurance;[27] however, no more than one third of indemnity plans routinely covered the most commonly used reversible method (i.e., oral contraceptives), making access to these methods financially prohibitive for some women.[46]

Contraception and Education in the Twentieth Century

Contraceptive use was the norm for American couples throughout the twentieth century, spurring the need for dissemination of information and education about contraception, especially to school-aged persons. In 1998, the U.S. public overwhelmingly supported the provision of services and of the dissemination of information about contraception in school-based sex-education courses.[60]

However, this support was not without opposition. Opponents to contraceptive education argued that the availability of contraceptives would cause school-aged children to become sexually active before they otherwise would have.[61] In 1999, sex education was taught in 93% of U.S. secondary public schools, but 28% of sex-education teachers emphasized that contraceptives were ineffective in preventing pregnancy and that condoms were ineffective in preventing STDs and HIV; 12% did not discuss the effectiveness of contraceptives or condoms at all, indicating that many young people received inadequate or inaccurate information in sex-education classes.[49]

Subgroup Patterns of Contraceptive Use at the End of the Twentieth Century

In 2002, the contraceptive methods used by women and men in the United States varied starkly across different life-stage and sociodemographic groups (Table 12.1). Those intending to have children in the future relied on nonpermanent methods of birth control, primarily the pill and other hormonal methods (60%) and the condom (27%); therefore, hormonal methods and the condom accounted for almost all contraceptive use of couples with women aged less than 25 years, most of whom planned to have children.

Similarly, most never-married couples, who tended to be young and to want children in the future, relied on hormonal methods and the condom, while sterilization was more common among currently married (45%) and formerly married women (58%). In contrast, 59% of men and women wanting not to have children in the future relied on contraceptive sterilization. The proportion relying on sterilization increased steadily with age, to 70% of couples in which the woman was aged 40–44 years. Of women who had never been married, 8% who relied on hormonal methods, sterilization, or the IUD also used condoms, as did 5% of formerly married women. These proportions more than doubled from 1988 through 1995 in response to growing concerns and public messages about the value of condom use in preventing HIV and other STDs.[28]

Poverty-status differences at the end of the century in contraceptive method choice reflect, in part, (1) earlier childbearing of poorer women and (2) a greater concentration of unmarried and nonwhite couples at lower economic levels. Thus, lower-income women using contraceptives were (1) most likely to have been sterilized

Table 12.1. Percentage of contraceptive users aged 15–44, by method, according to selected characteristics, 2002.

Characteristic	Total	Contraceptive Sterilization			Hormonal Methods			Condom	Other
		Total	Female	Male	Total	Pill	Long-acting		
Total	**100.0**	**36.2**	**27.0**	**9.2**	**37.1**	**30.6**	**6.5**	**18.0**	**8.7**
Childbearing intentions*									
Have (more) children	100.0	0.2	-	0.2	59.7	51.4	8.3	26.8	13.3
Have no (more) children	100.0	58.9	44.0	14.9	21.2	17.7	3.5	12.3	7.6
Age									
15–19	100.0	-	-	-	68.3	53.0	15.2	27.0	4.8
20–24	100.0	4.4	3.6	0.8	63.9	52.4	11.5	23.0	8.7
25–29	100.0	19.3	15.1	4.1	46.6	37.6	9.0	20.6	13.5
30–34	100.0	36.7	27.5	9.2	37.0	31.5	5.5	17.1	9.2
35–39	100.0	55.4	41.2	14.1	21.5	18.6	2.8	15.7	7.5
40–44	100.0	68.5	50.1	18.4	12.9	11.0	1.9	11.6	7.1
Union status									
Currently married	100.0	45.2	29.8	15.4	28.0	23.6	4.4	16.5	10.3
Cohabiting	100.0	28.4	25.3	3.0	44.1	33.2	10.9	18.0	9.5

Not cohabiting									
Formerly married	100.0	58.2	54.8	3.4	22.5	19.1	3.4	12.4	6.8
Never married	100.0	10.9	10.0	0.9	60.1	49.7	10.5	23.5	5.5
Poverty status									
<100%	100.0	42.5	38.1	4.5	34.3	22.7	11.6	15.0	8.2
100%–199%	100.0	40.0	33.9	6.1	33.0	24.4	8.6	16.9	10.1
200%–399%	100.0	38.9	26.4	12.5	34.3	29.6	4.8	17.8	9.1
400+%	100.0	25.1	14.7	10.4	46.3	42.4	3.9	21.1	7.5
Race/ethnicity									
Non-Hisp. black	100.0	41.3	38.9	2.4	33.1	22.5	10.6	19.9	5.7
Hispanic	100.0	38.1	33.7	4.4	32.3	22.0	10.3	18.4	11.2
Non-Hisp. white/other	100.0	35.7	24.1	11.6	39.4	34.5	5.0	16.6	8.2
Religion†									
None	100.0	30.0	22.9	7.1	40.2	31.2	9.1	21.9	7.8
Roman Catholic	100.0	33.2	24.4	8.8	37.8	31.6	6.3	18.1	10.8
Protestant	100.0	40.8	30.9	9.9	35.5	29.4	6.2	15.8	7.9

Sources: References 28 and 40.

*"Long-acting hormonal methods" includes only DMPA 3-month injectables.

†Data for women of other religions not shown because of small numbers.

themselves and least likely to have a partner who had had a vasectomy; (2) least likely to use the pill and most likely to use long-acting hormonal contraceptives, especially the injectable; and (3) less apt to rely on condoms (see Table 12.1).

Although reliance on contraceptive sterilization did not vary widely among Hispanic, black, and other women, the distributions between male and female sterilization were different: of Hispanic and black women, 34%–39% using contraception had been surgically sterilized, compared with only 24% of white women and other contraceptors. However, vasectomy was more common among partners of white and other women (12%) than among Hispanic (4%) and black (2%) contraceptors. During the first 70 years of the twentieth century, contraceptive use reflected the Roman Catholic Church's prohibition against use of any contraceptive methods except for periodic abstinence. However, this changed after the papal ratification of this prohibition in 1968, as many Catholics became more secular and turned away from the church's positions on behaviors such as contraception, abortion, and divorce. For example, the proportion of white, Catholic women married fewer than 5 years who had never used any form of contraception other than periodic abstinence declined from 80% among those married in 1951–1955 to 10% of those married in 1971–75. By 1975, only minimal differences were observed between Catholic and non-Catholic users of contraception, with the exception of sterilization. Among white married women using a contraceptive, 13% of Roman Catholics vs. 18% of non-Catholics were contraceptively sterilized.[62] In 2002, Roman Catholic women were still less likely than Protestant women using contraception to have been contraceptively sterilized (24% vs. 31%). Catholic and non-Catholic women were almost equally likely to be using other types of methods, however (see Table 12.1).

Accidental Pregnancy

Contraceptive Use—Effectiveness

Life-table methods of measuring contraceptive effectiveness were developed in the mid-1960s by Robert Potter and have remained the standard way of presenting data and comparing methods and subgroups of users. This approach corrects problems encountered with the Pearl index (see Fertility Control in the First Half of the 1900s: Withdrawal, Douche, and Condom) by calculating a separate failure rate for each month following onset of method use and combining measures together to yield a cumulative proportion of women who experienced an accidental pregnancy within x months of beginning use.[63]

Although most contraceptive methods are reliable when used correctly and consistently, a substantial number of users experience accidental pregnancy in spite of their attempts to use available methods, either because of method failure or because the method was used inconsistently or incorrectly. Patterns of actual method use from the mid-1980s through the mid-1990s indicated that one in eight women relying on reversible contraceptives became pregnant within the first 12 months of use (Table 12.2).[64]

The IUD and hormonal methods are the most effective reversible methods in use (≤7.5% pregnancy rate in the first 12 months of use). Methods linked to intercourse and

Table 12.2. Percentage of women experiencing an accidental pregnancy during the first 12 months of method use, by selected characteristics.

Characteristic	Percent Pregnant
Total	12.5
Method	
Injectable/implant/IUD	3.5***
Pill	7.5***
Diaphragm	13.1
Condom (ref.)	13.7
Periodic abstinence	22.9***
Withdrawal	24.5***
Spermicide	27.6***
Age	
<18	12.4
18–19 (ref.)	14.0
20–24	15.2
25–29	11.6*
30–44	9.5***
Union status	
Married	10.0***
Cohabiting	21.2
Not in union (ref.)	13.6***
Poverty status	
<100%	20.5***
100–249% (ref.)	15.5
250+%	9.1***
Race/Ethnicity	
Black	18.1**
Hispanic (ref.) + A53 + A18 + A53	15.5
White/other	11.2***

Source: Reference 64.

$*p \leq .05; **p \leq .01; ***p \leq .001.$

nonmedical methods have much higher failure rates—13%–14% for the diaphragm and condom; however, 25%–28% of women became pregnant when relying on periodic abstinence, withdrawal, and spermicides used alone. These rates change only minimally when adjusted for the different characteristics of women relying on each method. Failure rates were consistently highest among couples in which the woman was age less than 25 years, cohabiting couples, women not in union, low-income women, and black or Hispanic women. These patterns generally occurred for all reversible methods, with subgroup failure rates of ≤5% among all persons using long-acting reversible methods (except cohabiting women), pill users aged 30–44 years, and those with family incomes at ≥250% of the poverty level. In contrast, use-failure rates exceeded 33% among (1) periodic abstinence users who were aged 20–24 years, cohabiting, and with low incomes; (2) withdrawal users who were cohabiting, poor, or black; and (3) spermicide users aged 18–24 years, who were cohabiting, low-income, and black.[64]

Unintended Pregnancy and Induced Abortion

Until the mid-nineteenth century, abortions performed early in pregnancy were permitted in the United States by traditional common law and were often performed by women themselves or by midwives. But concerns about women's health and movements of physicians to take control of medical practice led to laws that prohibited abortion in most circumstances.[65] By 1900, most abortions were illegal throughout the United States. However, women continued to have unintended pregnancies and to seek abortions from trained and lay providers and to self-induce abortion. Whereas affluent women were sometimes assisted by sympathetic physicians, most women turned to illegal, clandestine abortion procedures, which often posed health risks. In 1930, for example, 18% of all maternal deaths (2700 women) were reportedly caused by abortion.[66] Mortality from induced abortion decreased with the advent of antibiotics, from 1700 reported deaths in 1940 to 316 in 1950 (though deaths from abortion were underreported). The number had fallen to 193 reported deaths in 1965, but still accounted for 17% of all maternal deaths. Economically disadvantaged women and those who were nonwhite had particularly high rates of health complications from illegal abortions. During 1972–1974, the mortality rate from illegal abortion was 12 times higher among nonwhite women than white women. Many women who survived illegal abortions suffered substantial health complications, a primary cause of hospital admission for women. In New York City municipal hospitals in 1969, for every 100 deliveries, 23 admissions were made for incomplete (usually illegal) abortions, which were treated most commonly with dilation and curettage.

In its *Eisenstadt v. Baird* decision in 1972 legalizing contraceptive practice for unmarried persons, the U.S. Supreme Court defined a constitutional right to privacy broad enough to include "the right of the individual, married or single, to be free from unwarranted governmental intrusion into matters so fundamentally affecting a person as the decision whether to bear or beget a child." Some states passed liberal abortion laws in the late 1960s and early 1970s. However, the situation nationwide changed dramatically on January 22, 1973, when the Supreme Court ruled (in *Roe v. Wade* and *Doe v. Bolton*) that this fundamental right to privacy included the right to chose whether to have an abortion. The Court set forth a framework balancing the woman's right to choose abortion with the state's interest in protecting her health as well as the developing human life. It delineated (1) a period, roughly the first trimester of pregnancy, in which states were prohibited from interfering with decisions about abortion made by women and their physician; (2) a later period in which states could enact laws as needed to protect the health of pregnant women; and (3) a period after fetal viability during which states could prohibit all abortions not necessary to protect the life or health of the woman. Abortion mortality and morbidity fell to negligible levels as safe, legal services became available.[66] For women obtaining abortions during this time, the safer vacuum aspiration technique had begun to replace dilation and curettage for abortions performed during the first trimester of gestation. For women obtaining abortions later in their pregnancies, most abortions were increasingly performed via dilation and evacuation.

Safe and accessible abortion services continue to be used by many American women. Whether from contraceptive failure or nonuse, high proportions of women who became pregnant even near the close of the twentieth century had not planned their pregnancies. In 1994, an estimated 49% of pregnancies (excluding miscarriages) were unintended, at a rate of 45 per 1000 women aged 15–44 years (Table 12.3).[67] Unintended pregnancy rates were highest among women aged 18–24 years, those who were unmarried, and low-income and black women (who were more likely also to be economically disadvantaged and unmarried).

Only 7% of women at risk for unintended pregnancy were not current contraceptive users; however, these women accounted for 47% of all unintended pregnancies.[67] The 93% of women at risk who used contraceptives accounted for only 53% of all unintended pregnancies. Among women who experienced unintended pregnancies (miscarriages excluded), 54% ended their pregnancy with an induced abortion. The proportion was highest among women with unintended pregnancies who were aged ≥40 years, unmarried women, those with family incomes at ≥200% of the poverty level, and black women.

Information from women and medical personnel indicate that induced abortion was used throughout the twentieth century when contraceptive measures were ineffective or when a woman became pregnant when no method was used. However, because abortion was at times illegal, the level and patterns of this procedure were not documented. The most reliable estimates suggest that the abortion rate in the 1960s may have been as high as 26 per 1000 women aged 15–44 years.[68] The incidence of legal abortion rose from 16 per 1000 in 1973, the year of nationwide legalization, to 29 per 1000 in 1979–1983, then decreased to 23 per 1000 women aged 15–44 years in 1995, and to 21 per 1000 in 2000.[69]

By the year 2000, abortion services were provided by 1819 facilities located primarily in the larger metropolitan areas.[69] Most of these facilities were specialized: 25% were clinics in which at least half of patient visits were for abortion services; 71% of the 1.3 million abortions in 2000 were performed in this type of facility. Another 21% of providers were other clinics, accounting for 22% of procedures; 33% were hospitals, representing only 5% of all abortions; and 21% were private physician offices, which provided 2% of abortions. Only 13% of U.S. counties had any abortion provider, accounting for 66% of the population of women aged 15–44 years.[69] An estimated 8% of women having abortions in nonhospital facilities traveled more than 100 miles, and 16% traveled 50–100 miles to obtain abortion services.

The concentration of services in metropolitan areas and in specialized facilities reflects focused opposition against abortion services. At the close of the twentieth century, the issue of abortion was one of great tension in the United States, with advocates polarized on both sides. Opposition to abortion has led to extensive harassment of providers, including murders of physicians and other staff. In 2000, 80% of nonhospital facilities where ≥400 abortions were provided per year were picketed; 28% of facilities reported picketing with physical contact or blocking of patients,

Table 12.3. Estimated number of pregnancies (excluding miscarriages), percentage distribution of pregnancies, by outcome and intention, and selected measures of unintended pregnancy, all by characteristic, 1994**.

Characteristic	No. of Pregnancies	% distribution of Pregnancies				% of Births that were Unintended	% of Pregnancies that were	% of Unintended Pregnancies	Pregnancy Rate*		
		Intended Births	Unintended Births	Abortions	Total				Total	Intended	Unintended
Total	5,383,800	50.8	23.0	26.6	100.4	30.8	49.2	54.0	90.8	46.1	44.7
Age at outcome											
<15[†]	25,100	18.3	33.2	48.5	100.0	64.5	81.7	59.4	13.7	2.5	11.2
15–19	781,900	22.0	42.7	35.3	100.0	66.0	78.0	45.3	91.1	20.0	71.1
15–17	306,100	17.3	46.5	36.2	100.0	72.9	82.7	43.8	59.0	10.2	48.8
18–19	475,800	25.0	40.2	34.8	100.0	61.7	75.0	46.4	140.3	35.1	105.2
20–24	1,479,500	41.5	26.2	32.3	100.0	38.7	58.5	55.2	164.1	68.1	96.0
25–29	1,405,200	60.3	17.2	22.5	100.0	22.2	39.7	56.7	147.0	88.7	58.4
30–34	1,111,400	66.9	14.6	18.4	100.0	18.0	33.1	55.7	100.0	66.9	33.1
35–39	482,400	59.2	17.9	23.0	100.0	23.2	40.8	56.3	43.7	25.9	17.8
≥40[‡]	98,300	49.3	17.9	32.8	100.0	26.7	50.7	64.7	9.9	4.9	5.0
Marital status at outcome											
Currently married[§]	3,003,900	69.3	19.3	11.3	100.0	21.8	30.7	37.0	95.2	66.0	29.2
Formerly married	356,700	37.5	21.8	40.7	100.0	36.8	62.5	65.1	64.7	24.3	40.4
Never married	2,023,100	22.3	31.0	46.7	100.0	58.2	77.7	60.1	91.0	20.3	70.8

Poverty status

<100%	1,358,000	38.6	31.3	30.1	100.0	44.8	61.4	49.0	143.7	55.4	88.3
100–199%	1,292,500	46.8	27.7	25.4	100.0	37.2	53.2	47.9	115.2	53.9	61.2
≥200%	2,733,200	58.8	15.9	25.4	100.0	21.3	41.2	61.5	70.8	41.6	29.2

Race

White	3,981,700	57.1	21.2	21.6	100.0	27.1	42.9	50.4	82.7	47.3	35.5
Black	1,130,700	27.7	28.6	43.7	100.0	50.8	72.3	60.4	136.7	37.8	98.9
Other	271,400	50.0	22.0	28.0	100.0	30.5	50.0	56.0	93.9	46.9	46.9

Ethnicity

Hispanic	900,200	51.4	22.4	26.1	100.0	30.4	48.6	53.8	143.0	73.5	69.4
Non-Hispanic	4,483,600	50.7	22.6	26.7	100.0	30.9	49.3	54.1	84.6	42.9	41.7

Source: Reference 67.

*Pregnancy rates for this category are expressed as per 1000 women aged 15–44, except for rates for age groups.

†Denominator for rates is women aged 14.

‡Numerator for rates is women aged 40 and older; denominator is women aged 40–44.

§Includes separated women.

**Intention status of births is based on births in the five years before the 1995 interview.

18% were subject to physical vandalism, 15% experienced bomb threats, and 14% of facilities reported picketing of private homes of staff members.[70]

A Century of Change

Changes during the twentieth century in the technology of contraceptives profoundly affected the lives of women and men, effects that have resounded into the medical-care system, gender relationships, and families. Medical advances reduced infant and maternal mortality, assuring that most births would lead to healthy outcomes. Developments in contraceptive technology allowed substantially more reliable and effective control over fertility, and concomitant social changes reduced the typical desired family size and motivated and enabled women to become involved in higher education and the workforce in addition to motherhood. Contraceptive methods evolved from those linked directly to intercourse (e.g., withdrawal, douche, condom, diaphragm, and periodic abstinence) to systemic methods (e.g., oral contraceptives, sterilization, the IUD, implants, and injectable contraception), which required greater medical involvement and precipitated wide differentials in contraceptive use and fertility control. These differentials helped spur the development of a nationwide network of publicly supported family-planning clinics that could provide contraceptive care, other reproductive-health services, and primary-care services to many low-income women and adolescents. These services have dramatically narrowed socioeconomic differences in method use and in family size.

Advances in contraceptive methods and use have been tempered, however, by relatively high rates of unintentional pregnancy among persons using reversible methods. High rates of unplanned pregnancy, in turn, have resulted in high levels of induced abortion and contraceptive sterilization, often in the early reproductive years.

Challenges for the Twenty-First Century

Couples at the beginning of the twenty-first century have more options for birth control and more effective tools for achieving the timing and number of children they desire than did sexually active persons in previous generations. Therefore, their goals are much more precise and encompass not only preventing unintentional pregnancy, but also avoiding sometimes life-threatening diseases.

Despite advances in the field of reproductive health, existing challenges remain regarding family planning, and the following new challenges have emerged.

- Improving success at preventing unintended pregnancies (a goal spanning contraceptive technology, method attractiveness, and ease of use, as well as open and positive attitudes and ability to communicate about sexuality and pregnancy planning).
- Dealing with dual goals of preventing unintended pregnancy and STDs, either though dual-purpose methods or through dual use of one method to prevent pregnancy and another to prevent STDs (including HIV).
- Assuring easy access for all to a full range of contraceptive information, services, and supplies.

- Addressing men's roles in contraceptive use and pregnancy prevention and their own sexual and reproductive health needs given current methods and the future availability of systemic male methods.

The history of the last century and the importance of these new challenges assure that contraception and family planning will remain important topics of personal concern and public health into the twenty-first century.

References

1. Sex and America's Teenagers. New York: Alan Guttmacher Institute, 1994.
2. Coale AJ, Zelnik M. New Estimates of Fertility and Population in the United States. Princeton, NJ: Princeton University Press, 1963.
3. Centers for Disease Control and Prevention. Achievements in public health, 1900–1999: Family planning. *MMWR* 1999:48:1073–80.
4. Fulfilling the Promise: Public Policy and U.S. Family Planning Clinics. New York: Alan Guttmacher Institute, 2000.
5. Martin JA, Hamilton BE, Ventura SJ. Births: preliminary data for 2000. *Natl Vital Stat Rep* 2001:49.
6. Minino AM, Smith BL. Deaths: preliminary data for 2000. *Natl Vital Stat Rep* 2001:49.
7. Statistical Abstract of the United States: 1999. Washington, DC: U.S. Census Bureau, 1999.
8. Harlap S, Kost K, Forrest JD. Preventing Pregnancy, Protecting Health: A New Look at Birth Control Choices in the United States. New York: Alan Guttmacher Institute, 1991.
9. Coale AJ, Zelnik M. New Estimates of Fertility and Population in the United States. Princeton: Princeton University Press, 1963, 36.
10. U.S. Bureau of the Census. Historical Statistics of the United States, Colonial Times to 1970, Bicentennial Ed., Part 2. Washington, DC: Government Printing Office,1975, 50–51.
11. Ventura SJ, Martin JA, Curtin SC, Menacker F, Hamilton BE. Births: final data for 1999. *Natl Vital Stat Rep* 2001: 49.
12. Public Broadcasting Service. People & events: Anthony Comstock's chastity laws. On: American Experience: The Pill. Available at: http://www.pbs.org/wgbh/amex/pill/people events/e_comstock.html. Accessed 17 February 2005.
13. Craig PB. Margaret Sanger: the fight for birth control. Law Library of Congress: American Women. Available at: http://memory.loc.gov/ammem/awhhtml/awlaw3/d6.html. Accessed 17 February 2005.
14. Whelpton PK, Campbell AA, Paterson JE. Fertility and Family Planning in the United States. Princeton: Princeton University Press, 1966.
15. Ryder NB, Westoff CF. Reproduction in the United States. Princeton: Princeton University Press, 1971.
16. Westoff CF, Ryder NB. The Contraceptive Revolution. Princeton: Princeton University Press, 1977.
17. Westoff CF, Jones EF. Patterns of aggregate and individual changes in contraceptive practice. *Vital Health Stat* 1979:3.
18. Mosher WD, Bachrach CA. Contraceptive use, United States, 1982. *Vital Health Stat* 1986:23.
19. Himes NE. Medical History of Contraception. New York: Gamut Press, 1936. First published 1963.
20. Trussell J, Kost K. Contraceptive failure in the United States: a critical review of the literature. *Stud Fam Plann* 1987:18:237–83.

21. Dawson DA, Meny DJ, Ridley JC. Fertility control in the United States before the contraceptive revolution. *Fam Plann Perspect* 1980:12:76–86.

22. Kopp ME. Birth Control in Practice: Analysis of Ten Thousand Case Histories of the Birth Control Clinical Research Bureau. New York: McBride, 1934, 134.

23. Stone HM. *Medical Journal & Record*, 19 April 19 and 3 May 3 1933.

24. Westoff CF. The modernization of U.S. contraceptive practice. *Fam Plann Perspect* 1972: 4:9–12.

25. Bachrach CA. Contraceptive practice among American women, 1973–1982. *Fam Plann Perspect* 1984:16:253–59.

26. Darroch JE. Tabulations from the 1988 National Survey of Family Growth, 2003, unpublished tabulations.

27. Darroch JE. Tabulations from the 1995 National Survey of Family Growth, 2003.

28. Mosher WD, Martinez GM, Chandra A, Abma JC, Willson SJ. Use of contraception and use of family planning services in the United States: 1982–2002. *Adv Data* 2004:350.

29. Evolution and revolution: the past, present and future of contraception. *Contracept Rep* 2000:10:15–25.

30. Sanger's role in the development of contraceptive technologies. *The Margaret Sanger Papers Newsletter* 1993/4: 4. Available at: http://www.nyu.edu/projects/sanger/sanger's_role_in_contraceptive_technology.htm and http://www.fpnotebook.com/GYN14 .htm. Accessed 27 April 2003.

31. Richardson RH. Family planning in the southeastern United States. *Fam Plann Perspect* 1969:1:45–46.

32. Scrimshaw SCM. Women and the pill: From panacea to catalyst. *Fam Plann Perspect* 1981:13:254–56, 260–62.

33. Mosher WD. Contraceptive practice in the United States, 1982–1988. *Fam Plann Perspect* 1990:22:198–205.

34. Piccinino LJ, Mosher WD. Trends in contraceptive use in the United States: 1982–1995. *Fam Plann Perspect* 1998:30:4–10, 46.

35. Jones RK. Tabulations from the 2002 National Survey of Family Growth, 2005, unpublished tabulations.

36. Inman WHW, Vessey MP. Investigation of deaths from pulmonary, coronary, and cerebral thrombosis and embolism in women of child-bearing age. *Br Med J* 1968:2: 193–99.

37. Collaborative Group for the Study of Stroke in Young Women. Oral contraceptives and increased risk of cerebral ischaemia or thrombosis. *N Engl J Med* 1973:288:871–78.

38. Mann JI, Vessey MP, Thorogood M, Doll SR. Myocardial infarction in young women with special reference to oral contraceptive practice. *Br Med J* 1975:2:241–45.

39. Collaborative Group for the Study of Stroke in Young Women. Oral contraceptives and stroke in young women: associated risk factors. *JAMA* 1975:231:718–22.

40. Jones EF, Beniger JR, Westoff CF. Pill and IUD discontinuation in the United States, 1970–1975: The influence of the media. *Fam Plann Perspect* 1980:12:293–300.

41. Hatcher RA, Trussell J, Stewart F, Stewart GK, Kowal D, Guest F, et al. Contraceptive Technology. New York: Irvington Publishers, 1994.

42. Tatum HJ, Schmidt FH, Phillips D, McCarty M, O'Leary WM. The Dalkon Shield controversy: structural and bacteriological studies of IUD tails. *JAMA* 1975:231:711–17.

43. Forrest JD. The end of IUD marketing in the United States: What does it mean for American women? *Fam Plann Perspect* 1986:18:52–55, 57.

44. Ory HW, Forrest JD, Lincoln R. Making Choices: Evaluating the Health Risks and Benefits of Birth Control Methods. New York: Alan Guttmacher Institute, 1983.

45. Forrest JD. Acceptability of IUDs in the United States. In: Bardin CW, Mishell DR Jr, eds. Proceedings from the Fourth International Conference on IUDs. Boston: Butterworth-Heinemann, 1994.

46. Uneven & Unequal: Insurance Coverage and Reproductive Health Services. New York: Alan Guttmacher Institute, 1994.

47. MacKay AP, Kieke BA, Koonin LM, Beattie K. Tubal sterilization in the United States, 1994–1996. *Fam Plann Perspect* 2001:33:161–64.

48. Sonfield A, Gold RB. States' implementation of the Section 510 Abstinence Education Program, FY 1999. *Fam Plann Perspect* 2001:33:166–71.

49. Darroch JE, Landry DJ, Singh S. Changing emphases in sexuality education in U.S. public secondary schools, 1988–1999. *Fam Plann Perspect* 2000:32:204–11, 265.

50. Landry DJ, Darroch JE, Singh S, Higgins J. Factors associated with the content of sex education in U.S. public secondary schools. *Perspect Sex Reprod Health* 2003:35: 261–69.

51. Beasley JD. View from Louisiana. *Fam Plann Perspect* 1969:1:2–15.

52. London GD. Past, present, future: an interview. *Fam Plann Perspect* 1969:1:18–22.

53. Center for Family Planning Program Development. Family planning services in the U.S.: a national overview, 1968. *Fam Plann Perspect* 1969:1:4–12.

54. Rosoff JI. Family planning, Medicaid and the private physicians: survey of a failure. *Fam Plann Perspect* 1969:1:27–32.

55. Population and Family Planning—The Transition from Concern to Action. Report of the President's Committee on Population and Family Planning. Washington, DC: Government Printing Office, 1968.

56. Dryfoos JG. Family planning clinics—a story of growth and conflict. *Fam Plann Perspect* 1988:20:282–87.

57. Frost JJ, Frohwirth L, Purcell A. The availability and use of publicly funded family planning clinics: U.S. trends, 1994–2001. *Perspect Sex Reprod Health* 2004: 36:206–15.

58. Frost JJ. Public or private providers? U.S. women's use of reproductive health services. *Fam Plann Perspect* 2001:33:4–12.

59. Landry DJ, Forrest JD. Private physicians' provision of contraceptive services. *Fam Plann Perspect* 1996:28:203–9.

60. Kaiser Family Foundation. Sex in the 90s: 1998 National Survey of Americans on Sex and Sexual Health,1998. Available at: http://www.kff.org/womenshealth/1430-index.cfm. Accessed 24 January 2004.

61. Dailard C. Sex education: politicians, parents, teachers and teens. *Guttmacher Rep Public Policy,* 2001:4:9–12.

62. Westoff CF, Jones EF. The secularization of U.S. Catholic birth control practices. *Fam Plann Perspect* 1977:9:203–7.

63. Trussell J, Kost K. Contraceptive failure in the United States: a critical review of the literature. *Stud Fam Plann* 1987:18:237–83.

64. Ranjit N, Bankole A, Darroch JE, Singh S. Contraceptive failure in the first two years of use: differences across socioeconomic subgroups. *Fam Plann Perspect* 2001:33:19–27.

65. Mohr JJ. Abortion in America: The Origins and Evolution of National Policy. New York: Oxford University Press, 1978.

66. Gold RB. Abortion and Women's Health: A Turning Point for America? New York: Alan Guttmacher Institute, 1990.

67. Henshaw SK. Unintended pregnancy in the United States. *Fam Plann Perspect* 1998: 30:24–29, 46.

68. Tietze C. Induced Abortion: A World Review, 1983. New York: The Population Council,1983.

69. Finer LB, Henshaw SK. Abortion incidence and services in the United States in 2000. *Perspect Sex Reprod Health* 2003:35:6–15.
70. Henshaw SK, Finer LB. The accessibility of abortion services in the United States, 2001. *Perspect Sex Reprod Health* 2003:35:16–24.

Suggested Reading

Himes NE. Medical History of Contraception. New York: Gamut Press, 1936, 1963.
Mohr JJ. Abortion in America: The Origins and Evolution of National Policy. New York: Oxford University Press, 1978.
Reagan L. When Abortion Was A Crime: Women, Medicine, and Law in the United States, 1867–1973. Berkeley: University of California Press, 1997.
Tone A. Devices and Desires: A History of Contraceptives in America. New York: Hill and Wang, 2001.

13

Teaching Birth Control on Tobacco Road and Mill Village Alley: Race, Class, and Birth Control in Public Health

JOHANNA SCHOEN

In 1937, Boston philanthropist and birth control activist Dr. Clarence J. Gamble, heir of the soap firm Procter & Gamble, approached North Carolina public health officials to discuss the marriage between contraceptive research and a public health birth control program. Gamble had developed a spermicidal foam powder, which, if applied to a moist sponge and inserted into the vagina before intercourse, promised to provide an easy birth control technique (Fig. 13.1). Looking for a rural area in which to test his contraceptive, he offered to pay the salary of a nurse for birth control work if the North Carolina State Board of Health promised to promote the use of his foam powder through local public health centers. In March 1937, Gamble employed Frances R. Pratt as his nurse and Pratt set out to organize local birth control clinics. "It was like manna from the sky," one social worker rejoiced.[1]

This article analyzes the history of public health birth control programs between the 1930s and the 1970s. Throughout the twentieth century, American health and welfare policies in general, and reproductive health policies in particular, were shaped by two contradictory forces: a progressive, democratic impulse that sought to give everybody an equal start in life, and a conservative distrust of any program aimed at helping the poor. Hoping to provide all with an equal chance, health and welfare officials established programs for poor whites and blacks across the South. They did so, however, within a larger political context of deep suspicion toward any services for the poor.[2]

279

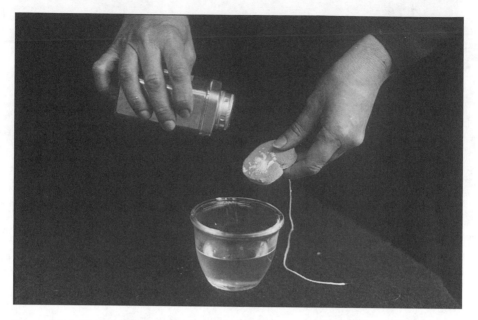

Figure 13.1. Sponge and foam powder. (Courtesy of Countway Medical Library.)

The tension between progressive health and social policies and a generally tight-fisted approach to public assistance provided the context in which North Carolina's reproductive health policies were developed and implemented. The progressive spirit of the New Deal was the backdrop for the establishment of North Carolina's public health birth control program in 1937, and the War on Poverty in the 1960s was accompanied by the implementation of progressive family planning programs. Throughout the period under discussion, family planning advocates understood the ability to control reproduction to be a fundamental right of all women, regardless of their capacity to pay for medical services. This democratic attitude was not limited to family planning programs, but extended to the passage of a voluntary sterilization law and the reform of the state's abortion law during the 1960s. Together, these policies significantly increased women's reproductive control. At the same time, however, the creation of a state welfare system during the Great Depression went hand in hand with the establishment of a eugenic sterilization program under the Department of Public Welfare. And the expansion of the welfare state in the 1950s and 1960s brought with it a significant increase in eugenic sterilizations and coercive family planning programs. Even the liberalization of the state's abortion law was motivated in part by the hope that access to abortion would lead to a reduction in births among welfare recipients.

Economic, eugenic, and humanitarian concerns motivated public health professionals in the 1930s to establish birth control services for the poor. As federal and state governments began to provide family planning through public health clinics and traveling birth control nurses, a patchwork of services emerged to address the contraceptive needs of poor women. Public, private, and nonprofit organizations participated in the establishment of a range of birth control services. Researchers, supported by national birth control organizations and private philanthropies, established contraceptive field trials.[3]

Clinics existed on a continuum between two extremes. On one end were clinics that saw contraceptives as an integral part of public health services which, if offered along with pre- and postnatal care and increased supervision of the state's midwives, would improve the health of mothers and infants. Spacing children, officials at these clinics held, was essential to women's health. By the 1960s, some clinics even expressed the belief that women had a right to reproductive control. On the other end of the continuum were clinics that offered contraceptives to the exclusion of general health services. Supporters of these clinics held that general health care services would divert funds needed more urgently for birth control work. These programs stressed quantity over quality by providing only basic services to a larger number of women. In the 1930s and 1940s, such clinics offered simple contraceptives to reach as many women as possible. Simple contraceptives did not require a physician for fitting but could be distributed by visiting nurses or through the mail, and used with minimal sanitary facilities. By the 1960s, such clinics moved to the use of contraceptives outside women's control. (See Chapter 12.)

Most of the women who took advantage of state-supported birth control programs welcomed the services, participated in them, and helped shape the contraceptive programs. Neither minority nor poor white clients of the birth control programs necessarily experienced the contraceptive offers as a form of state control. Nor did they see eye-to-eye with the largely white, middle-class professionals who ran the services. Instead, they had their own agendas often unanticipated by health and welfare officials.

Infant and Maternal Health in the Early Twentieth Century

High rates of infant and maternal mortality alerted health professionals in the early twentieth century to the need for improved infant and maternal health. In 1915, around 10% of all infants in the U.S. birth registration area—but 20% of infants of color—died before they were 1 year old. Approximately 6 white and 10 nonwhite women died for every 1000 live births between 1900 and 1930.[4] Mortality rates were exacerbated by the general ill health of poor women who often suffered from long-lasting and debilitating injuries that resulted from frequent pregnancies, deliveries, and abortion without sufficient medical care.[2,5,6]

The inaccessibility of medical care even in cases of serious disease contributed to high infant and maternal mortality. Medical resources, while plentiful enough, were not distributed according to need, but rather according to patients' ability to pay for services. For instance, while New York, a relatively wealthy and urbanized state, boasted 1 physician for every 621 persons, in extremely poor rural counties the physician-to-population ratio sometimes exceeded 1 to 20,000 and some had no practicing physicians at all.[2,5,7]

Patients who had access to medical care often encountered doctors and nurses lacking basic skills. Early twentieth-century reports indicted the quality of American medical education in general and obstetrics in particular. More childbearing women died from improper obstetrical operations than from infections caused by midwives.[8–10] One critical physician accused his colleagues of frequently hastening labor, needlessly intervening in the delivery, and disregarding the need for sterility. Careless physicians, he warned, not only contributed to maternal and infant mortality but also hurt the reputation of the entire medical profession.[11]

In the early twentieth century, state boards of health adopted a variety of measures to improve infant and maternal health. Together with officials from the U.S. Children's Bureau, for instance, North Carolina's health officers and physicians developed a series of responses ranging from the establishment of infant and maternal health centers to the regulation of midwives.[3] Since too-frequent and too-early pregnancies also contributed to women's poor health and high infant mortality rates, health officials concluded that birth control instruction had to be part of an integral program for maternal and infant health.

While health and welfare professionals considered birth control essential, they assumed that poor women lacked both the intelligence and motivation to use a diaphragm, the most effective contraceptive in the 1930s. The diaphragm was a "rich-folks' contraceptive," relatively expensive and difficult to use without privacy, running water, and full explanation of fitting—luxuries not available for many Americans.[12,13] As birth control nurse Doris Davidson explained to Mrs. Barclay, field director of the American Birth Control League (ABCL),

> We all know the ever-present need for a simpler method for unintelligent, illiterate, lazy and poverty-stricken patients. Although the diaphragm method may provide greater safety in the hands of the intelligent patient, it often acts in just the opposite way in the hands of the unintelligent patient, no matter how carefully she may have been instructed. This type of patient, (and I am referring to the low-intelligent strata found by the hundred in North Carolina, South Carolina, Tennessee and West Virginia) can learn a thing one moment and unlearn it the next with bewildering rapidity. Often by the time the poor creature has arrived back in her home, she is uncertain about technique and therefore hesitant in applying it. . . . If we are going to help this low-grade patient, do we not have to meet them on their own level?— give them something which is EASY for them to apply, and which they can readily understand?[14]

Researchers hoped to develop a birth control method so easy to employ that it could be used by patients who had neither the desire, the education, the privacy, nor the sanitary facilities to carry out more complicated procedures. Contraceptive foam powders and jellies met these conditions, and had the additional advantage of making pelvic examinations, which were assumed to deter many women from seeking contraceptive advice, unnecessary. Although it was unclear whether simpler methods were as effective as the diaphragm, many researchers considered it more important to reach a large number of women than to provide the most reliable contraceptive. As Davidson continued to explain: "There is the important problem of reaching *more* patients in a given time. With simpler methods, the reaching of greater numbers is assured. . . . If the jelly method or the sponge-foam method does not insure as high a degree of protection *per se*, the scales would be balanced, and more than balanced on the other hand because greater *numbers* of patients would be reached and protected."[14]

Researchers' emphasis on the simplicity of the method meant, however, that research was both driven by stereotypes about poor women and further reinforced these stereotypes. The drive to develop both cheaper and more "effective" contraceptives led to continued emphasis on a reduction of the birth rate rather than on the improvement of women's health and self-determination. In fact, the bias in favor of simpler birth control methods worked as a strong counterforce to the development of health and support services that might increase women's reproductive control. The development of simpler contraceptives was driven by the desire to help solve problems of poverty and poor health rather than to provide women with greater self-determination.[15]

Testing Contraceptives

Around the country, contraceptive field trials drove the development of public health birth control programs. In 1923, Robert Latou Dickinson, a New York gynecologist who lobbied his colleagues to promote contraceptive and sex education, joined Margaret Sanger in establishing the institutional frameworks for the distribution and testing of contraceptives. Together, they founded the National Committee on Maternal Health (NCMH) and the Birth Control Clinical Research Bureau (BCCRB) and began to systematically test the efficiency of contraceptive products.

During the 1930s, when a vast array of commercial contraceptive products flooded the market, testing greatly expanded. Under the auspices of the NCMH, Clarence J. Gamble and others like him established birth control programs in some of North America's poorest regions. With the help of nurses and local doctors, such trials tested foam powder in North Carolina and Puerto Rico; condoms in the Appalachian Mountains; contraceptive jelly in Logan County, West Virginia; and in the 1950s, the birth control pill in Kentucky and Puerto Rico. Health professionals followed each other's progress, exchanged formulas, and recommended or discouraged the use of one product over another. Researchers commented on each other's tests and negotiated with doctors, nurses, and women over the policies and practices of contraceptive trials.[3,16] Scholars have often condemned such testing for exploiting poor women as research subjects. Noting that these trials usually offered unreliable (and sometimes dangerous) contraceptives to women who were insufficiently informed about the risks and lacked access to alternative birth control methods, historians have remarked on the race and class politics involved.[17,18] Others have acknowledged concerns about such trials but argued that they were part of accepted medical procedure at the time.[13,19,20]

With the permission of state health officers, North Carolina's birth control program was expanded rapidly between 1937 and 1939. Frances Pratt traveled from county to county seeking to convince local public health officials to incorporate the distribution of contraceptive foam powder and sponges into their regular health department activities. Health officials who agreed to cooperate made a request for funding to the State Board of Health. Health officials received free supplies of foam powder and were asked to collect data on the acceptability and reliability of the powder. Although clinics were free to advise women in other methods, all but one clinic offered foam powder only.[21,22] Pratt instructed county public health nurses in the procedure who in turn held birth control clinics for mothers at public health departments. By March 1938, the State Board of Health operated 36 birth control clinics in 33 of the state's one-hundred counties and had reached 641 women. One year later, the state had 62 centers in 60 counties, serving 2000 patients, and by 1946, a total of 93 counties participated in the contraceptive tests (Fig. 13.2). Of 478 birth control clinics reported in the United States in December 1938, 97 were public health department clinics and more than half of those were located in North Carolina.[23,24]

Public health officials across the country stressed the medical and eugenic contributions of birth control. To be eligible for the programs, women had to be indigent.[25–29] In addition, public health nurses were to evaluate potential clients for a family history of insanity, feeblemindedness, and epilepsy; look for the presence of syphilis, gonorrhea, and tuberculosis; and consider whether a mothers' physical condition might improve with family planning. Patients had to be married and, if they were in basically good health, already have several children—usually three or four. Women with medical problems making pregnancy dangerous were considered ideal patients. The North Carolina Health Bulletin portrayed women who "pleaded for contraceptive advice" as victimized by health hazards "to which they are exposed by contraceptive innocence." Articles described patients with epilepsy, with "13 pregnancies and only 4 living children," with "10th pregnancy and bedridden with cardio-renal disease" at the age of 26, as well as patients who had been inmates of mental institutions or whose husbands were convicted criminals or suffered from alcoholism or chronic diseases.[25]

Whatever the health-related benefits, health and welfare professionals made it clear that public birth control services also made economic sense. The prolonged nature of the Great Depression and rising government spending for relief led many to worry about the creation of a permanent relief class. George H. Lawrence, professor of social work at the University of North Carolina and a fervent advocate of birth control, warned in an early call for support that

> relief families are reproducing out of all proportion to the general population. . . . [L]eaders in every field are becoming more verbal and outspoken. "Isn't it true that

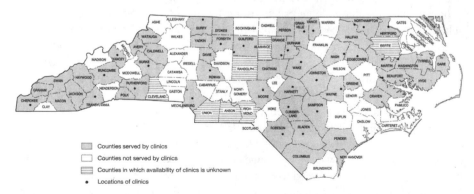

Figure 13.2. North Carolina counties with birth control services, 1939.

relief families as a group have an extremely high birth rate?" "Isn't the government feeding and maintaining large numbers of families whose outstanding characteristic is that they are producing more babies than ever before?" "Doesn't this mean increased dependency, more suffering, and an even greater tax burden?" "Doesn't this state of affairs add to the despair of such families and create a situation where it is less probable that they can be rehabilitated?"[30]

Controlling the birth rate of families on relief promised to keep the growing welfare state in check.

Some supporters might have found the birth control program appealing as a form of population control. One article suggested that the birth control program was targeting the poor and uneducated. "The South," author Frank Gilbreth announced, "is teaching birth control on tobacco road and mill village alley."[31] Another much-cited 1939 article recounted that one county health officer in North Carolina did not think his county needed contraception. As the author reported: "He was asked to check his vital statistics. When he discovered that Negroes were accounting for 85% of the births he quickly changed his mind."[32] The meaning of this exchange is far from clear, however. We know neither why state health officials sent county health officers to check their vital statistics nor what county health officials saw when they read those statistics. Health officials might have thought about race or they might have been concerned with high infant and maternal mortality rates. The only thing we know is that the journalist recounting this incidence thought about race.

Most health officials thought it unnecessary to provide any services for African Americans. As a result, African Americans were more likely to be underserved than to be the target of population control programs.[2,6] While by November 1939, two thirds of North Carolina's counties had one or more birth control centers, the counties with a high African-American population had fewer centers than the rest of the state. Of the nine counties in which African Americans made up more than 50% of the population (1940 census), three had no birth control clinics; of the nine counties in which 45–50% of the population was black, five had no birth control program; and of the 18 counties in which African Americans made up 35%–45% of the population, seven had no birth control clinics. Some officials cited white clients' refusal to attend the same facilities as blacks as an excuse for excluding African Americans from services. Others offered segregated services in the hope that such accommodation to local customs would attract the largest number of clients.[33] In times of scarce resources, however, health officials not only deemed any allocation for African Americans unnecessary but feared it would provoke opposition. When, in 1939, the Birth Control Federation of America (BCFA) offered North Carolina health officials funds to sponsor a birth control pilot project for the black community, the state director of infant and maternal health Dr. Cooper declined. "A public health program limited to the Negro race will most certainly stimulate opposition to the entire project."[34] In other words, contraceptive programs were a valued service, and like all other valued services, they were reserved disproportionately for whites.

Prejudices about black women's lack of intelligence frequently reinforced health officials' belief that funding birth control programs in black communities was a waste of money altogether. Many philanthropists and health professionals believed that African Americans lacked the intellectual capacity to use any form of birth control. Elsie Wulkop, a social worker working with Gamble to establish small contraceptive field trials, commented on the attempt of birth control education among African Americans: "It impresses me as being almost like trying to get sheer animals to conform."[35] Even sympathetic professionals regularly assumed that African Americans were not interested in birth control and would not avail themselves of the methods because they were too complicated or that patients would not accept or carry outrecommendations.[35-39] Frequently, such attitudes provided an excuse for the absence of programs.

Although black women found it harder to gain access to birth control, their greater poverty and poor health made frequent pregnancies even more dangerous and meant that they were yet more likely than whites to need contraceptive services. Black mothers died at twice the rate of white mothers. Out of 250,000 black babies born alive each year in the early 1940s, more than 22,000 died in their first year—a rate 60% higher than that of white babies. Syphilis, which caused 25% of the 18,000 stillbirths among African Americans each year, and tuberculosis were five to six times as prevalent among blacks than among whites.[2,40-42] Frequent pregnancies, deliveries, and abortion without sufficient medical care increased miscarriages and other "female troubles" and contributed to high maternal and infant death rates. "The Negro," black physician Dorothee Ferebee warned, "is saddled with problems of disease, poverty, and discrimination which menace not only his welfare, but the welfare of America. The existing medical and socio-economic problems of the Negro race are, therefore, problems of the nation."[41] Pregnancy spacing, Ferebee promised, "will do much towards general welfare improvement and is a major step towards health and happiness."[41]

Aware of the tremendous health and contraceptive needs of black women, Margaret Sanger secured funding to launch an educational campaign among African Americans. In 1938, she convinced Albert Lasker, a medical philanthropist, to donate $20,000 for the establishment of a Division of Negro Services (DNS) within the BCFA. From the very beginning, however, Sanger and the federation clashed in their visions of the so-called Negro Project. Sanger envisioned a broad grass-roots campaign under the direction and advice of African Americans that would educate black communities about birth control, allowing them to start their own services independently from potentially hostile whites.[43] Once out of Sanger's hands, however, the project became, according to historian Linda Gordon, a "microcosm of the elitist birth-control programs whose design eliminated the possibility of popular, grass roots involvement in birth control as a cause."[12] Federation officials and Gamble did more than resist African-American control over the project. Gamble argued explicitly for the need to control the reproduction of poor African Americans. "The mass of Negroes, particularly in the South, still breed carelessly and disastrously, with the result that the increase among Negroes, even more than among whites, is from that portion of the population least intelligent and fit, and least able to rear children properly."[12] Rather than invest in a grass-roots education campaign, the BCFA followed Gamble's advice in establishing so-called demonstration clinics. Such clinics, in offering birth control services to black women, could serve as a kind of social science laboratory, demonstrating that even African Americans could be taught how to use birth control successfully and confirming the value of birth control in improving health conditions among blacks.[44,45]

In 1940, the BCFA launched demonstration clinics in eastern South Carolina's Berkeley County and in Nashville, Tennessee. Economic and health conditions of African Americans were poor in both locations. Berkeley County had a population of 27,000, 70% black; the majority of these were tenant farmers with an average cash income of less than $100 per year. Illiteracy rates were high, nobody subscribed to a magazine or newspaper, and very few homes had a radio. Since the typical home was more than five miles from a paved road and during the rainy season homes were nearly inaccessible, most residents lacked access to Berkeley County's public health clinics.[42,46-48] Nashville—home to Meharry Medical School, which trained over 50% of the nation's black physicians—had a death rate among African Americans twice as high as that of the white population. Rather than establish new services, the DNS demonstration clinics expanded previously existing services in the hopes of reaching larger numbers of African Americans. Over the course of the following 2 years, the two Nashville clinics, staffed by black physicians, averaged a total of six monthly clinic sessions and advised a total of 638 women, while Berkeley county nurses held an average of eight monthly clinic sessions and advised 1008 women. Both projects relied mainly on the sponge and foam powder method, although both also advised some women in the use of contraceptive jelly.[42,49,50]

The birth control services had a profound impact on many women in Nashville and Berkeley County. For most patients, these services represented their first contact with the medical profession, and the physical examinations they received revealed a number of serious health conditions. Pelvic disorders, syphilis, and anemia were common and many of the patients were referred to family physicians or hospital clinics for further treatment.[42,49,51] These findings mirrored those in other parts of the country. Data of the Harlem Clinic, for instance, indicated that about 50% of their patients were found to need medical or surgical treatment.[52]

Health officials and the BCFA considered the demonstration project a success. By the end of the testing period, 520 women in Berkeley and Lee County and 354 women in Nashville had succeeded in preventing pregnancy during the previous 12 to 18 months. Women, officials in South Carolina reported, cooperated fully with the program and were so eager and grateful that health officials had trouble meeting the demand for services.[42] Since the Nashville women were on average 24 years old and had already had an average of 3.89 pregnancies with 3.12 living children, many felt strongly about the prevention of further pregnancies. The final report praised the two demonstration projects for proving

> that properly guided child spacing measures can be practiced by even the most disadvantaged groups and that they will: bolster maternal and child health, reduce high death rates among mothers and children, check the spread of venereal and other diseases, help lift the family standard of living . . . [and] raise the health standards of the whole community. . . . The cost of extending public health programs to include child spacing services is minute when weighed against the possible ultimate price of impaired health, delinquency, dependency, and death.[42]

Despite this glowing evaluation, the sudden cancellation of at least the Berkeley County demonstration project indicates that white health officials continued to view contraceptive and medical services to African Americans as dispensable. While it is unclear what happened to the demonstration project in Nashville, Robert Seibels, the director of the South Carolina program, concluded at the end of 18 months that he had demonstrated the success of the Berkeley County clinic and discontinued support of the project. Remarking on the achievements of the program, the report concluded: "the majority [of the 302 remaining patients] could have been kept active if there had been sufficient field force to keep in touch with them and see that they were supplied with materials."[42] With Seibels's termination of services, however, field force and supplies were no longer available and the 302 women were left with only those rudimentary services that had proved so inadequate prior to the establishment of the demonstration clinic. By 1942, a report indicated that only 14 of 52 public health clinics in South Carolina had met with BCFA representatives in the previous 3 years to discuss the contraceptive program. Between 1939 and 1942, public health officials had referred fewer than five patients per county annually to contraceptive clinics. Only half of these patients had, to the knowledge of local officials, received satisfactory attention.[53]

Women who requested birth control information agreed with health officials on the potentially devastating social and economic consequences of having too many children. Their requests for birth control testified to the physical strain of constant childbearing. As one mother wrote,

> Since I married I've done nothing but have babies. . . . I do think there's a limit for it, for my health has begun to fail fast, I have congested ovaries and with my first baby my womb lacerated terribly bad. That is giving me lots of trouble now. . . . And too my legs and thighs hurt almost constantly. I don't know why unless it is caused from "coitus interruptus" as that method is used lots. We know it is dangerous, but I've tried suppositories, condoms, douche, a pessary, and everything I've heard of but none have kept me from conceiving. My husband and I are only normal beings.[54]

Mothers described a wide variety of physical ailments that they attributed to constant pregnancies and childbearing, and they complained of the social isolation and economic hardship they experienced when having to take care of many children: "I have done nothing but . . . keep house and do the routine work that goes with that . . . I'm completely shut in. I never go to the church, Sunday school, visiting, shopping, or anywhere except occasionally to see my mother and father who are very old and feeble. . . . I have never rebelled at motherhood and no one on earth is more devoted to their home and children than I am. . . . I feel like I've had enough children."[54]

Often scared of more pregnancies, women had struggled for years to prevent conception. One study of clients of the Farm Security Administration (FSA) found that almost half of the women questioned had previously used birth control.[53] Withdrawal was the most common method. Others used one-size diaphragms, contraceptive jelly, salt in capsules, Lysol douches, or something procured from a Sears-Roebuck catalogue or a traveling peddler. Success rates, however, were low.[13,55] The average number of pregnancies for contraceptive users was 3.57, nonusers had had an average of 3.67 pregnancies.[55] Women in their twenties and early thirties only reported 0.1 child fewer with use of contraceptives. Most of the contraceptive devices were notoriously unreliable. Finding themselves pregnant, women frequently turned to illegal abortions in their quest for reproductive control.[3]

Patients thus appreciated the contraceptive advice and took advantage of contraceptive services even if they were aware of officials' condescending attitude. They negotiated with health-care providers over the contraceptives offered and used the services for their own purposes, not because they necessarily agreed with health officials on the value of contraception. Public health nurse Lena Hillard, who distributed condoms and contraceptive foam powder to every resident of Watauga County, North Carolina, reported that the women she approached were eager for birth control information (Fig.13.3). Indeed, despite the fact that condoms suffered from a bad reputation, about 50% of the households visited agreed to participate in the trial. Interest rose even more with the American entry into World War II. "Since the rubber shortage," one report noted, "we can hardly keep Trojans! I wouldn't be surprised if our patients aren't hoarding them."[56]

Frequently, women not only appreciated the birth control services offered but also behaved as educated consumers, complaining about side effects, comparing contraceptives, and demanding one birth control method over another. Having learned from neighbors and from Hillard herself that Hillard distributed not only condoms but also foam powder and jelly, women regularly demanded the contraceptive of their choice, regardless of research protocol.[57–59] While such demands could reflect women's personal preferences, patients also responded to recommendations from

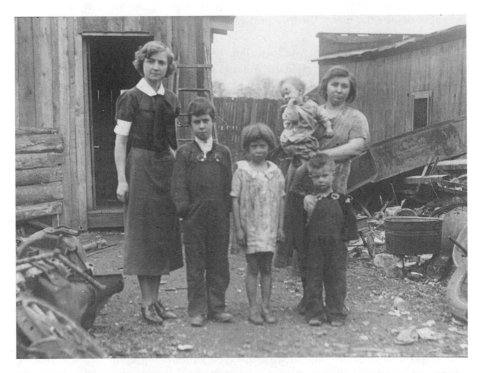

Figure 13.3. Birth control nurse Lena Hillard with a client and her children, late 1930s. (Courtesy of Countway Medical Library.)

neighbors and friends. Figuring that it was more important to help women prevent conception than to fulfill formal requirements of a field trial, Hillard and her assistant occasionally deviated from the protocol, allowing women to continue the use of condoms rather than switch to foam powder.[60,61]

Other times, however, both the nurses and patients felt painfully restricted by trial regulations. Hillard, who discovered that her own reputation and trustworthiness were closely tied to the quality of the birth control method she distributed, found the fact that she had to distribute an unreliable contraceptive so unbearable that she contemplated quitting her work. The news of method failure traveled quickly, and immediately influenced women's choices. After finding four of her foam powder patients pregnant, Hillard complained to Gamble that such results would make it difficult for her to convince women to use foam powder. "There are many cases that can not easily forgive a nurse who gives a poor material for such a very, very important purpose," she reminded Gamble. "It is very tragic for some mothers to get pregnant," she continued. "In all cases they have been nice to me but I had rather have them not so nice and keep the confidence they have had in me. Won't you reconsider the matter [of abandoning the foam powder tests and switching to a different method]? If you don't I may quit and raise babies and rabbits. . . . Maybe it is time for me to quit when we can't agree any more."[62] Even women who had trouble using the method consistently or who had become pregnant despite the use of birth control did not necessarily give up on contraceptive use. Reports of the Nashville clinic indicate, for instance, that a quarter of women who had gotten pregnant despite the use of birth control came back after delivery for refitting of the diaphragm.[42]

A nurse's control over her work was limited by the goals of researchers directing the programs. Gamble's interest in the Watauga project was not the prevention of pregnancies, but the testing of contraceptives. "It is disappointing to hear the pregnancies are developing in the group of mothers using foam powder," he responded to Hillard.

I don't think, though, that the time has yet come to switch to another method. . . . It's very important to have enough mothers and enough time in your series. In previous tests it has never been possible to say whether the pregnancies were due to failure to use the method or failure of the method to protect. . . . If the foam powder is found to be an unsatisfactory method that will protect a lot of mothers from being given it. If it turns out reasonably well it may make it possible to furnish many mothers protection who otherwise wouldn't have any.[63]

Assumptions about poor women's inability to use contraceptives properly pervaded the contraceptive services and tainted health authorities' interaction with clients. Despite the fact that many of the methods were in experimental stages, researchers and health officials tended to blame patients for the failure of contraceptive methods rather than to question the effectiveness of a given contraceptive. In fact, the research protocol at the Watauga study specified that Hillard should record method failure as a failure of the patient even if the patient claimed to have used the method consistently and correctly: "If the patient conceived while using contraception, that is, without having stopped [the use of the contraceptive], then she 'failed' whether she used it regularly or not."[64] Although clients repeatedly complained to county health officials about a high rate of failure and unpleasant side effects of the foam powder, and the majority of clinics eventually switched to diaphragms, State Health Officer Roy Norton concluded in 1957 that the main cause of failure was neglect or carelessness by the patient.[65] Health professionals' prejudices and lack of trust and interest in clients contributed to a lack of interest in patients' well-being, ultimately raising the risk of jeopardizing women's health.

If mothers feared the use of unreliable contraceptives, many feared the termination of field tests even more. For those women for whom field tests represented their only access to birth control, the completion of a trial could have devastating consequences. Lena Hillard reported of one mother who had falsely heard that Hillard had stopped doing birth control work. "She told her husband that she would simply catch a hen and take it to the store and sell it in order to get money to buy some Trojans. . . . It is true that a lot of our mothers are not financially able to pay $.50 for three Trojans. Yet, it is encouraging to see that some will be willing to sacrifice their chickens and eggs in order to stop babies from coming."[66]

Researchers rarely addressed the ethical issues involved in the termination of contraceptive trials. Gamble and Gilbert Beebe, a demographer hired by Gamble to help with the design of contraceptive field tests, were not only unconcerned with women's access to birth control after completion of the tests, but they saw it as their responsibility to cease distribution of contraceptives. Beebe assured public health authorities in North Carolina:

> When the experiment reaches a conclusion, the present service will terminate having provided useful data for health officers and others interested in contraceptive service from the standpoint of methods. What the Board of Health might then undertake in the area would, of course, be a matter for the Board to decide. . . . The public health responsibilities in North Carolina lie with the Board, with yourself and others of official position. It goes without saying that we have no right, and I may say that we have no desire, to operate a service which you feel threatens your work.[67]

Indeed, Gamble frequently withdrew funding when he had met his research objectives.[68] This half-hearted approach to contraceptive services was the rule rather than the exception. Health professionals who sponsored birth control services repeatedly changed their minds about these services and terminated financial support for a variety of reasons.[12,67,69,79]

But not all researchers showed such a lack of concern for women's ability to prevent conception. Occasionally, researchers acknowledged that contraceptives had become central to women's lives and felt responsible for the reproductive futures of women who had been willing to test their products. When Raymond Squier of the National Committee for Maternal Health made preparations for the conclusion of a contraceptive jelly trial in Logan County, West Virginia, he planned for the continuation of birth control advice to trial participants. The Logan County trials ran from June 1936 to August 1939 and were the largest field trials of a chemical contraceptive ever completed in the United States, involving 1345 women.[16] Squier reported to local health authorities in Logan County, West Virginia:

> Although our project has been scientific, as an experiment in population, not for contraceptive services as such, we are keenly aware that we have been instrumental

in acquainting a number of women with what virtually is a new way of life, so far as control of reproduction is concerned. In other words, there are women in Logan County who through us have come to rely upon contraceptive jelly for the spacing or avoidance of pregnancy, and who want to have the availability of this material continued. We think, and hope that you will agree, that it is humane and proper that such women continue to use this material if they so desire.[71]

Squier went on to suggest that the NCMH supply every physician in Logan County with free supplies of contraceptive jelly to distribute to women who asked for it. Physicians were encouraged to charge women 25 cents per tube, to be retained by the physician in appreciation of their cooperation. Such a fee, Squier noted, would "induce a desirable psychological effect on the applicants."[71] It is an ironic sign of the delicate relationship between private physicians and contraceptive researchers that the women who had lent their bodies for testing were now asked to pay a fee for the jelly while Logan County's private physicians received what amounted to a financial reward for tolerating birth control.

A lack of interest concerning birth control and, occasionally, outright opposition stifled a number of public health birth control programs. Many public health officers never requested birth control and indicated on questionnaires that they were "not interested" in the service. Others opposed the distribution of contraceptives through public health services as governmental intrusion into the medical profession or dismissed the dissemination of birth control as immoral. Some doctors worried that birth control would lead women to betray their role as housewives and mothers. "Let them have children, that's what they're here for," one physician responded to Virginia South's birth control campaign in West Virginia and Kentucky, threatening to have her indicted for discussing birth control in public. Health professionals opposed to the dissemination of birth control could effectively boycott the entire program by refusing to refer patients for contraceptive advice, withholding contraceptive information, or misinforming patients.[72–77] Opposition to state-supported birth control also came from the U.S. Children's Bureau and the U.S. Public Health Service. Supporting the birth control movement, Children's Bureau officials feared, would jeopardize already-existing programs for infant and maternal health. Officials of both agencies threatened states with the withdrawal of federal funds if they established state-supported birth control programs.[73,78]

In the end, however, health officials' fear of opposition hurt the birth control program most. To guard themselves against opposition and possible retaliations from the Children's Bureau, health officials frequently refused to publicize birth control programs in any meaningful way.[79,80] As a result, potential clients never learned about the existence of the services, and clinics ran far below their capacity.[3,81] Moreover, officials frequently separated the distribution of birth control from maternal and child health services. By doing so, they changed the very condition which had integrated birth control services into a general health program for mothers. Women in need of medical services now had to be referred to a different clinic. Staff lacking commitment to issues of maternal health were less likely to make such referrals. In addition, many clinics were poorly housed and offered inadequate medical services.[65] Some nurses and health officers, to be sure, continued to view their contraceptive work as an important contribution to maternal health. Others, however, attracted more by the eugenic and economic promises of birth control, lost sight of the health aspects, and made the control of dependent populations a goal in itself.

The limited outreach of many programs and officials' lack of dedication frustrated philanthropists such as Gamble. The establishment of clinics in more than 60 counties in 3 years, Gamble admitted to North Carolina officials in 1940, was a real accomplishment. But, he warned: "we really haven't reached every mother, and until then I won't be content . . . in spite of North Carolina's multiple distributing centers the number of mothers instructed in the last year had been less than in Texas where the public health system had given no help. . . . The limitation of the number of mothers instructed may . . . come from the fact that not enough mothers know that the service is available."[82]

In March 1940, he ended his financial support, and Pratt resigned as a birth control nurse. After Gamble's withdrawal from the program, county health officers tried to secure money from other sources. Some sought appropriations from their county commissioners; others obtained donations from local individuals and organizations or took money from their regular health department contingency funds. A few clinics had patients pay whatever they could. The program continued to grow until the late 1940s, and then began to dwindle for lack of funds.[65,83] When Gamble ceased support, health officials reported 3233 planned parenthood patients. The number rose to 4441 patients in 1948 and then fell to almost half the number in the late 1950s.

Structural changes in the mid-1940s contributed to a waning interest in public health birth control programs. Many health professionals were drafted for military service, and farmers abandoned their communities for the armed forces or urban wartime industries. Public health services were left with only rudimentary staff and many of the programs and initiatives introduced during the New Deal suffered considerable cutbacks. As the American economy prepared for war, the lingering effects of the Great Depression dissipated. Increasing hospital regulation of obstetrics practices, antibiotics to treat infection, transfusions to replace blood lost by massive hemorrhaging, and prenatal care to identify many potential high-risk cases improved maternal health while control of infectious diseases lowered infant mortality rates.

Finally, by the end of the decade, physicians had successfully replaced midwives. World War II produced a large demand for hospital care. Trying to meet a medical care crisis in the vicinity of military bases, legislators, in 1942, passed the Emergency Maternal and Infant Care program (EMIC) to provide free hospital, maternal, and infant care for dependents of servicemen and bring hospitals up to minimum standards. Women who previously delivered at home could now do so in the hospital. By the end of 1946, EMIC had handled almost 38,000 maternity cases in North Carolina alone.[2] And although EMIC ceased in 1947, the passage of the Hill-Burton Act in 1946 continued this trend by providing funds for the establishment of a national hospital system and public health centers. Greater access and the growth of group hospitalization plans meant that Southerners of both races began to enjoy access to modern hospital care that they had never known before.[2] By 1950, 88% of deliveries nationwide took place in the hospital.[4] With the majority of women now seeking the advice of physicians during pregnancy and delivery, physicians' professional interests that had driven their initial involvement in the free distribution of birth control waned.

The Re-emergence of Family Planning in the 1960s

As health professionals' interest in contraceptive services declined, family planning captured the attention of public welfare officials. World War II had helped to pull the United States out of the Depression, but the rising economic tide did not carry all. Pockets of deep poverty persisted as many of the most vulnerable, especially women, children, and the elderly, continued to need help. During the 1950s and 60s, Aid for Dependent Children (ADC), after 1962 known as Aid to Families with Dependent Children (AFDC), expanded dramatically, serving 803,000 families in 1960 compared with 372,000 in 1940. At the same time, unwed mothers replaced widows as the stereotypical ADC recipients. Federal pressure to include formerly excluded minorities into the program, as well as climbing fertility and divorce rates and a rising unemployment rate among women, contributed to the growth of the ADC program. These changes made poverty a politically volatile topic during the 1950s and 1960s. As payments to ADC mothers and their children skyrocketed in the 1950s, many believed that a high number of births by unwed ADC mothers was to blame.[84,85] Welfare officials looked to birth control for a solution to persistent welfare dependency. State supported family planning programs became central to this effort.

The new attention to family planning was accompanied both by changes in contraceptive technology and a shift in emphasis from family planning to population control. The development of the birth control pill and the intrauterine device (IUD) introduced a generation of contraceptives that separated the use of birth control from sexual activity. Contraception became easier and more reliable than ever before. Family planning programs across the country found that the inclusion of oral contraceptives in particular led to an exponential rise in the number of patients.[86,68] In Alabama, for instance, the rate of new patients quadrupled in 18 months.[86] At the same time, fears of overpopulation reinforced the view that poor women were irresponsible in their use of birth control. By the early 1960s, newspapers across the country linked the threat of world communism to a growing world population.[3] Population control at home and abroad promised social and political stability around the world. With this shift in focus, the federal government began to encourage the extension of family planning services to all women. In 1965, amendments to the Social Security Act required that state health departments extend services, including family planning, to all areas of the country. Grants were available for rural poverty pockets and distressed urban areas. The passage of the 1967 Social Security bill mandating federal expenditures for family planning signified the federal government's commitment to a domestic family planning policy.[87] In 1970, the federal government expanded family planning programs further when it passed the Family Planning Services and Population Research Act mandating the development of family planning programs on the state level.

Efforts to establish family planning services in the 1960s originated in public welfare departments or privately funded public health initiatives. Under the leadership of Wallace Kuralt, who served as director of the Mecklenburg County Department of Public Welfare from 1945 to 1972, Charlotte, North Carolina, was, in 1960, the first city to inaugurate a birth control program under the tutelage of the welfare department. In the mid-1960s, Tulane University pediatrician Joe Beasley founded Family

Planning Incorporated (FPI) to offer comprehensive family planning services in Louisiana.[88] Between 1965 and 1972, FPI became a national and international model of privately delivered public health services and comprehensive family planning programs to the poor.

Both Beasley and Kuralt espoused the rights of women to control their reproduction. "The inability of a woman to control her fertility," Beasley argued, "deprives her of a real right and a real power."[88] Choice, Kuralt argued, "is not only freedom to choose the method of family planning, but freedom to participate or not participate."[89] Both programs highlighted women's reproductive plans and recognized that contraceptive services needed to be integrated into comprehensive medical and social services. Patients received contraceptive counseling, sex education, annual breast and pelvic exams, and screening for cervical cancer. The Louisiana clinic also began to offer an annual physical exam, transforming the family planning clinic into clients' family doctor. If necessary, clinics referred clients for further treatment or to infertility specialists. Most likely staff members also helped some patients secure abortion services.[88] Clinics adopted a "cafeteria type of approach," letting patients choose among a variety of contraceptives. Both programs hired outreach workers who advertised clinic services in their respective communities. Patients with medical problems or missed appointments received particularly close follow-up. Finally, clinics offered help with transportation and baby-sitting, taught family life education, including better diet and housekeeping practices, distributed food, and invented recipes for preparing foodstuffs into nourishing meals.[88,90–92]

Such a comprehensive approach attracted an unprecedented number of clients. In Louisiana's Orleans Parish alone, the clinic had registered 17,459 families by 1969, 85% of patients remained active after 18 months.[88] Since no other statewide program existed in the United States at that time, it is difficult to compare the Louisiana program with other efforts. Mecklenburg County's service reached about 50% of the public welfare caseload.[89] Women frequently approached social workers to ask about the family planning program and request the pill.[89,92–94] Within 3 years, the Mecklenburg County family planning clinic was serving 800 women between the ages of 14 and 47; 2 years later, the number had climbed to 2200 women, and by September 1965, 3388 women had registered for the clinic. Such success proved wrong those officials who assumed that poor women were unwilling or unable to use contraceptives consistently. "Our experience and modern methods of Planned Parenthood," Kuralt exulted,

> have demonstrated the fallacy of a great many myths that circulate in our society today. The women of poor families do know when they want to stop having children. These women do have concern for their children; they are capable of participating, and they will take advantage of modern planned parenthood methods when they become acquainted with the methods and become convinced that this is a method that will meet their particular needs. . . . We are happy to say that we have had no complaints of any source about our program and we have nothing but "happy customers."[95]

Notwithstanding Beasley's and Kuralt's success, some health and welfare officials remained convinced that poor women were unable or unwilling to prevent conception. "I tried the [birth control] pills," the health director of North Carolina's Robeson

County complained. "I know these people and they don't take them like they ought to."[96] To these professionals, improvements of the IUD in the 1960s seemed to signal a new era in the goals family planning programs could achieve. By taking control out of women's hands and putting it into the hands of physicians who had to insert and remove the plastic coil, the IUD could "solve the problems of over population in the lower social groups in our state."[13,97] To some, reducing poverty became synonymous with preventing births to ADC-recipients.

Particularly in areas with significant minority populations, white policymakers were receptive to programs that promised to reduce the birth rate of its nonwhite population. In North Carolina's Robeson County, for instance, welfare officials decided to offer *only* the IUD in a family planning program "aimed at holding down the number of children born into poor families, especially those receiving welfare grants."[96,98] And in Louisiana, politicians of the racist State's Rights Party came to the spirited defense of Beasley's birth control program.[88] Some welfare officials tied the receipt of social services to women's participation in family planning. Although such policies were illegal, the North Carolina Department of Public Welfare decided in 1968 to require women on AFDC to receive birth control instruction.[99] After 6 months, welfare officials were forced to drop the requirement.

The focus on reducing poverty renewed the separation of contraceptive advice from general health care services and resulted in clinic personnel who frequently failed to give patients adequate attention. One report stated: "Many indigent women in North Carolina are given contraceptive service . . . and then are never rechecked if even followed outside the clinic. For many there is no information about their continued use of contraception or even about the occurrence of complications or dissatisfaction."[81]

Although lack of access rather than coercive policies continued to be the more common problem, the new prominence that family planning gained in the 1960s created tensions between white supporters of the new programs and many African Americans.[100] The low participation of white clients in some programs seemed to bolster the charge of racial genocide regardless of whether segregation resulted from the targeting of black clients or from the continued refusal of white women to visit integrated services.[88,101] With the rise of black militancy, all family planning programs came under suspicion. In 1968, black militants burned down a family planning clinic in Cleveland and forced the temporary closing of family planning clinics in Pittsburgh.[88,102] One prominent black Pittsburgh physician charged all government-supported birth control programs with being "an organized plot to cut down the Negro birthrate."[102] While not representative of general black attitudes, such charges were sure to capture the headlines. Aware that supporters of public contraceptive programs exploited racial stereotypes to promote the distribution of birth control, public health and welfare officials were jittery about the exposure of racist rhetoric. Some denied charges of racial genocide. Others gained the support of black clients who fought for the reopening of clinics.[102] In Louisiana, Beasley promoted one critic into top management and hired others for the clinics. Family Health was already a racially and economically integrated workplace. At one time, FPI employed over 1000 people; 81% of these were women and 52% members of racial minorities, largely from disadvantaged neighborhoods the program served. Members of these groups accounted for 78% of all management and professional positions. While the integration of critics into already existing programs could successfully enhance diversity and ensure that weak points might receive improvement, in Louisiana such co-optation aggravated already existing tensions between an increasingly remote managerial staff on the one side and family planning advocates and their clients on the other, eventually leading to the closing of the program.[88,103,104]

Despite the politicized nature, however, by the late 1960s government-supported family planning programs were there to stay. As Kuralt's and Beasley's programs demonstrated, President Lyndon B. Johnson's Great Society allowed family planning activists to link federally funded contraceptive programs to local antipoverty programs and to secure support for the delivery of birth control through both government agencies and private organizations. While federal programs remained uncoordinated and frequently underfunded, and local programs continued to be subject to the political fate of the particular institutions delivering services, family planning had become established policy.[87] With the rise of the women's health movement in the late 1960s, a new group of activists framed the demand for family planning increasingly in the context of women's reproductive rights, including access to abortion as well as protection from sterilization abuse and coercion to use family planning.

Summary and Conclusion

In the 1930s, public health professionals launched birth control programs as part of a comprehensive public health response to poor infant and maternal health. Health officials hoped to reduce infant and maternal mortality rates and improve infant and maternal health by offering mothers the opportunity to space the birth of children further apart. Distributing contraceptives was one part of a well-rounded maternal health program which also included pre- and postnatal care and the provision of basic gynecological services.

But offering birth control to poor women also seemed attractive for economic and eugenic reasons. The distribution of birth control to the poor, officials hoped, would reduce the birth rate of those currently on relief, curb the growth of the dependent population, and help to control poverty. Whatever their individual beliefs, officials recognized that economic and eugenic arguments were particularly powerful in attracting support for the birth control program.

Once implemented, public health birth control services straddled the divide between offering women reproductive control and seeking to control women's reproduction. Whether the services increased or limited women's reproductive autonomy depended on the extent to which officials integrated contraceptive advice into more general health and social services. Merely providing women with contraceptive supplies was insufficient. Health problems, a lack of education, and the absence of a support network often proved powerful obstacles to women's successful use of birth control. To truly increase women's reproductive control, birth control clinics needed to offer sex education, medical care, and ongoing support and follow-up. Moreover, clinics had to be accessible to working women and those living in remote rural areas.

While many programs were able to offer women the health and contraceptive services necessary, others were fraught with race and class prejudices. Stereotypes about poor and minority women's presumed inability to properly prevent conception pervaded both the research and development of new contraceptives and the delivery of contraceptive services. Throughout the twentieth century, most research on contraceptive technology was driven by the assumption that poor women lacked the intelligence and motivation to use existing contraceptive devices. As a result, researchers neglected considerations of women's self determination in favor of long-lasting anti-fertility methods that required little or no user participation. During the 1930s and 1940s, such a focus resulted in contraceptive field trials which swamped poor and minority women with inexpensive and often unreliable birth control methods. By the 1960s, research had turned to the development of methods outside of women's control. Contraceptive devices such as the IUD or Norplant removed control over the method from women and placed it into the hands of physicians who became responsible for insertion and removal. As development of birth control devices progressed, the potential for abuse inherent in new methods increased. While women still had control over the methods used in field trials during the 1930s and 1940s and could stop the use of contraceptives any time they wanted, they now had to rely on physicians to remove the IUD or Norplant.

While reproductive health policies were designed to provide an equal chance for all, such policies also found support because they promised to lighten the state's burden from the "socially useless."[105] The state seemed to acknowledge access to birth control, and later to sterilization and abortion, as basic citizenship rights. But these rights came with a responsibility: health and welfare officials expected women to have children within marriage and to limit the number of children they bore according to their families' financial means. Those unable or unwilling to exercise this responsibility placed themselves outside the body politic.[106,107] If the birth control program was for those responsible and intelligent enough to take advantage of it, coercive family planning policies were for those unable to control themselves.

Although clients were not blind to the race and class prejudices which underlay many family planning programs, they valued the contraceptive information, took advantage of the services offered, and bargained with authorities over the conditions of contraceptive advice. Clearly, some women suffered negative consequences from their participation in the contraceptive trials or found the attitude of health and welfare professionals so humiliating that they decided to forgo the contraceptive advice. Others, however, found that the birth control advice introduced them to a new way of life—one unthreatened by frequent pregnancy and childbearing. They used the services to improve their quality of life and found allies in local health authorities who lobbied in their interest.

Women's lack of access to decent health and contraceptive services, their poverty, their race, and gender significantly influenced their decision to participate in contraceptive field trials or take advantage of even imperfect birth control programs. Their choice was conditioned by their lack of other alternatives. They took advantage of the services in a social and economic context which denied them access to safe, effective, convenient and affordable methods of birth control and equitable social, political, and economic conditions under which to make choices.[108,109] Some people have more social space to make decisions than others. Public family planning services could play a crucial role in leveling the playing field by providing much needed access for poor and minority women.

References

1. Waddill EP to [Moore H], 5 April 1937. Clarence J. Gamble Papers, Countway Medical Library [hereafter CJG-CML], Box 23, File 408.
2. Beardsley EH. A History of Neglect: Health Care for Blacks and Mill Workers in the Twentieth-Century South. Knoxville: University of Tennessee Press, 1987, 13, 22, 174, 178, 247.
3. Schoen J. Choice and Coercion: Birth Control, Sterilization, and Abortion in Public Health and Welfare. Chapel Hill: University of North Carolina Press, 2005.
4. Leavitt JW. Brought to Bed: Childbearing in America, 1750–1950. New York: Oxford University Press, 1986, 25–26, 171, 174, 194.
5. Grey MR. New Deal Medicine: The Rural Health Programs of the Farm Security Administration. Baltimore: Johns Hopkins University Press, 1999.
6. Smith SL. Sick and Tired of Being Sick and Tired: Black Women's Health Activism in America, 1890–1950. Philadelphia: University of Pennsylvania Press, 1995.
7. Committee on the Costs of Medical Care. Medical Care for the American People: The Final Report of the Committee on the Costs of Medical Care. publication no. 28. Chicago: University of Chicago Press, 1932.
8. Borst CG. Catching Babies: The Professionalization of Childbirth, 1870–1920. Cambridge, MA: Harvard University Press, 1995, 101–16.
9. Flexner A. Medical Education in the United States and Canada. Washington, DC: Carnegie Foundation for the Advancement of Teaching, 1910 (reprint 1960, Washington, D.C.: Science and Health Publications).
10. Williams JW. Medical education and the midwife problem in the United States. *JAMA* 1912:58:1–7.
11. State Board of Health. Infancy and maternal mortality as it applies to the general practitioner. [n.d., 1933–1935], North Carolina State Archives [hereafter SBH-NCSA], 1924–1935, Dr. G.M. Cooper's File, Box 28.
12. Gordon L. Woman's Body, Woman's Right: A Social History of Birth Control in America, rev. ed. New York: Penguin, 1990.
13. Tone A. Devices and Desires: A History of Contraceptives in America. New York: Hill and Wang, 2001, 155.
14. Doris Davidson to Mrs. Barclay, 5 March 1937. CJG-CML, Box 190, File 2993.
15. Richter J. Vaccination Against Pregnancy: Miracle or Menace? London: Zed Books, 1996, chap. 4.
16. Reed J. From Private Vice to Public Virtue: The Birth Control Movement and American Society, rev. ed. Princeton: Princeton University Press, 1991.
17. Briggs L. Reproducing Empire: Race, Sex, Science, and U.S. Imperialism in Puerto Rico. Berkeley: University of California Press, 2002.
18. Marks L. A cage of ovulating females: the history of the early oral contraceptive pill clinical trials, 1950–1959. In: Chadarevain SE, Kamminga H, ed. Molecularizing Biology and Medicine: New Practices and Alliances, 1930s–1970s. Reading, UK: Harwood Academic Press, 1997, 221–47.
19. Watkins ES. On the Pill: A Social History of Oral Contraceptives, 1950–1970. Baltimore: Johns Hopkins University Press, 1998.
20. Lederer SE. Subjected to Science: Human Experimentation in America before the Second World War. Baltimore: Johns Hopkins University Press, 1995.

21. Pratt FR. Travel narrative, February 1940. CJG-CML, Box 25, File 432.
22. Pratt FR. Eighteen months of health department contraceptive work in North Carolina, 1 April 1937 to 1 October 1938. 1 October 1939, J.W.R. Norton Papers, Southern Historical Society, University of North Carolina [hereafter JWRN-SHC], Box 2, Misc. Papers.
23. Pratt FR. Outline developed in North Carolina State Board of Health for staff education programs for public health nurses in birth control work. 18 October 1939, CJG-CML, Box 24, File 424.
24. University News Bureau. Ninety-three counties now have contraceptive services. 24 May 1946, CJG-CML, Box 26, File 463.
25. Norton R. A Health Department birth control program. *Am J Public Health* 1939: 29:253.
26. Norton R. Planned parenthood. *The Living Age,* March 1940, 7.
27. Maternal Health Project. Second quarterly report, 15 November 1937. Planned Parenthood Federation of America I, Sophia Smith Collection [hereafter PPFA I], Series 3, Box 47, Folder: Birth Control, North Carolina, 1937–1942.
28. Morehead WC. Outline of talk. PPFA I, Series 3, Box 45, Folder: Birth Control, California, FSA Project, 1939–1941.
29. Maternal Health Project. First quarterly report, 15 July 1937. CJG-CML, Box 23, File 405.
30. Lawrence GH. Something ought to be done about it. 26 April 1935, JWRN-SHC. Box 2, Misc. Papers, File: Associations . . . Societies, Birth Control Federation of America.
31. Gilbreth FB. State takes lead in birth control clinic of South. *Raleigh News and Observer,* 30 June 1940.
32. Wharton D. Birth control: the case for the state. *Atlantic Monthly,* October 1939, 463–67.
33. Virginia F. South to [Cecil] Damon, 21 October 1937. CJG-CML, Box 14, Folder 269.
34. Roy Norton to Woodbridge E. Morris, 17 November 1939. JWRN-SHC, Box 2.
35. Elsie Wulkop to Clarence J. Gamble, 26 September 1936. CJG-CML, Box 7, Folder 135.
36. Frances R. Pratt to Clarence J. Gamble, 23 February 1937, CJG-CML, Box 23, File 403.
37. Moore H. Birth control for the Negro. 1937. PPFA I, Box 65, Folder 3.
38. Meeting of the South Atlantic Association of Obstetricians and Gynecologists, 10–11 February 1939. CJG-CML, Box 24, File 421.
39. Letter to Miss Pratt, undated, JWRN-SHC, Box 2.
40. Preliminary annual report of the Division of Negro Services. Margaret Sanger Papers, Sophia Smith Collection [hereafter MS Papers], SSC, Reel S 62.
41. Dorothy Boulding Ferebee. Project Reports, 29 January 1942. MS Papers, SSC, Reel S 20.
42. Better Health for 13,000,000. n.d. [June 1943]. PPFA I, Box 34, Folder 2.
43. Margaret Sanger to Clarence J. Gamble, 26 November 1939. MS Papers, SSC, Reel S 17.
44. Woodbridge E. Morris to John Overton, 6 February 1940. MS Papers, SSC, Reel S 17.
45. Woodbridge E. Morris to Albert D. Lasker, 21 November 1939. MS Papers, SSC, Reel S 17.
46. Minutes of Board of Directors Meeting of the Birth Control Federation of America. 7 December 1939. MS Papers, SSC, Reel S 62.
47. South Carolina, Moncks Corner, Berkeley County. 10 February 1940. CJG-CML, Box 36, File 601.
48. Preliminary annual report of the Division of Negro Services. MS Papers, SCC, Reel S 62.
49. Planned Parenthood. n.d. [1941] MS Papers, SCC, Reel S 62.
50. Minutes of the National Negro Advisory Council Meeting, 9 May 1940. MS Papers, SCC, Reel S 62.

51. Robert E. Seibels to Margaret Sanger, 29 January 1940. MS Papers, SCC, Reel S 17.
52. Race leaders endorse vitally important program: Planned Parenthood stressed in communities during observance of National Negro Health Week. *The New York Age*, 11 April 1942. MS Papers, SCC, Reel S 21.
53. No title [report on counties participation in maternal health program]. PPFA I, Series 3, Box 47. File: Birth Control, South Carolina, 1939–42.
54. Mrs. Edith Turner to Dr. Roy Norton, 8 December 1938, JWRN-SHC, Box 2.
55. Delp M. Baby spacing: a report on California and Arizona, March–August 1940. PPFA I, Box 44, Folder 4.
56. Sylvia Payne to Clarence J. Gamble, 9 February 1942, CJG-CML, Box 25, File 445.
57. Beebe G, Watauga County Project: Objectives, 17 August 1939. CJG-CML, Box 24, File 429.
58. Weekly Report on Project in Watauga County, 14 October 1939 to 11 December 1939. CJG-CML, Box 24, File 429.
59. Weekly Report on Project in Watauga County, 4 January 1940 to 7 December 1949. CJG-CML, Box 25, File 436.
60. Lena Hillard to Claire E. Folsome, 8 April 1942. CJG-CML, Box 25, File 445.
61. Sylvia Payne to Clarence Gamble, 17 November 1941. CJG-CML, Box 25, File 442.
62. Lena Hillard to Clarence J. Gamble, 14 July 1942, CJG-CML, Box 25, File 444.
63. Clarence J. Gamble to Lena Hillard, 9 August 1942, CJG-CML, Box 25, File 444.
64. Beebe G. Watauga County project: recording instructions, 19 August 1939. CJG-CML, Box 24, File 429.
65. Norton JWR. Twenty-one years' experience with a public health contraceptive service. *Am J Public Health* 1959:49:993–1000.
66. Lena Hillard to Youngs Rubber Corporation, 10 February 1941, CJG-CML, Box 25, File 442.
67. Gilbert Beebe to George Cooper, 18 May 1941. CJG-CML, Box 25, File 442.
68. Hutchins LG. Three decades of family planning in Appalachia. n.d. [1967]. North Carolina Fund [hereafter NCF-SHC], Folder 437, Southern Historical Collection, University of North Carolina-Chapel Hill.
69. LD to Catherine C. Banks, n.d. [1934], PPFA I, Box 58, Folder 6.
70. Lydia Allen Devilbiss to Margaret Sanger, 30 September 1936. MS Papers, SCC, Reel S 11.
71. Raymond Squier to L. L. Aultz, 7 June 1939. CJG-CML, Box 44, Folder 727.
72. Virginia F. South to Cecil Damon, 21 October 1937. CJG-CML, Box 14, File 269.
73. Hazel Moore, Memo to Clarence J. Gamble, 3 March 1938, CJG-CML, Box 24, File 418.
74. Virginia F. South to Cecil Damon, 1 October 1937. CJG-CML, Box 14, Folder 269.
75. Clarence J. Gamble to Dr. Hageman, 16 June 1941, CJG-CML, Box 25, File 442.
76. Morehead WC. May 1st—the pioneer year in farm security special rural projects. 8 May 1939, series 3, box 45, folder Birth Control, California, FSA Project, 1939–1941, PPFA-SSC.
77. Morehead WC. Nebraska: region VII. 27 January to 18 May, 1941, series 3, box 47, folder Birth Control, Nebraska, 1941, PPFA-SSC.
78. McCann C. Birth Control Politics in the United States: 1916–1945. Ithaca: Cornell University Press, 1994, 198–200.
79. G.M. Cooper to Dr. Cecil A. Demon, 25 January 1938, CJG-CML, Box 24, File 415.
80. Florence Rose to Margaret Sanger, 8 December 1942. MS Papers, SCC, Reel S 21.
81. North Carolina Public Health Department Family Planning Program: Historical Background, n.d. [1968]: 12, Ellen Black Winston Papers, University of North

Carolina – Greensboro [hereafter EBW-UNC-G], Box 9, File: Planned Parenthood — World Population, 1968–1973.

82. Clarence J. Gamble to Dr. Cooper, 12 August 1940, CJG-CML, Box 25, File 433.

83. Williams D, Williams G. Every Child a Wanted Child: Clarence James Gamble, MD, and His Work in the Birth Control Movement. Boston: Harvard University Press, 1978, 137–45.

84. Abramovitz M. Regulating the Lives of Women: Social Welfare Policy from Colonial Times to the Present. Boston: South End Press, 1988, 319, 321.

85. Bell W. Aid to Dependent Children. New York: Columbia Press, 1965, 40–56.

86. Jaffe FS. Family planning and rural poverty: an approach to programming of services. June 1967, p. 27, NCF-SHC, Folder 436.

87. Critchlow DT. Intended Consequences: Birth Control, Abortion, and the Federal Government in Modern America. New York: Oxford University Press, 1999, 50–111, 227.

88. Ward MC. Poor Women, Powerful Men: America's Great Experiment in Family Planning. Boulder, CO: Westview Press, 1986, 17, 23, 26, 30–31, 56–58, 62–65, 131–32.

89. Kirkpatrick JW, Winters A. Planned parenthood—a public welfare responsibility. Charlotte, Mecklenburg County Department of Public Welfare, May 1967, Appendix C, p. 3.

90. Shepherd J. Birth control and the poor: a solution. *Look*, 7 April 1984, 63–67.

91. Kuralt WH. A public welfare agency tries "prevention of dependency." *Public Welfare News* 1967:31:1–10.

92. Schoen J. Interview with Virginia Cloer, Dorothy Hicks, and Eleanor Anderson, Charlotte, NC, 11 June 1997.

93. Corkey EC.The birth control program in the Mecklenburg County Health Department, *Am J Public Health* 1966:56:40–47.

94. Interview with Murlene Wall, Charlotte NC, 19 June 1997.

95. Wallace H. Kuralt to Donald H. Winkler, 20 March 1964, Fred Alexander Papers, University of North Carolina-Charlotte [hereafter FAP-UNC-C].

96. Inman T. Birth control working in east. *Raleigh News and Observer*, 10 July 1963, 1–2.

97. More than 150 women try experimental birth control device. *Raleigh News and Observer*, 30 January 1964, 29.

98. Allen ES. Arkansas: results of the first three years. NCF-SHC, Folder 437.

99. Social work services in family planning: a course outline for the use of staff development personnel in public welfare. July 1967, CB-NA, 1967–68, Box 1143, File 4-4-1-1-9.

100. Birth control seen as aimed at Negroes. *Raleigh News and Observer*, 20 November 1968, 26.

101. Corkey EC. North Carolina: family planning in a rural maternity clinic. n.d. [1967]. NC Fund, Folder 437.

102. Caron SM. Birth control and the lack community in the 1960s: genocide or power politics? *Journal of Social History* 1998:31:545–69.

103. Richardson RH. Patterns and progress in the promotion of family planning in the Southeastern United States. Delivered at the 1969 Annual Meeting of the Population Association of America, 10 April 1969, EBW-UNC-G, Box 9, File: Planned Parenthood–World Population, 1968–1973.

104. Carl S. Shultz to Arthur J. Lesser, 29 July 1968, Children's Bureau, National Archives, 1967–1968, Box 1142, File 4-4-1-1-9 November 1968.

105. State adopts useable law for sterilization of defectives. *Public Welfare Progress* 1929:10:1.

106. Gordon L. Pitied but Not Entitled: Single Mothers and the History of Welfare. New York: Free Press, 1994, 287–306.

107. Fraser N. Struggle over needs: outline of a socialist-feminist critical theory of late-

capitalist political culture. In: Gordon L, ed. Women, the State, and Welfare. Madison: University of Wisconsin Press, 1990, 199–200.

108. Correa S, Petchesky RP. Reproductive and sexual rights. In: Sen G, Germain A, Chen L, eds. Population Policies Reconsidered: Health, Empowerment, and Rights.Cambridge, MA: Harvard University Press, 1994, 107–23.

109. Lopez I. Agency and constraint: In: Lampherc L, Ragone H, Zavella P, eds. Situated Lives: Gender and Culture in Everyday Life. New York: Routledge, 1997, 157–71.

Suggested Reading

Borst CG. Catching Babies: The Professionalization of Childbirth, 1870–1920; Cambridge, MA: Harvard University Press, 1995, 101–16.

Gordon L. Woman's Body, Woman's Right: A Social History of Birth Control in America; rev. ed. New York: Penguin, 1990.

Reed J. From Private Vice to Public Virtue: The Birth Control Movement and American Society; rev. ed. Princeton, NJ: Princeton University Press, 1991.

Schoen J. Choice and Coercion: Birth Control, Sterilization, and Abortion in Public Health and Welfare. Chapel Hill: University of North Carolina Press, 2005.

PART VII

ORAL AND DENTAL HEALTH: FLUORIDATION

14

Changing the Face of America: Water Fluoridation and Oral Health

BRIAN A. BURT

SCOTT L. TOMAR

During the early to mid-1900s, dental caries (i.e., tooth decay), usually associated with uncomfortable treatment and tooth loss, was one of life's unpleasant certainties. However, the dental health outlook for Americans growing up during the later part of the 1900s was quite different; national data obtained during this time tell the story. According to the first National Health and Nutrition Examination Survey of 1971–74 (NHANES I), one extracted permanent tooth occurred among each 1.6 persons aged 12–17 years.[1] By the mid-1980s, this average had dropped to only one lost tooth per 20 persons of the same age,[2] a 12-fold improvement. Incident cases of caries among persons in this age group also were down, and severity of the disease (measured as the average number of teeth affected per person) had dropped by 50%.[3] With the exception of vaccine-preventable childhood infectious diseases, few other public health problems have waned as quickly.

Substantial cohort improvements in oral health over a half-century are the result of many factors, including rising standards of living, better treatment technology, and more positive attitudes toward oral health. The wide scale exposure of Americans to fluoride has also played a crucial role. Fluoride changed the way people thought about dental health because fluoride's effects demonstrated that tooth decay and tooth loss were not inevitable.

Widespread exposure to fluoride began in Grand Rapids, Michigan, in 1945, where fluoride was first added to a public drinking water supply. The stage for that event was set by a series of epidemiologic studies of persons living in areas with naturally occurring fluoride in their drinking water. These studies led to the hypothesis that routine exposure to fluoride would reduce the prevalence and severity of caries—a hypothesis that was eventually proven correct. By the start of the twenty-first century, more than half of the U.S. population had access to fluoridated water, and virtually all mass-market toothpastes contained fluoride. Dentists currently use various fluoride materials in their practices, and because many food processing plants are located in areas with fluoridated water, processed food and beverages also provide fluoride.

This chapter traces the historical development of fluoride as a tool for preventing dental caries. The epidemiologic studies that contributed to knowledge regarding such prevention also are discussed.

Colorado Brown Stain

In 1901, Dr. Frederick McKay opened his dental practice in Colorado Springs, Colorado. A recent dental school graduate, McKay observed that many of his patients had an unusual blotching of the teeth that he had not learned about in school; local residents called the blotching Colorado brown stain. The cause of Colorado brown stain had not yet been elucidated. In 1908, McKay's curiosity prompted him to investigate the extent of this condition in the surrounding area.

Over the next few years, McKay found that Colorado brown stain was common in rural communities along the Continental Divide. It was found only in persons who had been born in these communities and those who had come to the area as infants. Because the stain seemed to be intrinsic and could not be polished off, McKay reasoned that it must be caused by exposure to an environmental agent during the period of enamel formation. He published his first description of what he called mottled enamel in 1916.[4]

McKay noted that mottled enamel was most prevalent among persons who obtained drinking water from deep artesian wells. By the 1920s, McKay had reached the conclusion that the etiologic agent had to be a constituent of the local groundwater,[5] despite the failure of chemical analyses to detect anything unusual. Empirical evidence of McKay's belief became apparent in Oakley, Idaho, where mottled enamel among local residents was endemic and severe. McKay found that children living on the outskirts of the city, who obtained water from a private spring, had no mottling. He advised the citizens of Oakley to abandon their old supply and tap this spring for a new source, advice that the community acted upon in 1925. After this year, children born in Oakley were unaffected by mottled enamel.[5]

McKay observed another unusual dental condition among persons living along the Continental Divide, and in 1928 he published data suggesting that the incidence of dental caries was reduced by the same waters that produced mottled enamel.[6] By 1930, the development of new methods of spectrographic analysis of water led to the identification of fluoride as the etiologic agent for endemic mottled enamel. The scientific community was immediately concerned because fluoride in high concentrations was known to have toxic effects in sheep and cattle. In 1931, H. Trendley Dean (shown in Fig. 14.1), the first dentist in the newly established National Institute of Health, was assigned to investigate fluoride levels in drinking water and the relationship between

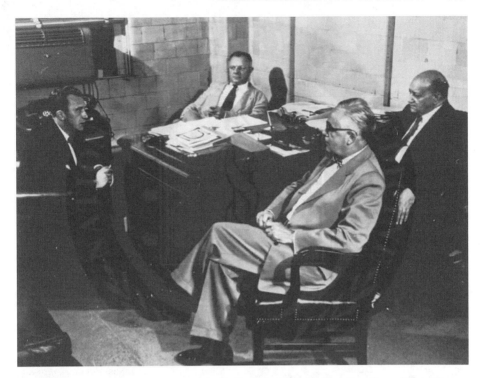

Figure 14.1. Fluoridation pioneers (clockwise from top): H. Trendley Dean, Elias Elvove, Frank J. McClure, and Francis A. Arnold, Jr. (From the National Library of Medicine, History of Medicine Collection. Available at: http://wwwihm.nlm.nih.gov/ihm/images/A/18/371.jpg. Accessed 15 June 2006.)

these levels and (1) mottled enamel and (2) the broader health issues related to fluoride consumption. Dean first mapped out the prevalence of mottled enamel in the United States by writing letters to seek the experiences of dental associations from regions across the country. Response was good, and he published his first map on the distribution of mottled enamel in 1933.[7] He then developed a seven-point, ordinal-scale index to classify the full range of mottled enamel, from the finest of lacy markings that characterized very mild fluorosis to the corroded, stained, and highly friable enamel seen in the most severe cases.[8] Figure 14.2 shows one of the charts Dean produced during this period of his research.

Dean began using the term *fluorosis* to replace *mottled enamel* in the mid-1930s.[9] He clinically examined thousands of children in many parts of the country using his fluorosis index and built up a substantial database. He grafted a numerical scale onto his original seven grades of severity, which he then used to compute a quantitative index of community fluorosis.[10] The ordinal nature of the numerical scale meant that the weighted means, which represented the community index scores, were of questionable validity. However, the index provided a useful relative measure for assessing the nature and extent of the fluorosis problem.

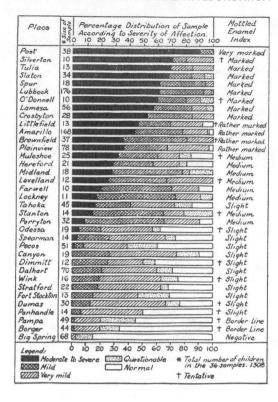

Figure 14.2. Graphical presentation, hand-drawn by Dean, to show the distribution of fluorosis severity related to fluoride concentration of the drinking water in Texas communities he studied. (From Dean HT, Dixon RM, Cohen C. Mottled enamel in Texas. *Public Health Rep* 1935:50:424–42.)

Researchers throughout the mid-1930s analyzed many drinking-water samples for minerals and other chemical constituents, but none apart from fluoride could be related to fluorosis.[9,11,12] Dean set out his criteria for a desirable fluoride concentration with respect to fluorosis. For public health purposes, Dean arbitrarily defined the minimal threshold of fluoride concentration in a domestic water supply as the highest concentration of fluoride incapable of producing a definite degree of mottled enamel in as much as 10% of the group examined.[9] By the mid-1930s, Dean had concluded that the minimal threshold level for fluoride was 1.0 ppm[13] and that fluorosis seen below that level, primarily resulting in questionable-to-mild fluorosis, was "of no public health significance."[11] Dean later referred to 1.0 ppm of fluoride as "the permissible maximum."[14]

Later in that decade, Dean condensed his original 1934 fluorosis index to one using a six-point ordinal scale by combining the categories of moderately severe and severe.[15] By 1942, Dean had documented the prevalence and severity of fluorosis for most of the United States.[16] His work primarily was descriptive, but it established the groundwork for the more analytical work to follow.

Waterborne Fluoride and Dental Caries

Toward the end of the 1930s, Dean's research shifted to focus on the relationship between waterborne fluoride and dental caries. Although severe caries was endemic in many areas, Dean observed that many persons affected by fluorosis had less caries than persons who were unaffected. The first report in which Dean commented on the inverse relationship between fluorosis and caries came in 1938, when he matched his fluorosis data from children in parts of South Dakota, Colorado, and Wisconsin with caries data from an earlier 26-state, etiologic survey.[17] The data suggested a relationship between mild fluorosis levels and low severity of caries.

Encouraged by these preliminary data, Dean chose four cities in central Illinois as study sites in which to test the hypothesis that consumption of fluoride-containing waters was associated with a reduced prevalence of dental caries. The cities of Galesburg and Monmouth, where Dean had already studied fluorosis,[11] provided residents with drinking water from deep wells; fluoride levels in this water were approximately 1.8 ppm. Residents of the nearby towns of Macomb and Quincy, however, used surface waters with an average fluoride level of 0.2 ppm. Clinical examinations of children aged 12–14 years, all with lifetime residence in their respective cities, demonstrated that the prevalence of caries in the towns with water that contained minimal amounts of fluoride was double that found in Galesburg and Monmouth,[18] providing more evidence to support a fluoride-caries hypothesis.

Although caries prevalence and severity were low in Galesburg and Monmouth, fluorosis remained problematic in both communities. Therefore, the next logical step was to define the lowest fluoride level at which caries prevalence was reduced. This was determined through a series of epidemiologic investigations that have become known collectively as the 21-cities study (see Fig. 14.3). The first part of the study consisted of clinical data from children aged 12–14 years with lifetime residence in eight suburban Chicago communities with various but stable fluoride levels in their drinking waters.[19] The project was expanded by adding data from 13 additional cities in Illinois, Colorado, Ohio, and Indiana.[20] City of residence was used as a proxy for fluoride exposure because naturally occurring fluoride in drinking water was virtually the only fluoride exposure of any significance for residents.

The results of the 21-cities study confirmed the association between fluoridated water and reduced prevalence and severity of caries.[19,20] Although the study could not establish a definitive cause-and-effect relationship because of its cross-sectional design, it demonstrated that such a relationship was highly probable. The data from this study led to the adoption of 1.0–1.2 ppm as the appropriate fluoride concentration in drinking water for temperate climates, a standard that remains in place in the United States. The data from the 21-cities study (shown in Fig. 14.3), also set the stage for a prospective test of the fluoride-caries hypothesis.

Early Studies with Controlled Water Fluoridation

In January 1945, the city of Grand Rapids, Michigan, began to fluoridate its water to levels of 1.0–1.2 ppm, the first U.S. city to do so. Newburgh, New York, began fluoridation in May 1945, and both cities took part in field trials to evaluate fluoridation's effectiveness. Other cities soon became involved in independent field trials in controlled fluoridation, including Evanston, Illinois, and Brantford, Ontario. In these trials, fluoride concentration in water was increased from negligible to 1.0–1.2 ppm.

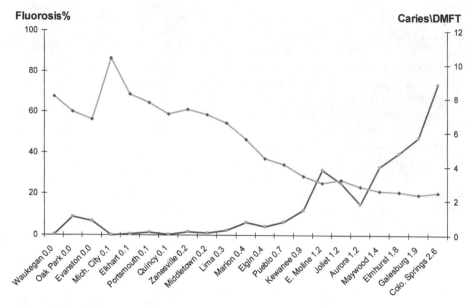

Figure 14.3. Data from the 21-Cities study, with the communities and the fluoride concentration of their drinking waters (in ppm F) along the x-axis, caries experience as the average number of teeth affected per child on the left y-axis, and fluorosis severity by mean scores from the Dean Fluorosis Index on the right y-axis. (From Dean HT, Jay P, Arnold FA Jr, Elvove E. Domestic water and dental caries. II. A study of 2,832 white children aged 12–14 years, of eight suburban Chicago communities, including *L. acidophilus* studies of 1761 children. *Public Health Rep* 1941:56:761–92; Dean HT, Arnold FA Jr., Elvove E. Domestic water and dental caries. V. Additional studies of the relation of fluoride domestic waters to dental caries experience in 4,425 white children aged 12–14 years of 13 cities in 4 states. *Public Health Rep* 1942:57:1155–79.)

The original fluoridation studies are sometimes called classic studies, although the term *pioneering* might be more accurate. In addition, these studies were referred to as longitudinal studies as they were being conducted; however, all of them were cross-sectional. By present-day standards of field trials, they were crude and exhibited design flaws. Sampling methods and dental examiners tended to vary from one year to another,[32] thereby creating the potential for bias and unnecessary random error. Methods of statistical analysis, by today's standards, were primitive; data from the control communities were largely neglected after the initial reports, and conclusions were based on the weaker historical controls.

Despite these design flaws, the magnitude of the reduced caries experience in these studies convinced dental and public health professionals to consider the critical role that fluoride might play in improving dental health. By the 1960s, caries severity had dropped sharply among residents of cities involved in the pioneer studies.[26–29] These pioneer studies also demonstrated that dental fluorosis occurred at the same incidence[30,31] that Dean had described earlier[16] (i.e., 7%–16% of the population had mild or very mild fluorosis when their fluoride exposure came from drinking waters with 1.0 ppm of fluoride).

Other cities slowly but steadily began to add fluoride to their water. By the 1960s, several large cities, including New York City and San Francisco, had begun to fluoridate. The numbers of people receiving fluoridated water grew sharply through the 1970s; by 1992, approximately 62% of Americans with public water supplies were receiving fluoridated water. By century's end, this proportion had grown to 66%.[21]

International Field Studies with Water Fluoridation

Evidence supporting the effectiveness of water fluoridation in preventing caries continued to accumulate from many parts of the world. Some of the most convincing evidence has come from Britain, where only about 15% of the population receives fluoridated drinking water. In Britain, the mean number of teeth affected by caries per child living in areas receiving fluoridated water is still about half of the mean found in nonfluoridated areas, in both primary and permanent teeth.[33–35] Similar results have been reported from Brazil,[36,37] Switzerland,[38] Australia,[39,40] New Zealand,[41] and Ireland, the only nation in the world where fluoridation is mandatory.[42]

The Role of Water Fluoridation in Preventing Dental Caries in the United States

Since around 1975, the caries prevalence and severity in U.S. children has declined steadily. However, the extent to which this decline is attributable directly to water fluoridation cannot be estimated precisely, for the following reasons:

- The development of fluoridated toothpaste and other dental products and the presence of fluoride in food and beverages processed with fluoridated water has presented Americans with many different exposures to fluoride.
- The mobility of the U.S. population means that most people have varied fluoride exposures at different times of life; therefore, finding true controls is difficult among U.S. residents.
- Documentation of lifetime exposure history to fluoridation is difficult because no biomarkers for lifetime exposure have been established and because data obtained from interviews can be unreliable.

Indirect estimates suggest that water fluoridation continues to benefit Americans despite increased exposure to other sources of fluoride. Data collected in a 1986–1987 national survey of school-aged children conducted by the National Institute of Dental Research (now the National Institute of Dental and Craniofacial research, or NIDCR) indicated that the proportion of the decline in caries attributable to water fluoridation was 18%. Among adults, an analysis of dental treatment insurance claims found that adults with exposure to high levels of fluoride had a lower probability of receiving a filling than did adults with no exposure.[44]

Fluoride and Caries Control: Establishing the Mechanisms of Action

Although it is now known that fluoride works best to prevent caries when a constant, low ambient level of fluoride is maintained in the oral cavity,[45] and that fluoride's action in preventing caries comes from a combination of several mechanisms (see Box 14.1), determining the way in which fluoride works to prevent caries has not been a straight-forward process. McKay's work in the early years of the twentieth century established that dental fluorosis was a pre-eruptive condition, a conclusion confirmed by later re-search. Therefore, when fluoride's role in caries prevention began to emerge, Dean and the other early researchers assumed that this, too, was a pre-eruptive phenomenon. Be-cause fluoride's affinity for calcified tissues was known, it became accepted that pre-eruptive absorption of fluoride into the hydroxyapatite crystals of the developing enamel must have served to make the enamel less acid-soluble. This assumption on flu-oride's mode of action was accepted uncritically for years. By the mid-1970s, however, enough evidence had been collected to cast doubt on the view that all of fluoride's ben-efits came from pre-eruptive action.[46] Caries severity could not be correlated with enamel fluoride levels, and the evidence was mounting for a primary role for fluoride in the demineralization-remineralization cycles at the plaque-enamel interface.[47]

By the end of the twentieth century, the topical effect of low-concentration fluo-ride (i.e., fluoridated water and fluoridated toothpaste) in enhancing remineralization in the early stages of the carious process was well understood.[48] Fluoride introduced into the mouth is partly taken up by dental plaque, from which it can be released in response to lowered pH.[49] Fluoride is taken up more readily by demineralized enamel than by sound enamel,[50] and the availability of plaque fluoride to respond to the acid challenge leads to the gradual establishment of more acid-resistant enamel during demineralization-remineralization cycles.[51-55]

Perhaps the most revealing study on how fluoride enhances remineralization came from the Tiel-Culemborg fluoridation study in the Netherlands.[56] Although

---

Box 14.1. The Principal Means by Which Fluoride Prevents the Formation of Initial Carious Lesions and Inhibits the Progression of Existing Lesions.

After teeth have erupted into the mouth:

1. Promoting remineralization and inhibiting demineralization of early carious lesions.
2. Inhibition of glycolysis, the process by which cariogenic bacteria metabolize fermentable carbohydrates.
3. Direct bactericidal action on cariogenic bacteria.

While teeth are still developing prior to eruption into the mouth:

4. Some reduction in enamel solubility in acid by pre-eruptive incorporation of fluoride into the hydroxyapatite crystal.

considerably fewer deep lesions (i.e., the type that require caries removal and the placement of a filling) occurred among persons living in fluoridated Tiel than in non-fluoridated Culemborg after 15 years of fluoridation, no substantial difference in initial enamel lesions (i.e., those that can repair themselves given a favorable intra-oral environment and do not require professional intervention) was observed between the two populations. The study demonstrated that early enamel lesions are less likely to progress to cavities in populations receiving fluoridated water than in those drinking nonfloridated water.

Fluoride in plaque also inhibits glycolysis, the process by which fermentable carbohydrate is metabolized by cariogenic bacteria to produce acid. Fluoride from drinking water and toothpaste concentrates in plaque, which contains higher levels of fluoride than does saliva.[57,58] However, saliva serves as a fluoride reservoir for plaque. Toothbrushing with a fluoride toothpaste causes the otherwise low salivary fluoride levels to rise 100- to 1,000-fold. This level soon drops back to low resting levels, during which saliva is a primary source of replenishing plaque fluoride.[59]

In addition to these mechanisms, high-concentration fluoride gels and varnishes, applied professionally in the dentist's office, have a bactericidal action on cariogenic bacteria in plaque.[60] These gels also leave a temporary layer of a calcium fluoride-like material on the enamel surface, which is available for release when the pH drops at the enamel surface.[61] At lower concentrations, caries-causing bacteria have been demonstrated to become less acidogenic through adaptation to an environment where fluoride is constantly present.[60,62–64] Whether this ecologic adaptation reduces the cariogenicity of acidogenic bacteria in humans remains unknown.[65]

Public Health Benefits of Water Fluoridation

Studies conducted in the 1970s and 1980s concluded that when water fluoridation ceases, so does the decline in caries experience.[66–68] However, more recent outcomes are not so clear-cut. In both Finland[69] and Germany,[70,71] the cessation of water fluoridation was followed by continued caries decline, or at least by stability in caries levels. Both of these studies were conducted in communities in which residents had widespread fluoride exposure from other sources; drinking water, once the sole source of fluoride, was just one of a number of exposures. Therefore, the effects of fluoridated water in these populations are not clearly identified.[72]

These data raise the question of whether water fluoridation is still needed, now that there are other convenient ways of maintaining ambient fluoride levels in the mouth. The answer is a clear affirmative, in the United States at least, for at least two reasons. First, the United States does not have school-based dental care as most European countries do, so that U.S. school children do not have regular fluoride exposure from these treatment services. In addition, not all children in the United States attend a dentist regularly and so do not receive regular professional fluoride attention. In many western European countries, by contrast, the school-based dental services mean that virtually all children attend a dentist regularly. For many children in the Unites States, especially those who are economically disadvantaged, water fluoridation remains the prime source of exposure to fluoride. Second, water fluoridation has been demonstrated to reduce dental health disparities that exist between socioeconomic groups.[40,73–79] Thus, water fluoridation is consistent with national efforts to reduce inequalities in health.

Multiple Fluoride Exposure

Into the twenty-first century, exposure to multiple fluoride sources has become the rule rather than the exception in the United States. Most persons now drink fluoridated water, brush their teeth with fluoride toothpastes, and receive professional fluoride applications by their dentists. Fluoride also can be obtained from many other sources. For example, fluoride is found in mouth-rinsing agents (including some over-the-counter mouthwashes), prescription dietary supplements for infants and young children, and processed foods and drinks.

This twenty-first-century phenomenon of multiple fluoride exposure is generally desirable, although dental fluorosis has become more prevalent in the United States in recent years,[80] most likely because of multiple and uncoordinated fluoride exposure. The goal of public health and dental professionals is to maximize the benefits from fluoride exposure in a cost-effective manner while avoiding dental fluorosis.

Opposition to Fluoridation

The fluoridation of water has been opposed by some people since it was first introduced in 1945. Although opponents are greatly outnumbered by proponents, they can influence public opinion and impede implementation of public health measures. Opponents to fluoridation question fluoridation's benefits, argue that fluoridation is neither necessary nor sufficient for good dental health, believe that fluoridation infringes upon individual rights, and believe that fluoridation of water presents health risks.[81]

The effectiveness of fluoridation in preventing dental caries was first formally questioned in 1959, when Sutton published criticisms of the methodology of the four original community fluoridation trials.[82,83] Sutton concluded that the methods used in the classic fluoridation trials were flawed and provided an inadequate basis for proceeding with fluoridation. Although the technical details and philosophical underpinning of Sutton's critiques were immediately challenged by dental researchers,[84–87] the effectiveness of fluoridation in preventing caries was again questioned by future opponents,[88,89] whose arguments were subsequently refuted on the basis of questionable data and outdated views of fluoride's anticariogenic mechanism.[90] Because arguments over the nuances of study design and analysis attract only minimal public interest, more recent opposition to fluoridation has focused on other issues,[81] including the claim that fluoride is neither necessary nor sufficient for healthy teeth.[89] Opponents have argued that some people can have good dental health without fluoridation, whereas others have extensive dental caries despite drinking fluoridated water. That logic, however, does not take into account the multifactoral etiology of dental caries and human variability.

Over the past five decades, opponents of water fluoridation have claimed that it increases the risk for many diseases and conditions, including cancer, Down syndrome, heart disease, osteoporosis and bone fracture, AIDS, low intelligence, Alzheimer's disease, and allergic reactions.[91] Recent comprehensive reviews, however, have concluded that no clear evidence supports an association between fluoridation and these adverse health outcomes,[92–95] and most of the American public continues to support fluoridation of their water.[96]

Cost of Fluoridation

The economics of water fluoridation were examined in a recent systematic review.[97] Costs of fluoridation per person varied widely in the seven reviewed studies that included 75 water systems, with much of the variation apparently resulting from economies of scale—that is, cost per person falls as the number of people served by the water system rises. The median cost per person per year ranged from $2.70 among 19 systems each serving ≥5000 people, to $0.40 among 35 systems serving ≥20,000 people. Five studies included sufficient data to calculate a cost-effectiveness ratio (i.e., net cost per tooth surface spared from decay). Community water fluoridation was cost-saving in all studies—that is, it saved more money than it cost. Few public health measures achieve this status. Using recent data on treatment costs, and assuming the highest amortized cost per person of fluoridation and an annual caries incidence rate of 0.06 surfaces/person, water fluoridation would, on average, save more than it cost even in small communities (i.e., 5000 to 20,000 residents).

Conclusion and Challenges for the Twenty-First Century

Water fluoridation is one of the major public health achievements of the twentieth century. The concept of adding fluoride to public water systems came from patient and logically sequenced epidemiology; the use of fluoride in various vehicles is supported by a sound scientific base. Fluoridated water is consumed by most Americans, and fluoride is added to almost all toothpaste products, resulting in the elevation of oral health among Americans to the highest level in history.

Despite the substantial decline in the prevalence and severity of dental caries in the United States during the last century, this largely preventable disease is still common. Based on findings from the 1999–2000 National Health and Nutrition Examination Survey, 59% of U.S. children have experienced dental caries in their permanent teeth by age 15.[98] Further reductions in caries prevalence likely will require approaches that complement water fluoridation, including evidence-based caries risk assessment and management targeted to high-risk communities and persons.

Among the most striking results of water fluoridation is the change in public attitudes and expectations regarding dental health. Tooth loss is no longer considered inevitable, and an increasing proportion of U.S. adults are retaining most of their teeth for a lifetime.[99] The oldest post-World War II baby boomers will reach age

60 years in the first decade of the twenty-first century, and more of that birth cohort will have a relatively intact dentition at that age than any generation in modern history. This trend means that there will be more teeth than ever at risk for caries among persons age 60 years and older. In the next century, water fluoridation will continue to help prevent caries among these older Americans, most of whom have come to expect relatively good dental health. Although the proportion of the U.S. population drinking fluoridated water increased fairly quickly from 1945 into the 1970s, the rate of increase has been much lower in recent years. This slowing in the expansion of fluoridation is attributable to several factors: (1) many of the U.S. public water systems that still are not fluoridated tend to serve small populations, which increases the per capita cost of fluoridating; (2) adoption of water fluoridation often requires political processes that make it difficult to institute this public health measure; and (3) the public, some scientists, and policy makers often perceive that dental caries is no longer a public health problem or that fluoridation is no longer necessary or effective. These barriers present serious challenges to expanding fluoridation in the United States in the twenty-first century. To help overcome these challenges, public health professionals at the national, state, and local levels will need to enhance their promotion of fluoridation and commit the necessary resources for equipment, personnel, training, and health education.

References

1. U.S. Public Health Service, National Center for Health Statistics. Decayed, Missing, and Filled Teeth among Persons 1–74 Years—United States. DHHS publication no. (PHS) 81-1673, Series 11 No 223. Washington, DC: Government Printing Office, 1981.
2. U.S. Public Health Service, National Institute of Dental Research. Oral Health of United States Children. NIH publication no. 89-2247. Washington, DC: Government Printing Office, 1989.
3. Burt BA, Eklund SA. Dentistry, Dental Practice, and the Community, 5th ed. Philadelphia: Saunders, 1999, 216.
4. Black GV, McKay FS. Mottled teeth—an endemic developmental imperfection of the teeth heretofore unknown in the literature of dentistry. *Dent Cosmos* 1916:58:129–56.
5. McKay FS. Mottled enamel: the prevention of its further production through a change of water supply at Oakley, Idaho. *J Am Dent Assoc* 1933:20:1137–49.
6. McKay FS. The relation of mottled enamel to caries. *J Am Dent Assoc* 1928:15:1429–37.
7. Dean HT. Distribution of mottled enamel in the United States. *Public Health Rep* 1933:48:703–34.
8. Dean HT. Classification of mottled enamel diagnosis. *J Am Dent Assoc* 1934:21:1421–26.
9. Dean HT, Elvove E. Studies on the minimal threshold of the dental sign of chronic endemic fluorosis (mottled enamel). *Public Health Rep* 1935:50:1719–29.
10. Dean HT, Dixon RM, Cohen C. Mottled enamel in Texas. *Public Health Rep* 1935:50:424–42.
11. Dean HT, Elvove E. Some epidemiological aspects of chronic endemic dental fluorosis. *Am J Public Health* 1936:26:567–75.
12. Dean HT, Elvove E. Further studies on the minimal threshold of chronic endemic dental fluorosis. *Public Health Rep* 1937:52:1249–64.
13. Dean HT. Chronic endemic dental fluorosis (mottled enamel). *JAMA* 1936:107:1269–72.

14. Dean HT, McKay FS. Production of mottled enamel halted by a change in common water supply. *Am J Public Health* 1939:29:590–96.

15. Dean HT, Elvove E, Poston RF. Mottled enamel in South Dakota. *Public Health Rep* 1939:54:212–28.

16. Dean HT. The investigation of physiological effects by the epidemiological method. In: Moulton FR, ed. Fluorine and Dental Health. Washington, DC: American Association for the Advancement of Science, 1942, 23–31.

17. Dean HT. Endemic fluorosis and its relation to dental caries. *Public Health Rep* 1938:53:1443–52.

18. Dean HT, Jay P, Arnold FA Jr, McClure FJ, Elvove E. Domestic water and dental caries, including certain epidemiological aspects of oral *L. acidophilus*. *Public Health Rep* 1939b:54:862–88.

19. Dean HT, Jay P, Arnold FA Jr., Elvove E. Domestic water and dental caries. II. A study of 2,832 white children aged 12–14 years, of 8 suburban Chicago communities, including *L. acidophilus* studies of 1,761 children. *Public Health Rep* 1941:56:761–92.

20. Dean HT, Arnold FA Jr., Elvove E. Domestic water and dental caries. V. Additional studies of the relation of fluoride domestic waters to dental caries experience in 4,425 white children aged 12–14 years of 13 cities in 4 states. *Public Health Rep* 1942:57:1155–79.

21. Centers for Disease Control and Prevention. Populations receiving optimally fluoridated public drinking water—United States, 2000. *MMWR* 2002:51:144–47. Available at: http://www.cdc.gov/OralHealth/factsheets/fl-stats-us2000.htm. Accessed 15 June, 2006.

22. Dean HT, Arnold FA Jr., Jay P, Knutson JW. Studies on mass control of dental caries through fluoridation of the public water supply. *Public Health Rep* 1950:65:1403–8.

23. Ast DB, Finn SB, McCaffrey I. The Newburgh-Kingston caries-fluorine study. I. Dental findings after three years of water fluoridation. *Am J Public Health* 1950:40:716–24.

24. Blayney JR, Tucker WH. The Evanston dental caries study. *J Dent Res* 1948:27:279–86.

25. Hutton WL, Linscott BW, Williams DB. The Brantford fluorine experiment: interim report after five years of water fluoridation. *Canada J Public Health* 1951:42:81–87.

26. Arnold FA Jr, Likins RC, Russell AL, Scott DB. Fifteenth year of the Grand Rapids fluoridation study. *J Am Dent Assoc* 1962:65:780–85.

27. Ast DB, Fitzgerald B. Effectiveness of water fluoridation. *J Am Dent Assoc* 1962:65: 581–58.

28. Blayney JR, Hill IN. Fluorine and dental caries. *J Am Dent Assoc* 1967:74:233–2.

29. Hutton WL, Linscott BW, Williams DB. Final report of local studies on water fluoridation in Brantford. *Canada J Public Health* 1956:47:89–92.

30. Ast DB, Smith DJ, Wachs B, Cantwell KT. The Newburgh-Kingston caries-fluorine study. XIV. Combined clinical and roentgenographic dental findings after ten years of fluoride experience. *J Am Dent Assoc* 1956:52:314–25.

31. Russell AL. Dental fluorosis in Grand Rapids during the seventeeth year of fluoridation. *J Am Dent Assoc* 1962:65:608–12.

32. Arnold FA Jr, Dean HT, Knutson JW. Effect of fluoridated public water supplies on dental caries incidence. Results of the seventh year of study at Grand Rapids and Muskegon, Mich. *Public Health Rep* 1953:68:141–48.

33. Booth IM, Mitropooulos CM, Worthington HV. A comparison between the dental health of 3-year-old children living in fluoridated Huddersfield and non-fluoridated Dewsbury in 1989. *Community Dental Health* 1992:9:151–57.

34. Evans DJ, Rugg-Gunn AJ, Tabari ED. The effect of 25 years of water fluoridation in Newcastle assessed in four surveys of 5-year-old children over an 18-year period. *Br Dent J* 1995:178:60–4.

35. Thomas FD, Kassab, JY, Jones BM. Fluoridation in Anglesey 1993; a clinical study of dental caries in 5-year-old children who had experienced sub-optimal fluoridation. *Br Dent J* 1995:178:55–59.
36. Cortes DF, Ellwoood RP, O'Mullane DM, Bastos JR. Drinking water fluoride levels, dental fluorosis, and caries experience in Brazil. *J Public Health Dent* 1996:56:226–28.
37. Lawrence HP, Sheiham A. Caries progression in 12- to 16-year-old schoolchildren in fluoridated and fluoride-deficient areas in Brazil. *Community Dent Oral Epidemiol* 1997:25:402–11.
38. Marthaler TM. Water fluoridation and results in Basel since 1962: health and political implications. *J Public Health Dent* 1996:56:265–70.
39. Slade GD, Davies MJ, Spencer AJ, Stewart JF. Associations between exposure to fluoridated drinking water and dental caries experience among children in two Australian states. *J Public Health Dent* 1995:55:218–28.
40. Slade GD, Spencer AJ, Davies MJ, Stewart JF. Caries experience among children in fluoridated Townsville and unfluoridated Brisbane. *Aust NZ J Public Health* 1996:20:623–29.
41. Treasure ET, Dever JG. The prevalence of caries in 5-year-old children living in fluoridated and non-fluoridated communities in New Zealand. *NZ Dent J* 1992:88:9–13.
42. O'Mullane D, Whelton HP, Costelloe P, Clarke D, McDermott S, McLoughlin J. The results of water fluoridation in Ireland. *J Public Health Dent* 1996:56:259–64.
43. Brunelle JA, Carlos JP. Recent trends in dental caries in US children and the effect of water fluoridation. *J Dent Res* 1990:69:723–27.
44. Grembowski D, Fiset L, Milgrom P, Conrad D, Spadafora A. Does fluoridation reduce the use of dental services among adults? *Med Care* 1997:35:454–71.
45. Featherstone JDB. Prevention and reversal of dental caries: role of low level fluoride. *Community Dent Oral Epidemiol* 1999:27:31–40.
46. Levine RS. The action of fluoride in caries prevention; a review of current concepts. *Br Dent J* 1976:40:9–14.
47. Clarkson BH. Caries prevention–fluoride. *Adv Dent Res* 1991:5:41–45.
48. Koulorides T. Summary of session II: Fluoride and the caries process. *J Dent Res* 1990: 69:558.
49. Tatevossian A. Fluoride in dental plaque and its effects. *J Dent Res* 1990:69:645–52.
50. White DJ, Nancollas GH. Physical and chemical considerations of the role of firmly and loosely bound fluoride in caries prevention. *J Dent Res* 1990:69:587–94.
51. Chow LC. Tooth-bound fluoride and dental caries. *J Dent Res* 1990:69:595–600.
52. Ericsson Y. Cariostasis mechanisms of action of fluorides; clinical observations. *Caries Res* 1977:11(suppl 1):2–23.
53. Kidd EA, Thylstrup A, Fejerskov O, Bruun C. Influence of fluoride in surface enamel and degree of dental fluorosis on caries development in vitro. *Caries Res* 1980:14:196–202.
54. Thylstrup A. Clinical evidence of the role of pre-eruptive fluoride in caries prevention. *J Dent Res* 1990:69:742–50.
55. Thylstrup A, Fejerskov O, Bruun C, Kann J. Enamel changes and dental caries in 7-year-old children given fluoride tablets from shortly after birth. *Caries Res* 1979:13:265–76.
56. Groeneveld A. Longitudinal study of the prevalence of enamel lesions in a fluoridated and a non-fluoridated area. *Community Dent Oral Epidemiol* 1985:13:159–63.
57. Hamilton IR. Biochemical effects of fluoride on oral bacteria. *J Dent Res* 1990:69:660–67.
58. Singer L, Ophaug RH, Harland BF. Dietary fluoride intake of 15–19-year-old male adults residing in the United States. *J Dent Res* 1985:64:1302–5.
59. Rölla G, Ekstrand J. Fluoride in oral fluids and dental plaque. In: Fejerskov O, Ekstrand J, Burt BA, eds. Fluoride in Dentistry. Copenhagen: Munksgaard, 1996, 215–29.

60. Bowden GHW. Effects of fluoride on the microbial ecology of dental plaque. *J Dent Res* 1990:69:653–59.
61. LeGeros RZ. Chemical and crystallographic events in the caries process. *J Dent Res* 1990:69:567–74.
62. Bowden GHW, Odlum O, Nolette N, Hamilton IR. Microbial populations growing in the presence of fluoride at low pH isolated from dental plaque of children living in an area with fluoridated water. *Infect Immun* 1982:36:247–54.
63. Marquis RE. Diminished acid tolerance of plaque bacteria caused by fluoride. *J Dent Res* 1990:69:672–75.
64. Rosen S, Frea JI, Hsu SM. Effect of fluoride-resistant microorganisms on dental caries. *J Dent Res* 1978:57:180.
65. Van Loveren C. The antimicrobial action of fluoride and its role in caries inhibition. *J Dent Res* 1990:69:676–81.
66. Künzel W. Effect of an interruption in water fluoridation on the caries prevalence of the primary and secondary dentition. *Caries Res* 1980:14:304–10.
67. Lemke CW, Doherty JM, Arra MC. Controlled fluoridation: the dental effects of discontinuation in Antigo, Wisconsin. *J Am Dent Assoc* 1970:80:782–86.
68. Stephen KW, McCall DR, Tullis JI. Caries prevalence in northern Scotland before, and 5 years after, water defluoridation. *Br Dent J* 1987:163:324–26.
69. Seppä L, Karkkainen S, Hausen H. Caries frequency in permanent teeth before and after discontinuation of water fluoridation in Kuopio, Finland. *Community Dent Oral Epidemiol* 1998:26:256–62.
70. Künzel W, Fischer T. Rise and fall of caries prevalence in German towns with different F concentrations in drinking water. *Caries Res* 1997:31:166–73.
71. Künzel W, Fischer T, Lorenz R, Bruhmann, S. Decline of caries prevalence after the cessation of water fluoridation in East Germany. *Community Dent Oral Epidemiol* 2000:28:382–89.
72. Lewis DW, Banting DW. Water fluoridation: current effectiveness and dental fluorosis. *Community Dent Oral Epidemiol* 1994:22:153–58.
73. Carmichael CL, Rugg-Gunn AJ, Ferrell RS. The relationship between fluoridation, social class and caries experience in 5-year-old children in Newcastle and Northumberland in 1987. *Br Dent J* 1989:167:57–61.
74. Evans DJ, Rugg-Gunn AJ, Tabari ED, Butler T. The effect of fluoridation and social class on caries experience in 5-year-old Newcastle children compared with results over the previous 18 years. *Community Dent Health* 1996:13:5–10.
75. Jones CM, Taylor GO, Whittle JG, Evans D, Trotter DP. Water fluoridation, tooth decay in 5 year olds, and social deprivation measured by the Jarman score: analysis of data from British dental surveys. *Br Med J* 1997:315(7107):514–17.
76. Jones CM, Worthington H. The relationship between water fluoridation and socioeconomic deprivation on tooth decay in 5-year-old children. *Br Dent J* 1999:186:397–400.
77. Provart SJ, Carmichael CL. The relationship between caries, fluoridation and material deprivation in five-year-old children in County Durham. *Community Dent Health* 1995:12:200–3.
78. Riley JC, Lennon MA, Ellwood RP. The effect of water fluoridation and social inequalities on dental caries in 5-year-old children. *Int J Epidemiol* 1999:28:300–5.
79. Treasure ET, Dever JG. Relationship of caries with socioeconomic status in 14-year-old children from communities with different fluoride histories. *Community Dent Oral Epidemiol* 1994:22:226–30.
80. Szpunar SM, Burt BA. Trends in the prevalence of dental fluorosis in the United States: a review. *J Public Health Dent* 1987:47:71–79.

81. Martin B. Scientific Knowledge in Controversy: The Social Dynamics of the Fluoridation Debate. Albany, NY: State University of New York Press, 1991.
82. Sutton PRN. Fluoridation: Errors and Omissions in Experimental Trials. Melbourne: Melbourne University Press, 1959.
83. Sutton PRN. Fluoridation: Errors and Omissions in Experimental Trials, 2nd ed. Melbourne: Melbourne University Press, 1960.
84. Galagan D. Comments on: Sutton PRN. Fluoridation: errors and omissions in experimental trials. *Aust Dent J* 1960:5:44.
85. Grainger RM. Comments on: Sutton PRN. Fluoridation: errors and omissions in experimental trials. *Aust Dent J* 1960:5:45–46.
86. Blayney JR. Comments on: Sutton PRN. Fluoridation: errors and omissions in experimental trials. *Aust Dent J* 1960:5:44–45.
87. Dunning JM. Biased criticisms of fluoridation. *Nutr Rev* 1960:18:161–65.
88. Colquhoun J. New evidence on fluoridation. *Soc Sci Med* 1984:19:1239–46.
89. Diesendorf, M. The mystery of declining tooth decay. *Nature* 1986:322:125–29.
90. Burt BA, Beltran ED. Water fluoridation: a response to critics in Australia and New Zealand. *J Public Health Dent* 1988:48:214–19.
91. Review of Fluoride Benefits and Risks: Report of the Ad Hoc Committee on Fluoride of the Committee to Coordinate Environmental Health and Related Programs. Washington, DC: U.S. Department of Health and Human Services, Public Health Service, 1991.
92. Allukian M, Horowitz AM. Effective community prevention programs for oral diseases. In: Gluck GM, Morganstein WM, eds. Jong's Community Dental Health, 5th Ed. St. Louis, MO: Mosby, 2003, 237–76.
93. National Research Council. Health Effects of Ingested Fluoride. Washington, DC: National Academy Press, 1993.
94. Locker D, Lawrence H, Jokovic A. Benefits and Risks of Water Fluoridation: An Update of the 1996 Federal-Provincial Sub-committee Report. Toronto: Ontario Ministry of Health, Public Health Branch and Health Canada, First Nations and Inuit Health Branch, 1999.
95. McDonagh MS, Whiting PF, Wilson PM, Sutton AJ, Chestnutt I, Cooper J, Misso K, Bradley M, Treasure E, Kleijnen J. Systematic review of water fluoridation. *Br Med J* 2000:321:855–59.
96. American Dental Association Survey Center. 1998 Consumers' Opinions Regarding Community Water Fluoridation. Chicago: American Dental Association, 1998.
97. Truman BI, Gooch BF, Sulemana I, Gift HC, Horowitz AM, Evans CA Jr, Griffin SO, Carande-Kulis VG. The Task Force on Community Preventive Services. Reviews of evidence on interventions to prevent dental caries, oral and pharyngeal cancers, and sports-related craniofacial injuries. *Am J Prev Med* 2002:23(1S):21–54.
98. U.S. Department of Health and Human Services. Healthy People 2010 progress review: oral health. Available at: http://www.healthypeople.gov/data/2010prog/focus21/. Accessed 26 January 2005.
99. Centers for Disease Control and Prevention. Public health and aging: retention of natural teeth among older adults—United States, 2002. *MMWR* 2003:52:1226–29.

Suggested Reading

Martin B. Scientific Knowledge in Controversy: The Social Dynamics of the Fluoridation Debate. Albany, NY: State University of New York Press, 1991.
Review of Fluoride Benefits and Risks: Report of the Ad Hoc Committee on Fluoride of the Committee to Coordinate Environmental Health and Related Programs. Washington, DC: U.S. Department of Health and Human Services, Public Health Service, 1991.

15

The Task Is a Political One: The Promotion of Fluoridation

GRETCHEN ANN REILLY

"I'd like to add a word to the topic which was assigned me," Al Schottelkotte told the audience at a public health conference in 1955. "On your program it reads: 'How a Community Loses—Case History of Cincinnati.' I'd like to amend that to read: 'How a Community Loses, *Temporarily*—Case History of Cincinnati.' "[1] Schottelkotte went on to explain why the Cincinnati fluoridation campaign, which he had chaired, had failed to convince Cincinnati voters to support fluoridation in 1953. In the November elections that year, Cincinnati citizens had voted 76,612 to 55,904 against fluoridating the city's water supply. He noted that pro-fluoridationists had not expected the vocal opposition that arose or the general apathy and ignorance of voters, but he was upbeat about the chances of fluoridation being approved in the future. He ended his presentation optimistically: "We haven't quit yet. . . . Someday I'd like to come back and give you a case history of how a city came back and approved this fine dental health program when it got a second chance."[1]

Al Schottelkotte never got the chance. Six years later, Sidney Weil, chairman of the 1960 Cincinnati fluoridation campaign, stood before another audience at a dental health conference and explained why Cincinnati voters had rejected fluoridation once again. The repeated failure of the pro-fluoridationists in Cincinnati was not unusual. Throughout the United States, in the 50 years that fluoridation has been promoted, pro-fluoridationists in many cities have found their efforts to enact the measure thwarted by a vocal opposition able to convince local elected officials and voters to reject fluoridation.

It was not simply that the opposition to fluoridation questioned the scientific evidence in support of fluoridation; anti-fluoridation arguments proved difficult to counter because they went beyond the realm of scientific debate to include sweeping philosophical and social concerns. Likewise, the anti-fluoridation movement was a coalition of various groups and individuals. Both anti-fluoridationists and pro-fluoridationists used the term *anti-fluoridationist* but anti-fluoridationists (often referred to in this chapter as "antis") varied widely in their objections and perspectives on fluoridation.

Initially pro-fluoridationists (in this chapter, often referred to as "pros") focused on running a standard public health campaign. In the face of continuing failures, pro-fluoridationists' perspective on their campaigns and their tactics evolved over time. Their efforts to promote fluoridation and the opposition they faced serve as a cautionary tale to scientists and public health professionals about the power of politics over science. The lessons pro-fluoridationists learned could easily be applied to other examples of the clash between accepted scientific beliefs and public opinion, such as the controversies surrounding irradiated and genetically modified foods, and the alleged connection between vaccination and autism.

The Initial Promotion of Fluoridation

Even as various organizations initiated independent field trials of fluoridation in the 1940s, a small group of Wisconsin dentists, such as Dr. John G. Frisch of Madison, Wisconsin, were already agitating for the fluoridation of all public water supplies in Wisconsin. They believed that further study of fluoridation was unnecessary because studies in the 1930s had proved that naturally fluoridated water safely and effectively prevented dental decay. These dentists identified themselves with earlier Wisconsin Progressives such as Robert M. LaFollette, Sr., who had put Wisconsin on the leading edge of social legislation. They believed Wisconsin could take the lead in adopting fluoridation because the state's Progressive tradition, especially regarding public health measures such as tuberculosis control and pure food laws, made the citizens of Wisconsin more receptive to a strong state role in promoting public health. Rather than wait for the results of the field trials, these dentists began promoting fluoridation across the state at the meetings of dental societies, city councils, and civic organizations.[2]

They discovered that their efforts to promote fluoridation were hindered by the reticence of national organizations like the U.S. Public Health Service (USPHS) and the American Dental Association (ADA), both of which argued that they could not recommend fluoridation for the general public until field trials were completed. Fluoridation's opponents in Wisconsin pointed to the USPHS and ADA's position to support their argument that it was too soon to begin fluoridating public water supplies. In response, throughout the 1940s, the Wisconsin dentists lobbied the USPHS and the ADA aggressively to change their stance. By 1949, when preliminary reports from the field trials in Grand Rapids, Michigan, showed a significant reduction in dental decay among children drinking fluoridated water, the USPHS re-evaluated its position. In 1950, it endorsed fluoridation for the general public, and within months, the ADA followed suit.[2]

The Wisconsin pro-fluoridationists believed then that the way was clear for widespread fluoridation; they never expected resistance to the measure from outside the public health profession. But in 1950, in Stevens Point, Wisconsin, their efforts to initiate fluoridation through a vote by the city council were thwarted by three local citizens, who mustered enough signatures to demand a local referendum on the issue. Through the public opinion section of the local newspaper, the Stevens Point opposition stressed that fluoride was a poison that made the water taste bad and cited scientists and dentists who questioned the safety and effectiveness of fluoridation. For the first time, the pro-fluoridationists encountered aggressive opposition that used name-calling and theatrics to highlight their arguments. After a tumultuous referendum campaign, voters in Stevens Point resoundingly rejected fluoridation. Encouraged by this success, the Stevens Point anti-fluoridationists mailed letters opposing fluoridation to mayors, aldermen, newspapers, and prominent citizens throughout Wisconsin.[2]

With the endorsement of the measure by national organizations, public health reformers and dentists nationwide began pushing for fluoridation in their communities, and individuals in those communities began to contact the Stevens Point anti-fluoridationists for assistance and advice on how to oppose fluoridation. From these early contacts sprang a network of opponents to fluoridation, sharing information, opposition materials and tactics, turning fluoridation from a public health issue into a political issue.[2]

Before 1951, fluoridation had been adopted only in Wisconsin and isolated communities in New York, Michigan, and Texas, but between 1951 and 1952, communities throughout the Midwest began to consider fluoridation. From 1953 to 1955, awareness of fluoridation spread, leading to adoptions in the South, East, and in areas of the Midwest that had not previously considered fluoridation.[3,4]

Yet 1953 proved to be the peak year for the adoption of fluoridation; with 378 communities nationwide adopting the measure. After 1953, communities continued to initiate fluoridation, but with decreased frequency. More troubling to pro-fluoridationists, referenda on fluoridation became more frequent. In 1952 only one in seven cities considering the measure held a referendum on fluoridation; by 1954 one out of every three cities put the measure to a public vote.[4,5] Pro-fluoridationists discovered that fluoridation was more likely to be accepted when the decision fell to an administrative body, such as a public water board or city council. When voters were given an opportunity to decide the issue, more often than not, the fluoridation proposal would be defeated. Of those cities that voted on fluoridation, at least 60% rejected it.[4,5]

After 1955, the rate of adoption continued to drop steadily. Fluoridation spread primarily in areas with communities that had already adopted it, which served as positive examples for neighboring communities; few new adoptions occurred in areas that did not already have fluoridated communities. In part, this was because opposition had solidified, and negative publicity about fluoridation had increased. At the same time, those communities most accepting of new health innovations had already initiated fluoridation. By 1960, 1850 communities had fluoridation programs, including two thirds of the major cities in the United States. Yet only 17% of smaller cities and towns had adopted fluoridation; consequently, only about one fourth of Americans were drinking fluoridated water in 1960.[6,7]

Because regulating public water supplies was generally a local issue, anti-fluoridation organizations were primarily small local groups; but because a national network formed to support these groups, anti-fluoridation campaigns were strikingly consistent. National organizations sold self-published books, flyers, and brochures in bulk quantities to local anti-fluoridation groups. Nationally prominent antis offered their services as lecturers or debaters for a modest fee, and gave advice and support to local organizations. The movement even supported a national periodical, *The National Fluoridation News*, which was published from 1955 until 1988.

A Coalition of Opponents

The opponents of fluoridation were never a unified group; rather, they were a shifting alliance of organizations and individuals who objected to fluoridation for a wide range of reasons. The movement included research scientists, medical and dental professionals, alternative health practitioners, health food enthusiasts, Christian Scientists, conservatives, and occasionally environmentalists and consumer groups. Each of these groups had distinct objections to fluoridation.

Antis from the medical and dental professions, including research scientists and alternative health practitioners such as chiropractors and homeopathic doctors, usually objected to fluoridation for medical and scientific reasons, most of these springing from the idea that fluoride was a dangerous poison. Medical opponents argued that fluoridation caused cancer, heart disease, and kidney damage, among other ailments. Scientists often charged that not enough testing had been done, based on the fact that USPHS had endorsed fluoridation before the studies in Newburgh, Sheboygan, and Grand Rapids had been completed. Other medical professionals insisted that enough testing had been done, but that those tests had confirmed that fluoride was one of the most dangerous substances on earth. They also argued that fluoridation was ineffective or dangerous because the dosage delivered through the water supply could not be controlled. Some insisted that there were safer ways of administering fluoride to children, either through fluoride tablets, fluoridated bottled water or milk, or drops. Still others claimed tests had shown that fluoridation was ineffective because it only delayed dental decay.[8-11]

The core medical objections to fluoridation were very consistent over time: antis invariably claimed fluoridation caused a range of diseases and ailments, and severe allergic reactions, such as rashes and intestinal problems. Beyond these perennial concerns though, antis' medical objections often responded to public opinion and new scientific discoveries. Specific new accusations often appeared when a disease or ailment grasped the public's attention, then faded away as either interest in that disease diminished or as medical research disproved any link to fluoride. Examples of this include sudden infant death syndrome (SIDS) and acquired immune deficiency syndrome (AIDS).

In the case of SIDS, prior to 1969, antis never suggested that fluoride caused crib death, a term generally used to describe the condition before it became known as SIDS. After 1969, however, when SIDS was named and recognized as a disease, reference to SIDS began to appear in anti-fluoridation literature. Typical of these references was an article in the *National Fluoridation News* in 1971, which theorized that excessive concentrations of fluoride in baby formula, both from the manufacturing process and the use of fluoridated water, might be a cause of SIDS.[12,13]

Antis expressed concern about SIDS for only a relatively short time in the 1970s, for a number of reasons. SIDS research by the late 1970s had determined that the mechanism of death in SIDS cases was most likely an obstruction in the infant's airway, ruling out allergic reactions and poison—the antis' explanation—as the primary cause of death. Moreover, by the 1980s, baby formula manufacturers had begun removing fluoride from their formulas, eliminating the conjectured connection between SIDS deaths and excess fluoride consumption.[14]

In the case of AIDS, after its discovery in the early 1980s, a few antis began to associate fluoride with the disease, although they never went so far as to say fluoride directly caused AIDS.[15] They usually suggested that fluoride might be an underlying cause of AIDS by damaging the immune system, leaving the body vulnerable to a virus that had always existed but before had been easily destroyed by the body. Antis supported this argument with statistical data showing that New York City, San Francisco, and Miami—the three major American cities with the highest number of AIDS cases—were all fluoridated cities, while the three major American cities with lower rates—Newark, New Jersey, Houston, and Los Angeles—were not fluoridated. Although not a common argument against fluoridation, the accusation that fluoride was linked to AIDS never faded away, as SIDS claims did, because vocal minorities, both inside and outside the scientific community, have sustained the controversy about the cause of HIV, preventing fluoridation's role from being ruled out decisively. Arguments linking fluoride and AIDS appeared not only in anti-fluoridation literature, but also in books focused solely on AIDS. One such book, *AIDS: Hope, Hoax and Hoopla*, explored a range of alternative theories regarding AIDS and gave as much credence to the fluoride theory as to suggestions that AIDS was a result of germ warfare or a new strain of syphilis.[16]

The antis' argument could incorporate the mainstream theory of AIDS as well. Speculated one anti: "Fluoride had already been proven to be a suppressor of . . . [the immune system]. Does the AIDS virus cause the immune system to be destroyed or does an immune system already destroyed by other causes render the body incapable of resisting the AIDS virus?"[17] The AIDS link has remained a part of the anti-fluoridation movement up to the present; most recently anti-fluoridationists have been expressing concern that AIDS patients and HIV-positive persons are more susceptible to fluoride poisoning.[18–20]

Other arguments against fluoridation also shifted to reflect new concerns in American society. Environmental arguments had always been part of the anti-fluoridationists' objections: in the 1950s antis had cited the dangers of excessive fluoride in the environment as a reason not to fluoridate water supplies. Beginning in the 1960s, though, the environmental arguments became more specific, more detailed, and more common, and anti-fluoridationists with environmental credentials joined the movement and related fluoridation to the broader environmental movement. As American society became more sensitive to environmental issues, antis increasingly depicted fluoride as a pollutant: both as an industrial waste emitted by factories and as an additive in water supplies that as run-off and effluent contaminated rivers and oceans.[21–24]

Gladys Caldwell was an example of an anti-fluoridationist attracted to the movement because of environmental concerns. Her book, *Fluoridation and Truth Decay*, published in 1974, was a landmark anti-fluoridation book, in that it was the first book to deal extensively with fluoride as a pollutant.[21] Unlike previous writers, Caldwell was critical not just of fluoride in drinking water or in the environment as a pollutant but also of its presence in consumer goods such as aerosol sprays, gasoline, produce, and meats. She called for strict government limits on the amount of fluoride in drinking water and in the general environment. While earlier authors had used stories of industrial fluoride pollution to illustrate the dangers of water fluoridation, Caldwell used stories about smog-damaged citrus groves and pine forests in California to argue that industrial discharge of fluoride, not just water fluoridation, must stop.[21]

Consumer advocates also joined the anti-fluoridation movement in the late 1960s and 1970s, claiming that fluoridation was a fraud and a misuse of tax funds.[25] These antis argued that fluoridation constituted fraud because people were being convinced to spend tax money or pay higher water rates for the privilege of receiving an ineffective and highly toxic chemical in their drinking water. They were especially critical of the use of federal funds to promote fluoridation. The most notable consumer supporter of the anti-fluoridationist cause was consumer advocate Ralph Nader. Although he did not actively fight against fluoridation, throughout the 1970s he provided ammunition for antis by questioning publicly the cost-effectiveness of fluoridation, expressing concern about the environmental impact of fluoridation, and criticizing the hostility of pro-fluoridationists toward anyone who questioned the measure.[25]

Those who opposed fluoridation for religious reasons, mostly Christian Scientists, were a very small part of the movement. The religious argument against fluoridation was based on the premise that fluoridation was a medication. According to these antis, since their religion forbade the use of medication, drinking fluoridated water would be a sin. Moreover, they claimed, it was unconstitutional for governments to enact fluoridation, with or without the consent of voters, because it violated these religious groups' First and Fourteenth Amendment rights to practice their religion.[2,26]

Federal and state courts nationwide, however, repeatedly rejected these arguments. The Missouri State Supreme court in 1961 noted that the local water supply naturally contained .5 ppm fluoride, yet Christian Scientists had not objected to drinking it.[27] An Oregon court ruled in 1955 that even if fluoridation violated Christian Scientist beliefs, the First Amendment did not bar fluoridation. In its ruling, the Court distinguished between the freedom to believe, which was protected, and the freedom to practice those beliefs, which could be limited by the public interest, and ruled that fluoridation was in the public interest.[27]

The Christian Science Church spoke out officially against fluoridation in the 1950s, but did not play an important role in opposing fluoridation. Although Christian Scientists in general were not a large or vocal segment of the anti-fluoridation movement, their argument, usually presented in terms of America's tradition of religious tolerance, was often repeated by non-Christian Scientists. Anti-fluoridationist William Cox, in his book *Hello, Test Animals . . . Chinchillas or You and Your Grandchildren?* explained their position: "There are people that do not believe in medication. That is their religion. Whether they're right or not, I don't know. But I do know that it's up to us to protect their right to believe the way they want to believe. . . ."[28] In 1980, the argument that fluoridation violated the rights of Christian Scientists was eliminated when an official letter from the Christian Science Church to an Illinois court affirmed "that the Church recognizes the greater public interest fluoridation serves, and does not take a stand that would deprive others of health care that they feel desirable and necessary."[29]

Nonreligious philosophical arguments against fluoridation were primarily put forth by political conservatives. Conservatives insisted that fluoridation was an infringement of individual liberties. Whenever fluoridation was enacted, either through government decree or voter referendum, individuals in the community who objected to fluoridation were forced to drink fluoridated water. Fluoridation violated an individual's right to choose what to put into his body.[30–32]

Anti-fluoridationists' views regarding tooth decay and the role of government in ensuring public health and safety were crucial to this argument. Antis insisted that fluoridation was not like other mandatory public health measures, such as chlorination, to which pro-fluoridationists regularly compared it. Chlorination was meant to kill germs in the water, not affect or alter the body of the individual consuming the water, as fluoridation did. Chlorination was meant to prevent communicable and often lethal diseases, prevention of which was a legitimate responsibility for governments, but fluoridation was treating a noncommunicable disease that was not life-threatening, and thus not a legitimate concern for governments.[33]

Conservative antis warned that fluoridation was only the first step in a growing expansion of government control over an individual's life, part of a trend in America toward socialism or totalitarianism. Fluoridation was a form of socialized medicine because the government, rather than a doctor, was prescribing medication. It was a dangerous expansion of government authority, wrote one anti: "I say that fluoridation of city water is a subtle way to promote socialized dentistry. . . . If the government is given further responsibility in prescribing for public health, that responsibility can lead to only one thing—yes, to socialized medicine."[34] Others defined it as socialized medicine because tax revenues were paying for that medication and the machinery to administer it.[35] Antis in the 1950s and 1960s used the term "socialized medicine;" by the 1970s and 1980s they were using the term "compulsory mass medication," but the underlying fears were the same.[33]

Conservatives also labeled fluoridation "totalitarian" because the government was forcing individuals to ingest a medication, regardless of whether the individual wanted or needed it. Worse, antis warned, fluoridation was only the first step in extending government control over individual health; once the precedent was set for using public drinking water to medicate the population, the government would argue for the addition of birth control medication, or sedatives or an "anti-hostility" drug.[36,37] For these antis, fluoridation's safety or effectiveness was irrelevant; what mattered was that its usage was a threat to personal liberties.

A small portion of conservatives in the 1950s believed that fluoridation was literally a Communist plot to destroy America.[38–41] Unlike other conservatives, who believed that fluoridation would lead to communism through the gradual erosion of American values, or who related fluoridation to totalitarianism philosophically, these conservatives warned that fluoridation was an actual weapon in a communist conspiracy backed by the Soviet Union. They completely rejected the pro-fluoridationists' version of fluoridation history, and insisted that its origins were sinister. Some of these antis claimed that Soviet scientists during World War II had used fluoridation to control political prisoners or had added fluoride to Poland's drinking water to help pacify the population during the Soviet invasion of 1939. Others claimed that the National Socialists (Nazis) in Germany had used fluoridation in conquered territories to cause sterility in the local population, or in concentration camps to kill their victims or reduce them to mindless slaves. The Soviets had gained knowledge about fluoride through meetings with the German General Staff during the brief period between the Nazi-Soviet Nonaggression Pact of 1939 and the German invasion of the Soviet Union in June 1941. Another version of this story claimed that the Soviets learned the secret of fluoride when they invaded eastern Germany in the final days of the war.[38–41]

The Communist-conspiracy antis did not all agree on the origins of fluoridation or the specifics of the communists' plot. Some believed the threat was posed by saboteurs who would use the fluoridation machinery at water treatment plants to deliver a lethal dose of fluoride to the unsuspecting public.[42] Others believed fluoride would poison its victims slowly, causing mental weakness, cancer, or sterility, and when the United States no longer had enough healthy young men to defend itself, the Soviet Union would invade.[43]

Other antis did not necessarily believe fluoridation was a communist plot, but reflecting the inclusive nature of the movement, they occasionally mentioned the communist conspiracy theory in the 1950s. For example, the Lee Foundation for Nutritional Research offered for sale reprinted material outlining the communist conspiracy theory, even though those materials did not correspond with the organization's stated mission of disseminating facts relating to nutrition.[44] Sometimes, in mentioning the communist connection, other antis suggested that fluoridation would be a convenient weapon for the communists, even if it was not necessarily promoted expressly by the communists for that purpose.[45,84]

Communist-conspiracy antis were a product of their times: their arguments were only important in the anti-fluoridation movement in the 1950s during the McCarthy era. By the 1960s, these antis had faded from the movement, and national anti-fluoridation leaders were advising their audience not to claim fluoridation was a communist plot. "In the first place," cautioned Frederick B. Exner in 1963, "it is not . . . and if you say it is, you are successfully ridiculed by the promoters. It is being done, effectively, every day. . . . Some of the people on our side are the fluoridators' 'fifth column.' "[46] Although Exner rejected the communist-conspiracy argument, he did not suggest that believers in the theory should be expelled from the movement, and he refrained from attacking them, except to point out that they were hurting the movement. Mainstream anti-fluoridationists seldom argued publicly that those believing in the communist conspiracy should be excluded from the movement, nor did they belittle them as crackpots as pro-fluoridationists did.[1,46,47]

The broader anti-fluoridation movement may have been tolerant of communist-conspiracy antis partly because many mainstream antis also believed there was a conspiracy behind the promotion of fluoridation, although they identified different groups as being responsible. Possible conspirators included the aluminum industry, the sugar industry, big business in general, or the federal government. Antis, in particular some environmental antis, claimed the aluminum industry needed an easy way to dispose of fluoride, a waste product of aluminum production, and were promoting fluoridation either to create an artificial demand for what was otherwise a difficult chemical to dispose of, or to lessen the pressure on them to stop releasing fluorides from their factories into the environment. Others claimed that the sugar industry hoped that widespread fluoridation would prevent tooth decay without requiring people to cut back on their consumption of refined sugar. Some antis cast their nets wider: corporate America in general was behind fluoridation because fluoride was a waste product of numerous industries, from fertilizer production to brick making. Others argued that the federal government was promoting fluoridation as a way of expanding its power. Typical of the coalition nature of the movement, antis varied widely on their views regarding the conspiracy behind the promotion of fluoridation, yet were still able to work together.[33,48–51]

The Pro-fluoridationists' Response

Pro-fluoridationists were surprised by the strength and success of the anti-fluoridation movement in the 1950s, and struggled both to explain and combat anti-fluoridationists' victories. "It is shocking, but true," noted a pro-fluoridationist in 1957, "that many people, even after they listen to professional advice—carefully, competently and intelligently given—blithely ignore it in favor of what they have been told and frightened into by someone with no professional background whatsoever."[52] Pro-fluoridationists in the 1950s identified the controversy as a conflict between science and the irrational. One pro-fluoridation commentator described his side as "the front lines, defending scientific thought against hysteria, confusion and unreason" and their opponents as "those who are basically enemies of all scientific progress."[52] The general consensus was that fluoridation would soon triumph. Pro-fluoridationists took comfort in likening the opposition to the opponents of pasteurization, chlorination, and vaccination, who eventually had become insignificant.[53]

Pro-fluoridationists in the 1950s clearly expressed an aversion to politics when promoting fluoridation. Pro-fluoridationist Charles Metzner's opinion, expressed in his 1957 article "Referenda For Fluoridation," was typical of the attitude at the time. He noted that "a referendum changes the situation from educational to political," a problem because "members of the profession are at a disadvantage in politics. . . . Many of us do not speak easily in and to the public, cheap appeals do not come quickly to mind, we are not good at mudslinging, and do not know how to organize a door-bell campaign."[54] Schottelkotte, the chairman of the unsuccessful 1953 Cincinnati fluoridation campaign, bluntly noted "the failure of the physicians and dentists, for the most part, to realize that they were in a political slugging match in the referendum . . . not a scientific discussion. For instance, a suggestion that they get volunteers to the polls on Election Day with suitable handbills was not even given serious consideration. But the opponents were there with their rat poison stuff."[1]

Prominent pro-fluoridationist historian Donald McNeil was the exception to this. In his 1957 book *The Fight for Fluoridation*, he insisted that fluoridation was a political issue, not simply a scientific question; more provocatively he argued that pro-fluoridationists were responsible for turning it into a political issue. In writing about one of the first major fluoridation referendum fights, McNeil stated that pro-fluoridationists "believed the public officials should accept the advice of the scientific experts. . . . Yet in asking public officials to adopt the measure, the advocates were engaging in political methods. Opponents merely carried the campaign one step further by appealing to the source of the officials' power—the people."[2]

Articles in professional journals on how to promote fluoridation expressed faith in the eventual acceptance of fluoridation; their primary suggestion was educating the public.[53,56] One writer confidently stated that "if public education has been well done, one need not fear a referendum."[54] Any rejection of fluoridation by voters, or reversal of the decision to fluoridate, was explained as evidence that the education process had not been thorough enough.[54] Beyond this though, articles in the 1950s were short on practical advice. Pro-fluoridationist commentators vaguely called for education of the public: "This means more than a repetition of the facts when we are asked to present them. It means we must take the initiative and present the facts about fluoridation as part of our daily health education activities."[53] These authors advised pro-fluoridationists to involve local leaders and others interested in health or the water supply and to create a public committee to spearhead the education campaign.[54]

Pro-fluoridationist writers in the 1950s were also ambivalent about the role dentists should play in fluoridation campaigns. One author listed a dentist's responsibilities as promoting fluoridation, supplying factual information about fluoridation, determining the need for fluoridation in a community, and evaluating the results of fluoridation.[55] His definition of promotion was extremely narrow: practicing dentists should see that their local and state dental societies unequivocally endorsed fluoridation and encourage their state boards of health to adopt a pro-fluoridation policy. Public health dentists were expected to "help develop close, cooperative teamwork in the health department, particularly between the dental and engineering staffs" and to notify "state and local medical and dental societies on the current status of fluoridation."[55] One writer suggested that "leadership should be in the hands of broad public figures whose position is pertinent to the issues."[54] He recommended asking a prominent physician, a well-known engineer, even industrialists or union leaders to lead the local campaign, but made no mention of asking anyone in the dental community to lead. This same author suggested that the defeat of fluoridation was caused in part by the position of dentists in society: "that position appears too high for many people, the very great many in the lower strata, so that they do not conveniently meet and listen to dentists, but not so high that his [the dentist's] transmitted word is accepted without question."[54] In a sense, the limited role for dentists fit with the idea that a fluoridation campaign should focus on education. If the only reason fluoridation was defeated was a lack of education, then to achieve fluoridation, all dentists had to do was educate the public so that citizens would demand fluoridation. Dentists need not take a strong leadership role in pushing for fluoridation.

As resistance to fluoridation continued though, pro-fluoridationists found these attitudes and ideas did not fit their real life experiences or adequately explain their continued failures. By the 1960s, most pro-fluoridation writers had come to agree with McNeil that fluoridation was a political fight, and to insist that pro-fluoridationists needed to run a political campaign. Pro-fluoridationist sociologist William Gamson asserted that education should be secondary, that "the task—is a political one—that of winning a referendum. The traditional arsenal of political techniques is appropriate and proponents, if they expect to win, should frankly accept that they are propagandizing, not simply educating."[54] McNeil, in an article entitled, "Political Aspects of Fluoridation" published in the *Journal of the American Dental Association*, insisted that pro-fluoridationists "must meet the anti-fluoridationists on their own ground—on the political hustings, using political methods, and striving for a political victory."[58]

As writers began to acknowledge that fluoridation was a political issue, they began to offer practical suggestions on how to fight politically. Their recommendations included contacting public officials through their dentists before the opposition had been aroused, door-to-door canvassing, placing placards reading "We Support Fluoridation" in private dental and medical offices, and sending flyers to parents of school-aged children. Writers suggested that pros should make arrangements to call people on Election Day to remind them to vote, drive people to the polls, and even to offer baby-sitting services to potential pro-fluoridation voters. Pros were advised to give their organizations a positive sounding name, such as "Citizens' Committee for Fluoridation" or "Committee for Our Children's Teeth."[7,58–62]

Education was still an important component of these newer campaigns: always pros stressed informing the electorate, not simply getting them to blindly support fluoridation. Leonard Menczer, dentist and director of the Hartford, Connecticut, Bureau of Dental Health, noted that Hartford's fluoridation campaign included fluoridation fact books distributed by the health department, a reference guide for public school teachers, efforts to keep public libraries stocked with pro-fluoridation materials, and the mailing of materials on fluoridation to all newly elected public officials. However, the stress on education did differ from the 1950s' emphasis in one significant way. Repeatedly the authors of these articles, many writing about their own experiences, spoke of the need for long-term education programs that continued even after a community adopted fluoridation. Writers presented evidence that an extensive education campaign did not necessarily lead to widespread public acceptance of fluoridation. Menczer acknowledged that even after a 9-year education program in his community, antis were still able to collect enough signatures on petitions to demand another referendum.[6,61–63] "Actually, the battle is never won," Menczer wrote, "and our fight continues against that small vocal group of misguided persons, 'the emotional descendants of those who saw catastrophe in smallpox vaccination, chlorination of water supplies, pasteurization of milk, and other sensible public health measures.' "[62]

The earlier uncertainty over the dentists' role fell by the wayside. In article after article, authors stressed the role of dentists in the campaign. Weil, chairman of the unsuccessful 1960 Cincinnati campaign, cited the lack of support from the medical and dental profession as one reason the campaign failed.[64] Menczer put it bluntly: "we ought not to wait for others to undertake programs—that we, as dentists, are well equipped to initiate and carry on, . . . We ought to exert the leadership in our communities that is expected of us by our confreres of the health professions and by the public we serve."[62] Pro-fluoridationists encouraged dentists to contribute to the campaigns not only by informing patients that they supported fluoridation and serving in speakers' bureaus but also by including pro-fluoridation notices in the bills they mailed patients and keeping pro-fluoridation materials in their waiting rooms.[58,61–63] As one writer noted: "It is only fair that the dentists of the community do their share."[59]

Pro-fluoridation authors in the 1960s wrote about their own personal experiences, rather than just abstractly talking about promoting fluoridation. Menczer understood the importance of articles about real experiences when he wrote in 1962: "All through our efforts . . . we borrowed from the experiences of other communities and developed a few original actions of our own. This then justifies the time and effort that goes into writing up experiences and, equally important, reading the written work and extracting therefrom that which is most suitable to one's own local use."[62] Pro-fluoridationists, such as Weil, the chairman of Cincinnati's 1960 campaign, even wrote about their failures, and honestly critiqued their efforts. These articles, which served as a way of pooling and exchanging information on how best to promote fluoridation, would become increasingly important when pro-fluoridationists in the 1970s and 1980s drew heavily on past experiences to shape their campaigns.[7,61–65] Public health dental professor David Rosenstein noted in a 1978 pro-fluoridationist article that "the insight that these reports provide into the operations of past fluoridation campaigns is useful to fluoridationists planning future campaign strategies."[66]

Pro-fluoridation Successes

Pro-fluoridationists' efforts at the community level led to a surge in communities adopting fluoridation between 1965 and 1970. New York City initiated fluoridation, and several states passed laws mandating fluoridation. In opinion polls, approval of fluoridation did grow, from 65% in 1959 to 77% in 1968, but fluoridation still lost more referenda than it won, and was even defeated in communities where only a few years earlier it had won. In reality, opinion polls were meaningless; after a community went through an emotionally charged fluoridation campaign, people who had approved of fluoridation in the abstract were no longer certain that they wanted it in their own communities.[67]

In the 1970s and 1980s, pro-fluoridation literature increased in political sophistication: instead of general recommendations that organizers form committees, authors now presented detailed descriptions of committee structure, with numerous subcommittees having specific tasks and goals. They recommended steering volunteers to subcommittees where their talents would be most useful, or seeking outside help, such as asking lawyers to volunteer for the legal subcommittee. Elected officials and newspaper editors were to be kept in line through pressure from fluoridation supporters in the community. Not only should dentists and doctors insert pro-fluoridation information into their mail to patients, pro-fluoridationists were also instructed to persuade insurance companies, political parties, unions, and hospitals to include pro-fluoridation materials in their regular mailings. The speakers' bureau became an important tool for both educating and seeking volunteers: many pro-fluoridation writers recommended it become a permanent organization, offering presentations on proper dental care, during which fluoridation would be discussed. Pro-fluoridation writers also stressed the importance of a positively worded, clearly phrased ballot, which avoided value-laden words like *mandatory*—one in which the voter chose *yes* for fluoridation—and timing the ballot for a general election or presidential election, when voter turnout would be greatest. Other advice built on earlier recommendations. Not only should a pro-fluoridation committee have a positive name, the name should not include words like *Ad Hoc* or *Temporary*, which might give voters the wrong impression.[67]

Suggestions for dealing with newspapers and television stations became more numerous and specific. No longer were pros told simply to have good relations with newspapers and television stations. Instead they were given specific advice on how to manage the media coverage of the campaign. For example, during public hearings, a pro-fluoridationist was to watch over each media representative, to prevent anti-fluoridationists from giving them false information. Pro-fluoridationists were instructed to plan events or issue press releases on "slow" news days in order to get the best coverage.[68–73]

Some of the advice could be labeled preemptive—actions that pro-fluoridationists could take before their public campaign began. Pro-fluoridationists were advised to approach the local elected officials, nonelected administrators, newspaper editors, television and radio station managers, and various community leaders before any opposition materialized and educate them about fluoridation. If possible, their direct support was to be enlisted, but if not, pro-fluoridationists were to warn these individuals about the anti-fluoridationists' tactics. Pros were instructed to encourage the science or health reporter of the local newspaper to write a favorable article about fluoridation before it became locally controversial, so that the opposition would be less likely to demand an article that presented their views.[69–73]

During the 1970s and 1980s, pro-fluoridationists adopted on a limited basis two alternatives to campaigns for community fluoridation: regional campaigns to promote fluoridation and the promotion of school-based fluoridation programs. These alternatives arose from the growing awareness among pros that some communities and areas had special hurdles to overcome before fluoridation could be implemented. In large urban areas, such as Boston, and in areas where many communities formed one municipal water district, such as the San Francisco Bay area of California, concerted lobbying efforts before regional water utility boards or area-wide political campaigns were needed to initiate fluoridation. In other cases, regional or state-wide fluoridation campaigns were needed to counteract renewed efforts by anti-fluoridationists to stop fluoridation through state laws barring it or state-wide referenda to prevent it.[69,74–76]

Pro-fluoridationists also became aware that for some communities even a sophisticated political fluoridation campaign would not be successful because of unique economic, political, or social conditions. Studies of smaller communities without fluoridation found that many were hindered by a small tax base, a decentralized or antiquated water system, or a complicated local political system. For communities with these problems, many pros advocated financial assistance from state and federal governments, state legislation requiring fluoridation, or school-based fluoride mouth rinse programs, which studies in the 1960s had shown were effective. Approval of the procedure by the Food and Drug Administration in 1974 encouraged pro-fluoridationists to promote mouth-rinse programs as an option when community fluoridation seemed unobtainable.[77–79]

Community fluoridation was still the favored method among pro-fluoridationists, but a small shift in attitude had occurred. In the 1950s, only anti-fluoridationists had suggested school-based programs as an alternative to community fluoridation, but once pro-fluoridationists acknowledged that some communities might never get fluoridation, school-based programs became acceptable to pros. Pro-fluoridationists did not believe school-based programs hindered the adoption of community fluoridation. "To my knowledge," wrote one of these pros, "this result has not materialized. There are, however, several communities that have begun community fluoridation after a fluoride rinse or tablet program had been started."[79] As late as 1980, pro-fluoridationists took comfort from the fact that, with only a few exceptions, anti-fluoridationists did not object to school-based programs because they were voluntary and required parental consent. By 1985 this had changed, and anti-fluoridationists were aggressively attacking school-based programs with the same arguments they had used against community fluoridation.[79,80]

Pro-fluoridationists in the 1970s and 1980s repeatedly stressed how long and difficult a fluoridation campaign could be. One pro warned that "the closer you get to success, the harder the antis will work to defeat you."[79] Pro-fluoridation commentators emphasized that anti-fluoridationists were as strong or stronger than ever, and that local pro-fluoridation committees needed to be vigilant against anti-fluoridation efforts and continue community education long after winning their victory. In contrast to earlier pro-fluoridationists, who envisioned an end to resistance, pro-fluoridationists in the 1970s did not. "Clearly the controversy about fluoridation is far from over," wrote one pro-fluoridationist, "We can expect that efforts will continue to be made to remove fluoride from public water supplies and to prohibit communities from adding fluoride to their water supplies."[66] The message, that fluoridation campaigns were hard, was not defeatist; rather, the attitude was that winning a fluoridation referendum was hard, but not unachievable.[66,68,71,80]

The Controversy Today

In the 50 years that fluoridation has been controversial, pro-fluoridationists' understanding of their mission has evolved: where once they believed they were simply promoting a public health measure, they came to see a fluoridation campaign as both an educational and a political campaign.

Each year, in communities across the country, pro-fluoridationists and anti-fluoridationists face off over the issue. On November 5, 2002, 10 communities voted on fluoridation. Of those, eight rejected it.[81] One of those communities was Billings, Montana, where voters rejected the measure for the third time in 35 years.[81] In Washoe County, Nevada, also one of the eight, a local anti-fluoridationist was quoted in the *Reno Gazette-Journal* celebrating their success: "I am so pleased that people have seen through the deception and voted to stop dumping toxic waste into our water supply."[82] Despite the longevity and successes of the opposition, pro-fluoridationists have continued to advocate fluoridation; the Washoe County referendum was in response to the lobbying efforts of the local pro-fluoridationist organization, Northern Nevada Citizens for Healthy Smiles. In spite of, or perhaps because of, pro-fluoridationists' persistence, as of December 2000, 66% of the U.S. population has access to fluoridated water.[83] Locked in a struggle over the content of America's drinking water, neither side appears to be weakening or willing to concede defeat.

Acknowledgments

The author wishes to thank Dr. Leo Ribuffo for his support and guidance.

References

1. Schottelkotte A. How a community loses—case history of Cincinnati. 23 March 1955, Box. 2, Donald R. McNeil Collection (M63-231), WHSM, Madison, WI.
2. McNeil DR. The Fight for Fluoridation. New York: Oxford University Press, 1957.
3. McClure FJ. Water Fluoridation: The Search and the Victory. Bethesda, MD: National Institute of Dental Research, 1970.
4. Crain RL. Fluoridation: the diffusion of an innovation among cities. *Social Forces* 1966: 44:467–76.
5. Roemer R. Water fluoridation: public health responsibility and the democratic process. *Am J Public Health* 1965:55:1337–48.
6. Knutson JW. Fluoridation: where are we today? *Am J Nurs* 1960:60:196–98.
7. Buckman S. How citizens can help the community health team achieve fluoridation. *J Am Dent Assoc* 1962:65:630–38.
8. Six ways to mislead the public. *Consumer Reports* 1978:43:480–82.
9. Spira L. Poison in your water. *American Mercury* 1957:85:67–75.
10. Spira L. The Drama of Fluorine: Arch Enemy of Mankind. Milwaukee, WI: Lee Foundation for Nutritional Research, 1953.
11. Waldbott GL. A Struggle with Titans. New York: Carlton Press, 1965.
12. Sheft C. Startling true facts on fluoridation. *National Fluoridation News* 1971:6:17.
13. Sheft C. Fluoride: the environmental pollutant and health hazard. *National Fluoridation News* 1977:1:23.
14. Bergman AB. The Discovery of Sudden Infant Death Syndrome. New York: Praeger, 1989.
15. Supervisor seeks probe. *National Fluoridation News* 1984:2:30.
16. Culbert M. Aids: Hope, Hoax and Hoopla. Chula Vista, CA: Robert W. Bradford Foundation, 1989.
17. Jansen I. Fluoridation: A Modern Procrustean Practice. Antigo, WI: Isabel Jansen/Tri-State Press, 1990.
18. Fluoride Action Network, Sutton PRN. Is the ingestion of fluoride an immunosuppressive practice? Available at: http://www.fluoridealert.org/immune-system.htm. Accessed January 2005.
19. Health Way House, Bennett, E. The fluoride debate, question 25, does drinking optimally fluoridated water cause AIDS? Available at: http://www.fluoridedebate.com/question25.html. Accessed January 2005.
20. Relfe, S. Chronological history of health, 1978–1994. Available at: http://www.relfe.com/history_3.html. Accessed January 2005.
21. Caldwell G, Zanfagna PE. Fluoridation and Truth Decay. Reseda, CA: Top-Ecol Press, 1974.
22. Franklin BGT, Franklin E, Clark L. It's a vicious cycle. *National Health Federation Bulletin* 1966:12:24–25.

23. Waldbott GL, Burgstahler AW, Mckinney HL. Fluoridation: the Great Dilemma. Lawrence, KS: Coronado Press, 1978.
24. Pollution cases souring. *National Fluoridation News* 1965:4:11.
25. Nader questions PHS policy. *National Fluoridation News* 1970:2:16.
26. Crain RL, Katz E, Rosenthal DB. The Politics of Community Conflict: The Fluoridation Decision. New York: Bobbs-Merrill Co. 1969.
27. Butler HW. Legal aspects of fluoridating community water supplies. *J Am Dent Assoc* 1962:65:653–58.
28. Cox WR. Hello, Test Animals . . . Chinchillas or You and Your Grandchildren? Milwaukee, WI: Lee Foundation for Nutritional Research, 1953.
29. Loe H. The fluoridation status of US public water supplies. *Public Health Rep*1986:101:160.
30. Moolenburgh H. Fluoride—the freedom fight. *National Fluoridation News* 1987–88:3:32.
31. Koziar EG. Letter to the editor. *New York Times*, 22 April 1974.
32. Exner FB. Government by laws, not by men. *National Fluoridation News* 1968:5:14.
33. Courtney P. How Dangerous Is Fluoridation? New Orleans, LA: Free Men Speak, 1971.
34. Swendiman GA. The argument against fluoridating city water. ca. 1951, Wis Mss 13 PB, Folder 25, Edward A. Hansen Collection, WHSM, Madison, WI.
35. Herrstrom WD. Americanism Bulletin No. 18. October 1951, Wis Mss 13 PB, Folder 25, Edward A. Hansen Collection, WHSM, Madison, WI.
36. Bottled water outlook rosy. *National Fluoridation News* 1969:5:15.
37. Exner FB. Why fluoridating water supplies is dangerous. In: Rorty J, ed. The American Fluoridation Experiment. New York: Devin-Adair Co., 1957.
38. Bronner EH, et al. Just one turn on one valve and!!/ spare the pigs. ca. 1952. Wis Mss 27 PB, Folder Anti-Fl. Material, Alex Wallace Collection, WHSM, Madison, WI.
39. Severance RM. Copy of a personal letter to a leading citizen of Saginaw, dated 5 January 1954. File 1953, 16 March, Box 204, Folder 1, Rollin M. Severance Collection, WHSM, Madison, WI.
40. U.S. House Committee on Interstate And Foreign Commerce. Hearings on H.R. 2341, a bill to protect the public health from the dangers of fluorination of water, 25–27 May 1954. Washington, DC: Government Printing Office, 1954.
41. Western Minute Men USA. Red scheme for mass control: some new ideas on the fluoridation conspiracy. *American Mercury* 1959:89:134–35.
42. The fluorine folly. 10 March 1952, Wis Mss 13 PB, Folder 25, Edward A. Hansen Collection, WHSM, Madison, WI.
43. Can flouridation [sic] of your water supply cause cancer?" *Freemen Speak*, 15 January 1955.
44. Lee Foundation for Nutritional Research. Price list. 1954, Wis Mss 13 PB, Folder 43, Mrs. Merlin Meythaler Collection, WHSM, Madison, WI.
45. Bealle MA. The great fluoride hoax: reprints from issues of *American Capsule News*. n.d. Box 1, Folder 9, Naturopathy Collection (M0759), Series I, Stanford University, Stanford, CA.
46. Exner FB. Fluoride vs. freedom. *National Health Federation Bulletin* 1963:9:23–34.
47. Machan DC. N. H. F. convention notes. *National Health Federation Bulletin* 1962:8:4–8.
48. Gotzsche AL. The Fluoride Question: Panacea or Poison? Briarcliff Manor, NY: Stein & Day, 1975.
49. Hill JH. Documented history of fluorine. ca. 1957. SC 923, Ethel B. Dinning Collection, WHSM, Madison, WI.
50. Robinson AS. PTA leaders and our Bill of Rights: letter to the editor, *Tallahassee Democrat*. ca. 1953. Unprocessed records #M71-022, Rollin M. Severance Collection, WHSM, Madison, WI.

51. Rorty J. Introduction. In: Rorty J, ed. The American Fluoridation Experiment. New York: Devin-Adair Co., 1957.
52. Dublin LI. Water fluoridation: science progresses against unreason. *The Health Education Journal* 1957:15:246–50.
53. Wertheimer F. Can facts successfully overcome the opposition to water fluoridatrion?" *Bull Am Assoc Public Health Dent* 1953:13:31–38.
54. Metzner C. Referenda for fluoridation. *The Health Education Journal* 1957:15:168–75.
55. Downs R. The dentist's responsibility in community water fluoridation programs. *Am J Public Health* 1952:42:575–78.
56. Schisa E. The role of the public health nurse in the community water fluoridation program. *Am J Public Health* 1953:43:710–11.
57. Gamson WA. The fluoridation dialogue: is it an ideological conflict? *Public Opinion Quarterly* 1961:25:526–37.
58. Mcneil DR. Political aspects of fluoridation. *J Am Dent Assoc* 1962:65:659–63.
59. Bishop E. Publicity during a fluoridation campaign. *J Am Dent Assoc* 1962:65:663–67.
60. Erlenbach M. Fluoridation: Organizing a community in support of water fluoridation. *J Am Dent Assoc* 1962:65:639–42.
61. Plaut T. Community organization and community education for fluoridation in Newton, Massachusetts. *J Am Dent Assoc* 1962:65:622–29.
62. Menczer LF. Fluoridation: analysis of a successful community effort– challenge to state and local dental societies. *J Am Dent Assoc* 1962:65:673–79.
63. Sebelius C. Fluoridation: the health department's challenge: the Tennessee story. *J Am Dent Assoc* 1962:65:648–52.
64. Weil S. Fluoridation: analysis of an unsuccessful community effort. *J Am Dent Assoc* 1962:65:680–85.
65. Chrietzberg J. Georgia's water fluoridation program. *J Am Dent Assoc* 1962:65:643–47.
66. Rosenstein D, Isman R, Pickles T, Benben C. Fighting the latest challenge to fluoridation in Oregon. *Public Health Rep* 1978:93:69–72.
67. Newbrun E. Achievements of the seventies: community and school fluoridation. *J Public Health Dent* 1980:40:234–46.
68. Faine RC, Collins JJ, Daniel J, Isman R, Boriskin J, Young KL, Fitzgerald CM. The 1980 fluoridation campaigns: a discussion of results. *J Public Health Dent* 1981:41:138–42.
69. Boriskin J, Fine J. Fluoridation election victory: a case study for dentistry in effective political action. *J Am Dent Assoc* 1981:102:486–91.
70. Isman R. Fluoridation: strategies for success. *Am J Public Health* 1981·71·717–21.
71. Barrett S. Fluoridation campaign tips. In: Barrett S, Rovin S, eds. The Tooth Robbers. Philadelphia, PA: G. F. Stickley, 1980, 67–82.
72. Domoto P. Victory in Seattle. In: Barrett S, Rovin S, eds. The Tooth Robbers. Philadelphia, PA: G. F. Stickley, 1980, 83–87.
73. Boriskin J. Winning a fluoridation campaign. In: Barrett S, Rovin S, eds. The Tooth Robbers. Philadelphia, PA: G. F. Stickley, 1980, 89–101.
74. Leukhart CS. An update on water fluoridation: triumphs and challenges. *Pediatr Dent* 1979:1:32–37.
75. Allukian M, Steinhurst J, Dunning JM. Community organization and a regional approach to fluoridation of the greater Boston area. *J Am Dent Assoc* 1981:102:491–93.
76. Evans Jr. CA, Pickles T. Statewide antifluoridation initiatives: a new challenge to health workers. *Am J Public Health* 1978:68:59–62.
77. Lantos J, Marsh L, Schultz R. Small communities and fluoridation; three case-studies. *J Public Health Dent* 1973:33:149–59.

78. Silversin J, Coombs, J, Drolette M. Achievements of the seventies: self-applied fluorides. *J Public Health Dent* 1980:40:248–57.
79. Horowitz A. An agenda for the eighties: self-applied fluorides. *J Public Health Dent* 1980:40:268–74.
80. Easley MW. The new antifluoridationists: who are they and how do they operate? *Am J Public Health* 1985:45:133–41.
81. Fluoride Action Network, Jones M. Communities which have rejected fluoridation since 1990. Available at: http://www.fluoridealert.org/communities.htm. Accessed August 2003.
82. Morales P. Results for Washoe tobacco, fluoride measures. *Reno Gazette-Journal*, 5 November 2002.
83. Centers for Disease Control and Prevention. Populations receiving optimally fluoridated public drinking water—United States, 2000. *MMWR* 2002:51:144.
84. Herrstrom WD. 75 reasons why community water supplies should not be fluoridated. ca. 1957. Joseph B. Lightburn Collection, West Virginia University Library, Morgantown, WV.

Suggested Reading

Martin, B. Scientific Knowledge in Controversy: The Social Dynamics of the Fluoridation Debate. Albany, NY: SUNY, 1991.
McClure FJ. Water Fluoridation: The Search and the Victory. Bethesda, MD: National Institute of Dental Research, 1970.
McNeil DR. The Fight for Fluoridation. New York: Oxford University Press, 1957.

PART VIII

VEHICULAR SAFETY

16

Drivers, Wheels, and Roads: Motor Vehicle Safety in the Twentieth Century

ANN M. DELLINGER
DAVID A. SLEET
BRUCE H. JONES

The public health problem of motor-vehicle-related death and injury emerged in the twentieth century. Over the last 100 years, substantial gains in driver behavior, vehicle safety, and road design were made to improve motor-vehicle travel despite dramatic increases in motorization, shifting demographics, and changing social patterns. This chapter defines the modern public health problem of motor-vehicle travel; outlines local and federal government and private industry efforts to reduce the incidence of death and injury attributable to motor vehicles, addresses issues specific to certain groups of motorists (e.g., motorcyclists and older drivers), and discusses the challenges that likely will persist into the twenty-first century.

Motor Vehicle Safety

At the beginning of the twentieth century, motor-vehicle travel was a novelty. Today, it is a necessity. In 1900, an estimated 8000 automobiles were registered in the United States. By 2000, more than 226 million vehicles were registered and 190 million drivers were licensed. As the number of vehicles and drivers increased, so did deaths and injuries on the road—from 1.0 motor-vehicle death per 100,000 population in 1900 to 26.7 in 1930.[1] The rapid increase in death and injury from 1910 through 1930 prompted R. B. Stoeckel, then commissioner of motor vehicles in Connecticut, to declare "road trauma" a public health problem.[2]

343

At the century's end, motor-vehicle-related deaths constituted about one third of all injury-related deaths representing the loss of more than 40,000 lives, about half of them aged less than 35 years.[3] In the past 100 years, more than 2.8 million persons have died and nearly 100 million persons have been injured on U.S. roads and highways.[4] Despite these statistics, the annual death rate has declined dramatically over the twentieth century, from 21.7 deaths per 100 million vehicle miles traveled in 1923 (the first year that data were available) to 1.55 in 2000—a 93% reduction (Fig. 16.1).[1] The reduction of death rates caused by motor-vehicle crashes in the United States represents a substantial public health success in injury prevention.

In contrast to other public health problems of the early twentieth century, injuries and deaths resulted from the development and rapid adoption of a new technology—the motor vehicle. The motor vehicle represented a major improvement over other modes of personal travel (e.g., the horse and buggy), and improvements in manufacturing made cars more affordable. Over the years, an increasing number of vehicles were registered and drivers were licensed, increasing the number of roads and miles traveled and increasing exposure to the potential risk for crashes.[5] In 2000, 174 times as many vehicles and 96 times as many drivers were traveling on U.S. roadways than were doing so in 1913. Likewise, by 2000, the number of miles traveled in motor vehicles climbed to a level 20 times higher than that reached in the mid-1920s.[1] The dramatic decline in death rates per 100 million vehicle miles traveled (VMT) can be

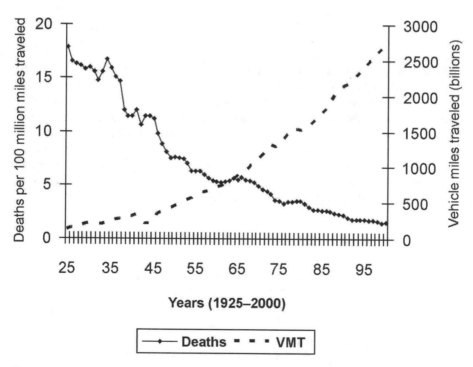

Figure 16.1. Motor vehicle deaths per vehicle miles traveled and annual vehicle miles traveled, 1925–2000—United States. (National Safety Council. Injury Facts. 2002 Edition, Itasca, IL.)

attributed to improvements in safer behavior, safer vehicles, and safer roads. However, the public health indicator, as measured by deaths per 100,000 population, has followed a more varied course. Nevertheless, since 1966, a steady decline in motor-vehicle-related death rates can be observed (Fig. 16.2).

The adverse public health consequences of increased motorization in the first few decades of the twentieth century (from four or five deaths per 100,000 population in 1913 to more than 12 in 1920) led President Herbert Hoover in 1924 to convene the first National Conference on Street and Highway Safety. This was the first in a series of presidential initiatives to create a uniform set of traffic laws designed to prevent collisions.[6] During 1924–1934, physicians and health workers were called in to participate in a national program, and formal committees were developed in all areas of traffic safety. However, traffic deaths continued to climb as the number of drivers and vehicles exposed to risk increased faster than the countermeasures designed to keep them safe. In 1934, a total of 36,101 traffic-related deaths were reported, a rate of 28.6 per 100,000 population. These numbers prompted President Franklin D. Roosevelt to enlist the cooperation of the governors in each state to reduce the traffic-injury problem (Box 16.1). By 1936, President Roosevelt had convened an Accident Prevention Conference that focused on vehicle safety and called for slower speeds, better lighting, and stronger auto body frames.[7,8]

These federal efforts, however, were not reflected in the mortality statistics. By 1937, motor-vehicle death rates had reached an all time high of 31 deaths per 100,000,

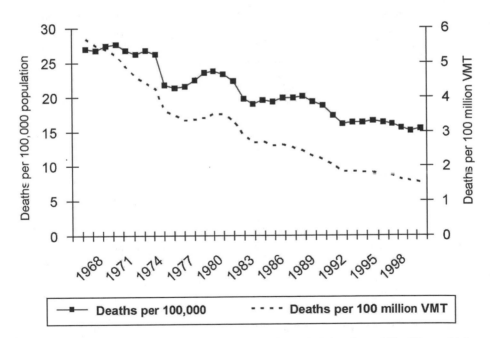

Figure 16.2. Motor vehicle death rates per 100,000 population and per 100 million vehicle miles traveled, 1966–2000—United States. (National Safety Council. Injury Facts. 2002 Edition, Itasca, IL.)

Box 16.1. In a Plea for State Cooperation to Reduce Injuries to Motor Vehicle Occupants, President Franklin D. Roosevelt Sent This Historic Letter to the Governors of the 48 States.

January 23, 1935.

Honorable Eugene Talmadge,
Governor of Georgia,
Atlanta, Georgia.

My dear Governor Talmadge:

I am gravely concerned with the increasing number of deaths and injuries occurring in automobile accidents. Preliminary figures indicate that the total of these losses during the year 1934 greatly exceeded that of any previous year. We should, as a people, be able to solve this problem which so vitally affects the lives and happiness of our citizens.

In order to assist in this, the Federal Government, through the Secretary of Commerce, has taken the leadership in developing remedial measures. Proposals for uniform State legislation have been worked out by the National Conference on Street and Highway Safety with the cooperation of responsible State officials and representatives of interested organizations from all parts of the country.

The remedies that need to be applied are thus available in form which appears to meet the unanimous approval of experienced judgment. The pressing problem is to secure universal application of these remedies which have proved effective where applied.

The responsibility for action rests with the States. There is need for legislation and for the organization of proper agencies of administration and enforcement. There is need also for leadership in education of the public in the safe use of the motor vehicle, which has become an indispensable agency of transportation.

With the legislatures of most of the States meeting during 1935, concerted effort for appropriate action in the States is most important.

Realizing the seriousness of the situation and the urgent need for attention to the problem, I am confident that you will desire to participate in this effort.

Yours very truly,

Franklin D. Roosevelt

and they remained at 18–26 deaths per 100,000 for the next quarter of the century. An exception to this was the period 1942–1944, when WWII led to a precipitous decline in motor-vehicle death rates. During these years, Americans were traveling less as fuel was scarce and resources and personnel were diverted to war efforts. After the war, deaths and death rates returned to prewar levels and then rose more than 30% during 1960–1969, to 27.7 per 100,000 population (Fig. 16.3).[1]

In response to rising motor-vehicle death rates in the early 1960s and the climate of social reform, in 1966 President Lyndon B. Johnson signed the National Traffic and Motor Vehicle Safety Act and the Highway Safety Act. These acts paved the way for an intensified effort by the federal government to set and regulate standards for

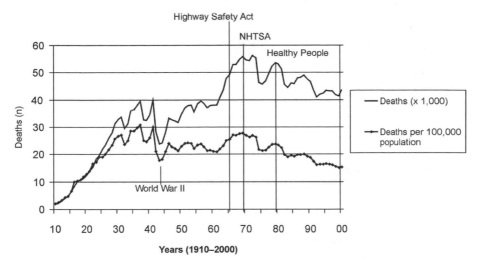

Figure 16.3. Motor vehicle related deaths and death rates in the United States, 1910–2000. (National Safety Council. Injury Facts. 2002 Edition, Itasca, IL.) Note: Highway Safety Act and National Traffic and Motor Vehicle Safety Act were passed and National Highway Safety Board established 1966. National Highway Traffic Safety Administration (NHTSA) established 1970. U.S. Public Health Service publications: *Healthy People* (1979) and *Objectives for the Nation* (1980).

motor vehicles and highways to improve safety.[9] This legislation led to the creation of the National Highway Safety Bureau (NHSB), which in 1970 became the National Highway Traffic Safety Administration (NHTSA). Beginning with 1968 models, these two acts gave the NHSB/NHTSA the authority to set safety standards for highways and new cars. A total of 19 standards were promulgated involving accident avoidance, crash protection, and post-crash survivability. These new standards related to braking, tires, windshields, lights, door strength, fuel systems, and transmission safety controls.[10] Automobile manufacturers initially were not required to develop new systems, but eventually they did so to comply with the standards. Elevated crash rates and injury deaths, along with research demonstrating the preventability and survivability of vehicle crashes, led the public health community to take an active role in promoting highway safety.[9,11,12] These mandates initiated many lifesaving changes in vehicle and highway design and motorist behavior. The establishment of the NHSB/NHTSA to provide national leadership in regulating highway safety was an important factor in the declining rates that followed (see Fig. 16.3).

Many of these gains in highway safety were attributed to the leadership of William Haddon, a public health physician and epidemiologist who became the first director of NHSB and the first administrator of NHTSA. He revolutionized the scientific approach to the prevention of motor-vehicle injuries by developing a conceptual framework rooted in public health.[13] Haddon's conceptual model, the Haddon Matrix (Fig. 16.4), recognized that like infectious diseases, injuries were the result of interactions between a host (person), an agent (motor vehicle), and the environment

	FACTORS			
	Human Factors	Agent/Vehicle Factors	Physical Environment	Sociocultural Environment
PHASES				
Pre-event				
Event				
Post-event				

Figure 16.4. Haddon Matrix.

(roadways). Haddon adapted the classic epidemiologic triangle that had been so successfully used in solving other public health problems to motor-vehicle-injury prevention. Haddon further described factors contributing to motor-vehicle injury as occurring during three phases: the pre-crash phase, crash phase, and post-crash phase.[14] NHTSA's strategic plan continues to employ the Haddon Matrix to focus on research related to driver factors, vehicle design, and roadway environments.[15]

The Redesign of Automobiles and Roads

As a result of the NHTSA regulations, manufacturers built vehicles (i.e., the agents of injury according to the Haddon Matrix) with improved safety features including head rests, energy-absorbing steering wheels, rollover protection, dual brakes, shatter-resistant windshields, and safety belts.[9,10] Multiple strategies were used to improve roads (i.e., environments) including better delineation of curves; the addition of edge and center line stripes and reflectors, breakaway signs and utility poles, and highway illumination; the use of barriers to separate oncoming traffic lanes, guardrails, and grooved pavement to increase tire friction in bad weather; the practice of channeling left-turn traffic into separate lanes; the addition of rumble strips; and the availability of crash cushions on exit ramps.[4,13,16] And with time, the behavior of drivers and passengers (i.e., the host factors) changed to reduce risk as people realized the importance of vehicle/person interactions (i.e., the host or human factors).[17,18] Enactment and enforcement of stricter traffic safety laws, reinforced by public education, led to personal safety choices (e.g., avoiding impaired driving, reducing speed, wearing helmets, and using child safety seats and safety belts).

Benefits associated with the NHTSA regulations were almost immediate. By 1970, motor-vehicle-related death rates were decreasing by both the public health measure (deaths per 100,000 population) and the traffic safety measure (deaths per vehicle miles traveled) (see Fig. 16.2). Safety standards (e.g., better braking and steering systems, head restraints, and occupant impact protection) made a substantial difference. Occupants riding in vehicles built according to these regulations experienced 20%–40% fewer fatalities than those in vehicles not meeting the standards.[10,13,19] The introduction of the National Maximum Speed Limit saved 3000–5000 lives in 1974 and 2000–4000 lives each year through 1983.[20] Fatality rates on the interstate highway system dropped to half that on other sections of the road system as a result of road improvements (e.g., divided traffic streams, controlled access, wide shoulders, and crash-absorbing barriers).[19]

Successful Collaborative Efforts

The consideration of motor-vehicle safety as a public health issue prompted initiation of programs by federal and state governments, academic institutions, citizen advocacy groups, community-based organizations, and the automobile industry. Since their creation in the 1960s, NHTSA and the Federal Highway Administration (FHWA) within the Department of Transportation have provided national leadership for traffic and highway safety efforts.[12] The FHWA began in 1893 as a small office in the U.S. Department of Agriculture, known as the Office of Road Inquiry, which was created to gather and disseminate information on road building. In the 1960s, this office became part of the Department of Transportation and has grown to employ 3500 staff members and have an annual budget of $26 billion. The FHWA oversees the Federal-aid Highway Program, which from its inception has been based on a state-federal partnership with states responsible for working with local governments to select, plan, design, and execute Federal aid projects. The FHWA's role is to assure that federal laws, standards, and regulatory requirements are satisfied while providing technical assistance to improve the quality of the transportation-road network.

In 1986, as a result of the Institute of Medicine report titled *Injury in America,*[21] Congress authorized and provided funding to establish a national injury prevention research program at the CDC. The CDC brought a public health framework and epidemiologic perspective to motor-vehicle injury prevention that included surveillance, risk factor research, intervention development, dissemination, program evaluation, and funding for state and local health departments to conduct motor-vehicle-injury prevention programs.[22,23] Examples of the CDC's contributions include: an early warning about the potential danger of passenger-side air bags, a description of child fatalities in alcohol-involved crashes, and establishment of a strong evidence base for the effectiveness of strategies for increasing safety belt and child safety seat use, and strategies for reducing alcohol impaired driving.

In response to laboratory tests that indicated that passenger-side air bags might be dangerous to infants in rear-facing child safety seats, the CDC published a warning on the potential interaction between these two safety technologies in 1993.[24] Although no fatalities among children related to this interaction were reported at the time, the CDC instructed parents and caregivers to properly restrain infants in the rear of the vehicle. This was followed in 1995 by a report that eight children died in otherwise survivable crashes because a passenger-side air bag deployed in the front seat where a child was sitting. Before the end of 2001, more than 100 deaths had been reported. The collaboration among several federal agencies (the CDC, National Transportation Safety Board [NTSB], the Society for Automotive Engineering, and NHTSA) helped bring this safety issue to the public's attention.[25] Subsequent research found that children

Table 16.1. Major highway safety legislation affecting public health.

1956	Enactment of the Federal-Aid Highway Act of 1956. This act was the first major legislation that began the trend toward building safer highways. It provided funds to develop programs and set standards for the interstate highway system and for upgrading existing roads. All federal-aid highway enactments since then have increased this trend.
1966	Enactment of the National Traffic and Motor Vehicle Safety Act of 1966 and the Highway Safety Act of 1966. These acts gave the National Highway Safety Bureau and the National Highway Traffic Safety Administration (in 1970) a legislative mandate to set and enforce safety performance standards for motor vehicles (codified under Title 49 of the United States Code, Chapter 301, Motor Vehicle Safety, and Title 23 U.S.C., Chapter 4, respectively). It provided grants to states and local governments to enable them to conduct highway safety programs and to conduct research on driver behavior and traffic safety. It also required the establishment of Uniform Standards for State Highway Safety Programs to assist the states and local communities in organizing their highway safety programs.
1973	Enactment of the 55 mph National Maximum Speed Limit (temporary).
1974	Enactment of the 55 mph National Maximum Speed Limit (permanent).
1982	Enactment of the Alcohol Traffic Safety Incentive Grant Program, Surface Transportation Assistance Act of 1982. This act provided incentive grants to states that adopted certain laws and programs to deter drinking and driving.
Mid-1980s	Congress and federal agencies began promoting the use of safety belts, and states began enacting laws on safety-belt use.
1984	DOT issued a rule mandating that passive restraints be phased in beginning with 1987 model year cars.
1984	Enactment of the National Minimum Drinking Age (NMDA).
1984	Enactment of legislation (included in NMDA law) providing incentive grants to states that adopted child safety-seat-use laws/programs.
1986	Mandatory safety belt use laws in 22 states and the District of Columbia.
1987	Enactment of the Surface Transportation and Uniform Relocation Assistance Act of 1987. This act permitted states to raise speed limits to 65 mph on rural interstates and certain other limited access highways.
1989	Enactment of Section 410 Drunk Driving Prevention Program Incentive Grants, part of the Omnibus Drug Initiative of 1989, later expanded in ISTEA legislation.
1991	Intermodal Surface Transportation and Efficiency Act of 1991 (ISTEA). This act included financial incentives and sanctions to encourage states to enact basic safety belt laws and to increase belt use and motorcycle-helmet use; it also increased the scope of the alcohol traffic safety grant program and made mandatory certain motor vehicle safety standards (including the installation of air bags).
1995	The National Highway Systems Designation Act of 1995. This act subjected states that do not consider a .02 BAC (or less) for drivers under age 21 to be driving while intoxicated to the withholding of federal-aid highway funds beginning in fiscal year 1999. In the fall of 1995, Congress lifted federal sanctions against states without helmet use laws, paving the way for state legislatures to repeal helmet laws.
1999	The Transportation Equity Act of the 21st Century (TEA-21) and the TEA-21 Restoration Act. Included in these acts are the following highway safety initiatives: federal-aid highway funds of states that do not establish a program to encourage states to enact Repeat Intoxicated Driver laws by FY 2002 would have funds transferred to the state's Section 402 State and Community Highway Safety grant program funds; established a new program of incentive grants to encourage states to increase safety belt use rates; established a new program of incentive grants to encourage states to implement child passenger protection programs; established a program to encourage states to adopt and implement effective programs to reduce highway deaths and injuries resulting from individuals riding unrestrained or improperly restrained in motor vehicles; and Open Container laws, a state which does not have an Open Container law by October 1, 2000,

Table 16.1. (*continued*)

	would be transferred to the state's Section 402 State and Community Highway Safety grant program.
2001	Enactment of .08 BAC legislation requiring states to lower permissible blood alcohol levels from .10% to .08% or face losing a portion of their highway safety funds.
2003	Department of Transportation Appropriations Bill: Directs NHTSA to improve ejection prevention performance, prohibits the trucking industry from conducting a pilot program using teenage truck drivers, and increases funding for the National Automotive Sampling System, a program that collects information on auto crashes and injuries.
2004	Enactment of Anton's Law. This directs the NHTSA to initiate rulemaking to establish performance requirements for child restraints, including booster seats, for the restraint of children weighing more than 50 pounds; it also requires NHTSA to submit a report to Congress on the development of a crash test dummy simulating a 10 year-old child; and it requires automakers to install lap and shoulder belt assemblies in all rear seating positions of passenger cars, including the center seat position. Includes funding to conduct research into child passenger safety issues.

aged less than 10 years seated in the front passenger position have a 34% increased risk of death in frontal crashes in vehicles with passenger-side air bags.[26]

The CDC studies also revealed that 64% of children killed by drinking drivers were riding in the same vehicle as the drinking driver.[27] Legislators in 38 states have imposed automatic child-endangerment charges on persons who transport children while driving impaired. The CDC and the Task Force on Community Preventive Services (an independent, nonfederal panel of community health experts) reviewed the scientific evidence for five community-based interventions that were implemented to reduce alcohol-impaired driving. The reviews revealed that 0.08% blood alcohol content (BAC) laws, minimum legal drinking-age laws, and sobriety checkpoints were effective interventions. Lower BAC laws specific to young or inexperienced drivers (i.e., zero tolerance laws) and intervention training programs for alcohol servers also were effective.[28] The CDC's systematic review of the effectiveness of 0.08% BAC laws for drivers was helpful in establishing 0.08% as the national standard. The review revealed that state laws that lowered the illegal BAC for drivers from 0.10% to 0.08% reduced alcohol-related fatalities by a median of 7%, which translated to approximately 500 lives saved annually. In October 2000, President Bill Clinton signed the Fiscal Year 2001 transportation appropriations bill, which included a requirement that all states pass the 0.08% BAC law by October 2003 or risk losing federal highway construction funds.

Collaboration among federal agencies is not the only factor contributing to the prevention of motor-vehicle injuries. State and local governments, with support from highway safety and public health agencies, have enacted, enforced, and evaluated laws in several areas that affect motor vehicle and highway safety, including, driver behavior, driver licensing and testing, alcohol policies, vehicle inspections, traffic regulations, public education, and special services to underserved populations. The motor-vehicle industry has contributed to prevention efforts through its own vehicle engineering and safety research. The insurance industry, through organizations such as the American Automobile Association and the Insurance Institute for Highway Safety (a nonprofit research and communications organization funded by auto insurers), has made substantial contributions to research and traffic safety activities. The Insurance Institute for Highway Safety conducts crash tests that evaluate the crashworthiness of vehicles and assigns safety ratings on the basis of crash performance.

Medical and other professional societies (e.g., the American Academy of Pediatrics and the Association for the Advancement of Automotive Medicine) have been active in advocacy for motor-vehicle injury prevention. Advocacy groups such as Mothers Against Drunk Driving (MADD) and the National SAFE KIDS Campaign focus their efforts on a variety of safety topics such as bicycle and pedestrian safety, child occupant protection, and air bag safety. Since 1966, these joint efforts of government and private agencies and organizations to reduce motor-vehicle fatalities have resulted in a 43% decrease in the rate of deaths per 100,000 population and a 72% decrease in deaths per VMT (see Fig. 16.2). These reductions translate into more than 250,000 lives saved and countless injuries averted in the past 30 years.[1]

Public Health Objectives in Motor-Vehicle Injury Prevention

In 1979, the U.S. Department of Health, Education, and Welfare (now the Department of Health and Human Services) identified motor-vehicle trauma as a major public health issue and developed specific objectives to reduce the burden by 1990.[29] The department's objectives were reviewed and expanded in 1990, and again in 2000, with a new set of goals and targets for the year 2010. In Healthy People 2010, 10 specific objectives are related to decreasing fatal and nonfatal motor-vehicle-related injuries and pedestrian traffic deaths and injuries, and increasing the use of safety belts and child restraints, use of motorcycle and bicycle helmets, increasing the number of states that have laws requiring graduated driver licensing for young drivers, and to increase the number of states with laws requiring bicycle helmets for riders.[30]

Public health activities have targeted several groups for aggressive prevention activities. These groups include alcohol-impaired drivers, young drivers, bicyclists and pedestrians, motorcyclists, and older drivers. Attention has also been paid to improve the use of effective occupant protection systems among all drivers and passengers (e.g., safety belts, child safety seats, and booster seats)—strategies that have been effective in preventing motor-vehicle-related injuries.

High-Risk Populations

Alcohol-Impaired Drivers

Alcohol-impaired driving has been a problem since the early days of the automobile. New York was the first state to pass an anti-drinking and driving law in 1910. The NHTSA began addressing this problem in earnest in the 1970s when they initiated 35 Alcohol Safety Action Projects designed to reduce drunk driving at the local level via enforcement, licensing, adjudication, and the dissemination of public information.

Although some were found effective, these projects did not change national levels of drunk driving. In 1980, the NHTSA began to address the problem of drinking and driving with a program that included general deterrence, prevention and intervention, and citizen activist support.[31]

That same year, MADD was formed in California, marking the beginning of a national movement to eliminate impaired driving. MADD brought this issue to the forefront of American consciousness and helped turn the popular view of drinking and driving from an accepted part of modern life to socially unacceptable criminal behavior. Responding to the grass-roots movement, in 1982 President Reagan appointed a National Commission of Drunk Driving to conduct an exhaustive study of the problem. Under the leadership of C. Everett Koop, the U.S. Public Health Service issued the first Surgeon General's report on drunk driving in 1989.[31]

Progress has been made as a result of these efforts. From 1982 through 2000, the percentage of motor-vehicle crash fatalities involving alcohol decreased 32%.[32] Several other countermeasures contributed to this decline, including new and tougher state laws, stricter enforcement, sobriety checkpoints, swift penalties, and an increased minimum legal drinking age.[31,33] Successful efforts to reduce drunken driving illustrate the effectiveness of health promotion approaches that combine public education with public policy, environmental control, advocacy, legislation, and law enforcement.[34]

Although all states now have laws to address drinking and driving, an estimated 123 million episodes of impaired driving occurred in 1993, and police made about 1.5 million arrests for impaired driving. Nearly 10 million drinking and driving episodes occurred among persons aged 18–20 years—persons who are too young to legally purchase alcohol.[35] In 2000, the 17,380 alcohol-related deaths still represented 41% of all traffic fatalities.[32] In addition, alcohol-related crashes resulted in $51 billion in economic costs in 2000, accounting for 22% of all crash-associated costs.[36]

Young Drivers and Passengers

Young drivers (i.e., those aged 16–20 years) have higher rates of death associated with motor vehicles than any other age group of drivers. Nighttime driving, driving with teenaged passengers, and alcohol-impaired driving are especially risky for young drivers. In 1964, Australia was the first country to introduce elements of graduated licensing. Graduated driver licensing (GDL) systems place restrictions on drivers (i.e., learner's permit phase, passenger limits, zero tolerance for alcohol, and nighttime driving restrictions) that are systematically lifted as young drivers gain driving experience and competence. In the United States, NHTSA developed a model GDL system, and in 1978, Maryland became the first state to enact a formal GDL system based on this model. California followed suit in 1983. The remaining states slowly implemented GDL laws; by the end of the 1990s, most states had some form of GDL legislation.[37]

Alcohol-impaired driving is a particularly important risk behavior for young drivers. At the same blood alcohol content, crash risk is higher for younger drivers than older drivers.[38] In 1984, Congress enacted the Federal "21" Minimum Drinking Age Act and the first of several incentive programs to encourage states to enact measures to counter driving while intoxicated. From 1982 through 2001, alcohol-related fatal-crash rates among drivers aged 16–20 years decreased almost 60%. This strong downward trend suggests that prevention measures specific to this age group (e.g., the implementation of the national minimum legal drinking age and zero alcohol tolerance laws for young drivers) have been effective.[39]

Research has shown the GDL approach is effective in reducing teenaged-driver crash risk: GDL studies conducted around the world have demonstrated 5%–16% reductions in crashes among teenaged drivers. Although additional research is needed to better understand which components of GDL are essential, it remains a promising solution for improving driver safety.

In 2000, motor-vehicle crashes led all other causes of death among Americans aged 16–20 years. Motor-vehicle crashes were responsible for 6041 deaths among persons in this age group in 2000; moreover, their occupant population-based death rates (14.9 deaths per 100,000) were more than double the national average (6.8 per 100,000).[3] Approximately 60% of deaths among teenaged passengers occur in vehicles driven by other teenagers.[40]

Motorcyclists

Motorcyclists benefited from the road improvements and general behavior changes that were promoted for all motor-vehicle drivers during the later part of the twentieth century. Per mile traveled, motorcyclists are about 18 times more likely than passenger car occupants to die in a crash, and three times more likely to be injured.[41,42] The advent of motorcycle helmets and laws requiring their use resulted in a decline in motorcycle fatalities. Before 1967, only three states had motorcycle helmet use laws. In 1967, the federal government began requiring states to enact motorcycle helmet use laws to qualify for certain federal safety program and highway construction funds. Within the next 2 years, 37 states enacted helmet use laws. By 1975, all but three states mandated helmets for all motorcyclists. However, state pressure to rescind these regulations led to their revocation by Congress in 1976, resulting in a change in helmet use laws in 20 states to include only coverage of young riders. Gradually, some of these states reinstated the stricter laws, and, by the end of the century, all but three states had some form of mandatory helmet-use legislation.[43]

Motorcycle fatality rates per registered vehicle have decreased from 91 per 100,000 registered motorcycles in 1978 to 64 per 100,000 registered motorcycles in 2000, a 30% decrease. However, 2862 motorcyclists died as a result of crashes in 2000, representing 7% of all motor-vehicle traffic deaths that year. Almost one third of deaths among motorcyclists could have been prevented by the use of motorcycle helmets. In states with mandatory or universal helmet use laws (i.e., laws for riders of all ages), virtually 100% of motorcyclists wear them. The NHTSA estimates that in 2000, helmets saved the lives of 631 riders; if all motorcyclists had worn helmets that year, an additional 382 lives could have been saved.[41,42]

In addition to promoting helmet use for all riders, motorcycle-injury prevention programs emphasize the hazards of riding a motorcycle while impaired by alcohol and the benefits of driver training and licensing requirements. Motorcycle drivers in fatal crashes have higher intoxication rates than any other type of driver (27% of fatal crashes for motorcycle drivers compared with 19% for passenger-vehicle drivers).[42] Future efforts to prevent deaths and injuries among motorcycle riders will need to address the changing characteristics of motorcycle enthusiasts. In the late 1990s, a shift in age distribution of motorcyclist fatalities occurred, with deaths declining in the youngest age groups (18–29 years) and increasing among riders aged ≥ 40 years. From 1997 through 2001, the number of fatalities in the $\geq$40 year age group increased by 79%.[44]

Older Drivers

Research into the safety of older drivers (i.e., those aged $\geq$65 years) began in the late 1960s and early 1970s and was motivated by the changing demographics of the U.S. population. During the twentieth century, the population of persons aged $\geq$65 years increased 11-fold.[45] By the year 2000, approximately 35 million people aged $\geq$65 years lived in the United States; this number is expected to double by the year 2030.[46] In addition, more older persons operated vehicles during the last third of the twentieth century. The proportion of older adults with driver's licenses increased from 45% in 1970 to 78% in 2000.[47]

In 1985, the American Automobile Association Foundation for Traffic Safety convened a panel of experts to discuss the needs and problems of older drivers, and in 1986, the Transportation Research Board convened a panel to review the design and operation of the transportation system and to recommend improvements for an aging population.[48] Congress, as part of the Surface Transportation Assistance Act of 1987, requested a comprehensive investigation into the factors that might inhibit the safety and mobility of older drivers and the means to address these factors. The Department of Transportation developed a long-range strategy to accommodate the aging population, and the NHTSA and FHWA embarked on developing older-driver programs. By 1998, the FHWA had published the *Older Driver Highway Design Handbook* to provide highway designers and engineers practical information linking declining functional capabilities among older drivers to specific roadway features. For example, the handbook recommended protected left turns (i.e., the use of separate traffic signals) because of the over-representation of deaths in left-turn crashes among older drivers.[49] In fatal two-vehicle crashes involving a younger and older driver, older drivers were three times more likely to be struck and six times more likely to be turning left at the time of the crash.[50]

Adjusting for their amount of travel, older drivers have crash rates more than three times that of younger drivers.[50] The population-based rate of motor-vehicle-related fatalities for persons aged $\geq$65 years was greater than 20% higher than the national average for the general driving population at the end of the century.[1] From 1990 through 2000, the number of traffic fatalities among persons aged $\geq$70 years increased nearly 10%, from 4844 in 1990 to 5335 in 2000.[51] Assisting older adults in successfully balancing safety and mobility will be an important future challenge for traffic safety and public health. This can be accomplished through changes directed toward the three levels of the Haddon Matrix, including changes to the vehicle (i.e., safety belts that are easier to reach and attach), the roadway (i.e., signs that are easier to read), and driver behavior (i.e., improved functional assessments for older adults to identify those who should no longer drive and alternative transportation options for those who stop driving).

Occupant Protection

Safety Belts

Safety belts were first available in 1955 as optional equipment in new automobiles.[52] These early safety belts were lap belts for front-seat occupants only. In 1962, New York passed the first law requiring safety belts for front-seat occupants, beginning in 1965 model-year cars. By 1968, federal law required safety belts for the front seats of all passenger cars, and in 1974, the NHTSA required three-point (lap and shoulder) belts for drivers and front-seat passengers. Consumers did not readily adopt this new safety feature and use-rates fluctuated from 10% to 15% through the mid-1980s. Moreover, when federal regulation required automobile manufacturers to phase-in safety belt interlock systems that prevented the engine from starting unless occupants were buckled up, the public outcry was so strong that Congress soon repealed the ruling.

When 31 states passed belt use laws during 1984–1987, use climbed above 40%. By 2000, 49 states (all but New Hampshire) and the District of Columbia had belt-use laws. Nationwide use rates increased from about 11% in 1981 to 71% in 2000,[50] and averaged around 80% in 2004. Additional efforts are needed to influence the remaining 20% of the U.S. population who do not use safety belts regularly. In states that have primary belt use laws (i.e., laws enabling police officers to stop motorists exclusively for a belt violation), belt-use rates average 17% higher than states with secondary enforcement (i.e., police officers must have another reason to stop the driver).[53]

When used properly, safety belts are the most effective injury-prevention intervention currently available. Lap-shoulder belts reduce the risk of death to car occupants by approximately 45%–55% and to light truck occupants by 60%–65%.[1,36] Safety belts also save money. In 2000, belt use saved $50 billion in medical care, lost productivity, and other injury-related costs.[36] Safety belts combined with air bags offer the greatest protection.

Child Safety Seats and Booster Seats

Safety belts do not fit children well until they are approximately 8 years old (or 4 feet, 9 inches tall). The inadequate fit decreases the effectiveness of safety belts among young children and has led to special restraint devices for infants (i.e., rear-facing child safety seats), toddlers (i.e., forward-facing child safety seats), and young school-aged children (i.e., booster seats). As with safety belts, public adoption was slow in the absence of legislation mandating use of these seats. In 1977, Tennessee became the first state to enact a child safety-seat law. By the close of the twentieth century, all states had child passenger protection laws in place, but they varied widely in age and size requirements and the penalties imposed for noncompliance. For example, some states do not require children to ride restrained if they are in out-of-state vehicles or if the child is in the back seat.[54]

Child safety seats and booster seats save lives and prevent injury. In the event of a motor vehicle crash, safety seats are 71% effective in preventing death among infants and 54% effective among children aged 1–4 years; booster seats are 59% effective in preventing injury.[55] Actual use of child restraints varies by age. In 2002, observational surveys estimated safety seat use at 99% for infants and 94% for children aged 1–4 years.[56] Although these figures seem high, of the 529 passengers less than 5 years of age killed in 2000, 47% were completely unrestrained at the time of the crash,[57] suggesting that children who are riding unrestrained (1% of infants and 6% of toddlers) are at an increased risk of a motor-vehicle crash. A recent systematic review of interventions to increase child safety-seat use concluded that mandatory-use laws, seat distribution combined with education programs, incentive and education programs, and community-wide information combined with enhanced enforcement campaigns were effective in increasing use.[58]

Although booster seat cushions have been used in Sweden and Australia since the mid-1970s, their promotion and use in the United States has lagged behind.[59] In some areas, use rate among children aged 4–8 years was less than 20% at the turn of the century.[60] Many programs to encourage booster seat use and move child passengers to the back seat (the safest position for children to ride) are conducted by state or local public health departments in conjunction with voluntary agencies and advocacy groups (e.g., SAFE KIDS). A variety of activities are conducted by these programs, including outreach campaigns, parent education, provider education, hotlines, discount coupons, and seat distribution.

Car crashes kill 10 times as many children as all childhood vaccine-preventable illnesses. The passage of a universal child-restraint attachment law (to simplify attachment of the child safety seat to the vehicle) and legislation requiring children who have outgrown their child safety seats to ride in booster seats should help protect these vulnerable passengers.

Challenges for the Twenty-First Century

Despite substantial gains in motor-vehicle injury prevention during the twentieth century, crashes and the injuries they inflict will remain a major public health issue into the twenty first century. Motor-vehicle crashes are the leading cause of death for persons aged 1–34 years. They lead all other injuries as a cause of death in the United States, accounting for one third of all injury deaths. In 2000, motor-vehicle crashes lead to 41,821 deaths, 3.2 million nonfatal injuries, and more than 6.4 million police-reported crashes,[50] costing an estimated $231 billion dollars. This estimate can be translated into $820 for every person living in the United States and 2.3% of the U.S. gross domestic product.[36]

For the driving public, motor-vehicle travel will contribute to a number of cross-cutting health problems in the future, from personal safety to environmental pollution. These problems will only increase with time as a result of increased travel, population growth, an aging society, and our growing reliance on cars for everyday living.

Conflict has always existed between the goals of mobility and the goals of safety; this balance must be continually reevaluated. For example, although the national 55 mile-per-hour speed limit was instituted to conserve fuel, it also resulted in fewer crashes and fewer crash deaths. When fuel availability increased, so did speeds and road deaths, illustrating the trade-off between one aspect of mobility (speed) and traffic safety; the public was not willing to maintain restricted mobility even in light of substantial safety benefits.

Changes in behavior and technology will present new challenges for public health. Aggressive driving, the increased use of cellular phones, and travel telematics (e.g., in-vehicle fax machines, Internet access, and global positioning systems) are emerging threats to motor-vehicle safety. Expected rises in traffic volume and congestion, and changes in the vehicle fleet (e.g., a greater proportion of sports utility vehicles, or SUVs) all present new safety challenges that will require innovative solutions.[19] Comprehensive, integrated public health surveillance systems will be necessary to provide data for setting priorities in motor-vehicle injury prevention in the midst of other competing health priorities.[61,62] One of the remaining obstacles to preventing motor-vehicle-related injuries is the public's misconception that injuries are accidents that occur by chance. While some progress has been made in changing the perception of injuries as predictable, preventable events, more must be done. Public health professionals need to frame motor-vehicle injuries in the context of other preventable diseases attributed to behavioral and environmental factors that are both predictable and preventable.

Public health agencies and organizations play a key role in the prevention of motor-vehicle injury. Health departments, which have the statutory responsibility for public health, provide community health services, deliver programs to undeserved populations, and typically are experienced in working with a broad range of community groups and agencies,[63] form a national infrastructure to address motor-vehicle-associated problems (e.g., alcohol-impaired driving, safety-belt use, and young driver safety). Public health agencies are increasing their attention to motor-vehicle-related injuries alongside heart disease, cancer, and stroke as preventable public health problems that respond well to targeted interventions.[64] Worldwide, motor vehicle injury prevention is recognized as an important global public health problem by the World Health Organization (WHO),[65] and World Health Day 2004 was dedicated to preventing road traffic injury.[66]

Safe and accessible transportation can prevent injury and death, thus playing a fundamental role in promoting health. In the context of health objectives for the nation, transportation safety means better public health into the twenty-first century.

References

1. National Safety Council. Injury Facts, 2002. Itasca, IL: National Safety Council, 2002.
2. Stoeckel, RB. The Problem of Prevention of Accidents Caused by the Use of Motor Vehicles. Johns Hopkins University, School of Hygiene and Public Health. De Lamar Lectures 1925–1926. Baltimore: Williams and Wilkins, 1927, 188.
3. Web-based Injury Statistics Query and Reporting System (WISQARS). 2003. National Center for Injury Prevention and Control. Available at: www.cdc.gov/NCIPC/WISQARS. Accessed September 2003.
4. Department of Health and Human Services, Public Health Service. Position papers from the Third National Injury Control Conference: Setting the National Agenda for Injury

Control in the 1990's. DHHS publication. no. 1992-634-666. Washington, DC: Government Printing Office, 1992.

5. Global Traffic Safety Trust. Reflections on the Transfer of Traffic Safety Knowledge to Motorizing Nations. Melbourne, Australia: Global Traffic Safety Trust, 1998.

6. American Public Health Association. Accident Prevention: The Role of Physicians and Public Health Workers. New York: APHA, 1961, 127.

7. Eastman JW. Styling vs. Safety: The American Automotive Industry and the Development of Automotive Safety 1900–1966. New York: University Press of America, 1984.

8. National Committee for Injury Prevention and Control. Injury prevention: meeting the challenge. *Am J Prev Med* 1989:5(3 suppl):123–27.

9. Transportation Research Board. Safety Research for a Changing Highway Environment. Special Report no. 229. Washington, DC: National Research Council, Transportation Research Board, 1990.

10. Crandall RW, Gruenspecht HK, Keeler TE, Lave LB. Regulating the Automobile. Washington, DC: Brookings Institution, 1986, 47.

11. Mashaw JF, Harfst DL. Regulation and legal culture: the case of motor vehicle safety. *Yale J Regulation* 1987:4:257–316.

12. Committee on Injury Prevention and Control, Institute of Medicine. Reducing the Burden of Injury: Advancing Prevention and Treatment. Washington, DC: National Academy Press, 1999.

13. Waller J. Injury Control: A Guide to Causes and Prevention of Trauma. Lexington, KY: D.C. Heath & Co., 1985.

14. Haddon W. The changing approach to the epidemiology, prevention and amelioration of trauma: the transition to approaches epidemiologically rather than descriptively based. *Am J Public Health* 1968:58:1431–38.

15. National Highway Traffic Safety Administration. Strategic Plan. Washington, DC: Department of Transportation, National Highway Traffic Safety Administration, 1998.

16. Rice DP, MacKenzie EJ, Jones AS, et al. Cost of Injury in the United States: A Report to Congress. San Francisco, CA: University of California, Institute for Health and Aging; Johns Hopkins University, Injury Prevention Center, 1989, 127–29.

17. Shinar, D. Psychology on the Road. New York: John Wiley & Sons, 1978.

18. Evans L. Traffic Safety and the Driver. New York: Van Nostrand Reinhold, 1991.

19. Graham JD. Injuries from traffic crashes: meeting the challenge. *Ann Rev Public Health* 1993:14:515–43.

20. Transportation Research Board. 55: A Decade of Experience. Special Report no. 204. Washington, DC: National Research Council, Transportation Research Board, 1984.

21. Institute of Medicine. Injury in America: A Continuing Public Health Problem. Washington, DC: National Academy of Sciences, National Research Council, Institute of Medicine, National Academy Press, 1985.

22. Bolen J, Sleet D, Johnson V, eds. Prevention of Motor Vehicle-related Injuries: A Compendium of Articles from the *MMWR*, 1985–1996. Atlanta: National Center for Injury Prevention and Control, Centers for Disease Control and Prevention, 1997.

23. Sleet DA, Bonzo S, Branche C. An overview of the National Center for Injury Prevention and Control at the Centers for Disease Control and Prevention. *Injury Prev* 1998: 4(4):308–12.

24. Centers for Disease Control and Prevention. Warnings on the interaction between air bags and rear-facing child restraints. *MMWR* 1993:42(14):280–81.

25. Centers for Disease Control and Prevention. Air Bag-associated fatal injuries to infants and children riding in front passenger seats-United States. *MMWR* 1995:4(45):845–47.

26. Braver ER, Ferguson SA, Green MA, Lund AK. Reductions in deaths in frontal crashes among right front passengers in vehicles equipped with passenger air bags. *JAMA* 1997: 278(17):1437–39.

27. Quinlan KP, Brewer RD, Sleet DA, Dellinger AM. Characteristics of child passenger deaths and injuries involving drinking drivers. *JAMA* 2000:283(17):2249–52.

28. Shults RA, Elder RW, Sleet DA, et al. Reviews of evidence regarding interventions to reduce alcohol-impaired driving. *Am J Prev Med* 2001:21(4S):66–88.

29. Department of Health, Education and Welfare. Healthy people: the Surgeon General's report on health promotion and disease prevention. DHEW publication no. 79-507111. Washington, DC: Public Health Service, 1979.

30. Department of Health and Human Services. Healthy People 2010, 2nd ed. With understanding and improving health and objectives for improved health. 2 vols. Washington, DC: Government Printing Office, 2000.

31. Department of Health and Human Services, Public Health Service, Office of the Surgeon General. Surgeon General's Workshop on Drunk Driving [Proceedings]. Washington, DC: 14–16 December 1988, Rockville, MD, 1989.

32. National Highway Traffic Safety Administration. Traffic safety facts, 2000. DOT HS 809 337. Washington, DC: Department of Transportation, National Highway Traffic Safety Administration, 2002.

33. Department of Health and Human Services, U.S. Public Health Service, National Institutes of Health. Ninth special report to the US Congress on alcohol and health. NIH publication no. 97-4017. Washington, DC: 1997.

34. Sleet DA, Wagenaar A, Waller P, eds. Drinking, driving, and health promotion. *Health Educ Q* 1989:16(3):329–447.

35. Liu S, Siegel PZ, Brewer RD, Mokdad, AH, Sleet DA, Serdula M. Prevalence of alcohol-impaired driving: results from a national self-reported survey of health behaviors. *JAMA* 1997:77(2):122–25.

36. National Highway Traffic Safety Administration. The economic impact of motor vehicle crashes 2000. DOT 809 446, Washington, DC: Department of Transportation, National Highway Traffic Safety Administration, 2002.

37. McKnight AJ, Peck RC. Graduated driver licensing: what works? *Injury Prev* 2002:8 (suppl II):ii32–ii38.

38. Zador PL, Krawchuk SA, Voas RB. Alcohol-related relative risk of driver fatalities and driver involvement in fatal crashes in relation to driver age and gender: an update using 1996 data. *J Stud Alcohol* 2000:61:387–95.

39. Centers for Disease Control and Prevention. Involvement by young drivers in fatal alcohol-related motor-vehicle crashes—United States, 1982–201. *MMWR* 2002:51(48): 1089–91.

40. Williams AF, Wells JK. Deaths of teenagers as motor-vehicle passengers. *J Safety Res* 1995:26(3):161–67.

41. Insurance Institute for Highway Safety. Fatality Facts, Motorcycles. Arlington, VA: Insurance Institute for Highway Safety, 2002.

42. National Highway Traffic Safety Administration. Traffic Safety Facts, 2000: Motorcycles. DOT HS 809 326. Washington, DC: Department of Transportation, National Highway Traffic Safety Administration, 2001.

43. Insurance Institute for Highway Safety. Helmet Use Laws as of 2003. Arlington, VA: Insurance Institute for Highway Safety, 2002.

44. Shankar UG. Recent trends in fatal motorcycle crashes. Paper no. 247. Washington, DC: National Highway Traffic Safety Administration, 2003.

45. Bureau of the Census. 65+ in the United States [Current Population Reports]. Washington, DC: Government Printing Office, 1996, 23–190.
46. Bureau of the Census. Population Projections Program, Population Division. Washington, DC: Bureau of the Census, 2003. Available from: URL: www.census.gov/population/ projections/nation/summary. Accessed September 2003.
47. Federal Highway Administration. Highway Statistics Summary to 2001. Washington, DC: Office of Highway Policy Information, Federal Highway Administration, Department of Transportation, 2002.
48. Transportation Research Board. Transportation in an Aging Society: Improving Mobility and Safety for Older Persons. Vol. 1. Special Report no. 218.Washington, DC: National Research Council, Transportation Research Board, 1988.
49. Staplin L, Lococo K, Byington S. Older Driver Highway Design Handbook. FHWA-RD-97–135.Washington, DC: Federal Highway Administration, Department of Transportation, 1998.
50. National Highway Traffic Safety Administration. Traffic Safety Facts, 2000: Overview. DOT HS 809 329. Washington, DC: Department of Transportation, National Highway Traffic Safety Administration, 2001.
51. National Highway Traffic Safety Administration. Traffic Safety Facts, 2000: Older Population. DOT HS 809 328. Washington, DC: Department of Transportation, National Highway Traffic Safety Administration, 2001.
52. Graham JD. Auto Safety: Assessing America's Performance. Dover, MA: Auburn House Publishing Company, 1989.
53. National Highway Traffic Safety Administration. Traffic Tech: Standard Enforcement Saves Lives—The Case for Strong Seat Belt Laws. Publication no. 191. Washington, DC: Department of Transportation, National Highway Traffic Safety Administration, 1999.
54. Insurance Institute for Highway Safety. Children Not Covered by Safety Belt or Child Restraint Laws. Arlington, VA: Insurance Institute for Highway Safety, 2002. Available at: www.highwaysafety.org. Accessed September 2003.
55. Durbin DR, Elliott MR, Winston FK. Belt-positioning booster seats and reduction in risk of injury among children in vehicle crashes. *JAMA* 2003:289:2385–40.
56. National Highway Traffic Safety Administration. Research Note: The Use of Child Restraints in 2002. DOT HS 809 555. Washington, DC: Department of Transportation, National Highway Traffic Safety Administration, 2003.
57. National Highway Traffic Safety Administration. Traffic Safety Facts, 2000: Children. DOT HS 809 324. Washington, DC: Department of Transportation, National Highway Traffic Safety Administration, 2001.
58. Zaza S, Sleet DA, Thompson RS, Sosin DM, Bolen JC, Task Force on Community Preventive Services. Reviews of Evidence regarding interventions to increase use of child safety seats. *Am J Prev Med* 2001:21(4S):31–47.
59. National Highway Traffic Safety Administration. Improving the Safety of Child Restraints Booster Seat Study: Report to Congress. DOT HS 809 54. Washington, DC: Department of Transportation, National Highway Traffic Safety Administration, 2002.
60. Ebel BE, Koepsell TD, Bennett EE, Rivara FP. Use of child booster seats in motor vehicles following a community campaign: a controlled trial. *JAMA* 2003:289(7):879–84.
61. Teutsch, SM. Consideration in planning a surveillance system. In: Teutsch SM, Churchill RE, eds. Principles and Practices of Public Health Surveillance. New York: Oxford University Press, 1994, 18–28.
62. Thacker SB, Stroup DF, Parrish RG, Anderson HA. Surveillance in environmental public health: issues, systems and sources. *Am J Public Health* 1996:86:633–38.

63. Sleet DA. Reducing Traffic Injuries in America: U.S. Objectives and Strategies. Proceedings of Inaugural Conference of Roadwatch. Perth, Australia: Road Accident Prevention Research Unit, University of Western Australia, Perth 1990, 31–46.
64. Sleet DA. Motor vehicle trauma and safety belt use in the context of pubic health Priorities. *J Trauma* 1987:27(7):695–702.
65. Peden M, Scurfield R, Sleet D, Mohan D, Hyder AA, Jarawan E, Mathers C. World Report on Road Traffic Injury Prevention. Geneva: World Health Organization, 2004.
66. Sleet DA, Branche CM. Road safety is no accident. *J Safety Res* 2004:35:173–174.

Suggested Reading

Doll L, Bonzo S, Mercy J, Sleet D, eds. Handbook of Injury and Violence Prevention. New York: Springer, 2006.
Elvik R, Truls V, eds. The Handbook of Road Safety Measures. Amsterdam: Elsevier, 2004.

17

The Nut Behind the Wheel: Shifting Responsibilities for Traffic Safety Since 1895

DANIEL M. ALBERT

In July 1997, National Highway Traffic Safety Administrator Ricardo Martinez testified in Congress that aggressive driving accounted for two thirds of the 41,907 highway deaths and more than 3 million injuries of the previous year. "A lot of the gains we've made through seat belt use and better car design are giving way to aggressive behavior," Dr. Martinez lamented.[1] Psychologist Leon James of the University of Hawaii testified next, telling the congressmen that he had a solution. "Dr. Driving," as he calls himself, testified that 53% of the drivers he studied suffered from road rage, a state of mind that leads to aggressive driving, from tailgating and honking to running another car off the road. James found that most sufferers are themselves the children of road-ragers and that, as with alcoholism and drug addiction, the first step to a cure is acknowledging the problem. He recommended using public schools, beginning in kindergarten, to teach "emotional intelligence" and develop a culture of good driving.[1,2]

To anyone who has studied the early history of traffic safety, the theme of the hearings—the responsibility of individual drivers for traffic safety—sounded familiar. The goal of the committee, to argue that more highways were needed to ensure safety, also harkens back to the pre-1960s world of traffic safety. Things were quite different when Ralph Nader and activist legislators blamed cars for traffic morbidity in the 1960s. Nader mocked what he called the "nut behind the wheel" approach, or the notion that bad drivers were responsible for crashes. Senator Abraham Ribicoff (for whom Nader worked) began hearings in 1965 into the failure of automakers to address safety in vehicle design. By 1966, a new regime based on engineering and the science of epidemiology had arisen. It did not take long, however, for societal pressures to reassert themselves, shifting responsibility back toward the errant driver.

Because driver-centered strategies have come back into vogue, it is especially useful to review the long history of efforts to control the driver. This chapter sets the science of safety within a historical context, revealing how permeable the boundary between science and society can be when dealing with a crucial and iconic machine, the car.

The Horseless Age

At the end of the nineteenth century, horses presented perhaps the most serious transportation-related threat to public health even as press accounts focused on rail-road and streetcar crashes. New York City had to cope with an estimated 2.5 million pounds of manure and 60,000 gallons of urine each day, along with 15,000 carcasses that had to be removed from its streets annually.[4] In addition, critics argued that the "brutish" horse was by nature a dangerous animal best replaced by a clean and compliant machine as soon as possible. The clean, progressive automobile, however, turned out to be far more dangerous than the horse. The first recorded motor vehicle fatality in the United States is that of Henry H. Bliss, who had just alighted from a streetcar when he was struck by a passing taxicab in 1899.[5,6] The highway death toll rose rapidly, from 26 in 1899 to 252 in 1905.

Because the initial cost of motor vehicles and their upkeep restricted ownership to the wealthy, early responses to traffic deaths took on an element of class warfare. Casualties were (like Bliss) typically on foot and most often were children of the poor and working classes who used city streets as play spaces.[6] Cities enacted speed limits as low as five miles per hour and child deaths sparked physical attacks in some cases. Similarly, because the early automobile was largely an urban phenomenon, a distinct urban-rural divide arose with farmers decrying the presence of "devil wagons in God's country."[7] Farmers organized opposition locally and some went so far as to fire on speeding motorists.[6,8] For their part, upper-class automobilists hoped to exercise social control over errant drivers through motor-journal moralizing against bad "motor manners."

It is difficult to speak of a coordinated industry response to traffic deaths in this period. The nascent automobile industry consisted of hundreds (or thousands, if one counts all of the small shops that assembled a converted carriage or two) of disparate car makers. Nevertheless, in 1902 the National Association of Automobile Manufacturers (NAAM) petitioned both houses of Congress to set federal vehicle-safety standards. Indeed, several bills calling for manufacturing standards were introduced into the Fifty-Ninth Congress (1905–1906) at the behest of the NAAM and the newly formed American Automobile Association. None made it out of committee.[9] Whereas in Europe national regulation became the norm, U.S. regulation of the automobile, road, and driver remained distinctly local. Courts at the state and national levels had found the automobile to be a "dangerous instrumentality" and therefore allowed cities to impose regulations such as speed limits. Yet courts upheld the equal right of the automobilist to use the public roads, and nothing like modern concepts of product liability came into play.[10]

Mass Production to World War I

Mass production of the Model T, begun in earnest in 1909, all but ended class warfare over the automobile, but it also contributed significantly to the increasing toll in death and injury. In the countryside, families rapidly joined the "haves" of motorized society, transforming their earlier hostility.[7,11] Municipalities were the first institutions to confront motor vehicle crashes comprehensively. Many cities were already coping with technologic challenges that taxed traditional forms of governance. Sewer and water systems, garbage collection, electricity, and trolley lines all had made cities resemble large-scale industrial enterprises. At the same time, in migration of African Americans from the rural South and waves of new immigrants from Eastern and southern Europe were reshaping urban life and culture. Native-born urban elites responded to the changing demographics in two ways that remain etched in our approach to traffic safety. They pressed for strict policing of "vices," and sought to dilute the voting power of immigrants by "reforming" city governments and relying on a new breed of technocrats to manage urban infrastructures.[12,13]

The automobile had a multifaceted association with vice—most clearly through its close association with alcohol consumption, juvenile delinquency, and illicit sexual activity. Myriad local and state vice laws were reinforced at the federal level with the 1910 White Slave Traffic Act (the Mann Act), and Prohibition in 1919.[14] Significantly, because it was based on Congress's right to regulate interstate commerce, the Mann Act specifically defined the transportation of women across state lines "for immoral purposes" as a crime. Indeed the automobile was said to stir improper sexual desires in women, and it was hysteria over "automobile bandits" that had led directly to the Mann Act. Worse even than the way the automobile facilitated consensual sex was its effect on the sex trade. "Automobile prostitution . . . is the bane of law enforcement," announced Bascom Johnson of the American Hygiene Association in 1919.[15] Easily stolen vehicles encouraged adolescent "joy riding," and automobiles provided young people an escape from parental control. Alcohol and automobile were linked early on, not only with regard to crash involvement but also because rum runners relied on them during Prohibition.

In addition to promoting vice laws, reform-minded city governments began to hire technocrats to manage city services and to reform police departments. Municipal managers created systems for managing new technologies, such as water and sewers, electrical networks, and streets. Cities had always had streets, of course, but in the motor age these multifunctional social spaces became traffic conduits, akin to the networks that distributed power, water, and communications.[16] Municipal managers—some of whom became specialized "traffic engineers"—worked hand in hand with metropolitan police forces to create codes of driver behavior. Because there was no victim directly associated with either vice crime or traffic violations, police relied on active surveillance to deter such crimes.[13,14] In these ways, the seemingly unrelated conflict between native-born progressives and new immigrants helped establish the initial regulatory response to the automobile hazard.

From a Return to Normalcy to the Great Depression

The population of 8.1 million motor cars expanded to 23 million during the 1920s. The vehicle fleet evolved from 90% fair-weather open cars to 90% all-season closed cars suitable for a daily commute. Police continued to enforce traffic law as vice law, and in so doing swamped the lower courts–a problem that persisted into the 1960s.[15,17–19] Travel by automobile was certainly growing safer, but pedestrians were still at grave risk and the public health consequences of motor traffic worsened.

Members of the National Safety Council, an industrial safety organization comprising state and local chapters, took the lead in confronting traffic crashes in the 1920s.[20,21] They had used worker education to reduce significantly the hazards of factory work, and they adapted their educational and propaganda techniques to do the same for street traffic. The NSC supported organizations such as the Institute of Traffic Engineers and what became the Northwestern University Traffic Institute (NUTI). The NUTI—which began life in Evanston, Illinois, the birthplace of temperance—became the fountain of modern, scientific traffic policing. During the 1920s, the NSC helped Franklin Kreml of the Evanston Police Department develop a system of scientific accident investigation and "selective enforcement" to target those moving violations said to cause crashes. Kreml created an Accident Investigation Squad and outfitted each squad car with a first-aid kit, bulky photographic equipment, measuring devices, a "decelerometer" to test the function of brakes and a typewriter for recording witness testimony. The police conducted compulsory vehicle inspections, issued so-called good-driver cards, and even established road blocks to root out drunk drivers. "All of this without any authority of law," Kreml recalled in a 1991 interview.[22] In 1933, Northwestern University President Walter Dill Scott, along with Kreml and the head of the local NSC chapter, helped found the NUTI, which institutionalized and disseminated nationally the work of the Evanston police.

Ostensibly, in 1924 the federal government began to confront the public health problems of motor traffic with the National Conference on Street and Highway Safety, known as the Hoover Conference. Yet the Hoover conference was less a pivotal moment in the history of traffic safety than a window into an existing network of traffic safety experts who had been working through voluntary associations for more than a decade. The federal government's role at this and two subsequent conferences prior to World War II was only to encourage and coordinate activities. Commerce Secretary Herbert Hoover couched his assault on traffic crashes primarily as a problem of inefficiency. Government officials—local, state, and federal—constituted the largest segment of conference participants. But virtually all those with an interest in roads attended, including motor vehicle manufacturers, farmers from the National Grange, railroad and streetcar companies, railroad worker unions, road builders associations, chambers of commerce, educators from the Parents and Teachers Association and the National Education Association, automotive and civil engineers, and representatives of the NSC. Pedestrians as a class had no representatives, but Hoover highlighted their importance, reminding attendees that "a very large portion of the

22,600 deaths and the 678,000 injuries [in 1923] happened to men, women, and children on foot."[23]

Among the attendees were industrial psychologists who put a scientific stamp on the conventional wisdom that "bad drivers" caused crashes—wisdom evident in early autoists' appeals to good manners. In 1929, psychologist and conference secretary Fred Moss summed up the era's engineering ethos when he noted that automobile and highway engineers had made cars and roads safer, but "unfortunately, the human engineer has not lock washers or cotter pins to hold the human 'nuts' in their proper position, the result being the fatal accidents that we read about daily."[24] Drawing on their experience testing soldiers during World War I, mental health professionals hoped to identify accident prone drivers. For example, industrial psychologist Alvah R. Lauer created a driving research laboratory at Iowa State University where he developed psychological assessments to help insurance companies grade drivers and thereby set premiums.

Although not represented at the Hoover conference, forensic psychiatrists were the first physicians to join the battle against crashes in the 1920s. They adapted their techniques for identifying the criminal tendencies of "mental defects" to the hunt for defective drivers. Overburdened municipal traffic courts employed forensic psychiatrists to evaluate a driver's mental health in accident cases or when faced with recidivism. The nation's leading Traffic Court Psychopathic Clinic was headed by Dr. Lowell Sinn Selling of the Detroit Recorder's Court. Publishing his studies in medical journals, he identified a host of traits, including excessive ego, feeblemindedness, and hysteria as markers of bad drivers.[23] Ultimately, mental health professionals called for viewing traffic crashes as a public health problem that could be eliminated through psychiatric intervention.[25,26]

A quantitative and qualitative analysis of the Detroit clinic's records and the published reports of forensic psychiatrists has revealed a distinct racial bias in their approach.[27] Just as police adapted their existing model of vice suppression to the problem of traffic law violations, forensic psychiatrists extended their model of crime prevention to the prevention of traffic crimes. In the fight on crime, medical professionals and the state sought to sterilize "mental defectives" who would otherwise breed offspring with a tendency toward crime and vice. The answer to criminality, declared the director of the Chicago Municipal Court Psychopathic Clinic in 1928, "is to reduce [the criminals'] number by a) regulating marriage, b) enforcing sterilization, c) adequate immigration laws."[28] Traffic court psychiatrists pursued an analogous strategy by denying or revoking licenses to such individuals, thereby purifying road society. The fact that judges were far more likely to send black Americans for examination by the Detroit Recorder's Court Psychopathic Clinic, and the fact that blacks were more than twice as likely as whites to be labeled poor risks as drivers, indicates the inherent racism of the modified eugenic strategy. Biases against nonwhite immigrants and the elderly show up as well in an evaluation of the clinic records.

Despite the rising death toll and a good deal of public discourse on the subject of crashes, the public in the 1920s was not particularly interested in the problem of traffic safety. Americans were more concerned with joining the motorized citizenry than reigning in the motor hazard.

From the Great Depression to World War II

The public attitude changed somewhat as death rates per population, death rates per vehicle mile traveled, and the overall death toll all spiked in the middle 1930s. Traffic crashes also symbolized the evident failure of scientifically led progress as surely as did the Great Crash of 1929. Even as they clung to their automobiles "as they clung to their self respect," the public focused a good deal of anxiety on the car as the king of consumer products and "capitalism's favorite child."[29-31] The Depression undermined the faith of many Americans in consumption, capitalism, and the promise of scientifically led technological progress.[32]

The unease directed at the automobile as source and symbol of a failed dream is reflected in the popular culture of the time. For example, Margaret Bourke White used the automobile as an ironic symbol of progress in her 1937 photograph of a bread line in Louisville, Kentucky.[33] Similarly, Grant Wood's 1935 painting *Death on the Ridge Road*—an image of an impending crash as a large, sleek car crests a hill into the path of an oncoming truck—is a commentary on the negative impact of car culture on rural life.[34,35] The most influential consideration of the traffic crash from the period is the 1935 *Reader's Digest* article "And Sudden Death"— the magazine's first attempt at original story telling.[36] It was a gory tale. The editors warned: "Like the gruesome spectacle of a bad automobile accident itself, the realistic details of this article will nauseate some readers."[37] Beyond the 1.5 million *Digest* subscribers (the largest subscription list in the nation), the story went out in 8 million reprints and had a series of spin-offs in magazines, newspapers, and on film.

Public polling (then a novel technique) showed why these artistic and journalistic representations resonated so strongly. A Gallup poll in 1936 asked, "Would you favor or oppose stricter penalties for violators of traffic laws?" More than 80% said they were in favor. Seventy percent agreed that drivers who caused accidents should be required to carry special markings on their cars—something akin to the Scarlet Letter. A majority favored compulsory vehicle testing, stricter licensing exams, and fully 90% of those asked favored harsh penalties for drunk drivers. Subsequent polls taken later in the decade showed a remarkable consistency of opinion.[38]

Public interest in combating crashes also is evident in the influence and even minor celebrity status traffic safety experts began to enjoy in the mid-1930s. *Fortune* magazine profiled Miller McClintock, whose Harvard-based Albert Russell Erskine Bureau of Street Traffic Research had developed traffic plans for several major cities, and who wrote the leading textbook on street traffic control.[39,40] *Scientific American* celebrated the work of the Detroit Recorder's Court clinicians in a feature entitled "Insanity at the Wheel."[41] Tales of the Evanston accident investigation squad worthy of the radio crime dramas of the day began to appear in popular magazines such as the *Atlantic Monthly* and *Forum*.[42-44] In *Atlantic Monthly*, one author enthused: "A new kind of detective has begun to unravel a comparatively new kind of crime in the United States. . . . Small boys will hold him in awe and weary men of affairs will regale themselves by reading of his sleuthing. . . . His prey includes storekeepers, dentists, clerks, housewives—the kind of people most of us are. The crimes in which he specializes are those which involve violations of the traffic laws."[45]

Public sentiment had measurable effects beyond mere poll numbers and media attention. Most states adopted driver licensing laws in the 1930s, and many of those with laws on the books added licensing exams.[46] Public school driver education mushroomed in this period, based on studies that showed a two- to threefold reduction in violations and crash involvement for graduates. The automobile insurance industry promoted driver education as a way to improve their bottom line, but support also came from the progressive education establishment, which used safety education to "give vitality to the work of the classroom" and help students develop attitudes necessary for successful modern living.[47–49]

At the height of the Great Depression, automakers and their suppliers responded to public concern by forming the Automotive Safety Foundation. Industry leaders had no newfound zeal for safety, but they did worry that safety crusaders could depress already weakened sales. Also, they wanted to bring the issue of safety to bear in their effort to promote a national network of superhighways. Supporters of highway building championed limited-access, grade-separated routes as safer alternatives to surface streets.[50] Traffic engineers also dreamed of highways in this period. Their cognitive model of traffic as a governable polity of drivers gave way to one that saw traffic as an inanimate fluid. In the new paradigm, congestion is inherently bad and improved volume and flow are inherently good.

Nevertheless, the enormous cost of building safe highways remained an obstacle. Until the economy emerged from depression and war, most superhighways remained mere plans. Through World War II traffic safety experts continued to rely on the far cheaper, if less effective, strategy of driver education and control.

Cold War Traffic Safety—A Golden Age?

In 1953 Congress officially chartered the National Safety Council, giving it the financial and institutional backing of the federal government. In 1954 President Eisenhower convened a White House Conference on Highway Safety and created the President's Action Committee for Traffic Safety to support NSC-coordinated work. Driver education reached the majority of high school students by the 1950s, despite critics who equated it with "underwater basket weaving."[51,52] Faced with the still chronic problem of overworked traffic courts, police turned to new tools such as the portable breath analyzer and the radar gun in order to circumvent the "unreliable" human element, including contradictory witnesses and juries unwilling to convict.[53,19] It may have seemed like a golden age for the existing network of traffic safety experts, but in retrospect one can see the seeds of their undoing. An emerging new breed of safety experts, borrowing a slur from the counter culture, began to criticize the "traffic safety establishment."[3] They promoted federal intervention, safer vehicles, an epidemiological approach to crashes, and administrative adjudication of traffic violations. They premised their reforms on the inevitability of traffic crashes.

The most significant change in the 1950s was the emergence of vehicle design for crash protection. There had been gadflies—a handful of physicians who treated traffic injuries and proposed fixes in the 1930s—but not until after World War II did the idea of making crashes more survivable catch on.[54] Hugh DeHaven, who pioneered the study of aviation crashes during World War II, created the Crash Injury Research project at Cornell University after the war. In 1951, with the help of the Indiana State Police and the NUTI, Cornell researchers turned their attention to automobile crashes.

Automotive engineers quickly responded to DeHaven's finding that car doors often flew open in a crash, fatally ejecting passengers, by quietly developing more secure door latches.[8] Domestic automakers created their own safety departments, though many in the industry continued to reject the premise that motor vehicles were inherently unsafe. Critics such as physician Paul Gikas countered, "This approach is not fatalistic—it is merely realistic."[55] Ford Motor Company went furthest in the pursuit of crash protection, supporting the Cornell studies and using safety as a selling point for 1956. The 1956 bread-and-butter Ford sedan could be purchased with interior padding, a shatter resistant, breakaway rear view mirror, and lap safety belts. The press and public reacted positively, with 43% of buyers choosing the safety upgrade. But in 1956 Chevrolet outsold Ford, leading industry executives to conclude that "safety doesn't sell."[9]

Absent leadership from industry, physicians and farsighted legislators took on unsafe vehicles. Significantly, personal experiences with automobile crashes—not constituent pressure—drew officials such as Senator Paul Douglas of Illinois, Alabama Congressman Kenneth Roberts, and Connecticut's Abraham Ribicoff to the quest for crashworthy cars. In contrast to the 1930s, federal officials in the 1960s became activists, or "policy entrepreneurs."[56,57] Despite a technocratic, nonconfrontational approach, domestic automakers resisted any form of regulation. By 1965, the only progress was a law requiring federally purchased vehicles to have certain safety features.[9]

NHTSA and a New Era of Traffic Safety

Undeterred, Ribicoff, with executive branch support in the person of Assistant Secretary of Labor for Policy Planning Daniel Moynihan, set his subcommittee to investigate automakers' spending on safety. The senators' pointed questions and the revelation of meager industry spending brought media attention. Behind many of the toughest questions was a young committee staffer named Ralph Nader, a pioneer of the consumer movement and product liability doctrine. Success for the reformers came on September 9, 1966, when twin acts created the National Highway Safety Agency and the National Traffic Safety Agency within the Department of Commerce. (These were consolidated into the National Highway Safety Bureau within a year and by 1970 had become the National Highway Traffic Safety Administration within the Department of Transportation.)

Dr. William Haddon, considered by many to be the father of scientific traffic safety, became the agency's first head. He developed the Haddon Matrix, which applies the classic epidemiological triangle to motor vehicle crashes (see Fig. 16.4). Haddon intentionally eschewed the traffic- safety establishment. For example, the agency rebuffed the Northwestern University Traffic Institute, the leader in traffic officer training. NHTSA officials also ignored the work the NUTI had been doing since

1942 with James P. Economos of the American Bar Association. In lieu of the ideas put forward by Economos, NHTSA pursued the administrative adjudication of traffic complaints and torts. Because there were no federal traffic laws, NHTSA used the carrot of federal highway grants to shape state laws. Economos called this use of the grant process "a serious encroachment by the executive branch of the federal government upon the judicial branch of the state court systems."[58]

Although the birth of NHTSA was indeed a watershed in the history of traffic safety, the long historical view reveals striking continuity. Traffic policing and driver education endured, and the automobile and insurance industries continued to shape the agenda as they had in the 1950s. More important, although an epidemiologic approach became ascendant under NHTSA, efforts to reduce traffic crashes remained deeply embedded in complex social realities.

The social context of traffic safety is abundantly clear in the story of the national speed limit. On January 2, 1974, in response to an Arab oil embargo, the president signed the Emergency Highway Energy Conservation Act, creating the 55-mile-per-hour national speed limit. Coincidentally, the limit was a crucial factor in the sharp decrease in traffic deaths. After the gas crisis passed, the national limit was kept in place as a safety measure, and with strict enforcement speeds did fall. But the law helped spark a collective sense that eluding the highway patrol was a noble sport. The CB radio enjoyed a brief vogue, and films such as *Citizen's Band* (1977), *Smokey and the Bandit* (1977), *Convoy*, (1978), and *The Last Chase* (1981) promoted a culture of highway outlaws.

Social context also explains the trouble NHTSA had with seat belts in the 1970s. Seatbelts had been among the first safety items the federal government required, but most Americans did not use them, despite a warning buzzer mandated in 1971. Industry encouraged public reluctance by denigrating safety belts as expensive and even dangerous. NHTSA tightened its grip by requiring an ignition interlock for the 1974 model year. The outcry from industry and the public was loud enough for Congress to intervene against safety regulators. Six congressmen introduced bills, including Washington's Senator Warren G. Magnusson, whose bill, passed in October 1974, "prohibits mandatory federal motor vehicle standards requiring a safety belt interlock system."[59-64] In fact, current U.S. law continues to require specifically that no safety belt warning may be used "except a buzzer that operates only during the 8-second period after the ignition is turned to the 'start' or 'on' position."[66]

Regulating Safety in the Age of Deregulation

The anti-regulatory 1980s saw NHTSA's budget slashed, allowing other parties such as the insurance industry and activists greater control over safety policy. The NHTSA budget was reduced 13% in the first year of the Reagan administration and by 1983 it had been cut in half.[66] The administration also rescinded the "passive restraint" standard NHTSA had developed in the 1970s to force automakers to install air bags. The federal government only restored the standard after losing a suit by consumer groups and the automobile insurance industry in 1983.[67]

In 1984, Transportation Secretary Elizabeth Dole compromised with the recalcitrant auto industry: she set an air bag deadline for model year 1990 but stipulated that the deadline would be lifted if states representing two thirds of the U.S. population enacted mandatory belt usage laws (MULs). Industry spent tens of millions of dollars lobbying states, and most passed MULs. Not only did these maneuvers delay an air bag standard until 1997, they also introduced yet another pretext for traffic stops, just as police use of racial profiling was gaining attention.

With the government reluctant to regulate industry, grass-roots activism emerged as a powerful force. In 1980, Candace Lightner, whose daughter died in an alcohol involved crash, founded Mothers Against Drunk Drivers (MADD). The organization soon had a membership in the hundreds of thousands and financial support from federal, state, and local governments. By 1982 the organization had 100 chapters. With the unimpeachable moral authority of mothers who had lost their children, the group created a public narrative of innocent victim and drunken villain. MADD's most significant achievement was to convince Congress and the president to withhold highway funds from states that did not set a minimum drinking age of 21—the same mechanism NHTSA had used to push for administrative adjudication. By 1975 the majority of states had set 18 as their minimum drinking age, aligned with the new minimum voting age set by the 26th Amendment of the U.S. Constitution. Reagan resisted infringing on states' rights, but Lightner gained the president's ear and his signature on the bill in 1984.

The new laws certainly paid off: from 1982 to 1987, the number of intoxicated drivers involved in fatal crashes fell by 17%; fatal crashes involving teenaged drivers fell by 34%.[68] But to many Americans, the "21" campaign also had the less measurable and more troubling effects. The crusade convinced courts to accept the legality of random police checkpoints to screen for drunk drivers.[69] In balancing public safety with the constitutional proscription against "unreasonable search and seizure," courts relied on statistics gathered by police and safety officials. The statistics used to support these rulings were not always frank. For example, the threshold for labeling a crash alcohol related is typically 10 times lower than the legal threshold for driving under the influence.[70]

Whatever the merits of the policy, the statistical legerdemain resembled that used by the erstwhile traffic safety establishment to support traffic engineering, selective enforcement, and driver education. Moreover, MADD conducted not a public health campaign but a moral crusade that echoed the Prohibition-era attack on automotive vice that had originally established the pattern of traffic law enforcement. For example, although men were roughly three times more likely to be victims of drunk driving, women figured more prominently in MADD publicity. Similarly, although MADD emphasized the tragedy of children dying at the hands of villainous drunk drivers, two thirds of children who die in alcohol-related crashes are in fact being driven by a drunk driver.[71] In other words, emotional appeals continued to play an important role in policy making even in the modern, epidemiological era.

Another corner of the old ways showed incredible resilience in the 1980s as well. NHTSA-funded studies to determine the effectiveness of public high school driver education, including a definitive study in DeKalb County, Georgia, that found that driver's education had no impact on accident involvement or violation frequencies.

These findings were supported by studies in Great Britain, Canada, Australia, and Scandinavia.[72–75] Paradoxically, because driver education tends to lower the age at which individuals obtain their licenses, the study showed a net increase in overall deaths and injuries. Some school districts dropped the popular class and some insurers eliminated the rate reduction they had offered for course completion.

By the end of the 1980s, however, driver's ed had rebounded. Proponents of driver's education classes argued that proving or disproving their effectiveness was almost impossible because accidents are such exceedingly rare events. Opponents such as Edward Tenney and Ralph Nader had argued since the 1960s that the otherwise useless class served only to line the pockets of textbook publishers and driving-simulator manufacturers.[3,51] A less conspiratorial explanation is that driver's ed still provides an ideal venue for life adjustment education and the promotion of good citizenship.[76,77] For example, the carrot of unhindered mobility and the threat of violent death make driver's education an ideal site for socializing adolescents and discouraging substance abuse. There has been a big change from the old language of moral rectitude to today's emphasis on healthy choices, but the message remains the same.

During the 1990s, with its budget still bumping along at little more than half its 1980 levels, NHTSA embraced driver behavior as the new frontier in traffic safety. The most significant reason for the return of attention to the driver is the great success achieved by the passive engineering advancements in vehicle and road design. Although they would continue to lobby against new safety regulations—indeed, against any new regulations in the 1990s—car makers had finally concluded that safety does in fact sell. This grudging acceptance is a function of many things, including government action, increased competition in a global vehicle marketplace, and consumer demand.[78] Just as decades before, when four-wheel brakes and electric starters became the norm, crumple zones, safety belts, and air bags are now embedded in vehicle design. Vehicle advertisements, particularly those for family vehicles, routinely tout government and insurance industry crash ratings and even show simulated crash tests.

The strategy once ridiculed as the "nut behind the wheel" concept of traffic safety returned to the fore as a central element of the balanced approach to 1990s traffic safety. Road rage, aggressive driving, and driver distraction are simply new terms for the age old bogeyman, bad driving. In part, the renewed emphasis on the driver reflects the same realities that shaped education-based worker safety efforts pioneered by the NSC. Education and deterrence remain far cheaper than increasingly complex vehicle and roadway engineering for safety while providing a tool of social control.

In the 1990s, the controversy over air bags highlighted the limits of passive engineering solutions. Federally mandated air bags began killing children in 1993. A series of interim solutions proved to be bureaucratic and public-relations nightmares. Interestingly, NHTSA ultimately adopted a behavioral solution alongside mandating improved technology. The government supported a recommendation that children always be placed in the back seat and with industry cooperation began a public safety campaign. As it did after the failure of safety belt interlocks, the agency recognized the limits of passive technology and shifted its focus from the machine to the user. Libertarians and other critics of the safety establishment had a field day.[79]

Perhaps the most troubling element of a renewed emphasis on driver behavior is the continuing racial bias in traffic law enforcement. Beyond the racism evidenced in municipal traffic court clinics, police have long used the traffic code for non-safety-related purposes, including targeting minorities. For example, during the famous 1956 civil rights bus boycott in Montgomery, Alabama, police used the traffic code to try to break the strike and arrest its leaders, including Martin Luther King.[80] Many in the African-American community long ago concluded that "driving while black" is itself a traffic offense, even though law enforcement has generated statistics supporting that claim only very recently.[81,82] Consent decrees involving the state police of New Jersey and the Maryland state police show that profiling is a widespread and ongoing problem.[83] Traffic code enforcement can, of course, serve as an effective dragnet; police enforcing the traffic code have caught killers from the Son of Sam (parking tickets) to the Oklahoma City Bomber (failure to display a license plate) and countless other dangerous criminals. Although concepts of vice have certainly changed, these uses and abuses of traffic law enforcement demonstrate that it continues to do more than merely promote motor traffic safety.

The Real Public Health Cost of the Automobile

The simple but often overlooked foundation of the chronic public health problem posed by the automobile is that Americans drive so much. One common public health strategy is to use education and regulation to reduce exposure to infectious agents or unhealthy environments. Reducing the number of vehicle miles traveled could easily become a useful part of the public health attack on injury and death from traffic crashes. Public health officials emphasize risk behaviors such as failing to wear a seat belt and driving under the influence of alcohol. But riding in automobiles—even being near automobiles—is itself a health hazard. Why not encourage people to drive less? The most obvious reason is that public health officials have internalized the traffic engineering ethos that developed around World War II—that mobility is a goal to be balanced against safety. But aside from a certain wanderlust, no one actually desires mobility per se. People want easy and broad access to the resources of daily life. Although today we must equate that access with automobility, history shows us compelling alternatives.

Certainly many powerful interests, such as automakers and home builders, and many individual Americans prefer automobile-dependant communities. Furthermore, the motor car and open road remain powerful icons in American culture. But the automobile's critics too have failed to examine traffic safety in historical context. For example, Deborah Gordon of the Union of Concerned Scientists (and now director of the Next Generation of Transportation Strategies Project at Yale University) argues that "environmental quality, energy efficiency, and aesthetics deserve as much attention in transportation policy debates as personal freedom, convenience, and safety."[84] Considering a reduction in VMTs as a way to reduce the death toll would move safety to the first half of Gordon's equation.

In this age of narrow expertise, public health officials may be timid about venturing into the wider world of transportation planning. But if transportation and land-use planning do indeed have a direct impact on morbidity and mortality, it makes sense for public health officials to engage these topics directly. History shows that motor traffic safety has always been a complex social undertaking rather than a merely technical or epidemiologic pursuit. Acknowledging and coming to terms with that complexity through historical study provides a more, not less, scientific picture of traffic safety.

The roads of the United States are now safer than those of most other nations. At great cost we have achieved the extremely low fatality rate of 1.5 deaths per every 100 million vehicle miles traveled. That encouraging news is offset by the fact that current trends show Americans driving more than 3 trillion miles by 2010. At that rate, more than 45,000 Americans—often very young Americans—will die in motor vehicle crashes and millions more will be injured each year.[85]

References

1. Wald ML. Anger cited in 28,000 road deaths a year. *New York Times*, 18 July 1997.
2. James L. Testimony before the Surface Transportation Sub-committee of the U.S. House of Representatives. Road rage: Causes and dangers of aggressive driving. Publication no. 105-34, 129–33. Available at: http://commdocs.house.gov/committees/Trans/hpw105-34.000/hpw105-34_0f.htm. Accessed 28 April 2006.
3. Nader R. Unsafe at Any Speed: The Designed in Dangers of the American Automobile. New York: Grossman Publishers, 1965.
4. Tarr JA. Urban pollution—many long years ago. *American Heritage* 1971:22(6):65–69, 106.
5. H. H. Bliss killed? *New York Times,* 15 September 1899.
6. McShane C. Down the Asphalt Path: The Automobile and the American City. New York: Columbia University Press, 1994.
7. Berger ML. The Devil Wagon in God's Country: The Automobile and Social Change in Rural America, 1893–1929. Hamden, CT: Archon Books, 1979.
8. Flink JJ. America Adopts the Automobile: 1895–1910. Cambridge, MA: MIT Press, 1970.
9. Eastman JW. Styling versus Safety. Lanham, MD: University Press of America, 1984.
10. Berry CP. Law of Automobiles. Chicago: Callahan & Company, 1921.
11. Kline RR. Consumers in the Country: Technology and Social Change in Rural America. Baltimore: Johns Hopkins University Press, 2000.
12. Langum DJ. Crossing over the Line: Legislating Morality and the Mann Act. Chicago: University of Chicago Press, 1994.
13. Monkkonen EH. Police in Urban America 1860–1920. Cambridge. Cambridge University Press, 1981.
14. Fogelson RM. Big-city Police. Cambridge, MA: Harvard University Press, 1977.
15. Burgess RL. Can you get a square deal in traffic court? *American Magazine,* 19 December 1932, 11.
16. McShane C. Transforming the use of urban space: a look at the revolution in street pavements, 1880–1924. *Journal of Urban History* 1979:5:291–96.
17. French PH. The Automobile Compensation Plan: A Solution for Some Problems of Court Congestion and Accident Litigation in New York State. New York: Columbia University Press, 1933.
18. Green L. Traffic Victims: Tort Law and Insurance. Evanston, IL: Northwestern University Press, 1958.
19. Kalven H, Zeisel H. The American Jury. Boston: Little Brown, 1966.
20. Stone RR. The History of the Industrial Safety Movement in the United States. Madison: University of Wisconsin, 1932.

21. Aldrich M. Safety First. Baltimore: Johns Hopkins University Press, 1997.
22. Leonard K, Roy M. Interview with Franklin M. Kreml, conducted 3 January 1991. Northwestern University Archives, Accession 283: 91–44, Tape 1, Side A.
23. Hoover H. First National Conference on Street and Highway Safety. Washington, DC: Department of Commerce, 1924.
24. Moss FA. Your Mind in Action: Applications of Psychology. Boston: Houghton Mifflin, 1929.
25. Raphael T, Lavine AC, Flinn HL, Hoffman LW. 100 traffic offenders. Ment Hyg 1929: 13:809–24.
26. Selling LS. The physician and the traffic problem. JAMA 1937:108:93–95.
27. Albert D. Psychotechnology and insanity at the wheel. JHBS 1999:35(3):291–305.
28. Annual Reports. Chicago: Municipal Court of Chicago, 1924–1928.
29. Lefebvre H. La vie quotidienne dans le monde moderne. Paris: Gallimard, 1968.
30. Lynd RS. Middletown in Transition. New York: Harcourt Brace, 1937.
31. Kennedy ED. The Automobile Industry: The Coming of Age of Capitalism's Favorite Child. New York: Reynal & Hitchcock, 1941.
32. Bix AS. Inventing Ourselves out of Jobs: America's Debate over Technological Unemployment, 1929–1981. Baltimore: Johns Hopkins University Press, 2000.
33. Bourke-White M. At the time of the Louisville flood. Life, 22,1937.
34. Wood G. Death on the Ridge Road. Williams College Museum of Art; 1935; oil on masonite; Accession No. 47.1.3.
35. Nash AJB. Death on the Highway: The Automobile Wreck in American Culture, 1920–1940. Minneapolis: University of Minnesota Press, 1983.
36. Heidenry J. Theirs was the Kingdom: Lila and Dewitt Wallace and the Story of the Readers Digest. New York: WW Norton, 1993.
37. Furnas JC. And sudden death. Reader's Digest 1935:27(160):21–26.
38. Gallup GH. The Gallup Poll: Public Opinion 1935–1971. New York: Random House, 1972.
39. Unfit for modern motor traffic. Fortune 1936:14:90 ff.
40. McClintock M. Street Traffic Control. New York: McGraw-Hill, 1925.
41. Boone AR. Insanity at the wheel. Sci Am 1939:161(4):199–201.
42. Forster AR. Safe streets sans sentiment Evanston, Ill. Rotarian 1937:50:45–47.
43. Peters RH. Death on the Highway I. Forum 1935:93:79–82.
44. Peters RH. Death on the Highway II. Forum 1935:93:179–83.
45. Billings C: Traffic crimes and criminals. Atlantic Monthly 1933:152:454–61.
46. Highway Statistics Summary to 1985. Washington, DC: U.S. Department of Transportation, Federal Highway Administration, 1985.
47. Payne EG. Education in Accident Prevention. Chicago: Lyons and Carnahan, 1919.
48. Payne EG. Contemporary accidents and their non-reduction. J Ed Soc 1937:11:21.
49. Tenney E. Highway Jungle: The Story of the Public Safety Movement and the Failure of Driver Education in the Public Schools. New York: Exposition Press, 1962.
50. Hoffman PG. Seven Roads to Safety: A Program to Reduce Automobile Accidents. New York: Harper & Brothers, 1939.
51. Cutter WA, Rogers VM. Driver education: the case for life. Am School Board J 1958:145: 23.
52. Key N. Status of Driver Education in the U.S. Washington: National Commission of Safety Education of the NEA, 1960.
53. Kalven H. The jury in auto cases: an invitation to research. Virginia Law Weekly 1956:8:1–4.
54. Eastman JW. Doctor's orders: the American medical profession and the origins of automobile design for crash protection, 1930–1955. Bull Hist Med 1981:55(3):407–24.

55. Gikas PW. Crashworthiness as a cultural ideal. In: Lewis DL, Goldstein L, eds. The Automobile and American Culture. Ann Arbor: University of Michigan Press, 1981:323–339.
56. Balogh B. Reorganizing the organizational synthesis: federal-professional relations in modern America. *Studies in American Political Development* 1991:(5):119–72.
57. Wilson JQ. The politics of regulation. In: Wilson JQ, ed. The Politics of Regulation. New York: Basic Books, 1980:357–394.
58. Economos JP, Steelman D. Traffic Court Procedure and Administration. Chicago: American Bar Association, 1983.
59. Buckley-S2863 J. A bill to amend the National Traffic and Motor Vehicle Safety Act of 1966 in order to provide that certain seatbelt standards shall not be required under such act; 1974.
60. Clark-HR16732. A bill to amend the National Traffic and Motor Vehicle Safety Act of 1966 with respect to certain seatbelt standards under such act; 1974.
61. Collins-HR9600. A bill to amend the National Traffic and Motor Vehicle Safety Act of 1966 to prohibit the Secretary of Transportation from imposing certain safety standards, and for other purposes; 1973.
62. Magnusson-S355. A bill to amend the National Traffic and Motor Vehicle Safety Act of 1966 to provide for remedies of defects without charge; 1974.
63. Moss-HR5529. A bill to amend the National Traffic and Motor Vehicle Safety Act of 1966 to authorize appropriations for the fiscal years 1974, 1975, and 1976, to provide for the recall of certain defective motor vehicles without charge to the owners thereof, and for other purposes; 1973.
64. Wyman-HR10277. A bill to amend the National Traffic and Motor Vehicle Safety Act of 1966 to prohibit the Secretary of Transportation from imposing certain seat belt standards, and for other purposes; 1973.
65. Public Law 103–272 § 30124, 1994.
66. Montero R. NHTSA Historical funding data file. Personal communication with the author, 7 February 2002.
67. *Motor Vehicle Manufacturers Association of the United States, Inc., et al. v. State Farm Mutual Automobile Insurance Co. et al.* 103 S. Ct. 2856, 1983.
68. Premature mortality due to alcohol related motor vehicle traffic fatalities—United States, 1987. *MMWR 1988*:37:753–755.
69. *Michigan Department of State Police et. al, Petitioners v. Rick Sitz et al.* 496 U.S. 444, 1990.
70. Lanza-Kaduce L, Bishop DM. Criminology: legal fictions and criminology: the jurisprudence of drunk driving. *J Criminal Law & Criminology* 1986:77:358–78.
71. Quinlan KP, Brewer RD, Sleet DA, Dellinger AM. Characteristics of child passenger deaths and injuries involving drinking drivers. *JAMA* 2000:17:2249–52.
72. Horneman C. Driver Education and Training: A Review of the Literature. Armidale, Australia: Roads and Traffic Authority, 1993.
73. Lund AK, Williams AF, Zador P. High school driver education: further evaluation of the DeKalb County Study. *Acc Analy and Prev* 1986:18(4):349–57.
74. Robertson LS, Zador, PL. Driver Education and Fatal Crash Involvement. Washington, DC: Insurance Institute for Highway Safety, 1978.
75. Mutch D. Collision course: what's happened since driver's ed hit the skids. *Washington Post,* 18 May, 1997:C1-C2.
76. Stock, JR, Weaver JK, Ray HW, Brink JR, Sadof MG. Evaluation of Safe Performance Secondary School Driver Education Curriculum Demonstration Project. Washington, DC: National Highway Traffic Safety Administration, U.S. Department of Transportation, 1983.

77. Robertson LS. Driver education: the mix of science and ideology. *Bull NY Acad Med* 1988:64(7):617–22.
78. Altshuler A, et al. The Future of the Automobile: The Report of MIT's International Automobile Program. Cambridge, MA: MIT Press, 1984.
79. Gladwell M. Wrong turn: How the fight to make America's highways safer went off course. *New Yorker,* 11 June 2001, 50–61.
80. Robinson JAG. The Montgomery Bus Boycott and the Women Who Started it: The Memoir of Jo Ann Gibson Robinson. Knoxville: University of Tennessee Press, 1987.
81. Maclin T. Can a traffic offense be DWB (driving while black)? *Los Angeles Times,* 9 March 1997: M2.
82. Meeks K. Driving While Black: Highways, Shopping Malls, Taxicabs, Sidewalks: How to Fight Back if You Are a Victim of Racial Profiling. New York: Broadway Books, 2000.
83. Institute on Race and Justice, Northeastern University Racial Profiling Data Collection Resource Center. Available from: http://www.racialprofilinganalysis.neu.edu2004. Accessed 3 February 2004.
84. Gordon D. Sustainable transportation: what do we mean and how do we get there? In: Sperling D, Shaheen SA. Transportation and Energy: Strategies for a Sustainable Transportation System. Berkeley: American Council for an Energy-Efficient Economy, 1995:1–11.
85. Highway statistics, 2002. Washington, DC: U.S.Department of Transportation, Federal Highway Administration, 2003.

Suggested Reading

Brottman, Mikita. Car Crash Culture. New York, N.Y.: Palgrave, 2002.
Gikas PW. Crashworthiness as a cultural ideal. In: Lewis DL, Goldstein L, eds. The Automobile and American culture. Ann Arbor: University of Michigan Press, 1981.
McShane C. Down the Asphalt Path: The Automobile and the American City. New York: Columbia University Press, 1994.
Welke, Barbara Young. Recasting American liberty: Gender, race, law, and the railroad revolution, *1865–1920.* Cambridge: Cambridge University Press, 2001.

PART IX

CARDIOVASCULAR DISEASE

18

Heart Disease and Stroke Mortality in the Twentieth Century

KURT J. GREENLUND

WAYNE H. GILES

NORA L. KEENAN

ANN MARIE MALARCHER

ZHI JIE ZHENG

MICHELE L. CASPER

GREGORY W. HEATH

JANET B. CROFT

Heart disease has been the leading cause of death in the United States since 1921, and stroke has been the third leading cause since 1938.[1] Heart disease and stroke account for most cardiovascular disease (CVD) deaths, and in 1998 they accounted for approximately 40% of all deaths in the United States and were substantial causes of disability and impaired quality of life. Although heart disease and stroke remain leading causes of death in the United States, age-adjusted death rates from all CVD have declined by 55% since 1950. This decline reflects an increased understanding of the causes of CVD, identification of the risk factors, developments in the treatment of heart disease and stroke and their major risk factors, and implementation of intervention and prevention programs. This chapter summarizes the trends in heart disease and stroke in the twentieth century, advances in the understanding of the risks for these diseases, and development of prevention and intervention programs to reduce the risks of developing and dying from heart disease and stroke.

Trends in Heart Disease and Stroke

During the past 100 years, the United States experienced both a dramatic rise and a dramatic decline in death rates from heart disease (Fig. 18.1). At the beginning of the twentieth century, heart disease was the fourth leading cause of death in the United States.[2] However, by 1921, heart disease had become the leading cause of death, and rates continued to increase into the 1950s. During this time, the percentage of deaths caused by cardiovascular diseases increased among persons of all ages, sexes, and races (categorized as white and nonwhite in the first half of the twentieth century).[2] In the latter half of the 1900s, however, CVD-associated deaths dramatically declined. Age-adjusted death rates per 100,000 persons (standardized to the 2000 U.S. population) for diseases of the heart (i.e., ischemic or coronary heart disease, hypertensive heart disease, and rheumatic heart disease) decreased from a peak of 586.8 in 1950 to 272.4 in 1998, an overall decline of 54%.[1,3] Age-adjusted death rates for ischemic or coronary heart disease (the most common form of CVD) continued to increase into the 1960s, but then declined to 172.8 by 1998. Age-adjusted death rates for stroke declined throughout the century, from 180.7 in 1950 to 59.6 in 1998, representing a 67% decline.[3]

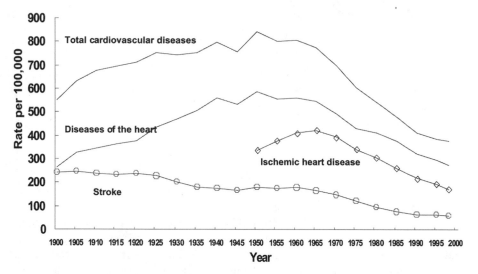

Figure 18.1. Age-adjusted mortality rates for total cardiovascular diseases, diseases of the heart, coronary heart disease, and stroke, 1900–1998. Rates are standardized to the 2000 U.S. population. Diseases are classified according to International Classification of Diseases (ICD) codes in use when the deaths were reported. ICD classification revisions occurred in 1910, 1921, 1930, 1939, 1949, 1958, 1968, 1979. Death rates prior to 1933 do not include all states. Comparability ratios were applied to rates for 1970 and 1975. (National Heart, Lung and Blood Institute. Morbidity & Mortality: 2000 Chartbook. Rockville, MD: U.S. Department of Health and Human Services, 2000; National Center for Health Statistics. Health, United States, 2001. Hyattsville MD: U.S. Department of Health and Human Services, 2001.)

Mortality data are the primary surveillance tool for monitoring heart disease and stroke. To assess trends in death rates over time, many factors must be considered, including reporting and classification of causes of death, selection of measurements for reporting, and reporting of demographic information. However, the categories for reporting and classifying deaths have changed over time, and these changes may influence trends in death rates. Numerous revisions have been made to the International Classification of Diseases (ICD; in 1910, 1921, 1930, 1939, 1949, 1958, 1968, and 1979), and causes of death are coded according to the version used during a particular year (Fig. 18.1). The ICD was last revised in 1999.

Other factors contribute to inconsistencies in reporting. All states did not begin to report deaths until 1933.[4] In addition, demographic information (e.g., age, sex, race, and ethnicity) are reported on death certificates by funeral directors based on observation or information with which they are provided, usually by family members. Therefore, assessment of trends by these demographics is dependent on the accuracy of the reporting.

Death rates per 100,000 persons are given in Figure 18.1 rather than actual numbers to account for the changing population size and the changing age distribution of the U.S. population. In 1940, the U.S. population was 132 million, which more than doubled to 270 million by 1998. Although rates per 100,000 persons have dramatically declined, the actual number of deaths caused by all cardiovascular diseases increased from 745,074 in 1950 to 948,572 in 1998 reflecting the population increase.[1,5] Deaths from ischemic heart disease increased from 321,003 in 1950 to 459,841 in 1998, and stroke deaths rose from 156,751 in 1950 to 158,448 in 1998.[3,5] However, had the rate for ischemic heart disease remained the same in 1998 as it was at its peak in the 1960s, an additional 684,000 ischemic heart disease deaths would have occurred.[1]

Death rates are also age-adjusted to a standard population to account for the differing age structure of the population over time. Crude rates (i.e., deaths per 100,000 population, not age-standardized) did not decline as dramatically after 1950. In 1940, the percentage of Americans aged ≥65 years was only 6.8%, but this percentage almost doubled to 12.7% by 1998. Traditionally, government statistics have used the 1940 standard population for age adjustment. However, the data presented in this chapter are adjusted to the 2000 U.S. population, which is the new standard in use. Compared with the 1940 U.S. standard population, the 2000 population age adjustment places more weight on deaths among persons aged ≥65 years because the number of persons in this age group is increasing. As a result, death rates using the 2000 population age adjustment are much higher than when adjusted to the 1940 standard. The overall age-adjusted trends using either adjustment, however, are similar to those shown in Figure 18.1.[1,3]

Overall rates mask differences in heart disease and stroke mortality by sex and race/ethnicity (Tables 18.1 and 18.2). Although rates of CVD are lower for women than men overall, more women than men have died of CVD in every year since 1984.[6] Data on race/ethnicity other than white and black have only recently been collected on death certificates.[3] Only 17 states collected data on Hispanic origin in 1985; however, by 1990, a total of 47 states (plus District of Columbia.) collected this data and encompassed greater than 99% of the Hispanic population. Death rates by race/ethnicity are

Table 18.1. Death rates from heart diseases,* by sex and race-ethnicity—United States, 1980–1998.

Group[†]	Rate per 100,000				
	1980	1985	1990	1995	1998
Women					
All, age-adjusted rate[§]	320.8	294.5	257.0	239.7	223.1
Crude rate	305.1	305.2	281.8	278.8	268.3
Caucasian, age-adjusted rate	315.9	289.1	250.9	233.6	217.6
Crude rate	319.2	321.8	298.4	297.4	286.8
African American, age-adjusted rate	378.6	357.7	327.5	309.3	291.9
Crude rate	249.7	250.3	237.0	231.1	224.6
American Indian-Alaska Native, age-adjusted rate	175.4	170.0	153.1	145.8	127.8
Crude rate	80.3	84.3	77.5	87.0	89.0
Asian and Pacific Islander, age-adjusted rate	132.3	149.4	149.2	153.2	120.9
Crude rate	57.0	60.3	62.0	68.2	67.3
Hispanic, age-adjusted rate	—	195.9	177.2	162.5	145.8
Crude rate	—	75.0	79.4	78.9	77.7
Men					
All, age-adjusted rate	538.9	488.0	412.4	372.7	336.6
Crude rate	368.6	344.1	297.6	282.7	268.0
Caucasian, age-adjusted rate	539.6	487.3	409.2	368.4	333.2
Crude rate	384.0	360.3	312.7	297.9	283.1
African American, age-adjusted rate	561.4	533.9	485.4	449.2	407.8
Crude rate	301.0	288.6	256.8	244.2	230.5
American Indian-Alaska Native, age-adjusted rate	320.5	280.5	264.1	230.5	219.5
Crude rate	130.6	117.9	108.0	110.4	113.2
Asian and Pacific Islander, age-adjusted rate	286.9	258.9	220.7	247.2	197.9
Crude rate	119.8	103.5	88.7	96.9	98.3
Hispanic, age-adjusted rate	—	296.6	270.0	246.8	213.8
Crude rate	—	92.1	91.0	87.5	84.9

Source: Reference 3.

*Codes 390–398, 402, 404–429 from the International Classification of Diseases, Ninth Revision.
[†]Rates for Caucasians, African Americans, American Indian/ Alaska Native, and Asian/ Pacific Islander include Hispanics. Rates for Hispanics include any race.
[§]Age adjusted to the 2000 U.S. standard population.

also dependent on accurate reporting of race/ethnicity on death certificates and on accurate population counts, which serve as the denominator for rates. An analysis examining the reporting of race/ethnicity and population counts suggests that heart disease-related death rates might be substantially higher for certain groups, particularly American Indians/Alaska Natives (21% higher) and Asians and Pacific Islanders (11% higher).[7]

Table 18.2. Death rates from stroke,* by sex and race-ethnicity—United States, 1980–1998.

Group[†]	Rate Per 100,000				
	1980	1985	1990	1995	1998
Women					
All, age-adjusted rate[§]	91.9	73.5	62.7	61.5	58.3
Crude rate	86.1	75.5	68.6	71.7	70.4
Caucasian, age-adjusted rate	89.2	70.9	60.5	59.5	56.6
Crude rate	88.8	78.4	71.8	76.0	75.0
African American, age-adjusted rate	119.8	99.4	84.0	81.0	75.3
Crude rate	77.9	68.6	60.7	60.4	57.9
American Indian-Alaska Native, age-adjusted rate	51.6	44.8	38.4	40.3	39.9
Crude rate	22.1	21.8	19.3	23.8	25.4
Asian and Pacific Islander, age-adjusted rate	61.0	54.8	54.9	53.4	45.6
Crude rate	26.5	23.3	24.3	24.9	26.4
Hispanic, age-adjusted rate	—	47.6	43.9	40.1	36.0
Crude rate	—	18.3	20.2	20.1	19.6
Men					
All, age-adjusted rate	102.4	80.2	68.7	66.3	60.1
Crude rate	63.6	52.5	46.8	48.0	46.3
Caucasian, age-adjusted rate	99.0	77.4	65.7	63.2	57.6
Crude rate	63.3	52.7	47.0	48.6	47.3
African American, age-adjusted rate	142.1	112.7	102.5	96.7	86.3
Crude rate	73.1	59.2	53.1	51.0	47.5
American Indian-Alaska Native, age-adjusted rate	66.9	48.6	44.3	44.6	34.0
Crude rate	23.2	18.5	16.0	20.1	16.6
Asian and Pacific Islander, age-adjusted rate	71.4	65.2	59.1	73.7	57.3
Crude rate	28.7	24.0	23.4	28.6	28.1
Hispanic, age-adjusted rate	—	57.5	46.5	48.5	43.1
Crude rate	—	17.2	15.6	17.2	17.4

Source: Reference 3.

*Codes 430–438 from the International Classification of Diseases, Ninth Revision.
[†]Rates for Caucasians, African Americans, American Indian/ Alaska Native, and Asian/ Pacific Islander include Hispanics. Rates for Hispanics include any race.
[§]Age adjusted to the 2000 U.S. standard population.

Whether the dramatic increase and then decline in death rates from CVD over the last century were true changes or caused by methodologic changes in mortality data over time has been investigated.[8] A 1979 national conference examined the trends in heart disease in the United States and other countries.[9] A conclusion was reached that the observed trends were real because the total mortality rate was also declining. Mortality trends in related causes of death (to which heart disease deaths might have been assigned) further suggested that changes in reporting of deaths did not account for the decline.[9]

Disease Epidemiology

Before the 1940s, knowledge about CVD was primarily obtained from clinical observation; cardiovascular epidemiology had not yet emerged as a focused endeavor. Early in the twentieth century, Sir William Osler and other clinicians noted from observation of their clinic populations that certain factors were associated with heart disease including advanced age, male gender, hypertension, and diabetes.[10] In 1912, James Herrick described the clinical features of acute myocardial infarction.[11] Researchers in the field of geographic pathology highlighted cross-country variation in heart disease and suggested that dietary patterns may contribute to this type of disease.[12-14] Intensive investigation into the CVD epidemic largely began in the 1940s after World War II. The first epidemiologic studies sought to identify factors associated with population or group differences and factors that increased heart disease risk among certain persons within populations. Landmark cross-population investigations included the Seven Countries Study by Ancel Keys,[15] which involved about 12,000 men in Finland, Greece, Italy, Japan, the Netherlands, Yugoslavia, and the United States—countries with differing rates of ischemic heart disease. The Ni-Hon-San Study of three cohorts of Japanese men living in Japan, Hawaii, and California examined factors related to population differences in heart disease (highest among those living in California) and stroke (highest among those living in Japan).[16] The Framingham Study in Massachusetts[17] and several worker-based studies in Chicago[14] examined factors associated with increased risk within study populations. Cross-country and cross-population studies were particularly important for highlighting lifestyle-related differences in the etiology of CVD. These studies established high blood cholesterol, high blood pressure, and smoking and dietary factors (particularly high dietary cholesterol, fat, and sodium intake) as primary risk factors for heart disease and stroke. (Chapter 19 provides information regarding the debate concerning the role of cholesterol in heart disease.) The risk factor concept (i.e., the association of particular biologic, lifestyle, and social conditions with increased risk for disease) evolved from CVD epidemiology[13,14] and highlighted the multi-factorial etiologies of heart disease and stroke. Interestingly, many of these studies are still active, some 50 years after they were initiated, and many have progressed beyond documenting mortality. For example, the Framingham study now also has a component examining heart disease and stroke in the offspring of the original participants.[18] The Chicago Western Electric study demonstrated that a low cardiovascular risk-factor profile in middle adult life is associated with lower Medicare costs in later adult life.[19] Study samples from several community-based epidemiologic studies have also been aggregated to examine genetic and non-genetic determinants of coronary heart disease (CHD), atherosclerosis, and cardiovascular risk factors in relation to family history.[20]

In the United States, the National Heart Institute (now the National Heart, Lung, and Blood Institute) was established by Congress in 1948 and began collaboration with the now well-known Framingham Heart Study. By 1959, the first major recommendations for reducing and preventing heart disease had been developed.[21,22] By the end of the twentieth century, epidemiologic studies of persons of all ages had identified risk factors and risk behaviors beginning in childhood and extending into older adulthood.[12,22]

In addition to commonly known risk factors, other factors related to heart disease and stroke included socioeconomic status, obesity, and level of physical activity. Early evidence offered by Osler suggested that heart disease was an affliction of the well-to-do in the United States during the first part of the century;[10] early epidemiologic studies supported this hypothesis.[23] However, by the end of the century, this trend had reversed, with lower socioeconomic classes having higher rates of heart disease.[24,25] The causes of such a socioeconomic shift in CVD are unknown. Some researchers suggest that upon identification of lifestyle-associated factors associated with heart disease and stroke, (i.e., dietary fat and cholesterol intake and tobacco use), persons with greater resources were better able to adopt healthier lifestyles associated with improved cardiovascular health than were those of lower socioeconomic status. The association of socioeconomic status with health also is shaped by the social context within which people live, including health-care access and utilization, the physical environment, and level of social support.

Adiposity and physical activity levels are associated with the development of heart diseases and stroke through their effects on certain risk factors (e.g., blood pressure and blood cholesterol levels). Results from studies examining the independent effects of these factors on CVD mortality have been mixed, however, partly because of differing definitions of obesity (e.g., weight relative to height, total body mass, central adiposity, and visceral versus subcutaneous fat) and physical activity (e.g., exercise levels, occupational activity, leisure time activity, housework, and aerobic versus strength training).[22,26,27] Nonetheless, researchers concur that these factors play a role in CVD mortality; many guidelines note the importance of obesity and physical inactivity to the development of cardiovascular diseases.[28,29]

Because death rates from stroke continually declined throughout the twentieth century, more epidemiologic research was devoted to heart disease than to stroke. However, many of the risk factors for stroke are similar to those for heart disease. Risk factors for stroke include hypertension, myocardial infarction, atrial fibrillation, diabetes, adverse blood lipids, asymptomatic carotid artery stenosis, cigarette smoking, alcohol use, physical inactivity, and dietary factors.[30] Risk for stroke in the United States also varies by geographic region; although the geographic variation in stroke mortality in the United States was not investigated until the 1960s,[22] high rates of stroke mortality among the southeastern states (known as the Stroke Belt) are now well recognized.

Approaches to Prevention

In response to the identification of risk factors for heart disease and stroke, intervention studies were conducted beginning in the mid-1900s to establish whether lowering risk-factor levels would reduce risk for CVD.[12–14] Studies in both Europe and the United States focused on diet, blood pressure, cholesterol, and multiple risk factors in both persons and communities.[22] Veterans Administration studies conducted in the 1960s demonstrated that lowering high diastolic blood pressure by medication resulted in fewer cases of stroke, cardiac failure, and worsening hypertension.[31,32] The National Diet-Heart Study initiated by the U.S. National Heart Institute in the early 1960s demonstrated the feasibility of dietary modification for primary prevention.[33] With the demonstration that risk factors could be modified, widespread community interventions were developed abroad (e.g., North Karelia, Finland) and within the United States (e.g., California, Minnesota, and Rhode Island).[34] The Centers for Disease Control and Prevention also carried out community demonstration projects in Missouri and South Carolina.[34] Population-based interventions and health promotion studies have been conducted in numerous settings, including schools, worksites, religious organizations, health-care settings, and entire communities. In 1996, evidence for the effectiveness of the various population-based programs that could be undertaken in community settings was reviewed.[35] As a result of population-based evidence, the theoretical background for health promotion was established to include both individual behavioral change as well as change at the community level.[36]

Recent efforts in prevention and risk reduction focus on the development of policy and environmental interventions that can influence populations and promote health (e.g., tobacco control, nutrition, and physical activity).[37-40] Over the past century, efforts to reduce the burden of heart disease and stroke have benefited from a combination of the high-risk approach (i.e., interventions aimed at persons with increased risk for heart disease and stroke) and the population-wide approach (i.e., interventions aimed at lowering risk for the entire community).[41] These approaches are complementary. Most heart disease and stroke events in a population with high rates occur among persons without extreme risk factor levels.[41] Therefore, whereas individual risk can be lowered by the high-risk approach, overall population risk may not be affected. Conversely, the population approach aimed at lowering average risk factor levels for the population will lower risk for the entire population and can result in the aversion of numerous deaths, although any particular person's risk may not be substantially influenced.[41] The combination of approaches has resulted in prevention and risk-reduction strategies through health promotion and risk behavior change; early detection, treatment and control; availability of more effective drugs for risk-factor control; improved technology for early detection; and health-care (e.g., preventive services) and environmental (e.g., tobacco regulations) policies that influence health outcomes.

Prevention strategies focus on all levels of risk, including prevention of the development of the risk factors, preventing a first event among persons with established risk factors, and preventing a subsequent event among persons with established cardiovascular disease. Several national programs aimed at the general public, patients and health-care providers combine the population and high-risk approaches; these programs include the National High Blood Pressure Education Program,[42,43] initiated in 1972, and the National Cholesterol Education Program, initiated in 1985.[44,45] In a 1993 report, the National High Blood Pressure Education Program emphasized the primary prevention of hypertension through interventions involving the general population and those aimed at persons in high-risk groups.[42] Strategies to accomplish this goal included public education on the role of lifestyle, education programs for the food industry and food service institutions, and education and support programs for health-care professionals. Like the National High Blood Pressure Education Program, the National Cholesterol Education Program guidelines for lowering blood cholesterol levels include a population approach and provide information regarding the detection and treatment of high blood cholesterol in individuals.[44] Strategies for individual and population change include public education and altering the availability, purchase, preparation, and consumption of particular foods. Recent recommendations from the third Adult Treatment Panel of the National Cholesterol Education Program included information regarding the assessment of disease risk based on the evidence from the major epidemiologic studies. Specifically, recommendations for assessing initiation of cholesterol treatment now include calculating a patient's 10-year risk of heart disease on the basis of blood pressure, treatment for high blood pressure, blood cholesterol levels, cigarette smoking status, age, and sex.[45] Persons with diabetes or previous CHD events are considered at high risk. A risk score is assigned to patients to motivate changes both in patient behavior and in treatments recommended by health-care providers.

The Centers for Disease Control and Prevention (CDC) established its National Center for Chronic Disease Prevention and Health Promotion in 1989; one of the priorities of this center was the promotion of cardiovascular health. At that time, few state health department funds were devoted specifically to heart disease and stroke; most federal government funds allocated to states for cardiovascular health prior to the late 1990s came from a general block grant that could be used for diverse public health problems. For example, hypertension detection programs were combined into the Preventive Health and Health Services Block Grant that began in the 1980s and is still providing funding into the twenty-first century.[46] In a 1994 survey, state health departments spent only about $1.05 per person on all chronic diseases, even though chronic diseases accounted for about 70% of all deaths.[47] About 77% of state health department funds for chronic diseases at that time came from state sources, and about 20% came from federal sources.[47]

In 1997, Congress designated funds through CDC for state health departments to address heart disease and stroke. In 1998, eight states received funding to develop capacity to build heart disease and stroke programs; funding was expanded to 11 states in 1999 and to 24 states in 2000. State-based activities through this program include (1) defining the heart disease and stroke problem within the state, (2) developing partnerships and coordination among concerned nongovernmental and governmental partners, (3) developing effective strategies to reduce the burden of heart disease, stroke and related risk factors with an overarching emphasis on heart-healthy policies and on physical and social environmental changes, (4) developing population-based interventions to address primary and secondary prevention, and (5) monitoring critical aspects of heart disease and stroke. These essential components and capacity-building activities for state health departments attempt to go beyond education and awareness efforts and emphasize policy and environmental strategies to promote cardiovascular health and disease prevention and control. Through these state-based programs, CDC aims to (1) increase state capacity by planning, implementing, tracking, and sustaining population-based interventions that address heart disease, stroke, and related risk factors; (2) conduct surveillance of CVD and related risk factors and assessment of policy and environmental supports for heart disease and stroke prevention within states; (3) identify promising practices to promote heart-healthy interventions in states; and (4) promote cardiovascular health in a variety of settings (health care, work site, schools, and community) through education, policy, systems, and environmental changes.[48]

Factors Contributing to the Decline in CVD Death Rates

Tracking trends in risk factors and in the provision of medical care is a surveillance tool used to monitor progress in reducing the burden of heart disease and stroke. Data regarding these trends are collected from several sources, including telephone and in-person surveys, examination surveys, and medical care records. Both public health prevention efforts and improvements in early detection, treatment, and care have resulted in the following beneficial trends (Table 18.3) that likely contributed to declines in heart disease and stroke mortality over the course of the twentieth century.

Table 18.3. Recent progress in risk factors and correlates of heart disease and stroke.

Risk Factors and Correlates	Baseline Year	Baseline Estimate	Follow-up Year	Follow-up Estimate
Percentage* of persons aged 20–74 years[†] with hypertension[§]	1960–1962	38	1988–1994	24
Percentage of hypertensive persons taking action to control their blood pressure (e.g., medication, diet, low salt, and exercise)	1985	79	1998	89
Percentage of hypertensive persons whose blood pressure is controlled	1976–1980	11	1988–1991	29
Percentage of hypertensive persons who are aware of their condition	1976–1980	51	1988–1991	73
Percentage of persons who are aware of their blood pressure values	1985	61	1990	76
Percentage of persons aged 20–74 years[†] with high blood cholesterol[¶]	1960–1962	33	1988–1994	20
Mean serum cholesterol levels (mg/dL), adults aged ≥18 years[†]	1960–1962	222	1988–1994	205
Percentage of persons with high cholesterol who are aware of their condition	1988	30	1995	60
Percentage of persons who ever had their cholesterol checked	1988	59	1998	72
Percentage of current smokers aged ≥18 years[†]	1965	42	1998	23
Percentage of persons aged 20–74 years[†**] who are obese	1960–1962	13	1988–1994	23
Percentage of calories in the diet from fat[††]	1976–1980	36	1988–1994	34
Percentage of calories in the diet from saturated fat[††]	1976–1980	13	1988–1994	12
Light to moderate physical activity ≥5 times per week	1990	23	1998	30
Number of physicians indicating cardiovascular diseases as their primary area of practice	1975	5046	1998	15,112

Sources: References 3, 43, 44, 53.

*Percentages are rounded.
[†]Age-adjusted to the 2000 U.S. population.
[§]Systolic pressure ∃140 mmHg, diastolic pressure ∃90 mmHg, or taking antihypertensive medication.
[¶]Serum cholesterol level ∃240 mg/dL (6.2 mmol/L).
[**]Body mass index ∃30 kg/m².
[††]Based on 1-day dietary recall.

- A decline in the prevalence of cigarette smoking among adults aged 18 years from 42% in 1965 to 23% in 1998.[3] Substantial public health efforts to reduce tobacco use began in 1964 after recognition of the association between smoking and CVD and between smoking and cancer in the first surgeon general's report on smoking and health.
- A decrease in mean blood pressure levels.[3,43] This decrease appears to have occurred throughout the blood pressure distribution[49]—not just among those with high blood pressure.
- An increase in the percentage of persons with hypertension who have the condition treated and controlled.[1,3] However, high blood pressure control rates have remained suboptimal.
- A decrease in mean blood cholesterol levels.[3]
- Changes in the American diet. Consumption of saturated fat and cholesterol has decreased since 1909.[50] Data from the National Health and Nutrition Examination surveys suggest that decreases in the percentage of calories from dietary fat and the levels of dietary cholesterol coincide with decreases in blood cholesterol levels.[51]
- Improvements in medical care, including advances in diagnosing and treating heart disease and stroke, development of effective medications for treatment of hypertension and hypercholesterolemia, greater numbers of specialists and health-care providers focusing on heart disease and stroke, an increase in emergency medical services for heart attack and stroke, and an increase in coronary-care units.[3,52] These developments have contributed to lower case-fatality rates, lengthened survival times, and shorter hospital stays for persons with heart attacks and strokes.[1,52] The establishment of coronary-care units in the 1960s had a substantial impact on in-hospital mortality, which decreased from approximately 30% in the 1960s to about 15% by the mid-1980s.[2]

Population-wide approaches have been implemented alongside medical advances in detection and treatment; therefore, apportioning out the relative contributions of public health versus medical aspects is difficult. Debate about the causes of the decline in heart disease and stroke mortality has been vigorous and contentious.[54–60] For example, whether the decline in mortality rates is the result of fewer incident cases (new cases) or fewer post-event deaths remains unknown because no national data exist to distinguish these cases. Changes in the incidence of heart disease would suggest the success of primary prevention, whereas fewer deaths among persons with existing heart or cerebrovascular disease would suggest the success of secondary prevention. Although medical advances (including hypertension treatment) substantially contributed to the decline in stroke mortality,[61] population-wide reductions in blood pressure levels and prevalence of hypertension have also had a major impact. An analysis of mean blood pressure levels by birth cohort among persons who participated in the U.S. National Health and National Health and Nutrition Examination Surveys from 1960 to 1994 revealed lower systolic and diastolic blood pressures with each decade of birth year and at the low, middle, and upper ends of the blood-pressure distribution.[49] These data suggest that blood pressure levels declined for the entire population (not solely among persons with high blood pressure) through prevention efforts.

Other recent studies suggest that both population-wide and high-risk approaches have significantly contributed to the decline of heart disease and stroke. Among almost 86,000 women in the Nurse's Health Study,[59] changes in lifestyle—particularly, reduction in smoking and improvement in diet—accounted for much of the decline in the incidence of coronary disease from 1980–1987 to 1992–1994. In a study that examined heart disease trends and determinants, more of the decline in coronary heart disease mortality in the 1980s was attributed to a reduction in coronary heart disease incidence rates (about two thirds) than to lower case-fatality (about one third).[60]

Further Challenges

Despite the remarkable progress that was made during the past century, heart disease and stroke remain substantial public health concerns. The success of reducing heart disease and stroke mortality has resulted in longer life expectancy, which in turn puts more people at risk for these conditions. Correspondingly, the absolute number of deaths from cardiovascular diseases has increased and likely will substantially increase in the coming years as persons in the baby boomer generation reach the age at which cardiac and cerebrovascular events become more common. However, mortality only captures a portion of the health burden imposed by heart disease and stroke. At least 50 million American adults have some form of cardiovascular disease, and more than 6 million inpatient cardiovascular procedures were performed in 1999.[6] In addition, heart disease and stroke are also leading causes of disability and impaired quality of life.[3,62] Estimated costs for morbidity and mortality from heart diseases and stroke, including health expenditures and lost productivity, were more than $360 billion in 2004.[63]

By the beginning of the twenty-first century, positive trends for some CVD indicators that were established over the course of the twentieth century had either slowed substantially, leveled off, or reversed. For example, the prevalence of obesity had increased among both children and adults,[3] and the percentage of adults reporting that they engage in recommended levels of physical activity remained at greater than 30% since 1985.[64] The decline in average cholesterol levels among U.S. adults was not as great in the 1990s as in earlier decades.[65] Nearly 70% of persons with hypertension do not have the condition controlled (i.e., do not maintain levels of <140/90 mm Hg),[43,66] and the decline in death rates for stroke has slowed in recent years.[1,3] Mean blood pressure levels have remained stable in the 1990s, and the prevalence of hypertension has increased slightly.[67]

Recognizing the lack of progress in controlling high blood pressure, the Joint National Committee on Prevention, Detection, Evaluation and Treatment of High Blood Pressure released new high blood pressure guidelines in 2004.[66] A new category of "prehypertension" was classified, consisting of persons with above-optimal blood pressure levels but not yet clinically hypertensive. This new category was based on recognition that persons with above-optimal blood pressure levels are more likely to develop hypertension than persons with optimal blood pressure levels. Almost 31/% of U.S. adults have prehypertensive blood pressure levels, and these persons are more likely to have at least one other adverse risk factor.[68] Therefore, preventive efforts through lifestyle changes are urgently advised.

Advances in medical treatment of hypertension and acute myocardial infarction combined with the aging of the U.S. population have also created a new population of high risk individuals. Heart failure has emerged as a major health concern for older adults[69] because adults who survive a myocardial infarction or other hypertension-related diseases remain at increased risk for chronic heart failure later in life. Future efforts must continue to promote the appropriate treatment of persons with hypertension, coronary heart disease, and heart failure to reduce the disability associated with chronic heart failure and to improve the quality of life of this elderly population.

Despite advances in medical technology and clinical intervention once a patient reaches the medical system, efforts must continue to educate the public to recognize and react immediately to cardiac and stroke events. Almost half of all cardiac deaths in 1999 occurred out-of-hospital (i.e., before emergency or hospital care could be rendered);[70] this proportion increased from 1989 to 1998.[71] Likewise, about half of stroke deaths occur before the person reaches the hospital.[72] These findings underscore the need for increased recognition of the signs and symptoms of heart attacks and stroke and increased access to emergency services in addition to prevention efforts.

Declines in heart disease and stroke have not been experienced by all groups equally. During 1980–1998, age-adjusted death rates from heart disease declined 38% among white men but only 21% among American Indian/Alaskan Native women.[3] Additionally, persons of lower socioeconomic status have higher mortality, morbidity, and risk factor levels for heart disease and stroke than persons of higher socioeconomic status;[24,25] rates of heart disease declined faster among higher social classes,[24] widening health disparity. Finally, declines in heart disease-related deaths have varied geographically. Areas with poorer socioeconomic profiles have been more likely to experience a later onset of the decline of heart disease mortality.[24]

Current and future efforts for federal health agencies include identifying disparities and developing programs in these communities or populations to eliminate disparities in health. For example, in collaboration with West Virginia University and the University of South Florida, CDC has developed a series of atlases of heart disease and stroke mortality among the five largest racial and ethnic populations in the United States (i.e., American Indians and Alaska Natives, Asians and Pacific Islanders, blacks, Hispanics, and whites).[73–75] The maps highlight the geographic, racial, and ethnic inequalities in heart disease and stroke mortality among men and women, and provide government agencies and their partners at the local, state, and national levels with information to tailor prevention programs and policies to the communities with the greatest burden of heart disease and stroke. Interactive maps derived from these atlases were also developed and are available on-line at http://www.cdc.gov/cvh. The REACH 2010 (Racial and Ethnic Approaches to Community Health) project is part of a federal initiative to eliminate racial and ethnic disparities in health, including heart disease and stroke. Begun in 1999, REACH 2010 is a two-phased demonstration project that supports community coalitions in designing, implementing, and evaluating community-driven strategies to eliminate health disparities. Each coalition comprises a community-based organization and three other organizations, of which at least one is either a local or state health department or a university or research organization. Fourteen projects funded by CDC focus on heart disease and stroke.[76] Similarly, the National Heart, Lung, and

Blood Institute (NHLBI) has funded 12 Cardiovascular Disease (CVD) Enhanced Dissemination and Utilization Centers (EDUCs) to conduct performance-based education projects to prevent and control CVD and promote heart-healthy behavior in high-risk communities.[77]

Public health challenges for the twenty-first century involve reducing or eliminating risk factors and preventing the development of adverse risk factors. Continued research and surveillance is needed to understand the determinants (i.e., social, psychological, environmental, physiologic, and genetic) of heart disease and stroke risk and to reduce their burden on society. In particular, research efforts and public health action are needed in the following topic areas:

- Reducing the racial and ethnic disparities in heart disease and stroke mortality.
- Increasing the ability to reach underserved groups with appropriate and effective public health messages.
- Promoting policy and environmental strategies that enhance healthy behavior and environments. Policy and environmental factors have been instrumental in reducing tobacco use and are feasible for impacting other factors associated with cardiovascular health.[78,79]
- Determining the relationship between genetics and disease. The association of genetic variants with heart disease and stroke, especially the interplay between genetic and environmental factors, may play increasingly important roles in the nation's efforts to prevent these conditions. Identification of genetic aspects of cardiovascular conditions may improve prevention efforts by helping to determine which medications or preventive efforts may be more effective for persons at high risk.
- Identifying new or emerging risk factors and determining their potential for public health intervention. Potential factors that recently have been identified as associated with CVD include (1) elevated concentrations of total homocyst(e)ine, fibrinogen, and C-reactive protein and (2) the presence of infectious agents (e.g., *Helicobacter pylori* and *Chlamydia pneumonia*). Research is needed to determine whether these factors are causally related to heart disease and stroke or whether they are markers related to other causal factors.
- Focusing on secondary prevention and reducing disability. An aging U.S. population and an increasing number of persons surviving life-threatening cardiovascular conditions requires public health programs to focus on issues such as disability and quality of life. Persons with existing cardiovascular conditions are at increased risk for future life-threatening events related to those conditions.
- Addressing the heart disease and stroke problem globally. The United States ranks 14th in coronary heart disease mortality for males and 11th for females among 27 industrialized countries, although the United States has one of the lowest stroke death rates.[1] Furthermore, cardiovascular disease is projected to be the number-one cause of death worldwide by the year 2020.[80] Although CVD death rates are higher in developed nations, about 70% of cases worldwide occur in developing nations;[81] developing countries face a double burden of infectious and chronic diseases. Therefore, international collaboration will be key to improving cardiovascular health to reduce the burden of heart disease and stroke worldwide.
- Enhancing national and state surveillance infrastructures to monitor changes and promote improvements in cardiovascular disease patterns. Major gaps remain in the ability to monitor state prevalence of hypertension, high cholesterol, control

of these two risk factors, and medication use and nonpharmacologic actions taken to improve these levels. Without these measures which require examination of sample populations within the state, health departments and their partners are unable to justify the need for programs, plan programs, target high risk populations, and demonstrate success. An additional gap is the inability of the nation, as well as states, to describe the number of new cases (incidence) with stroke, heart disease, hypertension, or high cholesterol. Legislative action will be necessary to mandate the reporting of acute myocardial infarctions and strokes by physicians and health systems—an effort that has been accomplished for specific infectious diseases and cancer.

The urgency of reducing the burden of heart disease and stroke has prompted increased efforts among medical and public health professionals, including disseminating surveillance data, expanding programs, updating guidelines, and improving medical care access and quality. By 2003, the CDC's state heart disease and stroke prevention program was expanded to 32 states and the District of Columbia. Additionally, in 2001, CDC established the Paul Coverdell National Acute Stroke Registry and funded pilot programs in eight states (California, Georgia, Illinois, Massachusetts, Michigan, North Carolina, Ohio, and Oregon) to assess acute stroke care in these states. Based on those results, in June 2004 CDC funded four state health departments (Georgia, Illinois, Massachusetts, North Carolina) to establish statewide Paul Coverdell National Acute Stroke Registries. Registry data will help state health departments and hospitals develop acute-care quality improvement plans to reduce death and disability from stroke and improve quality of life for survivors. CDC also supports several regional stroke networks, which allow state health departments and their partners to share and coordinate stroke prevention activities and advocacy strategies.[82] A challenge for the twenty-first century is to expand these prevention programs, stroke registries and partnership networks to all states. Similar state efforts are also needed to address the prevention and care of acute myocardial infarction and other heart diseases in hospitals.

In 2001, CDC also initiated development of A Public Health Action Plan to Prevent Heart Disease and Stroke.[83] The purpose of the plan is to chart a course for CDC and collaborating public health agencies, with all interested partners and the public at large, to help in promoting achievement of national goals for preventing heart disease and stroke over the next two decades—through 2020 and beyond. Key partners, public health experts, and heart disease and stroke prevention specialists developed and are beginning to implement targeted recommendations and specific action steps. The National Forum for Prevention of Heart Disease and Stroke was convened in 2003. The National Forum comprises more than 100 representatives from national and international organizations, from multiple sectors and constituencies and serves as the principal vehicle for implementing the *Action Plan.*

In conclusion, much has been learned through the dramatic rise and decline in heart disease and stroke mortality in the United States. At the same time, there is still much to be done to decrease the burden of heart disease and stroke for all persons and to eliminate disparities between racial/ethnic populations.

References

1. National Heart, Lung and Blood Institute. Morbidity & Mortality: 2000 Chartbook on Cardiovascular, Lung, and Blood Diseases. Rockville, MD: U.S. Department of Health and Human Services, National Institutes of Health, 2000.
2. Braunwald E. Shattuck Lecture: cardiovascular medicine at the turn of the millennium: triumphs, concerns, and opportunities. *N Engl J Med* 1997:337:1360–69.
3. National Center for Health Statistics. Health, United States, 2001 with urban and rural health chartbook. DHHS publication no. 01–1232. Hyattsville, MD: Department of Health and Human Services, Centers for Disease Control and Prevention No., 2001.
4. U.S. Department of Health, Education and Welfare. Diseases of cardiovascular system: death rates by age, race, and sex, United States, 1900–1953. *Vital Statistics-Special Reports* 1956:43(14).
5. Perrin EB, Lawrence PS, Fisher GF, et al. Mortality trends for leading causes of death, United States 1950–69. *Vital Health Stat* 1974:20(16).
6. 2000 Heart and Stroke Statistical Update. Dallas, TX: American Heart Association, 1999.
7. Rosenberg HM, Maurer JD, Sorlie PD, Johnson NJ, et al. Quality of death rates by race and Hispanic origin: a summary of current research, 1999. National Center for Health Statistics. *Vital Health Stat* 1999:2(128).
8. Stehbens WE. An appraisal of the epidemic rise of coronary heart disease and its decline. *Lancet* 1987:1:606–10.
9. Higgins MW, Luepker RV. Preface: trends and determinants of coronary heart disease mortality: international comparisons. *Int J Epidemiol* 1989:18(suppl):S1–S2.
10. Osler W. Diseases of the arteries. In: Osler W, MacCrae T, eds. Modern Medicine: Its Theory and Practice in Original Contributions by Americans and Foreign Authors. Philadelphia: Lea & Febiger, 1908.
11. Herrick JB. Clinical features of sudden obstruction of the coronary arteries. *JAMA* 1912: 59:2015–20.
12. Epstein FH. Contribution of epidemiology to understanding coronary heart disease. In: Marmot M, Elliott P, eds. Coronary Heart Disease Epidemiology: From Aetiology to Public Health. New York: Oxford University Press, 1992, 20–32.
13. Epstein FH. Cardiovascular disease epidemiology: a journey from the past into the future. *Circulation* 1996:93:1755–64.
14. Stamler J. Established major coronary risk factors. In: Marmot M, Elliott P, eds. Coronary Heart Disease Epidemiology: From Aetiology to Public Health. New York: Oxford University Press, 1992, 35–66.
15. Keys A. Seven Countries: A Multivariate Analysis of Death and Coronary Heart Disease. Cambridge, MA: Harvard University Press, 1980.
16. Worth RM, Kato H, Rhoads GG, Kagan K, Syme SL. Epidemiologic studies of CHD and stroke in Japanese men living in Japan, Hawaii, and California: mortality. *Am J Epidemiol* 1975:102:481–90.
17. Dawber TR. The Framingham Study: The Epidemiology of Atherosclerotic Disease. Cambridge, MA: Harvard University Press, 1980.
18. Wilson PWF, Garrison RJ, Castelli WP, Feinleib M, McNamara PM, Kannel WB. Prevalence of coronary heart disease in the Framingham Offspring Study: role of lipoprotein changes. *Am J Cardiol* 1980:46:649–54.
19. Daviglus ML, Liu K, Greenland P, et al. Benefit of a favorable cardiovascular risk-factor profile in middle age with respect to Medicare costs. *N Engl J Med* 1998:339:1122–29.
20. Higgins M, Province M, Heiss G. NHLBI Family Heart Study: objectives and design. *Am J Epidemiol* 1996:143:1219–28.

21. White PD, Sprague HB, Stamler J. A Statement on Arteriosclerosis, Main Cause of Heart Attacks and Strokes. New York: National Health Education Council, 1959.

22. Labarthe DR. Epidemiology and Prevention of Cardiovascular Diseases: A Global Challenge. Gaithersburg, MD: Aspen, 1998.

23. Cassel JC. Review of 1960 through 1962 cardiovascular disease prevalence study. *Arch Intern Med* 1981:128:890–95.

24. Kaplan GA, Keil JE. Socioeconomic factors and cardiovascular disease: a review of the literature. *Circulation* 1993:88:1973–98.

25. National Heart, Lung, and Blood Institute. Report of the Conference on Socioeconomic Status and Cardiovascular Health and Disease. Bethesda, MD: National Institutes of Health, National Heart, Lung, and Blood Institute. 6–7 November 1995.

26. Larsson B. Obesity and body fat distribution as predictors of coronary heart disease. In: Marmot M, Elliott P, eds. Coronary Heart Disease Epidemiology: From Aetiology to Public Health. New York: Oxford University Press, 1992, 233–41.

27. Seidell JC, Kahn HS, Williamson DF, Lissner L, Valdez R. Report from a Centers for Disease Control and Prevention workshop on use of adult anthropometry for public health and primary care. *Am J Clin Nutr* 2001:73:123–26.

28. Clinical Guidelines on the Identification, Evaluation, and Treatment of Overweight and Obesity in Adults: The Evidence Report. National Institutes of Health publication No. 98-4083. National Heart, Lung and Blood Institute, September 1998.

29. Physical Activity and Health: A Report of the Surgeon General. Atlanta, GA: U.S. Department of Health and Human Services, Centers for Disease Control and Prevention, National Center for Chronic Disease Prevention and Health Promotion, 1996.

30. Gorelick PB, Sacco RL, Smith DB, et al. Prevention of a first stroke: a review of guidelines and a multidisciplinary consensus statement from the National Stroke Association. *JAMA* 1999:281:1112–20.

31. Veterans Administration Cooperative Study Group on Antihypertensive Agents. Effects of treatment on morbidity in hypertension, I: results in patients with diastolic pressure averaging 115 through 129 mmHg. *JAMA* 1967:202:1028–34.

32. Veterans Administration Cooperative Study Group on Antihypertensive Agents. Effects of treatment on morbidity in hypertension, II: results in patients with diastolic pressure averaging 90 through 114 mmHg. *JAMA* 1967:213:1143–52.

33. The National Diet-Heart Study. *Nutrition Reviews* 1968:26(5):133–36.

34. Centers for Disease Control, Stanford University School of Medicine. Worldwide Efforts to Improve Heart Health: A Follow-up of the Catalonia Declaration: Selected Program Descriptions. Atlanta, GA: U.S. Department of Health and Human Services, Centers for Disease Control and Prevention, 1997.

35. Stone EJ, Pearson TA, eds. Community trials for cardiopulmonary health: directions for public health practice, policy and research. *Ann Epidemiol* 1997:7(suppl):S1–S120.

36. Green LW, Kreuter MA. Health Promotion Planning: An Educational and Environmental Approach, 2nd ed. Mountain View, CA: Mayfield, 1991.

37. Glanz K, Lankenau B, Foerster S, Temple S, Mullis R, Schmid T. Environmental and policy approaches to cardiovascular disease prevention through nutrition: opportunities for state and local action. *Health Educ Q* 1995:22:512.

38. Brownson RC, Matson Koffman D, Novotny TE, Hughes RG, Eriksen MP. Environmental and policy interventions to control tobacco use and prevent cardiovascular disease. *Health Educ Q* 1995:22:478.

39. King AC, Jeffery RW, Fridinger F, et al. Environmental and policy approaches to cardiovascular disease prevention through physical activity: issues and opportunities. *Health Educ Q* 1995:22:499.

40. Schmid TL, Pratt M, Howze E. Policy as intervention: environmental and policy approaches to the prevention of cardiovascular disease. *Am J Public Health* 1995: 85:1207.
41. Rose G. The Strategy of Preventive Medicine. New York: Oxford University Press, 1992.
42. National High Blood Pressure Education Program. Working group report on primary prevention of hypertension. National Heart, Lung, and Blood Institute, NIH. *Arch Intern Med* 1993:153:186–208.
43. The Sixth Report of the Joint National Committee on Prevention, Detection, Evaluation, and Treatment of High Blood Pressure. NIH publication no. 98-4080. Rockville, MD: U.S. Department of Health and Human Services, National Institutes of Health, National Heart, Lung, and Blood Institute, November 1997.
44. National Cholesterol Education Program. Second Report of the Expert Panel on Detection, Evaluation and Treatment of High Blood Cholesterol in Adults. NIH publication no. 93-3095. Rockville, MD: U.S. Department of Health and Human Services, National Institutes of Health, 1993.
45. Executive Summary of the Third Report of the National Cholesterol Education Program (NCEP) Expert Panel on Detection, Evaluation, and Treatment of High Blood Cholesterol in Adults (Adult Treatment Panel III). *JAMA* 2001:285:2486–97.
46. U.S. Department of Health and Human Services. Fulfilling State Priorities for Prevention: The Preventive Health and Health Services Block Grant. Washington, DC: Government Printing Office, 1998.
47. Centers for Disease Control and Prevention. Resources and priorities for chronic disease prevention and control, 1994. *MMWR* 1997:46:286–87.
48. Centers for Disease Control and Prevention. CDC State Cardiovascular Health Program. Available at: http://www.cdc.gov/cvh/stateprogram.htm. Accessed 28 February 2004.
49. Goff DC Jr, Howard G, Russell GB, Labarthe DR. Birth cohort evidence of population influences on blood pressure in the United States, 1887–1994. *Ann Epidemiol* 2001: 11:271–79.
50. Gerrior S, Bente L. Nutrient Content of the U.S. Food Supply, 1909–94. Home economics research report no. 53. Washington, DC: U.S. Department of Agriculture, 1997.
51. Ernst ND, Sempos CT, Briefel RR, Clark MB. Consistency between U.S. dietary fat intake and serum total cholesterol concentrations: the National Health and Nutrition Examination Surveys. *Am J Clin Nutr* 1997:66(suppl):965S–972S.
52. Higgins M, Thom T. Trends in CHD in the United States. *Int J Epidemiol* 1989:18(3suppl 1): S58–S66.
53. National Center for Health Statistics. Healthy People 2000 Final Review. USDHHS publication no. 01-0256. Hyattsville, MD: U.S. Public Health Service, 2001.
54. Goldman L, Cook EF. The decline in ischemic heart disease mortality rates: an analysis of the comparative effects of medical interventions and changes in lifestyle. *Ann Intern Med* 1984:101:825–36.
55. Rosamond WD, Chambless LE, Folsom AR, et al. Trends in the incidence of myocardial infarction and in mortality due to coronary heart disease, 1987 to 1994. *N Engl J Med* 1998:339:861–67.
56. McGovern PG, Pankow JS, Shahar E, et al. Recent trends in acute coronary heart disease: mortality, morbidity, medical care, and risk factors. *N Engl J Med* 1996:334: 884–90.
57. Hunink MG, Goldman L, Tosteson ANA, et al. The recent decline in mortality from coronary heart disease, 1980–1990: the effect of secular trends in risk factors and treatment. *JAMA* 1997:277:535–42.

58. McGinnis JM, Foege WH. Actual causes of death in the United States. *JAMA* 1993:270: 2207–12.

59. Hu FB, Stampfer MJ, Manson JE, et al. Trends in the incidence of coronary heart disease and changes in diet and lifestyle in women. *N Engl J Med* 2000:343:530–37.

60. Tunstall-Pedoe H, Kuulasmaa K, Mähönen M, Tolonen H, Ruokokoski E, Amouyel P. Contribution of trends in survival and coronary-even rates to changes in coronary heart disease mortality: 10-year results from 37 WHO MONICA Project populations. *Lancet* 1999:353:1547–57.

61. Whisnant JP. The decline of stroke. *Stroke* 1984:15(1):160–68.

62. Centers for Disease Control and Prevention. Prevalence of disabilities and associated health conditions among adults—United States, 1999. *MMWR* 2001:20:120–25.

63. Heart Disease and Stroke Statistics—2004 update. Dallas, TX: American Heart Association, 2003.

64. Pratt MC, Macera CA, Blanton C. Levels of physical activity and inactivity in children and adults in the United States: current evidence and research issues. *Med Sci Sports Exerc* 1999:31(11suppl):S526–S533.

65. Ford ES, Mokdad AH, Giles WH, Mensah GA. Serum total cholesterol concentrations and awareness, treatment, and control of hypercholesterolemia among U.S. adults. Findings from the National Health and Nutrition Examination Survey, 1999 to 2000. *Circulation* 2003:107:2185–89.

66. Chobanian AV, Bakris GL, Black HR, Cushman WC, Green LA, Izzo JL Jr, et al. Seventh Report of the Joint National Committee on Prevention, Detection, Evaluation, and Treatment of High Blood Pressure. *Hypertension* 2003:42:1206–52.

67. Hajjar I, Kotchen TA. Trends in prevalence, awareness, treatment, and control of hypertension in the United States, 1988–2000. *JAMA* 2003:290:199–206.

68. Greenlund KJ, Croft JB, Mensah GA. Prevalence of heart disease and stroke risk factors in persons with prehypertension in the United States, 1999–2000. *Arch Intern Med* 2004:164:2113–18.

69. Croft JB, Giles WH, Pollard RA, Keenan NL, Casper ML, Anda RF. Heart failure survival among older adults in the United States: a poor prognosis for an emerging epidemic in the Medicare population. *Arch Intern Med* 1999:159:505–510.

70. Zheng ZJ, Croft JB, Giles WH, et al. State specific mortality from sudden cardiac death—United States, 1999. *MMWR* 2002:51:123–26.

71. Zheng ZJ, Croft JB, Giles WH, Mensah GA. Sudden cardiac death in the United States, 1989 to 1998. *Circulation* 2001:104:2158–63.

72. Ayala C, Croft JB, Keenan NL, Neff LJ, Greenlund KJ, Donehoo RS, Zheng ZJ, Mensah GA. Increasing trends in pretransport stroke deaths—United States, 1990–1998. *Ethn Dis* 2003:13(suppl 2):S2131–S2137.

73. Casper ML, Barnett E, Williams I, Halverson J, Braham V, Greenlund K. Atlas of Stroke Mortality: Racial, Ethnic, and Geographic Disparities in the United States. Atlanta, GA: Centers for Disease Control and Prevention, 2003.

74. Barnett E, Casper ML, Halverson JA, Elmes GA, Braham VE, Majeed ZA, Bloom AS, Stanley S. Men and Heart Disease: An Atlas of Racial and Ethnic Disparities in Mortality, 1st ed. Morgantown, WV: Office for Social Environment and Health Research, West Virginia University, 2001.

75. Casper ML, Barnett E, Halverson JA, Elmes GA, Braham VE, Majeed ZA, Bloom AS, Stanley S. Women and Heart Disease: An Atlas of Racial and Ethnic Disparities in Mortality, 2nd ed. Morgantown, WV: Office for Social Environment and Health Research, West Virginia University, 2000.

76. Centers for Disease Control and Prevention. REACH 2010. Available at www.cdc.gov/reach2010/. Accessed 27 February 2004.
77. National Heart, Lung, and Blood Institute. Cardiovascular disease enhanced dissemination and utilization centers (EDUCs) awardees. Available at http://hin.nhlbi.nih.gov/educs/awardees.htm. Accessed 27 February 2004.
78. Fishman JA, Allison H, Knowles SB, et al. State laws on tobacco control—United States, 1998. *MMWR* 1999:48(3suppl):21–62.
79. McGinnis JM, Williams-Russo P, Knickman JR. The case for more active policy attention to health promotion. *Health Affairs* 2002:21:78–93.
80. Murray CJL, Lopez AD, eds. The Global Burden of Disease: Vol. 1. Boston: Harvard University School of Public Health, 1996.
81. World Health Organization. Cardiovascular diseases. Available at: www.who.int/ncd/cvd/index.htm. Accessed 11July 2001.
82. Centers for Disease Control and Prevention. The Paul Coverdell National Acute Stroke Registry. Available at: www.cdc.gov/programs/chronic5.htm. Accessed 27 February 2004.
83. A Public Health Action Plan to Prevent Heart Disease and Stroke. Atlanta, GA: U.S. Department of Health and Human Services, Centers for Disease Control and Prevention, 2003. Available at: www.cdc.gov/cvh. Accessed 27 February 2004.

Suggested Reading

Braunwald E. Shattuck lecture: cardiovascular medicine at the turn of the millennium: triumphs, concerns, and opportunities. *N Engl J Med* 1997:337:1360–69.
Marmot M, Elliott P, eds. Coronary Heart Disease Epidemiology: From Aetiology to Public Health. New York: Oxford University Press, 1992.

19

Dietary Policy, Controversy, and Proof: Doing Something versus Waiting for the Definitive Evidence

KARIN GARRETY

Controversies over diet and its relationship to health are never out of the headlines for long. At the beginning of the twenty-first century, a heated debate is in progress about the causes of the obesity epidemic sweeping the United States and some other nations.[1,2] The percentage of the population classified as obese in the United States jumped from 14.5% in 1971 to 30.9% in 2000.[3] Many commentators attribute the increase to simple overeating. In their view, Americans, spurred on by advertising and ever-increasing serving sizes, are ignoring dietary advice and consuming more calories than they are expending.[1,2,4] Others maintain that the problem is more complex. A few researchers claim that recent dietary advice,[5,6] which advocates restricting fats and increasing carbohydrate intake, is contributing to weight gain. According to them, dieters following stricter versions of this regime are upsetting the insulin-based physiological system that regulates blood sugar, appetite, and fat metabolism, with the result that they gain weight and often develop diabetes.[1,2] Alongside this recent skepticism about the wisdom of fat avoidance is a renewed interest on the part of mainstream medicine in the controversial Atkins diet—a high-fat, low-carbohydrate regime that was for decades relegated to the realm of quackery. Baffled and frustrated by obese but starving patients who fail to lose weight, some orthodox physicians have begun testing Atkins' claims,[7,8] much to the chagrin of those who find any questioning of the anti-fat message a danger to health.[9]

As these recent controversies illustrate, discussions about diet, disease, and health take place in a highly politicized arena. In an ideal world, scientific research would settle controversies, as the opposing parties would be forced to agree on hard and in-disputable facts. However, within the vast body of knowledge related to diet and disease, there are many contradictory claims and experimental results that are open to conflicting interpretations. Nonetheless, because of intense public, commercial, and political interest, health policy makers are under considerable pressure to come up with answers and advice. Although policy decisions draw on and lend legitimacy to some interpretations of the "evidence," other interpretations are often possible, and controversies erupt again. This chapter traces the development of one view of the healthy diet—a diet that is low in fats and high in carbohydrates. Although it became mainstream and widely accepted during the second half of the twentieth century, this diet was the subject of considerable controversy. It was primarily developed and promoted as a response to a disease that was rife in the decades after World War II—coronary heart disease (CHD). The rise of the low-fat diet is therefore closely bound up with attempts to "do something" about CHD at a population-wide level.

The chapter covers the period from the 1940s, when medical and lay awareness of the increasing incidence of CHD began to grow, to 1985, the year the National Cholesterol Education Program (NCEP) began its widespread and concerted effort to sell the anti-fat, anti-cholesterol message to the nation. This campaign marked a victory for advocates of fat reduction over skeptics who, for decades, continued to question the efficacy of low-fat diets as a means of preventing disease. To make sense of the scientific knowledge, its policy ramifications, and the controversy as a whole, it is useful to divide the knowledge linking fats, cholesterol, and heart disease into three separate but related hypotheses. These are (1) that higher serum cholesterol levels are associated in some way with an increased risk of CHD, (2) that serum cholesterol levels can be reduced by modifying the fat and cholesterol content of the diet, and (3) that a cholesterol-lowering diet will reduce the risk of developing cardiovascular disease. By the mid-1960s, scientists had established the validity of hypotheses 1 and 2. However, hypothesis 3 remained problematic. While scientists struggled to test its validity, public, commercial, and political interest in the link between diet and disease intensified, stimulating the creation of policy before the issue was resolved to everyone's satisfaction. The history of dietary policy in postwar America provides a fascinating insight into the way science, culture, economics, and politics intertwine with policy making in the field of public health.

Putting Cardiovascular Diseases on the Public Health and Medical Research Agenda

Although rates of CHD in the United States increased markedly during the first half of the twentieth century,[10] there was initially little public awareness of the disease. Lay people and medical organizations were still primarily interested in treating and preventing infectious diseases. In 1945, for example, a report on fund-raising by voluntary health agencies stated that the funds raised that year represented $94 for each case of infantile paralysis, $22 for each case of tuberculosis, $8 for cancer, and 3 cents for each case of heart disease.[11] Over the next 10 years, a group of cardiologists and medical research lobbyists worked diligently to raise the profile of cardiovascular diseases (CVD), or diseases of the circulation. Their efforts were closely bound with another highly successful campaign, led by wealthy philanthropists Mary and Albert Lasker, to increase funding for research into chronic diseases in general. The Laskers and their allies fervently believed that well-funded research would soon produce cures for CVD and cancer. In 1948, the federal government rewarded their efforts by establishing the National Heart Institute (NHI).[12–14] Funds for research rose steadily. Between 1950 and 1967, annual funding escalated from $16 million to $164 million.[14]

The American Heart Association (AHA) was also involved in these efforts. In 1946 the association, until then a private, professional body, voted in favor of becoming a national voluntary health agency, which allowed it to expand its public education and fund-raising activities.[15] It established a National Heart Week, and used newspapers, radio, magazines, Hollywood stars and community organizations to publicize heart disease and the need for more money for research. It distributed heart-shaped collection boxes to drugstores emblazoned with the slogan "Open Your Heart . . . Give to Fight the Heart Diseases, America's Number One Killer."[16,17] The 1949 campaign raised $2,850,000, and the 1950 campaign raised a further $4 million.[18,19] The association estimated that during its first 12 years as a voluntary health agency, it channeled nearly $50 million into research.[20]

Before 1950, scientific knowledge about the causes of CVD was indeed scanty. Early experiments with rabbits suggested some kind of link between diet and atherosclerosis. However, many scientists believed that these findings could not be extrapolated to humans.[21,22] During the 1930s and 1940s, scientists found higher levels of serum cholesterol in humans with various diseases of the kidneys and circulation.[23,24] Hints also began to emerge that serum cholesterol levels could be decreased by manipulating the diet. In the late 1940s patients with high blood pressure were often treated with a very strict rice-fruit diet, which contained no cholesterol and virtually no fat. Researchers observed that patients on this diet experienced substantial decreases in serum cholesterol levels.[25,26] They conducted experiments to investigate the comparative effects of vegetable and animal fats on serum cholesterol. However, results were confusing and contradictory.[27,28] They would remain so until the second half of the 1950s, when scientists redefined the problem in terms of fat saturation.

Early publicity reflected the uncertainty about the causes of cardiovascular diseases. In 1947, *Better Homes and Gardens* published an article titled "The 100% American Way to Die," which informed readers of the growing incidence of several forms of cardiovascular disease, including coronary thrombosis, stroke, hypertension, and rheumatic heart disease.[29] It canvased several theories of causation, including high-cholesterol foods. The section on cholesterol ended with a caution: "It's only a theory yet, nothing that should justify tampering with a good diet *unless your doctor himself tells you to*" [emphasis in original]. Instead, the advice given was vague and general, and based on an assumption that cardiovascular diseases were caused by some mixture of stress, overeating and lack of exercise: "calm down and get out into the sun," readers were advised, "instead of rushing and worrying and getting flabby and stuffing your paunch with the $3 dinner."[29]

Early Heart Disease Epidemiology: Ancel Keys
and the Framingham Heart Study

Of the many projects funded during the medical research boom of the 1950s, only a few stand out as having played pivotal roles in the development of knowledge about CHD and its causes. In 1951, Ancel Keys met a fellow physiologist from Naples who told him that the disease was not a problem in his home city. This stimulated Keys to set up a comparative study of the heart disease rates and diets of various socioeconomic groups in Naples, Madrid, and Minnesota. He found very little heart disease among the poorer populations of Naples and Madrid and attributed this to their diets, which contained little meat and few dairy products.[27] Keys presented these findings at two international congresses in 1952. In a memoir published in 1990, he wrote that the findings "were politely received but few were convinced that diet had anything to do with coronary heart disease."[30] At the time, dietary policies aimed to prevent deficiencies, not to deter excess. As milk, meat, and eggs supplied protein, iron, and valuable vitamins, they were considered healthy, not potentially pathogenic.[31]

The large gap between Keys's ideas and those of the majority of his colleagues is evident in a symposium on atherosclerosis published in the AHA journal *Circulation* in 1952.[32] In the symposium, Louis Katz, an eminent atherosclerosis researcher, said that he would only prescribe a low-fat, low-cholesterol diet for obese patients or for those who had already had two or more heart attacks, because "prohibitions should not be carelessly advocated until such time as it is clearly revealed that the prohibition has a great chance of being beneficial to the patient."[32] Keys, on the other hand, boldly asserted that "if mankind stopped eating eggs, dairy products, meats and all visible fats," atherosclerosis would become "very rare." His diet for atherosclerosis patients included skim milk, lean meat or fish, and "a boiled or poached whole egg for Sunday."[32] It would be at least another decade or two before other doctors would consider such a strict diet to be appropriate for heart disease patients.

In contrast to his later "seven countries" study,[33] Keys's early investigations were retrospective—that is, they compared variables at a single point in time, seeking to correlate possible causes with disease after the disease had manifested itself. Critics found it easy to question these studies because there was no guarantee that the putatively causal variables (for example, high-fat diet, high cholesterol levels) chronologically preceded the putative outcome.[34,35] To overcome these problems, epidemiologists devised prospective studies. In these, they chose persons, randomly or otherwise, and characterized them according to various criteria. A research team then periodically investigated the incidence of new disease among subjects, and determined causes of death in those who died between examinations. Epidemiologists argue that these studies are more rigorous because the characteristics of the persons under observation are measured before the disease appears.

In postwar America, epidemiologists set up many prospective studies.[36–41] The most famous and influential was—and is—the Framingham Heart Study. Begun in 1947, it was taken over by the newly formed NHI in 1949. The original aim was to study the incidence of heart disease over time in a defined community: the town of Framingham, about 20 miles from Boston. However, the new NHI directors decided that it could also be used to search for "constitutional and conditioning factors" (later known as risk factors) associated with the development of the disease. Accordingly, they expanded the range of personal and medical information to be collected.[42] The original cohort consisted of 2282 men and 2846 women aged 30–59 years; all were subjected to a thorough medical examination and questioning, then recalled every 2 years for re-examination. Causes of death were sought for those who died between examinations.[43] In 2006, the study was still collecting data on the remaining members of the original cohort, as well as their spouses and offspring.

Data from the first 4 years of the Framingham study did not appear until 1957,[44] and the risk factors that are now so well known did not become clear until the early 1960s. In the meantime, there was a great deal more publicity about CHD and its causes, much of it fueled by the work of Ancel Keys.

More Publicity and the First Battles over Policy

In the mid-1950s some sectors of the popular press became much less circumspect in their reports about the links between diet and heart disease. A 1954 *Newsweek* article reporting on a recent conference was titled "Fat's the Villain." Much of the article was taken up with descriptions of the retrospective country comparisons made by Keys and his colleagues. The author summarized the work with the claim: "A world survey of recently discovered facts shows that cardiovascular troubles are most common in countries where there is the most fat in the diet."[45] In December 1955 the *Reader's Digest* also published a flattering article describing Keys's research, and cautiously advocated dietary change.[46] The news-worthiness of CHD received a further boost in September 1955, when President Eisenhower suffered a heart attack.[47]

While publicity about heart disease and its possible links to fat consumption increased, the question of the effects of different types of fats on serum cholesterol levels remained unresolved. This issue was of great interest to sectors of the food industry, some of which were linked to scientific research through the Nutrition Foundation, an industry-funded research body.[48] In exchange for a membership fee, companies gained access to the latest knowledge about nutrition. Although the direction of research was decided by a Scientific Advisory Committee, it was open to influence by industry representatives. During the 1950s, member companies offered to donate an extra million dollars over and above their usual payments if the foundation would fund an intensive research effort into the effects of different types of fats on serum cholesterol.[48] The committee agreed. It was during this time that scientists managed to sort out the confusion by reframing the problem as one of fat saturation. The findings were consistent and noncontroversial. Despite some variation among persons, the lowest cholesterol levels were obtained by ingesting oils with high concentrations of polyunsaturated fatty acids.[49] Soon after these studies were published, the first polyunsaturated margarine appeared, and vegetable oil manufacturers began to claim that their products could prevent heart disease.[50,51]

The new findings quickly found their way into the popular press and stimulated another spate of articles on diet, cholesterol, and heart disease. By this time, Keys was no longer alone in advocating dietary change. In 1956 *Time* published this bold claim by New York nutritionist Norman Jolliffe: "No prudent person who has had, or wishes to avoid, coronary heart disease should eat a high-fat diet of the type consumed by most Americans. . . . Stress and strain, physical indolence, obesity, luxury living or tobacco play but a minor role."[52] Jolliffe and colleagues persuaded more than 1000 men in New York to join an Anti-Coronary Club in which they would abide by his dietary rules.[53] He hoped that within 5 years he would have enough data to prove the salutary effects of diets low in saturated fats.[52]

The public advocacy of low-fat diets troubled some of the more conservative members of the scientific profession. In May 1957 two researchers went public with a message of caution published in a *Newsweek* cover story titled "The Diet Mania— Do Fats Really Kill?" The article began: "Currently the dieters are swarming to a new fad—the anti-cholesterol or low-fat diet—though scientists have not yet reached any considerable measure of agreement as to whether such a diet does anything but harm."[54] The author asserted that cholesterol was "the mysterious compound around which one of medicine's most heated controversies is now raging" and contrasted the views of Keys and Jolliffe with those of Frederick Stare (a Harvard University nutritionist) and Irvine Page (a former president of the AHA). Page was particularly critical of Keys's country comparison studies. Foreign CHD statistics were unreliable, he said, because of "poor methods of reporting, understaffed health departments, and dubious autopsy proceedings." He claimed that there was not yet enough evidence to justify "wholesale tinkering with the American diet."[54]

Page and Stare were also the leading authors of the first AHA policy statement on diet and heart disease, published in *Circulation* in August 1957. Although some later accounts cite this report as the first policy statement advocating reductions in dietary saturated fat,[5] it was actually quite cautious and circumspect. The five authors expressed concern about a "flood of diet fads and quackery."[34] They noted that, "great pressure is being put on physicians to do something about the reported increased death rate from heart attacks in relatively young people." However, they warned, "some scientists have taken uncompromising stands based on evidence that does not stand up under critical examination."[34] They expressed skepticism about Keys's studies and warned against the extrapolation of results from formula dietary experiments to the general population. They argued that there was not enough evidence to "permit a rigid stand" on the link between diet and heart disease and concluded: "We are certain of one thing: the evidence now in existence justifies the most thorough investigation."[34]

Several leading scientific and medical organizations supported the conservative stance of the AHA, including the Research Council of the National Academy of Sciences,[55] the AMA Council on Foods and Nutrition,[56] and the Nutrition Foundation.[51] In December 1959, the Food and Drug Administration (FDA) issued a statement announcing that "the role of cholesterol in heart and artery diseases has not been established. A causal relationship between blood cholesterol levels and these diseases has not been proved." Therefore, advertising claims linking consumption of vegetable oils and margarine to a decreased risk of heart disease were "false and misleading."[57]

Changes in Policy

The late 1950s and early 1960s were pivotal years in the history of dietary policy. While the AHA and other organizations initially advised caution, Mary Lasker, the wealthy philanthropist and influential advocate of medical research, tried to persuade doctors to "do something" about cardiovascular disease, even in the face of imperfect knowledge.[12] A decade had passed since her lobbying efforts had helped establish the NHI, and she and her allies now turned their efforts to public education. In 1959, she persuaded eight physicians, including five former AHA presidents (erstwhile conservatives Page and Stare, among them), to issue a statement under the auspices of the National Health Education Committee, a committee she chaired. The statement outlined five "factors predisposing to arteriosclerosis": "heredity, overweight, elevated blood cholesterol level, elevated blood pressure and excessive cigarette smoking." People were advised to see their doctors if any of these factors were present.[58]

By now, generous funding for research was yielding results, and some aspects of the links among diet, cholesterol levels, and CHD were becoming clearer. In 1960, *Time* magazine reported that at the AHA's annual meeting, the "great cholesterol controversy" was beginning to subside, and that "even onetime skeptics were prepared to concede that abnormal quantities of fatty material in the blood should be regarded as one of the major factors in producing heart-artery disease."[59] Shortly after this, the AHA released another policy statement.[60] This time, it cautiously endorsed dietary change. The statement was formulated by an elite group of six scientists, including Page and Stare. However, the group now had two new members—Keys and another staunch supporter of dietary change, Jeremiah Stamler. The document began by announcing: "Current available knowledge is sufficient to warrant a general statement regarding the relation of diet to the possible prevention of atherosclerosis."[60] As supporting evidence it cited Keys's work, about which no doubts were raised, and animal and human dietary experiments. The AHA worded its recommendations carefully: "These and other research studies have given clues as to the prevention of atherosclerosis by dietary means. A reduction in blood cholesterol by dietary means, which also emphasizes weight control, may lessen the development or extension of atherosclerosis and hence the risk of heart attack or strokes. It must be emphasized that there is as yet no final proof that heart disease or strokes will be prevented by such measures."[60] The policy statement recommended dietary changes for overweight people, those who had already had a heart attack or stroke, men with a family history of heart disease, high cholesterol, high blood pressure and for those "who lead sedentary lives of relentless frustration."[60]

The AHA statement listed 23 references in support of its recommendations. Most described experiments in which cholesterol levels were reduced by modifying the diet. Others were epidemiologic studies linking high cholesterol levels or other variables with an increased risk of heart disease. In other words, the studies were concerned with the first two of the three hypotheses outlined above. Only two of the references discussed experiments designed to test the crucial final link in the chain: whether dietary change (through a reduction of cholesterol levels) could also reduce the incidence of cardiovascular disease. These studies were Jolliffe's Anti-Coronary

Club[61] and an English study with people who already had CHD.[62] Both papers described how the studies were set up, but were too recent to yield any data.

The Search for the Definitive Evidence

Before, during, and after the AHA's first cautious endorsement of dietary change, scientists continued to work toward the "definitive proof." Ideally, this would be an experiment demonstrating a reduction in the incidence of heart disease in people consuming a cholesterol-lowering diet. Some early studies were suggestive. In 1950 and 1951, John Gofman and colleagues published reports claiming that diet could reduce the incidence of further attacks in heart disease patients.[63,64] Lester Morrison, a doctor from Los Angeles, made similar claims on the basis of a 12-year study of 100 patients.[65] However, neither study held up well under later standards of methodology and reporting, and were not cited in the AHA's 1961 policy statement.

The 1950s and 1960s were decades of rapid change in the design of clinical trials.[66] What passed for a reasonable experiment in the 1950s was deemed to be full of errors by the end of the 1960s. For example, Jolliffe's Anti-Coronary Club recruited subjects with a previous history of heart disease, obesity, hypertension, or diabetes alongside those who were healthy. No thought was given to the establishment of a control group. The investigators tried to improve their study later by adding a retrospective control group and excluding men with a previous history of heart disease from the analysis. Results published in 1966 claimed that men who lowered their fat intake suffered less heart disease.[53] However, because of its flaws, the study did not qualify as the "definitive proof." The same was true of other early studies.[67]

During the 1960s, scientists did strive to set up a large, well-designed study that would finally settle the issue. In 1960 the NHI began funding a National Diet-Heart Study that involved many prominent researchers. Their aim was to investigate the effects of dietary change on normal, healthy men. However, they calculated that for such an experiment to yield a statistically significant result, they would need to enroll 100,000 subjects for 5 years[68]—a formidable task, but one that the scientists were determined to carry out. Because of the expense and sheer logistical difficulties, they spent several years conducting feasibility studies. Their report, published in 1968, claimed that the experiment was feasible, and recommended that the NHI carry it out as soon as possible.[69]

However, a few years later, an NHI task force recommended against a purely dietary study. Instead, it called for a Multiple Risk Factor Intervention Trial (MRFIT), designed to test whether a combined attack on smoking, high blood pressure, and cholesterol levels would prevent deaths from CHD.[70] Investigators began planning this experiment in 1971, and the results were published in 1982.[71] Scientists thus spent more than two decades designing and conducting a large trial of the cholesterol hypothesis. In the meantime, those concerned with promoting health found it difficult to wait. Instead, public, political, and commercial interest in the links between diet and disease mounted. More policies were formulated. By the time MRFIT produced a result, the urgency had passed.

The 1960s: More Controversy and More Policies

There is a fine line between scientifically respectable treatment and so-called fad-dism: the use of unproven remedies and preventative measures. Such practices are beyond doctors' control,[72] and orthodox medical organizations often warn against the use of fad diets—that is, diets outside the realm of official recommendations—for weight loss and/or health reasons.[73,74] Without definitive evidence of their effi-cacy, cholesterol-lowering diets in the early 1960s hovered on the edge of faddism. However, mounting suggestions of a positive correlation between high cholesterol levels and disease, and the possibility of lowering levels through diet, gradually made cholesterol-lowering diets a scientifically respectable, if still experimental, treatment for patients at high risk of heart disease.

The AHA's cautious endorsement in 1960 of cholesterol-lowering diets for high-risk patients may have been an attempt to regain control over knowledge linking diet to cardiovascular diseases.[75,76] Ironically, however, its equivocal tone encouraged the opposite effect. Its cautious endorsements and careful provisos were exploitable by both sides of the controversy. Vegetable oil companies tested the limits of the FDA ban on health claims by highlighting the AHA statement in advertisements. The National Dairy Council, on the other hand, seized on the disclaimer about "no final proof" to support its counter-claim that "The idea that replacing some 'saturated' fats with 'unsaturated' fats will help prevent heart disease is clearly unproved."[77]

In 1962, the Council on Foods and Nutrition of the American Medication Associ-ation (AMA) published a statement on "The Regulation of Dietary Fat" that, like the AHA report, cautiously endorsed dietary change for those at increased risk of heart disease.[78] It received wide coverage in the popular press.[75,76] The council was so dis-turbed by the enthusiastic media and lay response that it issued a press release titled "Latest Food Fad is Wasted Effort" that tried, once again, to regain control. It pointed out that laboratory tests were necessary to determine cholesterol levels and stressed that doctors should be in charge of any dietary change.[79,80] Again, vegetable oil companies and the dairy industry exploited the situation. Another round of claims and counter-claims created even more confusion.[81–83]

During the 1960s, the lobbyists whose efforts had initially helped to stimulate the massive research effort into the causes of cardiovascular disease became increas-ingly impatient with the scientists' equivocation. Mary Lasker and her allies used their influence in Congress and the NIH to push for comprehensive policies aimed at "conquering" heart disease. When these failed to materialize, they asked President Kennedy to establish a President's Conference on Heart Disease and Cancer.[84] Kennedy was assassinated before these efforts bore fruit. However, President John-son, a sufferer of CHD and personal friend of Lasker's, was a staunch ally of the health lobbyists. His Commission on Heart Disease, Cancer and Stroke was the sec-ond such commission established during his administration, after the Commission on the Assassination of President Kennedy.[85] In 1964, it produced a report recom-mending the establishment of new regional centers for research and treatment of cancer and heart disease, extra training for physicians, and education for the public.[86] The AMA opposed the effort, known as the Regional Medical Program, because it smacked of state intervention in medical practice.[87] The recommendations were watered down. Nevertheless, one outcome of the program did affect policy. An Inter-Society Commission on Heart Disease Resources brought together representatives from 29 medical organizations to formulate policies on prevention, diagnosis, treatment, and rehabilitation.[88]

All these activities—the articles in the popular press, the conflicting advertisements, the lobbying, and the commission—were indications of mounting interest in the relationship between diet and heart disease. The demands that something be done created problems for scientists, as developments in clinical trial methodology made it increasingly difficult for them to produce quick answers. Nevertheless, while the definitive proof of the efficacy of cholesterol-lowering remained elusive, investigations of other aspects of the links between cholesterol and CHD continued. During the 1960s, more epidemiologic studies were reported, including several from Framingham.[89–91] The studies affirmed a consistent positive correlation between serum cholesterol levels and risk of cardiovascular diseases.

In the mid-1960s, the AHA and the AMA decided to broaden their dietary recommendations to include people who did not already have heart disease.[92,93] Both statements cited new epidemiologic knowledge to justify the move to primary prevention. The AMA Council stated: "The observations regarding risk which support this position are derived chiefly from the Public Health Service Study in Framingham, Mass." However, it also noted: "it must be recalled that definitive proof that lowering serum cholesterol, or preventing a rise in serum cholesterol, will lower the morbidity and mortality associated with coronary heart disease, is still lacking."[92] Over the next decade, researchers continued to refine and expand their understanding of many aspects of CHD. Several more policy statements advising dietary change were published.[67,94] For a time, it seemed as though the cholesterol controversy had died down. It reignited, however, when the federal government re-entered the dietary policy arena in the 1970s.

Government Involvement in Nutrition Policy

Since 1917, when it issued its first set of dietary guidelines, the U.S. Department of Agriculture (USDA) has been the federal agency responsible for formulating and disseminating nutrition policies in the United States. For most of the century, the policies were aimed at preventing deficiencies, not deterring excess. Consumers were advised to choose foods from "protective" groups—dairy products, meat and eggs, fruits and vegetables, and so on. The first four editions of the USDA dietary guidelines, published between 1917 and 1946, recommended daily consumption of up to eight food groups, including fat. Such advice benefited the agriculture and food industries.[31] However, the new scientific knowledge linking fats and cholesterol to disease upset the comfortable relationship between food producers and nutrition policy makers. The USDA avoided provoking the wrath of industries selling foods containing saturated fats and cholesterol through two decades of controversy. The 1958 edition of the dietary guidelines did not mention fat at all, and the department refrained from publishing any more guidelines until 1980. The first U.S. government guidelines recommending reductions in fat and cholesterol intakes were highly controversial. They did not emerge from the USDA, but from a temporary body—the Senate Select Committee on Nutrition and Human Needs (SCN).[31,95]

The SCN was initially established in 1968 to tackle malnutrition due to poverty. In 1976, it turned its attention to what it called "diet related to killer diseases" and held hearings to "consider the role of diet in preventive health care and the degree to which diet contributes to the development of major diseases including heart disease, cancer and diabetes."[96–98] A few months later, the SCN released the first edition of *Dietary Goals for the United States*. Among the recommendations were some very provocative suggestions, including, "Decrease consumption of meat. . . . Decrease consumption of butterfat, eggs and other high cholesterol sources."[99]

The meat, diary, and egg industries had made some sporadic, but unsuccessful, attempts during the 1970s to challenge claims that their products caused disease.[100,101] Now, the alarm bells really rang. If *Dietary Goals* were adopted as official government policy, there could be changes to nutrition education, labeling and advertising laws, and the content of diets fed to millions of people, including schoolchildren, hospital patients, prisoners, and armed services personnel. Income price-support mechanisms might also be affected. Food industry lobbyists exerted pressure in Washington, and SCN hearings on the *Dietary Goals* were re-opened. Sessions were set aside to hear testimony from the meat and egg industries.[102,103]

Food industry lobbyists were able to accumulate numerous scientific statements expressing skepticism about the efficacy of dietary change.[104] The SCN revised the *Dietary Goals* and released a second edition in December 1977. Although some proponents of dietary change claimed that industry had exerted strong and illegitimate control over policy,[95,101] the changes were minor. The recommended daily allowances of fats and cholesterol were unchanged. Suggestions for food selection were reworded as follows: "Decrease consumption of animal fat, and choose meats, poultry, and fish which will reduce saturated fat intake. . . . Decrease consumption of butterfat, eggs and other high cholesterol sources. Some consideration should be given to easing the cholesterol goal for pre-menopausal women, young children and the elderly in order to obtain the nutritional benefits of eggs in the diet."[105]

Select Committees can act only in an investigative and advisory capacity and are not empowered to present legislation to Congress.[98] In order for *Dietary Goals* to affect government activities, it had to be taken up and used. Between 1977 and 1980, the situation was quite confused, as it was unclear which sector(s) of the federal health or agricultural bureaucracy, if any, would take responsibility for implementing policies aimed at reducing fat and cholesterol intake. For a time, there was a turf war between the USDA and the Department of Health, Education, and Welfare (DHEW) over nutrition research and policy. Some food activists and their political allies expected the DHEW to take a more proactive role in the dietary prevention of disease. However, scientists at the National Heart Lung and Blood Institute (NHLBI), as the NHI was now called, were in a bind. They were still engaged in two long-term and expensive experiments designed to provide the long-awaited definitive proof of the efficacy of lowering cholesterol levels. The results of MRFIT and a drug trial—the Lipid Research Clinics Coronary Primary Prevention Trial (LRC-CPPT)—would not be available until the early 1980s. Speaking out in favor of dietary change before then would be tantamount to anticipating the results of the trials.[9,106–108]

Although the NHLBI scientists were reluctant to speak out, three sets of dietary recommendations did emerge from various other corners of the federal bureaucracy during 1979 and 1980: a Surgeon General's Report titled *Healthy People*;[109] a joint USDA-DHEW document, *Dietary Guidelines for Americans*;[110] and a report from the Food and Nutrition Board (FNB) of the National Academy of Sciences called *Towards Healthful Diets*.[111] The first two of these advocated reductions in fat and cholesterol intakes, though the former used more emphatic language. The controversy that erupted around the documents followed a pattern that was, by now, quite familiar. Food activists praised *Healthy People* and blamed the meat industry for the more cautious wording of the *Dietary Guidelines*.[108] Meat industry representatives, on the other hand, repeated their claims that the link between diet and disease was still unproven.[112] Of the three statements, the FNB's *Towards Healthful Diets* caused the most uproar. The board had long taken a conservative position on the cholesterol issue.[55,113] Now, members expressed concern about what they saw as an excessive and unrealistic hope that nutrition could prevent diseases such as cancer and heart disease, which they believed were not primarily nutritional in nature. The board took a skeptical approach to the evidence linking saturated fats and cholesterol to heart disease, stating that "intervention trials in which diet modification was employed to alter the incidence of coronary artery disease and mortality in middle-aged men have generally been negative." It also claimed that "epidemiology establishes coincidence, but not cause and effect."[111]

By 1980, at least 18 organizations in the United States and elsewhere had formulated policies recommending dietary change.[114] The FNB was a very prestigious body, and its deviation from the prevailing viewpoint provoked much media interest.[75,76] The debate illustrated the degree to which diet had become a political issue.[114–116] Consuming less fat and cholesterol had become a "progressive," pro-health, pro-consumer cause—a means through which people could protest against corporate greed. On the other hand, political conservatives praised the FNB for taking a stance against the "Naderites" who "mope around Washington, D.C., proclaiming that everything we eat is unsafe."[117] However, although the conservatives were gathering momentum (the Reagan administration was about to begin), they were unable to gain the high moral ground on the cholesterol issue. Food activists pointed out that some of the FNB scientists had links to the egg, dairy, meat, and processed food industries.[114,118] The FNB's consumer liaison panel resigned in protest, and members of the board were required to justify their views in hearings before a House Agriculture Subcommittee.[116,119] After the FNB report, it was difficult for scientists to question the status of evidence in favor of cholesterol-lowering without being labeled dupes of those sectors of the food industry that profited from the sale of saturated fats and cholesterol.

The Large Trials and an End to Controversy

In 1982, the results of the Multiple Risk Factor Intervention Trial (MRFIT) were published.[71] Researchers had designed this trial to test the combined effects of diet, blood pressure medication, and smoking cessation in middle-aged men exhibiting multiple risk factors for heart disease. After screening, 12,866 men were enrolled for an average of 7 years. Despite careful planning, the results were not what the investigators had expected.[71] There was no statistically significant difference between the control and intervention groups in the primary end-point: death from CHD. In designing the trial, scientists had used Framingham data to predict a death rate of 29 per 1000 men in the untreated group and 21.3 per 1000 in the intervention group. However, the death rates were 19.3 and 17.9, respectively. The investigators gave several explanations. There were more deaths than expected among men taking blood pressure medication. Death rates from CHD across the nation had fallen, for reasons that were not clear. Finally, men in the intervention group had not changed their risk factors as much as expected, while many in the "untreated" group had made changes.[71] A report in the *New York Times*, based on interviews with men assigned to the control group, gives an insight into factors that affected the results. One of the men stated: "I said to myself I'm not going to be a part of the control group and kill myself for the sake of their statistics. . . . Once I realized that I had two risk factors, I made some modification."[120] Despite all the careful preparation, definitive proof of the effects of cholesterol-lowering on the incidence of coronary disease remained elusive.

The results of the other large NHLBI test of the cholesterol hypothesis were published in 1984.[121] The Lipid Research Clinics Coronary Primary Prevention Trial (LRC-CPPT) was a drug trial that enrolled 3806 middle-aged men in the top 5% of the risk profile for heart disease. After an average of 7.4 years of medication or placebo, there was slightly less heart disease in the treated group. This result was statistically significant, provided a one-sided test for significance was used.[121] This type of test assumes that the result of the experiment can only go one way—that is, that the treatment can only be beneficial. It is customary to use a two-sided test in clinical trials, thus allowing for the possibility that treatment may be harmful.[122]

Although the LRC-CPPT produced a marginal result, despite enrolling only middle-aged men at very high risk, the NHLBI claimed that it provided the long-awaited definitive proof of the efficacy of cholesterol-lowering drugs and diets in preventing CHD in the general population.[123] There was a lively debate over the interpretation of the results in the medical journals.[122,124–126] In addition to the unorthodox use of the one-tailed test, scientists questioned the validity of extrapolating the results to dietary recommendations for the whole population. The deaths of men in the treatment group also provoked concern. More men taking the drug had died from accidents, suicide, and violence than in the control group. According to some commentators, this warranted further investigation.[122,124–126]

The controversy in medical circles did not spill into the public arena. In the popular press, any lingering uncertainty had been clarified. *Time* magazine, for example, featured a cover story titled "Sorry, It's True. Cholesterol really is a Killer." It quoted leading NHLBI investigator Basil Rifkind: "It is now indisputable that lowering cholesterol with diet and drugs can actually cut the risk of developing heart disease and having a heart attack."[123] Not long after the LRC-CPPT results were published, scientists at the NIH organized a Consensus Conference on Lowering Blood Cholesterol to Prevent Heart Disease. Despite a few dissenting voices, the conference attendees produced a strong statement in favor of dietary change for everyone in the

United States over the age of 2 years.[127–129] It also recommended the establishment of a National Cholesterol Education Program to convince everyone in the United States of the importance of monitoring their cholesterol levels, and if deemed appropriate, reducing them through diet or drug treatment.[130]

Conclusion

By the end of the twentieth century, the anti-fat, anti-cholesterol message was widespread and well-entrenched.[5,6] From time to time, dissenters have argued that the evidence in favor of dietary change is less substantial than is commonly supposed.[131–133] However, so far these arguments have had little or no effect on policy. The institutional mechanisms in favor of fat and cholesterol restriction have become large and well-developed. Only time will tell if, when, and how policy will change. As CHD rates decline and the incidence of obesity increases, we may see a fundamental reassessment of what constitutes healthy eating, similar to that which occurred when medical attention shifted in the mid-twentieth century away from infectious diseases and vitamin deficiencies toward cancer and CHD. On the other hand, the rise in obesity may merely provoke policy makers into intensifying their anti-fat message.

The story of the controversies over fat, cholesterol, and CHD does not hold any easy lessons for the policy makers of the future. It provides, at best, a cautionary tale that illustrates the degree to which policies in the field of public health are inextricably bound up with social, political, and economic concerns. The recent trend toward evidence-based medicine seeks to deflect pressures and influence from these quarters by strengthening the link between policy and reliable scientific evidence.[133] However, it is unlikely that such efforts will be able to neutralize these pressures altogether. "Evidence" is often a slippery concept and hard to come by, and lay people, politicians, and others will continue to demand that scientists and policy makers do something about health problems in the community. Given the pressures, and the difficulties of obtaining definitive evidence, complex political imbroglios are bound to develop. There is no way to insulate medical science from the rest of society. While definitive evidence of efficacy is a powerful resource for legitimating policies, policy makers also need considerable political skills to appreciate and balance the conflicting pressures under which they work.

References

1. Taubes G. What if it's all been a big fat lie? *New York Times Magazine*, 7 July 2002: 22.
2. Larkin M. Little agreement about how to slim down the USA. *Lancet* 2002:360: 1400.
3. Flegal KM, Carroll MD, Ogden CL, Johnson CL. Prevalence and trends in obesity among U.S. adults, 1999–2000. *JAMA* 2002:288:1723–27.
4. Food and Drug Administration, Obesity Working Party. Report on obesity, 2004. Available at: http://www.fda.gov/oc/initiatives/obesity. Accessed 13 February 2005.
5. American Heart Association, Nutrition Committee. Dietary guidelines for healthy American adults. *Circulation* 1996:94:1795–1800.
6. U.S. Department of Agriculture, Department of Health and Human Services. Nutrition and your health: dietary guidelines for Americans. 5th ed. Home and Garden bulletin no.

232, 2000. Available at: http://www.usda.gov.cnpp/dietary-guidelines.html. Accessed 13 February 2005

7. Westman EC, Yancy WS, Edman JS, Tomlin KF, Perkins CE. Effect of 6-month adherence to a very low carbohydrate diet program. *JAMA* 2002:113(1):30–36.

8. Foster GD, Wyatt HR, Hill JO, McGuckin BG, Brill C, Mohammed BS, Szapary PO, Rader DJ, Edman JS, Klein S. A randomized trial of a low-carbohydrate diet for obesity. *N Engl J Med* 2003:348:2082–90.

9. Liebman B. The truth about the Atkins diet. *Nutrition Action* 2002:29:1–7.

10. Braunwald E. Shattuck lecture: Cardiovascular medicine at the turn of the millennium: triumphs, concerns and opportunities. *N Engl J Med* 1997:337:1360–69.

11. Pooling of funds urged in health report. *JAMA* 1945:129:1037.

12. Drew EB. The health syndicate. *Atlantic Monthly*, December 1967, 75–82.

13. Strickland SP. Politics, Science, and Dread Disease: A Short History of United States Medical Research Policy. Cambridge, MA: Harvard University Press, 1972.

14. Spingarn N. Heartbeat: The Politics of Health Research. Washington, DC and New York: Robert B. Luce, 1976.

15. Shepard WP. The American Heart Association as a national voluntary public health agency. *Circulation* 1950:2:736–41.

16. The American Heart Association prepares for intensified educational and fund-raising activities. *American Heart J* 1947:34:933–34.

17. National heart week. *American Heart J* 1948:35:528.

18. Gold awards given at annual dinner. *American Heart J* 1949:38:159.

19. $4 million raised in heart campaign. *Circulation* 1950:2:320.

20. News from the American Heart Association. *Circulation* 1960:21:477.

21. Weiss S, Minot GR. Nutrition in relation to arteriosclerosis. In: Cowdry EV, ed. Arteriosclerosis. A Survey of the Problem. New York: Macmillan, 1933, 233–48.

22. Leary T. Atherosclerosis: the important form of arteriosclerosis, a metabolic disease. *JAMA* 1935:105:475–81.

23. Davis D, Stern B, Lesnick G. The lipid and cholesterol content of the blood of patients with angina pectoris and atherosclerosis. *Annals Intern Med* 1937:11:354–68.

24. Boas EP, Parets AD, Aldersberg D. Hereditary disturbance of cholesterol metabolism: a factor in the genesis of atherosclerosis. *American Heart J* 1948:35:611–22.

25. Kempner W. Treatment of hypertensive vascular disease with rice diet. *Am J Med* 1948:4:545–77.

26. Keys A, Mickelsen O, Miller E, Chapman CB. The relation in man between cholesterol levels in the diet and in the blood. *Science* 1950.112.79–81.

27. Keys A, Anderson JT. The relationship of the diet to the development of atherosclerosis in man. In: Allen EV, ed., Symposium on Atherosclerosis. Washington, DC: National Academy of Sciences, National Research Council, 1954, 181–97.

28. Page IH. The Lewis A. Connor memorial lecture: atherosclerosis. an introduction. *Circulation* 1954:10:1–27.

29. Adams W. The 100% American way to die. *Better Homes and Gardens* 1947:26:32, 224–231.

30. Keys A. Recollections of pioneers in nutrition: from starvation to cholesterol. *J Am Coll Nutrit* 1990:9:288–91.

31. Hunt SM, Kaufman M. Applying nutrition science to the public's health. In: Kaufman M, ed., Nutrition in Public Health: A Handbook for Developing Programs and Services. Gaithersburg, MD: Aspen Publishers, 1990, 14–41.

32. Allen EV. Atherosclerosis: a symposium. *Circulation* 1952:5:98–100.

33. Keys A. Seven Countries. A Multivariate Analysis of Death and Coronary Heart Disease. Cambridge, MA and London, England: Harvard University Press, 1980.

34. Page IH, Stare FJ, Corcoran AC, Pollack H, Wilkinson CF. Atherosclerosis and the fat content of the diet. *Circulation* 1957:16:163–78.

35. Moore FE. Committee on Design and Analysis of Studies. *Am J Public Health* 1960:50: 10–19.

36. Doyle JT, Heslin AS, Hilleboe HE, Formel PF. Early diagnosis of ischemic heart disease. *N Engl J Med* 1959:261:1096–1101.

37. Zukel WJ, Lewis RH, Enterline PE, Painter RC, Ralston LS, Fawcett RM, Meredith AP, Peterson B. A short-term community study of the epidemiology of coronary heart disease. *Am J Public Health* 1959:49:1630–39.

38. Paul O, Lepper MH, Phelan WH, Dupertuis GW, MacMillan A, McKean H, Park H., A longitudinal study of coronary heart disease. *Circulation* 1963:28:20–31.

39. Chapman JM, Massey FJ. The interrelationship of serum cholesterol, hypertension, body weight, and risk of coronary disease. Results of the first ten years' follow-up in the Los Angeles Heart Study. *J Chronic Dis* 1964:17:933–49.

40. McDonough JR, Hames CG, Stulb SC, Garrison GE., Coronary heart disease among Negroes and whites in Evans County, Georgia, *J Chronic Dis* 1965:18:443–68.

41. Epstein FH, Ostrander LD, Johnson BC, Payne MW, Hayner NS, Keller JB, Francis T. Epidemiological studies of cardiovascular disease in a total community: Tecumsah, Michigan. *Ann Intern Med* 1965:62:1170–86.

42. Gordon T, Kannel WB. The Framingham, Massachusetts, study twenty years later. In: Kessler II, Levin ML, eds. The Community as an Epidemiological Laboratory. Baltimore: John Hopkins University Press, 1970, 123–44.

43. Dawber TR, Meadors GF, Moore FE. Epidemiological approaches to heart disease: the Framingham study. *Am J Public Health* 1951:41:279–86.

44. Dawber TR, Moore FE, Mann GV. Coronary heart disease in the Framingham study. *Am J Public Health* 1957:47(part 2):4–23.

45. Fat's the villain. *Newsweek,* 27 September 1954, 90–91.

46. Clark B. Is this the no. 1 villain in heart disease? *Readers Digest* 1955:67:130–36.

47. The president: a difficult time. *Newsweek,* 3 October 1955, 19–21.

48. King CG. A Good Idea: The History of the Nutrition Foundation. New York and Washington, DC: Nutrition Foundation, 1976.

49. Berryman GH. Nutrition and nutritional diseases. In: Rytand DA, Creger, WP, eds. Annual Review of Medicine, 1959. Stanford, CA: Annual Reviews Inc.,127–44.

50. Bello F. How good is Mr. Hurley's diet? *Fortune* 1959:60:129–34, 188–96.

51. Health claims by cooking oils due for censure. *Printers' Ink* 1959: 278:14–15.

52. Fats and heart disease. *Time,* 12 November 1956, 45–46.

53. Christakis G, Rinzler SH, Archer M, Winslow G, Jampel S, Stephenson J, Friedman G, Fein H, Kraus A, James G. The anti-coronary club: a dietary approach to the prevention of coronary heart disease—a seven-year report. *Am J Public Health* 1966:56: 299–314.

54. Clark M. Fats—not proved guilty. *Newsweek,* 20 May 1957, 33–35.

55. Heart report issued. *New York Times,* 8 May 1958, 74.

56. Council on Foods and Nutrition. Council activities. *JAMA* 1959:171:925–28.

57. Unsaturated fats and oils claims get back hand from FDA. *Oil, Paint and Drug Reporter* 1959:176:7, 62.

58. Plumb RK. 8 Physicians give advice on heart. *New York Times,* 22 January 1959, 33.

59. Two apples a day. *Time* 1960:76:73.

60. American Heart Association. Dietary fat and its relation to heart attack and strokes: report by the Central Committee for the Medical Community Program of the American Heart Association. *Circulation* 1961:23:133–36.

61. Jolliffe N, Rinzler SH, Archer A. Anti-coronary club: including discussion of effects of prudent diet on serum cholesterol levels of middle-aged men. *Am J Clin Nutr* 1959: 7:451–62.

62. Pilkington TRE, Stafford JL, Hankin VS, Simmonds FM, Koerselman HB. Practical diets for lowering serum lipids: a long-term study on out-patients with ischaemic heart disease. *Br Med J* 1960:23–25.

63. Gofman JW, Jones HB, Lindgren FT, Lyon TP, Elliott HA, Strisower B. Blood lipids and human atherosclerosis. *Circulation* 1950:2:161–77.

64. Jones HB, Gofman JW, Lingren FT, Lyon TP, Graham DM, Strisower B, Nichols AV. Lipoproteins in atherosclerosis. *Am J Med* 1951:11:358–79.

65. Morrison LM. Diet in coronary atherosclerosis. *JAMA* 1960:173:884–88.

66. Marks, HM. The Progress of Experiment: Science and Therapeutic Reform in the United States, 1900–1990. Cambridge UK: Cambridge University Press, 1997.

67. Inter-Society Commission for Heart Disease Resources. Primary prevention of atherosclerotic diseases. *Circulation* 1970:42:A55–A95.

68. Baker, BB, Frantz ID, Keys A, Kinsell LD, Page IH, Stamler J, Stare FJ. The National Diet-Heart Study: an initial report. *JAMA* 1963:185:105–6.

69. National Diet-Heart Study Research Group. The National Diet-Heart Study Final Report. AHA monograph no. 18. New York: American Heart Association, 1968.

70. A Report by the National Heart and Lung Institute Task Force on Arteriosclerosis, vol. 1. DHEW publication no. NIH 72–137. Washington, DC: National Institutes of Health, 1971.

71. MRFIT Research Group. Multiple Risk Factor Intervention Trial: risk factor changes and mortality results. *JAMA* 1982:248:1465–77.

72. Freidson, E. Professional Dominance: The Social Structure of Medical Care. New York: Harper and Row, 1970.

73. Beeuwkes, AM. Food faddism—a growing threat. *Postgraduate Medicine* 1960; 28: 75–81.

74. Stein K. High-protein, low-carbohydrate diets: do they work? *J Am Diet Assoc* 2000: 100:760–61.

75. Garrety K. Actor networks, social worlds and controversy: the case of cholesterol, dietary fat and heart disease. *Social Studies of Science* 1997:27:727–73.

76. Garrety K. Science, policy, and controversy in the cholesterol arena. *Symbolic Interaction* 1998.21.401–24.

77. Fat in the fire. *Time,* 26 December 1960, 33.

78. Council on Foods and Nutrition. The regulation of dietary fat. *JAMA* 1962:181:411–29.

79. Council warns against unsupervised dieting to lower cholesterol. *JAMA* 1962:182:36.

80. Darby WJ. Diet and coronary atheroma. *JAMA* 1962:182:1328–29.

81. Bart, P. Advertising: dairy men open counterattack. *New York Times,* 7 August 1962, 36.

82. Company answers AMA diet warning. *New York Times,* 14 October 1962, 14.

83. National Dairy Council. Physicians are asking us . . . what is the dairy industry doing about the question of diet and heart disease? (Advertisement) *JAMA* 1962:182:22.

84. Heart-Cancer Conference. *JAMA* 1961:176:26.

85. Wolanin TR. Presidential Advisory Commissions. Truman to Nixon. Madison: University of Wisconsin Press, 1975.

86. Langer E. U.S. medicine: LBJ Commission on Heart Disease, Cancer and Stroke offers sweeping recommendations. *Science* 1964:146:1662–64.

87. A national program to conquer heart disease, cancer and stroke. *JAMA* 1965:192: 299–301.
88. Hicks, N. Heart study group uses U.S. funds. *New York Times,* 16 December 1970, 37.
89. Cornfield J. Joint dependence of risk of coronary heart disease on serum cholesterol and systolic blood pressure: a discriminant function analysis. *Federation Proceedings* 1962: 21(suppl 2):58–61.
90. Dawber TR, Kannel WB, Revotskie N, Kagan A. The epidemiology of coronary heart disease: the Framingham enquiry. *Proc R Soc Med* 1962:55:265–71.
91. Kannel WB, Dawber TR, Friedman GD, Glennon WE, McNamara PM. Risk factors in coronary heart disease: an evaluation of several serum lipids as predictors of coronary heart disease. *Ann Intern Med* 1964:61:888–99.
92. Heart group urges all to eat less fatty food. *New York Times,* 9 June 1964, 71.
93. Council on Foods and Nutrition. Diet and the possible prevention of coronary atheroma: a council statement. *JAMA* 1965:194:1149–50.
94. Council on Foods and Nutrition. Diet and coronary heart disease. *JAMA* 1972:222:1647.
95. Nestle M. Food lobbies, the Food Pyramid and U.S. nutrition policy. *Int J Health Serv* 1993:23:483–96.
96. Congressional Information Service. CIS Annual 1976. Washington, DC: Government Printing Office, 1977.
97. Zebich ML. The politics of nutrition: issue definition, agenda-setting, and policy formulation in the United States. PhD thesis, University of New Mexico, 1979.
98. Porter DV. Nutrition policy making in the United States Congress. PhD thesis, Ohio State University, 1980.
99. U.S. Congress, Senate Select Committee on Nutrition and Human Needs. Dietary goals for the United States. 95th Congress, 1st Session, February 1977. Washington, DC: Government Printing Office, 1977.
100. Brody JE. FTC studies ads disavowing link of eggs to heart disease. *New York Times,* 7 January 1974, 15.
101. Hausman P. Jack Sprat's Legacy: The Science and Politics of Fat and Cholesterol. New York: Richard Marek Publishers, 1981.
102. Congressional Information Service. CIS Annual 1977. Washington, DC: Government Printing Office, 1978.
103. Congressional Information Service. CIS Annual 1978. Washington, DC: Government Printing Office, 1979.
104. U.S. Congress. Hearings Before the Select Committee on Nutrition and Human Needs of the U.S. Senate. 95th Congress, 1st Session. March 24, 1977. Response to the dietary goals for the United States: re: meat. Washington, DC: Government Printing Office, 1977.
105. U.S. Congress Senate Select Committee on Nutrition and Human Needs. Dietary goals for the United States, 2nd ed. 95th Congress, 1st Session, December 1977. Washington, DC: Government Printing Office, 1977.
106. Broad WJ. Jump in funding feeds research on nutrition. *Science* 1979:204:1060–64.
107. Broad WJ. NIH deals gingerly with diet-disease link. *Science* 1979:204:1175–78.
108. Broad WJ. Surgeon General says get healthy, eat less meat. *Science* 1979:205:1112–13.
109. U.S. Surgeon General. Healthy People. The Surgeon General's Report on Health Promotion and Disease Prevention. Washington, DC: Department of Health, Education and Welfare, 1979.
110. U.S. Department of Agriculture & Department of Health & Human Services. Nutrition and your health: dietary guidelines for Americans. Reproduced in *Nutrition Today* 1980:15:14–18.

111. Food and Nutrition Board of the National Academy of Sciences. Towards healthful diets. Reproduced in *Nutrition Today* 1980:15:7–11.

112. King SS. Federal role is expanding as advisor on nutrition. *New York Times* 6 February1980, C1, C8.

113. Schmeck, HM. Report prescribes exercise, less fat. *New York Times,* 11 July 1966, 1, 14.

114. Broad, WJ. Academy says curb on cholesterol not needed. *Science* 1980:208:1354–55.

115. Seligman, D. Fear of eating. *Fortune* 1980:101:45.

116. Wade, N. Food board's fat report hits fire. *Science* 1980:209:248–50.

117. Seligman, D. The food test. *Fortune* 1980:101: 41.

118. Altman, LK. Report about cholesterol draws agreement and dissent. *New York Times,* 28 May 1980, 16.

119. De Witt, K. Scientists clash on academy's cholesterol advice. *New York Times,* 20 June 1980, 15.

120. Friedland S. Heart study led to changes in life style. *New York Times,* 10 October 1982, K4.

121. Lipid Research Clinics Program. The Lipid Research Clinics Coronary Primary Prevention Trial results. I. Reduction in incidence of coronary heart disease. *JAMA* 1984:251: 351–64.

122. Kronmal RA. Commentary on the published results of the Lipid Research Clinics Coronary Primary Prevention Trial. *JAMA* 1985:253:2091–93.

123. Sorry, it's true: cholesterol really is a killer. *Time,* 23 January 1984, 32.

124. Enloe C. Coronary disease prevention should be individualized. *Nutrition Today* 1984: 19:12–14.

125. Rahimtoola, SH. Cholesterol and coronary heart disease: a perspective. *JAMA* 1985: 253:2094–95.

126. Olson RE. Mass intervention vs. screening and selective intervention for the prevention of coronary heart disease. *JAMA*1986:255:2204–7.

127. Consensus Conference. Lowering blood cholesterol levels to prevent heart disease. *JAMA* 1985:253:2080–6.

128. Oliver MF. Consensus or nonsensus conferences on coronary heart disease *Lancet* 1985: 325:1087–89.

129. Moore TJ. Heart Failure. New York: Random House, 1989.

130. Lenfant C. A new challenge for America: The National Cholesterol Education Program. *Circulation* 1986:73:855–56.

131. Mann GV, ed. Coronary Heart Disease: The Dietary Sense and Nonsense. London: Janus, 1993.

132. Ravnskov U. The Cholesterol Myths. Washington, DC: New Trends Publishing, 2000.

133. Cooper MJ, Zlotkin SH. An evidence-based approach to the development of national dietary guidelines. *J Am Diet Assoc* 2003:102(suppl 2):S28–S33.

Suggested Reading

Keys A. Recollections of pioneers in nutrition: from starvation to cholesterol. *J Am Coll Nutr* 1990:9:288–91.

Garrety K. Actor networks, social worlds and controversy: the case of cholesterol, dietary fat and heart disease. *Social Studies of Science* 1997:27:727–73.

PART X

TOBACCO AND DISEASE PREVENTION

20

Thank You for Not Smoking: The Public Health Response to Tobacco-Related Mortality in the United States

MICHAEL P. ERIKSEN
LAWRENCE W. GREEN
CORINNE G. HUSTEN
LINDA L. PEDERSON
TERRY F. PECHACEK

The recognition of cigarette smoking as a cause of disease and the subsequent reduction in tobacco use and associated mortality and death is a remarkable public health achievement.[1] During the last third of the century and following the release of the first surgeon general's report, smoking rates and per capita consumption of cigarettes declined by 50%,[2] and exposure to secondhand tobacco smoke was reduced dramatically.[3] As a result, more than 1 million deaths that would have been caused by tobacco were avoided, resulting in longer life expectancy and an improved quality of life for the American public.[4]

Unfortunately, this achievement came too late for millions of smokers. The Centers for Disease Control and Prevention (CDC) estimated that in the 30 years following the first surgeon general's report in 1964,[5] 10 million Americans died as a result of smoking.[6] Analyses done in the 1990s suggest that if current trends continue, another 25 million Americans will be killed by cigarette smoking, including 5 million children.[7] Thus, although much progress has been made (see Fig. 20.1), tobacco use continues to cause a substantial public health burden.

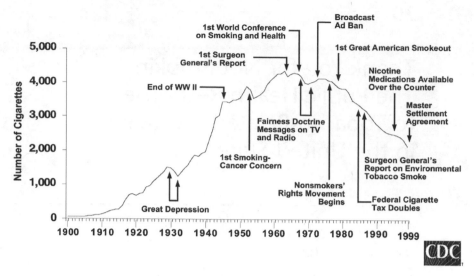

Figure 20.1. Adult per capita cigarette consumption and major smoking and health events—
United States, 1900–1999. (USDA; 1986–2000 Surgeon General's Reports.)

Changing Patterns in Tobacco Use and Disease

Tobacco consumption in the United States before the twentieth century included cer-
emonial use by Native Americans and the use of tobacco for pipes, hand-rolled cigarettes, cigars, and chewing tobacco by non-Native Americans. Cigarette smoking as
a highly addicting and habituated behavior is a twentieth-century phenomenon. The
introduction of blended tobacco that allowed deeper inhalation, the invention of the
safety match, and the introduction of mass production of cigarettes, coupled with
sophisticated distribution systems and unprecedented marketing efforts, led to the
rapid adoption of the cigarette smoking habit during the first half of the twentieth
century. In 1963, per capita consumption of cigarettes peaked prior to the release of
the First Surgeon General's Report the following year. With a growing awareness of
the danger of smoking came the first filter in the 1950s, which was designed to reduce the tar inhaled in the smoke. Later, low-tar cigarettes were developed, but their
design allowed smokers to compensate by smoking more intensely and by blocking
the filter's ventilation holes.[61] Paralleling the changes in cigarette design and smoking behavior, adenocarcinoma exceeded squamous-cell carcinoma as the leading
cause of lung cancer-related death in the United States.[62]

In the early twentieth century, lung cancer was rare. As cigarettes became increasingly popular, first among men and later among women, the incidence of lung
cancer reached epidemic levels. In 1930, the lung-cancer death rate for men was 4.9
per 100,000; by 1990, the rate had increased to 75.6 per 100,000.[13] In the 1940s and
1950s, epidemiologic studies involving substantial numbers of participants, including one study of male British physicians,[14] linked cigarette smoking to lung cancer.
In 1964, on the basis of approximately 7000 articles relating smoking and disease,

the Advisory Committee to the U.S. Surgeon General concluded that cigarette smoking is a cause of lung and laryngeal cancer in men, a probable cause of lung cancer in women, and the most important cause of chronic bronchitis in both sexes.[5] The committee stated that "cigarette smoking is a health hazard of sufficient importance in the United States to warrant appropriate remedial action."

In the years following the First Surgeon General's Report, tobacco use was implicated as the cause of diseases affecting nearly every vital organ system. In fact, the 2004 surgeon general's report concluded that "smoking harms nearly every organ of the body."[74] Diseases of the pulmonary and cardiovascular systems were most commonly associated with tobacco use, with heart disease, lung cancer, and respiratory diseases (including chronic obstructive pulmonary disease) occurring most frequently. Tobacco use was also recognized as a cause of stroke; artherosclerotic peripheral vascular disease; cancers of the larynx, oral cavity, esophagus, and pancreas; intrauterine growth retardation; low birth weight, and sudden infant death syndrome (SIDS).[11,12] The 2004 surgeon general's report also reviewed more recent data showing that smoking causes many other additional diseases including stomach cancer, acute myeloid leukemia, pancreatic cancer, and pneumonia among others. In 1995–1999, smoking caused an annual average of 155,761 deaths from cancer, 148,605 deaths from cardiovascular-related diseases, and 82,431 deaths from chronic lung disease; 55,600 deaths among persons who used tobacco were attributable to other causes.[9] Although other causes contribute to many of these diseases, tobacco makes the largest contribution to the death toll. Tobacco use exacerbates symptoms and multiplies the effects of the other contributing causes of diseases and conditions.

At the end of the twentieth century, smokers died more frequently from lung cancer (an average of 124,813 deaths annually for 1995–1999) than any other single disease caused by smoking.[9] In 1987, lung cancer surpassed breast cancer as the leading cause of cancer death among U.S. women;[15] by 2000, 27,000 more women were dying annually from lung cancer than from breast cancer.[12] Among men, nearly 90% of lung cancer is caused by cigarette smoking.[11]

As a result of these adverse health effects, an estimated one of every two lifetime smokers will have their lives shortened as a result of their use of tobacco products.[8] On average, smoking shortens the lives of men by 13.2 years and women by 14.5 years when compared with the life expectancy of a person who never smoked.[9] In addition, although 20–30 years can lapse between the initiation of tobacco use and the manifestation of life-threatening symptoms, death and disease caused by smoking is not limited to older age groups; certain symptoms (e.g., coughing spells, productive cough, and wheezing or gasping) and loss of full functioning begin to appear soon after habitual smoking is established.[10] Cigarette smoking is a major cause of death among persons 35–64 years of age; in this age group, smoking causes an estimated 42% of coronary heart disease deaths in men and 26% in women.[11]

In addition to smoking, the use of other forms of tobacco causes illness. Pipe and cigar smoking increases the risk of lip, oral, and lung cancer; smokeless (i.e., spit) tobacco causes oral cancer as well as other oral lesions.[17,18] Other tobacco products, popular internationally, most notably, kreteks (popular in Indonesia) and bidis (popular in India), can cause cancer and diseases of the heart and lungs.[19]

In addition to health risk for consumers of tobacco products, the adverse health effects for nonsmokers' exposure to environmental or secondhand smoke were documented. In 1986, a report by the U.S. Surgeon General concluded that exposure to secondhand smoke can cause disease, including cancer, in otherwise healthy adults.[20] In 1992, the U.S. Environmental Protection Agency (EPA) documented the effects of secondhand smoke on respiratory outcomes, especially among children.[21] Several groups subsequently concluded that secondhand smoke is a potent carcinogen.[22-24]

Populations categorized by factors such as income, occupation, and education levels differ in the use of tobacco and the frequency of associated diseases. In 1995, the age-adjusted rate of death per 100,000 U.S. residents from malignant diseases of the respiratory system age-adjusted deaths were 80.5 among black men compared to 53.7 among white men. Age-adjusted death rates for cerebrovascular disease also reflect a disparity in health outcomes; in 1992–1994, the rate was 53.1 per 100,000 among black men and 26.3 among white men.[16] The reasons demographic factors (e.g., race/ethnicity and socioeconomic status) profoundly affect patterns of tobacco use and health outcomes are complex. Some possible factors include racial discrimination, cultural characteristics and acculturation, stress, biologic elements, advertising practices, the price of tobacco products, and varying capacities of communities to mount effective tobacco-control initiatives. Ongoing research is needed to address these questions.

Decline in the Use of Tobacco

Given the broad acceptance of the cigarette and its diffusion throughout society, the dramatic reduction in smoking over the last three decades of the twentieth century is an extraordinary achievement. Reflecting the impact of multiple public health measures, the annual per capita cigarette consumption peaked at a high of 4345 cigarettes in 1963, the year before the release of the 1964 Surgeon General's Report, and decreased to 2030 cigarettes by the start of the twenty-first century,[2] a reduction of more than 50% since 1964.

Paralleling the reduction in per capita consumption, smoking prevalence among persons aged ≥18 years decreased from 43% in 1965 to 25.5% in 1990.[27] By the first quarter of 2004, prevalence had declined to 20.1%,[29] representing a reduction of more than 50% since the issuance of the 1964 Surgeon General's Report. In addition, the percentage of adults who had never smoked increased from 44% in the mid-1960s to 58% in 2004.[27,29] The number of American smokers declined by tens of millions from what would be expected had earlier rates continued. Progress since 1964, however, has not been experienced equally by all U.S. population groups.

Contrary to experiences in other parts of the world, in the United States, smoking rates differ only minimally by gender. However, race/ethnicity, socioeconomic status, age, and geographic region of residence continue to be predictors of tobacco use. By the end of the twentieth century, the percentages of adults smoking by race and ethnicity varied widely, from 36% of American Indians and Alaska Natives to 14% of Asians. A similar differential was seen for education, with persons having a General Educational Development (GED) diploma being five times more likely to smoke than those with a graduate degree; this differential may be increasing into the twenty-first century.[30]

The 1994 Surgeon General's Report, *Preventing Tobacco Use Among Young People*,[31] focused on smoking among youth and young adults. This report emphasized that smoking onset and nicotine addiction almost always began in the teen years, and it provided an early warning of an increase in tobacco use among young adults. After more than a decade of relatively stable rates among youth in the 1980s,[32] cigarette smoking began increasing rapidly among high school students in the early 1990s, peaked in the 1996–97 school year, and began a decline by the end of decade.[33] In 2000, smoking prevalence among high school seniors was 31%, a level comparable to the 1980 rate,[34] and since 2000 teenage smoking rates have fallen further.[73]

The relationships between rates of smoking among black and white youth changed throughout the century. In the late 1970s, rates were similar; however, during the 1980s and 1990s, white youth continued to smoke at relatively high rates and rates among black youth plummeted.[16] By the end of the 1900s, however, the difference in rates between black and white students lessened.[33] By 2000, rates between black and white middle-school students were comparable.[35]

The Use of Other Tobacco Products

Use of smokeless tobacco changed only slightly during 1970–1998, with a 5% prevalence in 1970 and 1998 for men, and a 2% and less than 0.5% prevalence, respectively, for women.[12] Smokeless tobacco use was highest among high school males, with a prevalence of 18.9% among whites, 6.4% among Hispanics, and 2.9% among blacks.[36] Rates were lower in the Northeast and higher in the South. Total consumption of cigars decreased from $8 billion in 1970 to $2 billion in 1993, but increased 68% to $3.6 billion in 1997.[37] In 1998, rates of cigar use were 8% for men and less than 1% for women.[12] However, among high school students in 2001, the prevalence of cigar smoking increased to 22.1% for boys and 8.5% for girls,[36] reflecting a disturbing pattern of use of alternative or novel tobacco products (particularly bidis and kreteks) among young persons.[35] Although rates of frequent use of cigars, smokeless tobacco, pipes, bidis, and kreteks among adolescents are low when compared with cigarettes,[35] when all forms of tobacco are combined, the range of tobacco use is 25%–40% for all demographic subgroups of high school students; these rates approach 50% for boys in the 12th grade.[36]

Shortly after the cancer risk associated with tobacco was described in 1964, substantial public health efforts were undertaken to reduce the prevalence of tobacco use. With the subsequent decline in smoking, the incidence of smoking-related cancers (including cancers of the lung, oral cavity, and pharynx) eventually declined, with the exception of lung cancer among women.[12] In addition, age-adjusted deaths per 100,000 persons (standardized to the 1940 population) for coronary heart disease decreased from 307.4 in 1950 to 134.6 in 1996 (25). During 1964–1992, approximately 1.6 million deaths that would have been caused by smoking were prevented.[4]

Changes in Strategies to Prevent Tobacco Use

Rather than a single event or policy, many public health forces can be credited for reducing smoking (Fig. 20.1). The dramatic reduction in tobacco use started with the
widespread dissemination of scientific information regarding the dangers of active
and passive smoking, followed by clinical strategies to help persons quit smoking,
and most recently by legal strategies to create disincentives for persons to begin or
continue to use tobacco. The tobacco industry was also held accountable for the
harm caused. All of these prevention efforts were conducted in an environment of
the continued marketing of cigarettes and other products by the tobacco companies,[38] creating a continual state of action and reaction between the tobacco industry
and public health organizations that has characterized the history of tobacco control.

Informational and Educational Strategies

With the publication of the first studies in the 1950s regarding the hazards of smoking,[11] and after the publication of the 1964 Surgeon General's Report,[5] tobacco-use
initiatives were primarily informational or educational. Educational strategies operated on the assumption that knowledge about the adverse health effects of tobacco
would lead to behavior change. The studies and reports documenting the adverse
health impact of secondhand smoke to nonsmokers triggered similar educational efforts.[20–24,39] Other initiatives created to inform the public about the dangers of tobacco
included the addition and subsequent strengthening of warning labels on tobacco
products and in tobacco advertising. Counter-marketing as an educational strategy began with the Fairness Doctrine in 1969, which required radio and television stations to
broadcast one cigarette counter-advertisement for every paid cigarette advertisement.[11] In 1970, counter-marketing became much more limited in scope after tobacco
advertising was removed from television and radio, but became more prominent again
in the early 1990s as a result of the development of California's comprehensive tobacco prevention and control program, which relied heavily on media messages.[40]
Most recently, the tobacco industry developed their own media campaign purportedly
to reduce youth smoking. However, there are no data supporting the effectiveness of
the tobacco industry campaign, and it might in fact have reduced the effectiveness of
other independent counter-marketing campaigns.[41]

During the twentieth century, the tobacco industry worked to influence public
opinion about smoking and to counter growing scientific information on the harm of
smoking. In 1954, cigarette companies sponsored advertisements disputing the evidence that smoking caused cancer.[42] The tobacco industry continued to deny any link
between their products and disease until 1998, when they acknowledged that public
health authorities had concluded that smoking was harmful; tobacco companies,
however, still disputed the link between secondhand smoke and disease. The tobacco
industry continues to promote the appeal, access, and affordability of tobacco products. In 2002, the U.S. cigarette companies spent $12.5 billion on marketing and pro-
moting cigarettes[43]—an 85% increase from 1998, amounting to an annual marketing
expenditure of more than $.80 for every pack sold. The magnitude of this expendi-
ture is not surprising given the rapid decline in total U.S. cigarette consumption

dropping from 465 billion cigarettes in 1998 to 390 billion in 2004,[2] which might have triggered tobacco companies to intensify efforts to attract more smokers. Successful efforts to reduce tobacco use must restrict the form, content, and magnitude of tobacco advertising.

Clinical Strategies

In the 1980s, clinical strategies for reducing tobacco gained momentum with the increased understanding of the addictive nature of nicotine.[44] In 1984, the Food and Drug Administration (FDA) began to approve medications to help smokers quit.[45] In the 1990s, strategies were developed to reach smokers with intensive counseling services (e.g., telephone quit-lines),[46] and clinical practice guidelines outlined the strong evidence base for effective clinical interventions.[47] However, despite the implementation of effective clinical strategies, the treatment of tobacco dependence is not fully integrated into routine clinical care, and effective treatments are neither widely available to all smokers nor covered under private and public insurance.

The Public Health Service guideline titled *Treating Tobacco Use and Dependence*,[47] published in 2000, documented that basic advice received from a health-care provider can increase cessation rates by 30%. If half of all U.S. physicians provided this advice to their smoking patients, a 30% increase would translate into more than 2 million additional smokers quitting each year.[50] Intensive counseling interventions and pharmacotherapy can double cessation rates when used individually, and the combination of both interventions is even more effective.[47] Clinical interventions are also highly cost-effective.[51,52] In a 2001 study in which 30 recommended clinical preventive services were prioritized on the basis of their impact, effectiveness, and cost-effectiveness, treating tobacco use among adults ranked second only to the vaccination of children against infectious diseases.[53] However, integrating routine tobacco-use treatment into the health-care system and increasing access to effective treatments proved challenging.

In 2001, the Task Force on Community Preventive Services found that reminder systems increase the provision of treatment services and those reminder systems together with provider training are even more effective.[54] The task force also found that both the use of effective treatments and cessation rates can be increased by reducing the out-of-pocket costs of treatment and making cessation counseling more convenient (e.g., by providing treatment through telephone cessation help-lines).[54]

Legislative, Regulatory, and Other Legal Strategies

One of the most effective means of reducing tobacco use is increasing the cost of tobacco use through increases in federal and state excise taxes. A 10% increase in the price of cigarettes can lead to a 4% reduction in the demand for cigarettes.[54] Low-income, adolescent, Hispanic, and non-Hispanic black smokers were most likely to stop smoking in response to a price increase.[55]

In the 1960s and 1970s, economic interventions focused on smokers "paying their way."[56] However, because of the link that had been established between cost of tobacco and reduction in cigarette smoking, raising the price of tobacco products became a primary tobacco-control strategy in the 1990s.[55] The accelerated use of this strategy is evident by comparing the average combined federal/state excise tax for 1910 ($0.025), 1982 ($.08), and 2002 ($0.60). In addition to federal and state excise taxes, some local jurisdictions independently taxed tobacco products. In 2002, New York City imposed an additional $1.50 tax on top of the state tax of $1.50, which increased the price of a pack of cigarettes to over $7.00.[58] The tobacco industry, however, has countered the effect of tax increases by absorbing the price increases, reducing prices, developing discount brands, providing coupons and other promotional discounts, and distributing free cigarettes.

With the further development of the science base for tobacco control and growing public demand for remedial action during the 1990s, legal, regulatory, and legislative strategies have assumed a larger role in tobacco prevention and control. However, tobacco products remain virtually unregulated, particularly given their harmful and addictive nature.

In 1938, the federal regulatory oversight of tobacco use began when the FDA asserted jurisdiction over tobacco products that were making health claims.[59] During the 1990s,[60] the FDA exerted authority over tobacco products but this authority was challenged by the tobacco industry. In 2000, the Supreme Court determined that Congress had not given explicit authority to FDA to regulate the sale and marketing of tobacco products. Overall, progress in federal tobacco regulation has been slow and difficult. Not only are tobacco products not subject to meaningful regulation, but they are also expressly exempted from regulation by various federal laws designed to protect consumers (e.g., the Consumer Product Safety Act).[59]

Despite the lack of federal legislation, private industry began to establish its own smoking-related policies. In 1970, airlines voluntarily adopted policies restricting smoking in flight. These policies were expanded in 1989 to impose mandatory total smoking bans on U.S. airlines. Restrictions on smoking in indoor areas expanded in 1998 to include all bars in California.[65] However, because much of the regulatory impetus for clean indoor air occurred at the local level, the industry countered by promoting preemptive legislation (i.e., legislation prohibiting localities from promulgating stronger regulations that those of the state) at the state level. By 2000, 30 states had preemptive legislation in place.[66]

Comprehensive Approaches

The combination of scientific documentation of harm, public advocacy, changing social norms and litigation, and disclosure of industry documents will, it is hoped, continue into the twenty-first century. However, future progress in reducing tobacco use will be accelerated only by (1) vigorous implementation of comprehensive tobacco-control interventions, (2) helping smokers quit, and (3) protecting nonsmokers from exposure to secondhand smoke. California, Massachusetts, Florida, Arizona, Oregon, and Mississippi have state-based interventions that have greatly accelerated reductions in tobacco use among both adults and children. These programs serve as models for other states. However, in 2000, only six states met the Centers for Disease Control and Prevention (CDC) minimum recommended funding levels for tobacco control programs,[66] and funding for many programs was cut to deal with state budget crises. As the twenty-first century unfolds, adequately funded and proven interventions will, it is hoped, be vigorously implemented in conjunction with continued declines in the social acceptability of tobacco use.[67]

The U.S. Department of Health and Human Services (HHS) has published reviews of the evidence supporting the effectiveness of certain tobacco-control interventions. In 1999, CDC published *Best Practices for Comprehensive Tobacco Control Programs*[67] to guide states in their tobacco-control efforts following the implementation of the Master Settlement Agreement. *Best Practices* provides the research and scientific evidence in support of nine key elements of a comprehensive tobacco control program, excluding regulatory and public policy efforts, to guide state spending on programmatic activities. *Reducing Tobacco Use: A Report of the Surgeon General,*[38] released in 2000, took a broader view of tobacco control, reviewing the evidence for programmatic work but also assessing the effectiveness of economic and regulatory strategies to reduce tobacco use. Also in 2000, the Public Health Service published an evidence-based guideline on effective clinical interventions to treat tobacco use and dependence.[47] Most recently, the Task Force on Community Preventive Services established rules of evidence to conduct rigorous reviews of the published literature on several health-care system and community tobacco-control strategies, including efforts to reduce exposure to environmental tobacco smoke, increase cessation of tobacco use, and prevent the initiation of such use.[54]

Although each tobacco-reduction strategy can reduce tobacco use, most practitioners and scholars recommend comprehensive approaches in which different program elements work in concert to reinforce a specific message.[38] These comprehensive programs should strive to reduce both the demand and the supply of tobacco products, although a recent review of the evidence concludes that demand-reduction strategies are more effective than those attempting to influence the supply of tobacco products.[68]

Conclusion

Tobacco is the only legal product that, when consumed as intended, kills both users and nonusers. Despite its lethal nature, tobacco is virtually unregulated and continues to be ubiquitously sold and marketed. The situation is particularly tragic given that the harm caused by tobacco has been known by the medical and public health communities, as well as by the tobacco industry, for nearly half a century, and that the means to reduce tobacco use are well known and relatively inexpensive and cost-effective.

The achievements of the last third of the twentieth century notwithstanding, much remains to be done. Approximately 47 million U.S. adults smoked cigarettes by the start of the twenty-first century[30]; half of those who do not quit will die from a disease caused by smoking. Once a socially accepted behavior, smoking is now the leading preventable cause of death for men and women in the United States. Tobacco is now responsible for more than one in five deaths (>440,000 per year) with an annual loss of over 5 million years of life.[9]

This burden need not continue. Tobacco use can be cut dramatically by putting in place those actions that have been proven to be effective. To accelerate efforts to reduce tobacco use, the United States has proposed specific objectives for the year

2010 in the publication *Healthy People 2010*. This document outlines the ambitious objective of reducing tobacco use by half for all population groups by 2010.[69] This objective can be achieved only if effective control activities are fully implemented.[70] Cutting smoking rates by half would save millions of lives and would prevent the expenditures of billions of dollars on treating diseases caused by smoking. State-based preliminary evidence is already demonstrating that sustained implementation of effective tobacco-control interventions not only can reduce smoking rates, but also save lives and dollars.[71,72]

Priorities for the future are clear. *Healthy People 2010* articulates a comprehensive tobacco control agenda to reduce adult smoking rates to 12% and teen smoking rates to 16% by the year 2010.[69] CDC's *Best Practices for Comprehensive Tobacco Control* provides guidance and cost estimates to states for implementing evidence-based and effective tobacco control programs.[67] The Task Force for Community Preventive Services reviewed the entirety of the scientific literature and concluded that there are a number of interventions that have strongly recommended based on the quality of the scientific evidence.[54]

Both the 2000 and 2004 Surgeon General's reports describe a clear vision for the future of tobacco control, with both reports calling for sustained and comprehensive efforts to reduce tobacco use and to continue to build the scientific foundation for tobacco control.[38,74] These reports note many future challenges including the continuing lack of tobacco product regulation, particularly during a period of the development of new tobacco technologies, purportedly providing lower exposure to harmful tobacco constituents. Objective and independent scientific analysis and a coherent regulatory framework are needed to responsibly address the tobacco control challenges of the twenty-first century.

References

1. Centers for Disease Control and Prevention. Achievements in public health, 1900–1999: Tobacco use: United States, 1990–1999. *MMWR* 1999:48:986–93.
2. U.S. Department of Agriculture. Tobacco Situation and Outlook Yearbook, TBS-2004, December 2004. Washington, DC: Economic Research Service/USDA, 2004. Available at: http://usda.mannlib.cornell.edu/reports/erssor/specialty/tbs-bb/2004/tbs2004.pdf. Accessed 8 May 2006.
3. Centers for Disease Control and Prevention. National report on human exposure to environmental chemicals. Atlanta, GA: Department of Health and Human Services, 2001. Available at: http://www.cdc.gov/nceh/dls/report/PDF/CompleteReport.pdf. Accessed 25 October 2002.
4. U.S. Department of Health and Human Services. For a Healthy Nation: Returns on Investment in Public Health. Washington DC : Public Health Service, 1994.
5. U.S. Department of Health, Education and Welfare. Smoking and Health: Report of the Advisory Committee to the Surgeon General of the Public Health Service. Public Health Service publication no. 1103. Washington DC: Public Health Service, Centers for Disease Control and Prevention, 1964.
6. Centers for Disease Control and Prevention. Smoking attributable mortality and years of potential life lost: United States, 1984. *MMWR* 1997:46:444–51.
7. Centers for Disease Control and Prevention. Projected smoking-related deaths among youth: United States, 1996. *MMWR* 1996:45:971–74.

8. Doll R, Peto R, Wheatley K, Gray R, Sutherland I. Mortality in relation to smoking: 40 years' observations on male British doctors. *Br Med J* 1994:309:901–11.

9. Centers for Disease Control and Prevention. Smoking-attributable mortality, years of potential life lost and economic costs: United States, 1995–1999. *MMWR* 2002:51:300–3.

10. Arday DR, Giovino GA, Shulman J, Nelson DE, Mowery P, Samet JM. Cigarette smoking and self-reported health problems among U.S. high school seniors, 1982–1989. *Am J Health Promotion* 1995:10:111–16.

11. U.S. Department of Health and Human Services. Reducing the Health Consequences of Smoking: 25 Years of Progress. A Report of the Surgeon General. DHHS Publication no. 89-8411. Rockville, MD: Public Health Service, Centers for Disease Control, 1989.

12. U.S. Department of Health and Human Services. Women and Smoking: A Report of the Surgeon General. Rockville, MD: Public Health Service, Office of the Surgeon General, 2001.

13. Wingo PA, Ries LA, Giovino GA, et al. Annual report to the nation on the status of cancer, 1973–1996, with a special section on lung cancer and tobacco smoking. *J Natl Cancer Inst* 1999:91:675–90.

14. Doll R, Hill AB. Lung cancer and other causes of death in relation to smoking: a second report on the mortality of British doctors. *Br Med J* 1956:2:1071–81.

15. Centers for Disease Control and Prevention. Mortality trends for selected smoking-related cancers and breast cancer United States, 1950–1990. *MMWR* 1993:42:863–66.

16. U.S. Department of Health and Human Services. Tobacco Use Among U.S. Racial/Ethnic Minority Groups—African Americans, American Indians and Alaska Natives, Asian Americans and Pacific Islanders, and Hispanics: Report of the Surgeon General. Atlanta, GA: Centers for Disease Control and Prevention, Office on Smoking and Health, 1998.

17. U.S. Department of Health and Human Services. Smokeless Tobacco or Health: An International Perspective. Smoking and Tobacco Control monograph no. 2. NIH publication no. 92-3461. Bethesda, MD: National Cancer Institute, 1992.

18. U.S. Department of Health and Human Services. Cigars: Health Effects and Trends Smoking and Tobacco Control monograph no. 9. NIH publication no. 98-4302. Bethesda, MD: National Cancer Institute, 1998.

19. Centers for Disease Control and Prevention. Bidi use among urban youth: Massachusetts, March-April 1999. *MMWR* 1999:48:796–99.

20. U.S. Department of Health and Human Services. The Health Consequences of Involuntary Smoking: A Report of the Surgeon General. Rockville, MD: Centers for Disease Control and Prevention, National Center for Chronic Disease Prevention and Health Promotion, Office on Smoking and Health, 1986.

21. Environmental Protection Agency. Respiratory Health Effects of Passive Smoking: Lung Cancer and Other Disorders. EPA/600/6-90/006F. Washington, DC: Office on Air and Radiation, 1992.

22. National Cancer Institute. Health Effects of Exposure to Environmental Tobacco Smoke: The Report of the California Environmental Protection Agency. Smoking and Tobacco Control monograph no. 10. NIH publication no. 99-4645. Bethesda, MD: U.S. Department of Health and Human Services, National Institutes of Health, 1999.

23. National Toxicology Program, National Institute of Environmental Health Science. National Toxicology Program Report on Carcinogens, 9th ed. Research Triangle Park, NC: National Institute of Environmental Health Science, 2000.

24. International Association of Research on Cancer. Tobacco Smoke and Involuntary Smoking: Summary of Data Reported and Evaluation. Monograph ol. 83. International Association of Research on Cancer, 2002. Available at: http://mongraphs.IARC.fr/htdocs/indexes/vol83index.html. Accessed 25 October 2002.

25. Centers for Disease Control and Prevention. Decline in deaths from heart disease and stroke—United States, 1900–1999. *MMWR* 1999:48:649–56.

26. Giovino GA, Henningfield JE, Tomar SL, Escobedo LG, Slade S. Epidemiology of tobacco use and dependence. *Epidemiol Rev* 1995:17:48–65.

27. Giovino GA, Schooley MW, Zhu BP, et al. Surveillance for selected tobacco-use behaviors—United States, 1900–1994. CDC surveillance summaries, 18 November 1994. *MMWR* 1994:43(SS-3):1–43.

28. Centers for Disease Control and Prevention. Cigarette smoking among adults—United States, 1998. *MMWR* 2000:49:881–84.

29. Centers for Disease Control and Prevention, National Center for Health Statistics. Early release of selected estimates based on data from the January–June 2004 National Health Interview Survey (Released 12/16/2004). Available at: http://www.cdc.gov/nchs/data/nhis/earlyrelease/200412_08.pdf. Accessed 9 March 2005.

30. Centers for Disease Control and Prevention. Cigarette smoking among adults—United States, 2000. *MMWR* 2002:51:642–45.

31. U.S. Department of Health and Human Services. Preventing Tobacco Use Among Young People: Report of the Surgeon General. Atlanta, GA: Centers for Disease Control and Prevention, National Center for Chronic Disease Prevention and Health Promotion, Office on Smoking and Health, 1994.

32. Johnston LD, O'Malley PM, Bachman JG. National Survey Results on Drug Use from the Monitoring the Future Study, 1975–1998. Vol 1: secondary school students. NIH publication no. 99-4660. Rockville, MD: National Institutes of Health, National Institute of Drug Abuse, 1999.

33. Centers for Disease Control and Prevention. Trends in cigarette smoking among high school students: United States, 1991–1999. *MMWR* 2000:49:755–58.

34. Johnston LD, O'Malley PM, Bachman JG. Smoking Among Teenagers Decreases Sharply and Increase in Ecstasy Use Slows. Ann Arbor, MI: University of Michigan News and Information Services, 2001.

35. Centers for Disease Control and Prevention. Youth tobacco surveillance—United States, 2000. *MMWR* 2001:50(SS-4):1–84.

36. Grunbaum JA, Kann L, Kinchen SA, et al. Youth risk behavior surveillance—United States 2001. CDC surveillance summaries, 28 June 2002. *MMWR* 2002:51(SS-04): 1–64.

37. U.S. Department of Agriculture. Tobacco Situation and Outlook Yearbook. U.S. Department of Agriculture. Washington, DC: Economic Research Service, TSB-240, 1997.

38. U.S. Department of Health and Human Services. Reducing Tobacco Use: A Report of the Surgeon General. Atlanta, GA: Centers for Disease Control and Prevention, National Center for Chronic Disease Prevention and Health Promotion, Office on Smoking and Health, 2000.

39. Hirayama T. Cancer mortality in nonsmoking women with smoking husbands based on a large-scale cohort study in Japan. *Prev Med* 1984:13:680–90.

40. Pierce JP, Gilpin EA, Emery SL, White MM, Rosbrook B, Berry CC. Has the California tobacco control program reduced smoking? *JAMA* 1998:280:893–99.

41. Farrelly MC, Healton CG, Davis KC, Messeri P, Jersey JC, Haviland ML. Getting to the truth: national tobacco countermarketing campaigns. *Am J Public Health* 2002:92:901–7.

42. Cummings KM, Morley CP, Hyland A. Failed promises of the cigarette industry and its effect on consumer misperceptions about the health risks of smoking. *Tobacco Control* 2002:11(suppl 1):I110–7.

43. Federal Trade Commission, Cigarette Report for 2002, issued 2004. Available at: http://www.ftc.gov/reports/cigarette/041022cigaretterpt.pdf. Accessed 8 May 2006.

44. U.S. Department of Health and Human Services. The Health Consequences of Smoking, Nicotine Addiction: A Report of the Surgeon General. Atlanta, GA: Public Health Service, Office on Smoking and Health, 1988.

45. Centers for Disease Control and Prevention. Use of FDA-approved pharmacologic treatments for tobacco dependence. *MMWR* 2000:49(29):665–68.

46. Zhu S, Stetch V, Balabanis M, et al. Telephone counseling for smoking cessation: effects of single-session and multiple-session interventions. *J Counsel Clin Psychol* 1996:64: 202–11.

47. Fiore MC, Bailey WC, Cohen SJ, et al. Treating Tobacco Use and Dependence: Clinical Practice Guideline. Washington, DC: U.S. Department of Health and Human Services, Public Health Service, 2000.

48. Shamasunder B, Bero L. Financial ties and conflicts of interest between pharmaceutical and tobacco companies. *JAMA* 2002:288:738–44.

49. Warner KE. What's a cigarette company to do? *Am J Public Health* 2002:92:897–900.

50. U.S. Department of Health and Human Services. How to Help Your Patients Stop Smoking: A National Cancer Institute Manual for Physicians. NIH publication no. 93-3064. Rockville, MD: National Institutes of Health, National Cancer Institute, 1993.

51. Cummings SR, Rubin SM, Oster G. The cost-effectiveness of counseling smokers to quit. *JAMA* 1989:261:75–79.

52. Cromwell J, Bartosch WJ, Fore MC, Hasselblad V, Baker T. Cost-effectiveness of the clinical practice recommendations in the AHCPR guideline for smoking cessation. *JAMA* 1997:278:1759.

53. Coffield AB, Maciosek MV, McGinnis M, et al. Priorities among recommended clinical preventive services. *Am J Prev Med* 2001:21:1–9.

54. Task Force on Community Preventive Services. Recommendations regarding interventions to reduce tobacco use and exposure to environmental tobacco smoke. *Am J Prev Med* 2001:20(suppl 2S):10–15.

55. Chaloupka FJ, Warner KE. The economics of smoking. In: Newhouse J, Culyer A, eds. The Handbook of Health Economics. Amsterdam, The Netherlands: Elsevier Science, 1999.

56. Manning WG, Keeler EB, Newhouse JP, Sloos EM, Wasserman U. The taxes of sin: do smokers and drinkers pay their way? *JAMA* 1989:261(11):1604–9.

57. Campaign for Tobacco Free Kids. Available at: http://tobaccofreekids.org/research/ factsheets/pdf/0097.pdf. Accessed 30 October 2002.

58. U.S. Department of Agriculture. Tobacco Situation and Outlook Yearbook. U.S. Department of Agriculture. Washington, D.C.: Market and Trade Economics Division, Economic Research. Service, TBS-2002, 2002.

59. Slade J, Henningfield J. Tobacco product regulation: context and issues. *Food and Drug Law Journal* 1998:53:43–74.

60. Food and Drug Administration. Regulations restricting the sale and distribution of cigarettes and smokeless tobacco products to protect children and adolescents: proposed rule analysis regarding FDA's jurisdiction over nicotine-containing cigarettes and smokeless tobacco products. *Federal Register* 1995:60(155):41314–787.

61. Centers for Disease Control and Prevention. Filter ventilation levels in selected U.S. cigarettes, 1997. *MMWR* 1997:46(44):1043–47.

62. Thun MJ, Lally CA, Flannery JT, Calle EE, Flanders WD, Heath CW. Cigarette smoking and changes in the histopathology of lung cancer. *J Natl Cancer Inst* 1997:89(21): 1580–86.

63. Warner KE, Slade J, Sweanor DT. The emerging market for long-term nicotine maintenance. *JAMA* 1997:278:1087–92.

64. Institute of Medicine. Clearing the Smoke: Assessing the Science Base for Tobacco Harm Reduction. Washington, DC: National Academy Press, 2001.
65. Bell C, Urbach D. Bartenders' pulmonary function after establishment of a smoke-free workplace. *JAMA* 1999:282(7):629.
66. Albuquerque M, Kelly A, Schooley M. Fellows JL, Pechacek TF. Tobacco Control State Highlights 2002: Impact and Opportunity. Atlanta, GA: Department of Health and Human Services, Centers for Disease Control and Prevention, Office on Smoking and Health, 2002.
67. Centers for Disease Control and Prevention. Best Practices for Comprehensive Tobacco Control Programs: August 1999. Atlanta, GA: U.S. Department of Health and Human Services, 1999.
68. Jha P, Chaloupka FJ, eds. Tobacco Control in Developing Countries. New York: Oxford University Press, 2000.
69. U.S. Department of Health and Human Services. Healthy People 2010, 2nd ed. Washington, DC: U.S. Government Printing Office, 2000.
70. Green LW, Eriksen MP, Bailey L, Husten C. Achieving the implausible in the next decade: tobacco control objectives. *Am J Public Health* 2000:90:337–39.
71. Centers for Disease Control and Prevention. Declines in lung cancer rates: California, 1988–1997. *MMWR* 2000:49:1066–69.
72. Fichtenberg CM, Glantz SA. Association of the California Tobacco Control Program with declines in cigarette consumption and mortality from heart disease. *N Engl J Med* 2000: 343:1772–77.
73. Johnston LD, O'Malley PM, Bachman JG, Schulenberg JE. Cigarette smoking among American teens continues to decline, but more slowly than in the past, 21 December 2004. *University of Michigan News and Information Services*. Available at: http://www.monitoringthefuture.org. Accessed 8 January 2005.
74. U.S. Department of Health and Human Services. The Health Consequences of Smoking: A Report of the Surgeon General. Washington, DC: Centers for Disease Control and Prevention, National Center for Chronic Disease Prevention and Health Promotion, Office on Smoking and Health, 2004.

Suggested Reading

Giovino GA, Henningfield JE, Tomar SL, Escobedo LG, Slade S. Epidemiology of tobacco use and dependence. *Epidemiol Rev* 1995:17:48–65.
Institute of Medicine. Clearing the Smoke: Assessing the Science Base for Tobacco Harm Reduction. Washington, DC: National Academy Press, 2001.

21

The First Surgeon General's Report on Tobacco: Science and the State in the New Age of Chronic Disease

ALLAN M. BRANDT

Historians are often in search of what they refer to as watersheds. The term derives from a geological description of a ridge dividing two drainage areas—a parting of the waters. For historians, a watershed is defined as a sharp divide in time, a historical event that indicates a dramatic and fundamental shift. The Surgeon General's *Report* of 1964—now known simply as the First Surgeon General's *Report*—marks just such a watershed in the history of public health. Following its publication in January 1964, both the science and the practice of public health were visibly transformed. Just as historians of public health in the nineteenth century look to John Snow's treatise *On the Mode of Communication of Cholera* (1849) as marking a radical shift in the understanding of disease, its causes, and prevention in the nineteenth century, the surgeon general's *Report* represents the most significant achievement of the twentieth.

The importance of the *Report*, however, is not as a typical scientific or medical breakthrough. Indeed, the committee that produced the report conducted no new research and relied exclusively on investigations that had culminated in the 1950s. By 1964, a number of other nations had issued reports concluding that smoking caused disease.[1,2] For historians of twentieth-century public health, nonetheless, it remains a central document marking the powerful transition from institutions and approaches that centered on infections to a critical reorientation to approaching chronic disease. Ultimately, the *Report* offered a compelling critique of biomedical reductionism. By insisting on the fact of multiple causalities, the *Report* did much to disrupt the characteristic reductionist ethos of mid-century science and medicine.

As the history of science and medicine demonstrates, all human knowledge in the sciences is provisional and subject to expansion and/or modification. But we nonetheless reach conclusions on which we base important judgments. In the case of the 1964 report, the depth of the review, the importance of the analysis of causality, and the momentous character of the conclusions were reflected on every page. The report brought—for all essential purposes—an end to a debate within contemporary medicine and science that had been stoked and sustained by powerful economic interests. In the dry prose of federal bureaucracy and modern science, the report succeeded in categorically identifying the substantial—even lethal—harms associated with the use of cigarettes.[3]

For the 70 million regular smokers in the United States, the *Report* offered very bad news. It found that the death rate from cancer of the lung was 1000% higher among men who smoked cigarettes than among those who didn't. The *Report* also cited chronic bronchitis and emphysema to be of far greater incidence among smokers, and it found that rates of coronary artery disease, the leading cause of death in the United States, were 70% higher among smokers. In short, cigarette smokers placed themselves at much higher risk of serious disease than did nonsmokers.[4,5]

But the *Report* went far beyond a mere statement of these sobering statistics—and the statistics themselves were not new, collected for more than a decade. The watershed of the *Report* is that it marks a dramatic new phase in modern public health, health policy making, and the role of the state. This break from earlier public health approaches is best captured in four central aspects of the *Report*. First, it legitimated population based studies that would offer the core methods of public health and medical assessments of causality and efficacy from that time. It insisted that public health and policy must be based upon medical and scientific evidence. Second, it marked the expansion of state responsibility for resolving critical scientific disputes of public interest. Never before had a government stepped in to adjudicate a scientific dispute in the name of public health. The *Report* made explicit that the public could not rely on industry for knowledge regarding crucial health decisions. Third, it signaled a central role for the state in the emergence of new approaches to health promotion and disease prevention in the second half of the twentieth century. In the face of the health transition in which chronic diseases would constitute the predominant causes of morbidity and mortality, the *Report* signaled a fundamental reorientation to new epidemiologic realities. And fourth, it led to the Office of the Surgeon General having central significance in identifying and promoting key public health issues.

Following this report, the American public would look to the Surgeon General's Office for expert assessments and advice about health and disease. As a result, the authority of the office would be substantially augmented. The *Report* underscores the fundamental relationships of science, public health, and the political process in the second half of the twentieth century.

Collecting the Data

From our contemporary vantage point, simple logic suggests that the threefold increase in lung cancer cases noted in 1946 over the previous three decades must be attributed to the dramatic rise in cigarette smoking.[6] What in retrospect seems an obvious conclusion, however, was anything but obvious to critical observers of the early to mid-twentieth century. Indeed, there were impressive biologic, sociocultural, methodologic, and scientific obstacles to arriving at this conclusion.

The development of modern epidemiologic technique occurred in the face of the severe limitations that other scientific approaches had in resolving critical questions about the potential harms of smoking. By mid-century the limitations of clinical observation and experimental methods to answer critical questions of causality—especially concerning the rising prevalence of systemic chronic diseases—had become increasingly apparent. For systemic diseases like cancers and heart disease that clearly were influenced by a multitude of endogenous and exogenous forces, isolating a single cause and demonstrating its mechanism—the central aspect of germ theory medicine and the biomedical paradigm it had established—would never be possible. The problem of the relationship of lung cancer to smoking starkly demonstrated the limitations of this model. No laboratory experiment could answer the fundamental questions about the health impact of smoking. The progenitors of this new epidemiology sought to develop systematic approaches to address these methodological constraints.[7]

By the late 1920s, researchers had begun to focus more precisely on the specific health consequences of smoking instead of the previously typical clinical evaluations of throat irritation and "smoker's cough." As early as 1928, researchers associated heavy smoking with cancer in a somewhat primitive epidemiologic study.[8] In 1931, Frederick L. Hoffman, a well-known statistician for the Prudential Insurance Company, tied smoking to cancer in a more sophisticated manner, but he also noted the difficulties of conducting epidemiologic studies in this area. The basic methodologic questions of statistical research—issues of representativeness, sample size, and the construction of control groups—all presented researchers with a series of complex problems.[9]

In 1938, Raymond Pearl, the Johns Hopkins population biologist, published one of the first significant statistical analyses of the health impact of smoking, noting that it was difficult to assess the risks of such behaviors in individuals, especially when the impact was not immediate and when many intervening variables also affected individuals' health. Therefore, he concluded, the only precise way to evaluate their effect on health was to employ statistical methods after collecting data on large groups. Comparing the mortality curves of smokers and nonsmokers, Pearl found that persons who smoked could expect shorter lives.[10] Although many research questions were left to be resolved, Pearl and other researchers had begun to consider the best ways to uncover proof of the relationship between lung cancer and smoking. The first case control study that showed the connection was published in Germany just a year later in 1939.[11,12]

In the late 1930s, surgeons also began to publish clinical reports linking cancer in their patients with their smoking habits.[13] Noted chest surgeons including Alton Ochsner in New Orleans and Richard Overholt in Boston drew attention to their observations that patients with advanced lung malignancies typically had smoked. Ochsner went so far as to prohibit his staff from smoking and came to be well known as an anti-tobacco advocate. Assessing the increase in cases of primary carcinoma of the lung, Ochsner and surgeon Michael DeBakey concluded: "In our opinion the increase in smoking with the universal custom of inhaling is probably a responsible factor, as the inhaled smoke, constantly repeated over a long period of time, undoubtedly is a source of chronic irritation to the bronchial mucosa."[14]

These early clinical observations of the impact of smoking are, in retrospect, quite impressive. Almost all the risks that would come to be attributed to smoking in the second half of the twentieth century had been well-documented—from a clinical perspective—in the first decades of the century. Even the risks of passive exposure to cigarette smoke had been well articulated. And yet, physicians and researchers could not easily move from such clinical observation to more powerful and generalizable assessments of the specific causal relationship of smoking to disease. Physicians such as Ochsner might well be convinced that tobacco had caused their patients' malignancies, but the larger question of cause and effect could not be definitively resolved on the basis of such anecdotal observations. Laboratory research and animal studies also pointed to cigarettes as a cause of disease. By the late 1940s, it was already known that prolonged exposure to certain industrial chemicals and vapors—chromate, nickel carbonyl, and radioactive dusts—could produce lung cancer. Some scientists now suggested that the inhalation of cigarette smoke might have similar effects. This hypothesis led to a series of epidemiologic studies of the risk of smoking.[15]

Beginning in the late 1940s, researchers began to devise studies that would directly assess the harms of cigarette smoking. These epidemiologic studies introduced the concept of large, population-based surveys as legitimate scientific method in itself. They focused attention on the definition of comparative risk and excess mortality. Implicit in such studies was a critique of the whole notion of specific causality, with researchers recognizing that there were literally hundreds of variables affecting the incidence of disease. Therefore they sought to design studies which, by including many persons, would be controlled except for a single variable; in this case, cigarette smoking.

Evarts Graham, a nationally known surgeon at Barnes Hospital in St. Louis, and Ernst Wynder, a medical student at Washington University, designed and implemented such a study in 1949. Graham, who had performed the very first pneumonectomy in 1933, was a heavy smoker himself, skeptical of the cigarette-lung cancer hypothesis. He initially speculated that if smoking was a cause of lung cancer it would occur more bilaterally (rather than in a single lobe). At a medical meeting in Chicago in 1940, he challenged Alton Ochsner's contention that there was a connection between smoking and lung cancer, noting that the sale of silk stockings had increased at a same rate as the sale of cigarettes and could just as well be connected to lung cancer. Following the meeting, he tempered this comment in a letter to Ochsner, calling it "facetious," but he still said, "there are still some things about bronchiogenic carcinoma that are difficult to explain on the basis of smoking."[16,17]

Even so, Graham agreed to support Ernst Wynder's endeavor to study the lung cancer-cigarette hypothesis. Wynder collected extensive data on a group of 684 patients with lung cancer located in hospitals throughout the United States. These patients were interviewed at length about their smoking practices and histories. Histological exams confirmed the diagnosis in all cases. This group was then compared to a "control group" of nonsmokers similar in age and other demographic characteristics.[18]

Wynder and Graham did note that lung cancer could occur among nonsmokers and that heavy smokers did not necessarily develop cancer. Therefore they reasoned that "smoking cannot be the only etiological factor in the induction of the disease." Nonetheless, they explained, "the temptation is strong to incriminate excessive smoking, and in particular cigarette smoking over a long period, as at least one important factor in the striking increase of bronchogenic carcinoma." They offered four reasons to support this conclusion. First, it was very unusual to find lung cancers among nonsmokers. Second, among patients with lung cancer, cigarette use tended to be high. Third, the distribution of lung cancer among men and women matched the ratio of smoking patterns by gender. And finally, "the enormous increase in the sale of cigarettes in this country approximately parallels the increase in bronchogenic carcinoma." On May 27, 1950, these results were reported in the *Journal of the American Medical Association*.[18]

That issue of the journal included another investigation by Morton Levin and colleagues that reached similar conclusions. In his commentary on research into the connection between cigarettes and lung cancer, Levin compared the current epidemiologic research on cigarette smoking to research on the smoking/lung cancer connection done in the preceding 20 years, arguing that the past work was "inconclusive because of lack of adequate samples, lack of random selection, lack of proper controls or failure to age-standardize the data."[19] In the case of the data gathered for his study, careful attention to "excluding bias" had been central: "in a hospital population, cancer of the lung occurs more than twice as frequently among those who have smoked cigarets for 25 years than among other smokers or nonsmokers of comparable age."[19]

At this point, Levin and colleagues were appropriately cautious in drawing causal conclusions, but nonetheless these new methodologic approaches would be central to resolving the hypothesis.

The New Epidemiology

Research across the ocean paralleled that in the United States—with even more rigorous consideration of method. Following World War I, A. Bradford Hill had become one of the most distinguished medical statisticians in Great Britain. Richard Doll, a physician, also possessed sophisticated training in statistics and epidemiologic methods. Under the auspices of the Medical Research Council, a unit of the recently created National Health Service in the United Kingdom, Hill and Doll initiated a case control study beginning in 1948. As their data from lung cancer patients and the control group came in, in late 1948 and early 1949, it became clear to them that cigarettes were the crucial factor in the rise of lung cancer. With data on almost 650 lung cancer patients, they concluded that they had in fact found cause and effect. Even without the sophisticated statistical analyses they would employ in their published writings, the findings were impressive: among the 647 lung cancer patients entered into Doll and Hill's study, all were smokers. They waited to publicize their results, however, until they had data on 1400 lung cancer patients, further strengthening their conclusions.[20]

Even so, Doll and Hill understood that it would be easy to dismiss such findings—as the industry would try—as "merely" statistical. As a result, they meticulously described the specific criteria that they had required before designating an "association" as a genuine causal relationship. First, they worked to eliminate the possibility of bias in the selection of patients and controls, as well as in reporting and recording their histories. Second, they emphasized the significance of a clear temporal relationship between exposure and subsequent development of disease. Finally, they sought to rule out any other factors that might distinguish controls from patients with disease. Their explicit search for possible "confounders" and their elimination marked a critical aspect of their arrival at a causal conclusion. They insisted on carefully addressing all possible criticisms and all "alternative explanations" for their findings.[21]

Two years later, in a follow-up report, they offered additional evidence for sustaining their finding that smoking caused lung cancer, carefully noting that their analysis had "revealed no alternative explanation."[22] Specifically, they addressed the "physical constitution" possibility, explaining that they had found "no evidence" that some people might simply be "prone to develop . . . the habit of smoking, and . . . carcinoma of the lung."[22] With such careful and critical assessment of alternative explanations for the rise in rates of lung cancer, Doll and Hill's conclusions took on great weight.

By late 1953, researchers had published at least five epidemiologic investigations, as well as other articles pursuing carcinogenic components in tobacco smoke and its impacts.[23] No single study would conclusively demonstrate the causal relationship between smoking and cancer. Rather, it was the aggregation of similar repeated studies with consistent findings that would build a convincing case. Although some of the epidemiologic methods were innovative, the scientists using them were careful to be thorough, and their methods were consistent with historically established scientific procedure and process. The studies had substantially transformed the scientific knowledge base concerning the harms of cigarette use. Unlike earlier anecdotal and clinical assessments, they offered new and path-breaking approaches to investigating and resolving causal relationships.

Still, critics raised a series of objections to these studies that needed to be addressed. Initially, the investigations of the early 1950s were based upon retrospective findings: persons with lung cancer were identified in hospitals and interviewed regarding their smoking practices; they were then compared to a similar group who did not smoke.[18,19,21,22] It was clear that there were a number of opportunities for bias in the construction of sample and control groups. For example, lung cancer patients might be expected to exaggerate their smoking habits. Given the methodological problems with retrospective studies, two major prospective studies on smoking and cancer were begun in 1951. Under the auspices of the British Medical Research Council, Richard Doll and Bradford Hill sent questionnaires on smoking practices to all British physicians (some 40,000). When members of the profession died, Doll and Hill obtained data concerning the cause of their deaths. The results were consistent with the earlier findings from the retrospective studies: physicians who smoked heavily had death rates 24 times higher than their nonsmoking colleagues.[24,25]

A second major prospective study conducted by E. Cuyler Hammond under the auspices of the American Cancer Society led to similar conclusions. An initial skeptic of the 1950 retrospective studies, Hammond found that total death rates among smokers were far higher than those for nonsmokers, and lung cancer deaths were 3–9 times as high—5–16 times as high among heavy smokers. Among those who smoked two or more packs a day, the death rates were 2.25 times as high as for men who had never smoked, a strong indication of a dose effect. Excess mortality was even higher for coronary artery disease than for lung cancer; rates for smokers exceeded those for nonsmokers by 70%. Quitting, Hammond found, reduced risk; formerly a heavy smoker, he himself now quit.[26] By 1960, a range of epidemiologic studies—both prospective and retrospective—had all arrived at consistent findings: cigarette smoking significantly contributed to lung cancer and coronary artery disease.[27] With the addition of Hammond's massive prospective study confirming these earlier studies, remaining skeptics found themselves holding on to shop-worn arguments.

Building Consensus

By the mid-1950s, groups of scientists made the effort to come together to analyze the collective findings on the risks of cigarettes. In 1956, at the urging of Surgeon General Leroy Burney, a study group on smoking and health was organized by the American Cancer Society, the American Heart Association, the National Cancer Institute, and the National Heart Institute. This group of distinguished experts met regularly to assess the character of the scientific evidence relating to tobacco and health. At that time, the group noted that 16 studies had been conducted in five countries, all showing a statistical association between smoking and lung cancer. In their 1957 published report, they concluded: "The sum total of scientific evidence establishes beyond reasonable doubt that cigarette smoking is a causative factor in the rapidly increasing incidence of human epidermoid carcinoma of the lung."[28] They also noted that the epidemiologic findings were supported by animal studies in which malignant neoplasms had been produced by tobacco smoke condensates. Further, human pathologic and histologic studies added evidence to strengthen the "concept of causal relationship."

In January 1959, another distinguished group of cancer researchers led by statistician Jerome Cornfield offered a substantive review of the available evidence linking cigarettes to lung cancer. This group carefully considered the range of alternative hypotheses to account for the significant rise in cases of, and deaths from, lung cancer. They concluded, "The consistency of all the epidemiologic and experimental evidence also supports the conclusion of a causal relationship with cigarette smoking. . . ."[27] Both reports stressed that the available findings were "sufficient for planning and activating public health measures."[27,28] Importantly, Cornfield and colleagues also noted that the persistent "debate" about the scientific findings regarding cigarette smoking was driven by the tobacco industry: "if the findings had been made on a new agent, to which hundreds of millions of adults were not already addicted, and on one which did not support a large industry, skilled in the arts of mass persuasion, the evidence for the hazardous nature of the agent would generally be regarded as beyond dispute."[27]

As Cornfield had explained, despite the impressive accrual of data—not only from epidemiology but from laboratory and clinical spheres—bringing the controversy to resolution would prove no easy matter. The industry worked assiduously to discount these findings, to augment scientific skepticism, and to reassure smokers through public relations, advertising, and the aggressive promotions of filter cigarettes.

As a result, even the most concerted efforts of the voluntary health organizations, the surgeon general, and other public agencies failed to bring closure to the controversy. This situation, in which powerful interests both shaped and clouded a scientific debate of public moment, ultimately required an important and unprecedented role for the surgeon general and the federal government. Resolving this crucial medical question ultimately required the intervention of the state for an independent and definitive reading and assessment of the scientific evidence. This was precisely what the surgeon general's committee would successfully achieve. A question that had arisen in doctor's offices and clinics now achieved its ultimate resolution in conference rooms in Washington. This circular route of resolution would indicate important characteristics in the modern history of medicine and public health now buffered by powerful economic and political forces of industry and commerce.

Constructing Controversy

Maintaining the idea of a scientific "controversy" was a crucial element in industry efforts to sustain their profits and market their product. By late 1953, executives from various tobacco companies were aware both of the scientific findings linking cigarettes and lung cancer and the public attention the findings were receiving. Wynder and Graham's 1953 research on tobacco tars and tumors in mice had proven to be especially alarming within the industry.[29] These executives well understood that this new scientific evidence constituted a full-scale crisis for their respective corporations.[30-33] In December 1953, the president of American Tobacco, Paul Hahn, called a meeting of all the major tobacco chief executives; only those from Liggett declined.[33] The purpose of the meeting was to develop a collaborative public relations plan in response to the new scientific evidence concerning the harms of cigarette use.[34]

The tobacco executives agreed to meet with John Hill of the New York public relations firm Hill and Knowlton in order to consider how best to shape their new strategy in this moment of crisis. Hill and Knowlton executives recommended that the industry executives come together and form the Tobacco Industry Research Committee (TIRC), publicly sponsoring new scientific research on tobacco and health.

From the outset the dual functions of TIRC, public relations and scientific research, were intertwined. The scientific program of TIRC had actually always been subservient to the goals of public relations.[35] Beginning in January 1954, the newly created TIRC would take the lead in forging the industry's response to the scientific evidence of tobacco's harms. That month the TIRC published "A Frank Statement to Cigarette Smokers," an advertisement that appeared in 448 newspapers in 258 cities. The "Frank Statement," as an act of public relations, fit well with the essential strategy that the tobacco industry would stick to over the next decade. Written by Hill and Knowlton executives who came to direct the day-to-day operations of the TIRC, it reassured smokers, promising them that the industry was absolutely committed to their good health. The statement announced: "we accept an interest in people's health as a basic responsibility, paramount to every other consideration in our business." Such reassurances became characteristic even as the scientific evidence indicting cigarettes grew in strength, sophistication, and professional acceptance.

Industry accounts of the scientific "controversy" consistently set up straw men, misrepresented the evidence that smoking causes disease, and ignored the progress being made in scientific research. For example, a serial publication entitled *Tobacco and Health* that the TIRC sent to doctors and dentists declared in 1958: "Continuing scientific research lends support to the position that too many unknowns exist today concerning lung cancer to warrant conclusions placing a major causative role on cigarette smoking. . . ."[36]

The TIRC never developed an approach to carcinogenesis and tobacco that could resolve the question of the harms induced by cigarette smoking. As one company executive explained confidentially in retrospect:

> Historically, the joint industry funded smoking and health research programs have not been selected against specific scientific goals, but rather for various purposes such as public relations, political relations, position for litigation, etc. Thus, it seems obvious that reviews of such programs for scientific relevance and merit in the smoking and health field are not likely to produce high ratings. In general, these programs have provided some buffer to the public and political attack of the industry, as well as background for litigious strategy.[37]

The Cigarette and Public Health

Even as the industry attempted to obscure scientific results on cigarettes and lung cancer, government agencies in the United States and abroad began to publicly recognize cigarettes' harms. In November 1959, U.S. Surgeon General Leroy E. Burney carefully evaluated the scientific evidence linking cigarettes to lung cancer. He revisited the epidemiologic data, as well as other confirmatory animal and pathological investigations. After a thorough assessment of current data, Burney came to the following conclusion, published as the official "Statement of the Public Health Service":

> The Public Health Service believes that the following statements are justified by studies to date:
>
> 1. The weight of the evidence at present implicates smoking as the primary etiological factor in the increased incidence of lung cancer.
> 2. Cigarette smoking particularly is associated with an increased chance of developing lung cancer. . . .[38]

For Burney, these findings meant that there were important and timely opportunities to prevent disease that merited governmental attention. Nonetheless, the TIRC continued to disparage such consensus statements. In response to Burney, the TIRC scientific director C.C. Little asserted, "scientific evidence is accumulating that conflicts with, or fails to support, the tobacco-smoking theories of lung cancer."[39]

In the next few years, the Medical Research Council of Great Britain, the Royal College of Physicians, the World Health Organization, and public health officials in the Netherlands, Norway, and the United States also publicly acknowledged that cigarette smoking caused lung cancer.[4,40-43] The Royal College of Physicians report, *Smoking and Health: Summary and Report of the Royal College of Physicians of London*, was a crucial step toward the medical and public legitimation of the link between cigarettes and disease.[42] E. Cuyler Hammond, director of the Statistical Research Section of the American Cancer Society, wrote the preface to the American edition. He noted the esteem of the Royal College and highlighted that "the reader is asked to accept nothing on faith." Emphasizing the huge amount of scientific research supporting the hazardous nature of cigarette smoking, Hammond explained that the report provided "evidence from which they [the readers] can draw their own conclusions concerning the effects of cigarette smoking."

By the time of the establishment of the Surgeon General's Advisory Committee on Smoking and Health in 1962, therefore, the character of the data on smoking and disease was considerably different than it had been in the early 1950s when the first major epidemiologic studies had appeared. The work of Wynder and Graham and Doll and Hill had not only been consistently replicated, it had also been considerably expanded through the deployment of new epidemiologic techniques as well as confirmatory animal and human pathologic investigations.

By the early 1960s, pressure was building for the U.S. Public Health Service (USPHS) to take some action against smoking. The voluntary health agencies—the American Lung Association and the American Heart Association—had proposed in June 1961 that President Kennedy appoint a commission to "study the widespread implications of the tobacco problem."[4] Although these health organizations and consumer groups had growing stature on Capitol Hill, Kennedy declined to respond. Apparently, he wished to avoid alienating Southern congressional delegations. Correspondingly, there was little enthusiasm in Congress, even though Senator Maurine Neuberger (D-Oregon) had proposed legislation also calling for a commission. It seemed likely the issue might be tabled when Kennedy was asked about the health controversy during a nationally televised press conference in 1962. His halting response revealed his surprise; he was clearly unprepared for the question: "The—that matter is sensitive enough and the stock market is in sufficient difficulty without my giving you an answer which is not based on complete information, which I don't have, and therefore perhaps we could—I'd be glad to respond to that question in more detail next week."[44,45]

Two weeks after this press conference, Kennedy's surgeon general, Luther Terry, publicly announced that he would establish a committee.[45,46]

If the Terry committee was to offer a rigorous and systematic assessment of the health implications of smoking, it was crucial that it appear to be above the fray. To establish the Advisory Committee, Surgeon General Luther Terry created a list of some 150 persons representing a number of fields and medical specialties from pulmonary medicine to statistics, cardiology to epidemiology. The Public Health Service then circulated the list to the American Cancer Society, the American Heart Association, the National Tuberculosis Association, the American Medical Association, and the Tobacco Institute, the tobacco industry's public relations arm since 1958 when the TIRC was renamed the Council for Tobacco Research (CTR). Terry allowed each group to eliminate any name, without any reason cited. Terry also eliminated persons who had already published on the issue or had taken a public position.

When word of this procedure for selecting the committee became public, objections were raised. Congressman Clark MacGregor wrote to Terry, "It has been suggested that several members of the commission were appointed on the basis of tobacco industry recommendations. If so, this would immediately suggest a conflict of interest destructive to the necessary unbiased study and recommendations of the commission."[47] But the selection process actually indicated Terry's political savvy. He had ensured that the report could not be attacked on the basis of its membership. Terry and his advisors at the Public Health Service clearly anticipated that the industry would eagerly seek to discredit any findings that suggested the harms of tobacco. At the outset, it would be impossible for the industry to later level charges of bias. And, tellingly, a number of committee members began their investigation as committed smokers. Three members of the committee smoked cigarettes, and two others occasionally smoked pipes or cigars. Photos of the committee meeting at the National Library of Medicine showed a smoke-filled room with a conference table littered with ashtrays. All 10 of the members were eminent physicians and scientists; eight were medical doctors, one was a chemist, and the other a statistician.[4,45] The selection process indicated Terry's commitment to a process that would eventuate in a genuine and definitive consensus.

Luther Terry was himself a former cigarette smoker who switched to a pipe just weeks before the 1964 report was released. He explained immediately after the release of the report, "I became increasingly more convinced that cigarettes were not good for me and frankly that I was not setting a good example for the American youth and the American public."[48] A native of Alabama, Luther Terry had a long record in the U.S. Public Health Service when Kennedy appointed him surgeon general in 1961, holding prominent positions at the National Heart Institute for the 11 years preceding that appointment.[49] Terry's first 10 selections all agreed to serve on the committee, indicating to him "that these scientists were convinced of the importance of the subject and of the complete support of the Public Health Service."[50]

The *Report* drew on the respective disciplinary strengths of the committee members. Walter J. Burdette was a prominent surgeon and chair of the Surgery Department at the University of Utah; John B. Hickman was chair of Internal Medicine at the University of Indiana; Charles LeMaistre was a pulmonary specialist and head of a very large cancer treatment center. The pathologists joining the committee were Emmanuel Farber, chair of Pathology at the University of Pittsburgh; Jacob Furth from Columbia, an expert on the biology of cancer; and Maurice Seevers, chair of the University of Michigan Pharmacology Department. Louis Fieser of Harvard University was an eminent organic chemist. Completing the committee were Stanhope Bayne-Jones, a bacteriologist, former head of New York Hospital, and dean of Yale Medical School; Leonard M. Schuman, epidemiologist at the University of Minnesota; and William G. Cochran, a Harvard University mathematician with expertise in statistical methods. By appointing this distinguished group, Terry assured that the advisory committee would be protected from political attacks and charges of bias and subjectivity.[50]

Terry immediately set the charge for the Advisory Committee, and he divided the work into two distinct phases. The first phase was to determine the "nature and magnitude of the health effects of smoking."[51] Committee members sought to arrive at a clinical judgment on smoking. As one public health official explained, "What do we [that is, the Surgeon General of the United States Public Health Service] advise our Patient, the American public, about smoking?" Terry promised that the report on these findings would be followed by phase II, proposals for remedial action. This separation into two phases was significant, for it kept the committee away from the political morass which swirled around the tobacco question. What Terry sought—and ultimately got—was a document that would be unimpeachable from a scientific point of view. This would be the ammunition that regulatory agencies and the Congress would need to create powerful public health policies relating to smoking and health.

In fact, Terry was probably aware that the so-called phase II would be left to other branches of the government. As Stanhope Bayne-Jones, a member of the committee later explained: "Phase II led, of course, into economic and legal considerations of great magnitude. What would be done would affect the industries, affect part of the national economy, affect international relationships, possibly disturb labor relationships as well as laboring individuals. It was so important from a governmental standpoint that I doubt whether any clear notion of ever undertaking phase II through this mechanism was envisioned under the Public Health Service.[52]

Terry astutely recognized that the Advisory Committee could only speak with authority about the scientific and medical nature of the health risks of smoking; he would leave the policy questions to the politicians. This, of course, is not to suggest that the *Report* was not a political document; indeed, its preeminent purpose was to provide sufficient medical authority to generate new public policies.[53]

At its first meeting in November 1962, the committee decided that it would base its assessment on a comprehensive review of the now considerable existing data; new research would delay too greatly the announcement of any conclusions. The committee met together nine times in just over a year. In between these meetings both committee members and staff worked concertedly to review, critique, and synthesize what had become a formidable volume of scientific work on tobacco. As Advisory Committee member Leonard Schuman later explained in an interview, what struck the committee was the "consistency of the findings" on lung cancer over the 30 case-controlled studies the committee examined. As he explained it, "the strength of the associations" was undeniable: "regardless of the methodology, regardless of the controls, regardless of the characteristics of the case samples . . . the outcome was the same."[50,54-56] The First Surgeon General's *Report* had the effect of ending any remaining medical and scientific uncertainty concerning the harmfulness of smoking. The weight of their conclusion, of course, did not mean that important scientific questions about tobacco no longer needed examination, but rather that the essential question—critical to the public's health—had been systematically and thoroughly investigated, and definitively resolved. At the press conference announcing the committee's findings, Terry was asked whether he would now recommend to a patient to stop smoking. His answer was an unequivocal yes.[57]

Legitimation of Epidemiologic Causality

The methodology behind this conclusion had required the committee to articulate explicit criteria on which to base their judgment. The resolution of the question—Do cigarettes cause disease?—had required important innovations in both the methodologic and epistemologic approaches in the medical sciences. Fundamental aspects of the production and legitimation of new medical knowledge were at stake. The authority of clinical medicine was deeply invested in the notion of individual experience and variability instead of generalized statistics. At the same time, notions of causality had come to center on experiment and visualization rather than more traditional population-based evaluative methods. As a result, the Surgeon General's Advisory Committee worked to define the specific approaches utilized to reach a causal conclusion.

In the Committee, William Cochran, the noted Harvard statistician, took the lead in organizing and drafting the report's single most critical chapter, "Criteria for Judgment." Most centrally, the committee labored over the issue of causality. What did it mean to say, for example, that cigarettes *caused* lung cancer? How should cause be distinguished from "associated with," "a factor," or "determinant?" The report sought to clarify this issue at the outset, noting: "the word 'cause' is the one in general usage in connection with matters considered in this study, and it is capable of conveying the notion of a significant, effectual, relationship between an agent and an associated disorder or disease in the host."

But members of the committee realized the complexity of saying simply that smoking causes cancer. Many persons could smoke heavily throughout their lives, and yet not develop lung cancer. Therefore they acknowledged the complexity of causal processes in medical science: "It should be said at once, however, that no member of this Committee used the word "cause" in an absolute sense in the area of this study. Although various disciplines and fields of scientific knowledge were represented among the membership, all members shared a common conception of the multiple etiology of biological processes. No member was so naive as to insist upon mono-etiology in pathological processes or in vital phenomena."[4]

And yet the members of the committee did not wish to give too much ground on what they considered a semantic argument. Therefore they concluded: "Granted that these complexities were recognized, it is to be noted clearly that the Committee's considered decision to use the words 'a cause' or 'a major cause' or 'a significant cause,' or 'a causal association' in certain conclusions about smoking and health affirms their conviction."[4]

Although the tobacco industry would consistently argue for an esoteric and unobtainable definition of *cause*, the Surgeon General's Committee understood that the public's health was at stake, and in the medical sciences, *cause* always required inference. The committee defined and utilized a clear set of criteria to evaluate the significance of a statistical association. Recognizing that the nature of inference as a process requires judgment, the committee sought to define this process specifically, outlining five specific conditions for judging causal relations:

1. Consistency of the Association. Comparable results are found utilizing a wide range of methods and data.

2. Strength of the Association. The cause and effect has a dose response, the greater the exposure, the more likely the effect.
3. Specificity of Association. The effect is typically and powerfully associated with the cause. (90% of all lung cancers were found to occur among smokers.)
4. Temporal Relationship of Associated Variables. The cause must precede the effect.
5. Coherence of the Association. There must be an overall logic to the cause and effect relationship.[4]

Through these five principles, the assessment of causality was part of a consistent and rational explanation. These criteria have become the basic orthodoxy for causal inference concerning disease since the time of the *Report*, integrating quantitative techniques with other confirmatory scientific and clinical data. Although the criteria themselves had been used in the past, never before had they been so systematically articulated in a consolidated fashion.

The Disinformation Campaign

Although epidemiologists and the Surgeon General's Advisory Committee cited a wide range of evidence beyond narrowly statistical findings, critics—especially those representing the tobacco industry—continued to portray the causal link as but a mathematical aberration. Given the categorical findings of the surgeon general's *Report*, the industry was forced to redouble its efforts to maintain the shroud of scientific controversy and uncertainty. They quickly developed an approach—dominated by their legal staffs—to neither deny nor confirm the findings. Their public message—though wearing thin—remained the need for more research; the "merely statistical" nature of the surgeon general's conclusion; and their eagerness for their customers to "keep an open mind." They also continued to insist on the need for experimental evidence to demonstrate causality.

In the face of massive research and the definitive review and conclusions of the Advisory Committee, the industry issued what had come to be its mantra: a call for more research: "After 10 years," said the Council for Tobacco Research (CTR) report, "the fact remains that knowledge is insufficient either to provide adequate proof of any hypothesis or to define the basic mechanisms of health and disease with which we are concerned."[58] The industry constructed a standard of proof, which they well understood could not be met. This was not a scientific strategy for reaching a conclusion; it was a socio-political strategy for inventing "controversy" in the face of scientific findings of crucial importance to public health and clinical medicine.

Researchers responded adamantly to the tobacco industry's unrealistic criteria. Ernst Wynder noted that calls for experimental evidence negated the potential for any conclusion: If you doubt statistics . . . you have already cut off every possible road to coming to an answer to the problem before you even start it."[62] Others reached similar conclusions. As Austin Bradford Hill explained in 1965: "All scientific work is incomplete—whether it be observational or experimental. All scientific work is liable to be upset or modified by advancing knowledge. That does not confer upon us a freedom to ignore the knowledge we already have, or to postpone action that it appears to demand at a given time. . . . "Who knows," asked Robert Browning, "but the world may end tonight?" True, but on available evidence, most of us make ready to commute on the 8:30 next day."[60]

In the face of such definitive conclusions, the tobacco industry could no longer rely solely on tactics questioning the contention that cigarettes were harmful, finding them much less effective than they were before 1964. The authoritative voice of the Surgeon General's Advisory Committee and the subsequent surgeon general's reports made it very difficult for the industry to argue that there was any remaining question about whether cigarettes were harmful.[45]

The New Role of the Federal Government

Following the release of the report, expectations ran high for substantial reductions in cigarette use among the American public. After a banner year in 1963, sales dropped off 15–20% in the 6 months immediately following the release of the report, but by 1965, the industry had already rebounded, reporting record sales. In that year the industry reported per capita consumption of 4318 cigarettes, and profits were the highest in the industry's history. By 1973, tobacco consumption had not declined appreciably from 1964 levels.[61-64]

Despite heightened expectations, the surgeon general's *Report* did not have a major effect in policy making. Legislative antismoking efforts had trouble withstanding tobacco interests. Congress did succeed in passing the Federal Cigarette Labeling and Advertising Act in 1965, but the legislation was limited in scope. The legislation established a National Clearinghouse on Smoking and Health and required that all packs of cigarettes carry a warning: "Caution: Cigarette Smoking May be Hazardous to Your Health." However, this warning was remarkably cautious indeed, reflecting the effectiveness of the tobacco lobby on Capitol Hill. Not surprisingly, the warning had little effect on sales, which continued to rise in 1966.

Although the report did not immediately reduce cigarette use or change governmental policy, it was nonetheless a pivotal document in the history of twentieth-century public health. In making such a powerful and definitive statement, the surgeon general's *Report*—and the subsequent efforts made by federal officials—created a new realm of public health action that has had powerful consequences. As A. Lee Fritschler pointed out in his analysis of smoking and federal policy making, the Surgeon General's Office provides a "combination of legitimacy and exposure" so central to making the harms of smoking an unquestioned fact. With 350,000 copies of the *Report* distributed in less than a year after its release, the Public Health Service quickly set as a goal the distribution of copies of the report to every medical student. They also planned by January 1965 to post a brief summary of the report in 50,000 pharmacies across the nation.[65]

In spite of the fact that the *Report* did not lead to the remedial actions that Luther Terry anticipated would constitute Phase II of his original charter, it did mark the expansion of the Surgeon General's Office as a sociopolitical entity. The 1964 report established the format that became the model for the subsequent 29 reports on smoking and its harms. Surgeons general since have been eager to use the authority of their office in a fashion resting heavily on Terry's experience. These reports, utilizing the methods and rhetorical strategies of the original 1964 report, were similarly important vehicles for shaping the policy context of subsequent tobacco regulation. Ultimately, additional surgeon general's reports would confirm the addictiveness of tobacco and the harmful impacts of secondhand smoke as well as greatly expanding our knowledge and understanding of the health consequences of smoking. These subsequent reports underscored the importance of analysis on smoking and health issues as well as the significance of the Office of the Surgeon General.

The most recent surgeon general's *Report*, issued in 2004, concluded that "smoking harms nearly every organ of the body." The report also reviewed more recent data showing that smoking causes many other additional diseases including stomach cancer, acute myeloid leukemia, pancreatic cancer, and pneumonia among others. From 1963 to 2002, per capita annual consumption of cigarettes among adults had fallen from 4345 to 1979. Nonetheless, smoking continues to cause some 440,000 premature deaths each year, remaining the leading cause of preventable disease and death in the United States. The report format also became a model for reports on numerous other health concerns as well.[66]

The *Report* marked the beginning of a revolution in attitudes and behaviors relating to cigarettes. In the last quarter century, half of all living Americans who have ever smoked have now quit. At the time of the 1964 report, 42% of all U.S. adults smoked; in 2002, only 23% were smokers.[67] According to the surgeon general's *Report* of 1989, approximately 750,000 smoking-related deaths had been avoided since 1964 because people had quit or not started smoking; today, this number is well over 1 million.[68] Terry's *Report* signaled the beginning of a profound change in the meaning of the cigarette and spurred new interest more generally in the relationship of behavior, risk, and health.

Following the release of the *Report* and the replication of its conclusions, the Surgeon General's Office and the federal government would assert new authority and responsibility for the most important health issues of our time. In this sense, the *Report* heralded the fundamental expansion of the role and function of the federal government characteristic of the Kennedy and Johnson administrations. With the Surgeon General's Advisory Committee and its report, the federal government established cigarette smoking as the pre-eminent public health issue of the second half of the twentieth century. In so doing, the government established new responsibilities and authority for science and health in the consumer culture. Inherent in the *Report* therefore were powerful notions of the possibility of the liberal state. From tobacco to HIV, the American public and indeed, the global community, would look to the surgeon general for scientifically validated public health policies. The first Surgeon General's *Report* remains a signal contribution not only in the history of tobacco, but for the history of public health.

References

1. Royal College of Physicians of London. Smoking and Health: Summary and Report of the Royal College of Physicians of London on Smoking in Relation to Cancer of the Lung and Other Diseases. New York and London: Pitman Publishing Company, 1962.
2. World Health Organization. Epidemiology of Cancer of the Lung: Report of a Study Group. Geneva: WHO Technical Reports 192, 19603–13.
3. Burnham JC. American physicians and tobacco use: two surgeons general, 1929 and 1964. *Bull Hist Med* 1989:63:1–31.
4. U.S. Department of Health, Education, and Welfare. Surgeon General's Report, Smoking and Health: Report of the Advisory Committee to the Surgeon General of the Public Health Service. PHS publication no. 1103. Washington, DC: Government Printing Office, 1964.
5. The smoking report. *New York Times*, 12 January 1964, E12.
6. Cigaret smoking causes lung cancer. *NEA Journal* 1946:35:2.
7. Susser M. Epidemiology in the United States after World War II: the evolution of technique. *Epidemiol Rev* 1985:7:147–77.
8. Lombard HL Doering CR. Cancer studies in Massachusetts: 2. Habits, characteristics, and environment of individuals with and without cancer. *N Engl J Med* 1928:196:481–87.
9. Hoffman FL. Cancer and smoking habits. *Annals of Surg* 1931:93:50–67.
10. Pearl R. Tobacco smoking and longevity. *Science* 1938:37:216–17.
11. Muller FH. Abuse of tobacco and carcinoma of the lungs (trans.) *JAMA* 1939:113:1372.
12. Proctor RN. The Nazi War on Cancer. Princeton: Princeton University Press, 2000, 194–98.
13. Ochsner A. My first recognition of the relationship of smoking and lung cancer. *Prev Med* 1973:2:611–14.
14. Ochsner A, DeBakey M. Symposium on cancer: primary pulmonary malignancy, treatment by total pneumonectomy: analysis of 79 collected cases and presentation of 7 personal cases. *Surg Gynecol Obstet* 1939:68:435.
15. Cantor D. Cancer. In: Bynum WF, Porter R, eds. Companion Encyclopedia of the History of Medicine. Vol. I. New York: Routledge, 1993, 556.
16. Evarts A. Graham to Alton Ochsner, 28 October 1940. Graham Papers, St. Louis: Washington University.
17. Wilds J, Harkey I. Alton Ochsner: Surgeon of the South. Baton Rouge: Louisiana State University Press, 1990, 180.
18. Wynder EL, Graham EA. Tobacco smoking as a possible etiologic factor in bronchiogenic carcinoma: a study of 684 proved cases. *JAMA* 1950:143(4):336.
19. Levin, ML, Goldstein H, Gerhardt PR. Cancer and tobacco smoking: a preliminary report. *JAMA* 1950:143(4):336–37.
20. Doll R. Conversation with Sir Richard Doll. Journal interview no. 29. *Br J Addict* 1991:86:370.
21. Doll, R, Hill AB. Smoking and carcinoma of the lung: preliminary report. *Br Med J* 1950:221(ii):739–48.
22. Doll, R, Hill AB. A study of the aetiology of carcinoma of the lung. *Br Med J* 1952:225(ii):1271,1283.
23. Sadowsky DA, Gilliam AG, Cornfield J. The statistical association between smoking and carcinoma of the lung. *J Natl Cancer Inst* 1953:13:1237–58.
24. Doll, R, Hill AB. The mortality of doctors in relation to their smoking habits: a preliminary report. *Br Med J* 1954:228(i):1451–55.

25. Doll R, Hill AB. Lung cancer and other causes of death in relation to smoking: a second report on the mortality of British doctors. *Br Med J* 1956:2:1071–81.
26. Hammond EC, Horn D. Smoking and death rates report on forty-four months of follow-up of 187,783 men. I: total mortality. *JAMA* 195810:1159–72.
27. Cornfield J, Haenszel W, Hammond EC, Lilienfeld AM, Shimkin MB, Wynder EL. Smoking and lung cancer: recent evidence and discussion of some questions. *J Natl Cancer Inst* 1959:22(1):173–203.
28. Strong FM, Bing RJ, Dyer RE, et al. Smoking and health: joint report of the study group on smoking and health. *Science* 1957:124:1129–33.
29. Tursi FV, White SE, McQuilkin S. Lost empire: the fall of R.J. Reynolds Tobacco Company. *Winston-Salem Journal,* 2000, 51.
30. Hilts PJ. Smokescreen: The Truth Behind the Tobacco Industry Cover-up. Reading, MA: Addison-Wesley Publishing, 1996, 4.
31. Kluger R. Ashes to Ashes. New York: Alfred A. Knopf, 1996, 152.
32. Sobel R. They Satisfy: The Cigarette in American Life. Garden City, NY: Anchor Books, 1978, 167–69.
33. Wynder EL, Graham EA, Croninger AB. Experimental production of carcinoma with cigarette tar. *Cancer Res* 1953:13:855–58.
34. Hoyt WT. A brief history of the Council for Tobacco Research. Council for Tobacco Research. Lorillard, 1984, 1. Available at: http://legacy.library.ucsf.edu/tid/tpg3aa00. Bates no. 515847269/7336.Accessed 1 May 2006.
35. Glantz SA. The Cigarette Papers. Berkeley: University of California Press, 1996.
36. Tobacco Information Committee. Tobacco and health. American Tobacco. 2 January 1958. Available at: http://legacy.library.ucsf.edu/tid/utg70a00. Bates no. MNAT00515648/5651.
37. Spears AW, Judge CH. Confidential: brief review of the organizations contributing to research into tobacco. Lorillard. 24 June 1974. Available at: http://legacy.library.ucsf.edu/tid/lmf20e00. Bates no. 01421596/1600.
38. Burney, LE. Smoking and lung cancer: a statement of the Public Health Service. *JAMA* 1959:71:1835–36.
39. Laurence WL. Science in review: controversy on lung cancer and smoking flares up again over the statistics. *New York Times,* 6 December 1959, E11.
40. Council, British Medical Research. Tobacco smoking and cancer of the lung: statement by British Medical Research Council. *Br Med J* 1957:234:1523–24.
41. World Health Organization. Epidemiology of Cancer of the Lung: Report of a Study Group. Geneva: WHO Technical Reports, 1960, 192.
42. Royal College of Physicians of London. Smoking and Health: Summary and Report of the Royal College of Physicians of London on Smoking in Relation to Cancer of the Lung and Other Diseases. New York and London: Pitman Publishing Company, 1962.
43. Berridge V. Science and policy: the case of postwar British smoking policy. In: Lock S, Reynolds L, Tansey EM, eds. Ashes to Ashes: The History of Smoking and Health. Amsterdam and Atlanta, GA: Editions Rodopi B.V., 1998, 149–50.
44. Transcript of the president's news conference on foreign and domestic matters. *New York Times,* 24 May 1962, 16.
45. Fritschler AL. Smoking and Politics: Policy Making and the Federal Bureaucracy. Englewood Cliffs, NJ: Prentice Hall, 1989, 39–41, 44, 89.
46. Fritschler AL, Neuberger MB. Smoke Screen: Tobacco and the Public Welfare. Englewood Cliffs, NJ: Prentice-Hall, 1963, 62–64.
47. MacGregor to Terry (memo), 9 November 1962. NARG 90, SGAC,.College Park, MD: National Archives.

48. Interview with Surgeon General Luther Terry on Today Show. Tobacco document #TDO-217-37. Tobacco Institute. TIMN0114289/4293. Available at: http://www.tobaccodocuments.org/view.cfm?docid=TIMN0114289/4293&source=SNAPTI&ShowImages=yes. Accessed 18 December 2001.

49. Pearson R, Dr. Luther Terry, former surgeon general, dies. *Washington Post*, 31 March 1985, B6.

50. Terry, LL. The surgeon general's first report on smoking and health: a challenge to the medical profession. *NY State J Med* 1983:83:1254–55.

51. The nature, purpose and suggested formulation of the study of the health effects of smoking, phase I. Typescript (1962). National Archives Manuscripts, Record Group 90, Washington, DC, Records of the Surgeon General's Advisory Committee.

52. Bayne-Jones S. Oral History Memoir. National Library of Medicine, Bethesda, MD, 1108.

53. Hamill PVV to Schuman L, March 5, 1963. National Archives Manuscripts, Record Group 90, Washington, DC, Records of the Surgeon General's Advisory Committee.

54. Interview with Leonard M. Schuman. Richard Kluger interviews concerning Ashes to Ashes, Vol. 2, 15 July 1988. Ness Motley documents . Available at: http://tobaccodocuments.org/ness/76600.123.html. Accessed 1 May 2006.

55. Breslow L. Some Sequels to the Surgeon General's Report on Smoking and Health: Thirty Years Later. *Ann Epidemiol.* 1996;6:372–375.

56. Schuman LM. The origins of the report of the Advisory Committee on Smoking and Health to the Surgeon General. *J Public Health Policy* 1981:2(1):19–27.

57. Hunter M. Smoking banned at news parley. *New York Times,* 12 January 1964, 66.

58. Little CC. Tobacco industry says indictment of cigarrets isn't backed by data. *Wall Street Journal,* 17 August 1964, 5.

59. Reiser SJ. Smoking and health: congress and causality. In: Lakoff SA, ed. Knowledge and Power. New York: The Free Press/MacMillan, 1966, 293–311.

60. Hill AB. The environment and disease: association or causation? *Proc R Soc Med* 1965:58:300.

61. Tobacco industry's peak year: 523 billion cigarettes smoked. *New York Times*, 1 January 1964, 29.

62. Cigarette sales decline sharply. *New York Times*, 30 June 1964, 41.

63. Has the smoking scare ended? *U.S. News and World Report*, 18 October 1965, 46.

64. Total and per capita manufactured cigarette consumption—United States, U.S. Department of Agriculture, 1900–1995. National Center for Chronic Disease Prevention and Health Promotion, Tobacco Information and Prevention Source. Available at: www.cdc.gov/tobacco/research_data/economics/consump1.htm. Accessed 1 May 2006.

65. Talks by Surgeon General Luther Terry in Miami Beach, Sunday 29 November 29 1964. Tobacco document no. TDO-21646. Available at: http://www.tobaccodocuments.org/view.cfm?docid=TIMN0114118/4121&source=SNAPTI&ShowImages=yes. Accessed 18 December 2001.

66. U.S. Department of Health and Human Services. The Health Consequences of Smoking: A Report of the Surgeon General. Washington, DC: Centers for Disease Control and Prevention, National Center for Chronic Disease Prevention and Health Promotion, Office on Smoking and Health, 2004, 8.

67. Centers for Disease Control and Prevention. State-specific prevalence of current cigarette smoking among adults—United States, 2002. *MMWR* 2004:52(53):3.

68. U.S. Department of Health and Human Services. Reducing the Health Consequences of Smoking; 25 Years of Progress: A Report of the Surgeon General. Rockville, MD: Public Health Service, Centers for Disease Control, 1989.

Suggested Reading

Fritschler AL. Smoking and Politics: Policy Making and the Federal Bureaucracy. Englewood Cliffs, NJ: Prentice-Hall, 1989.

Lock S, Reynolds L, Tansey EM, eds. Ashes to Ashes: The History of Smoking and Health, Amsterdam and Atlanta, GA: Editions Rodopi B. V., 1998.

22

Epilogue: Public Health at the Dawn of the Twenty-First Century

JEFFREY P. KOPLAN
STEPHEN B. THACKER

The extraordinary accomplishments in the field of public health during the twentieth century changed the focus of what public health professionals do in the field and how they do it. But the changes that are described in the chapters of this book set the stage for what will no doubt be an even more dramatic, and in many ways unpredictable, vision of health in the year 2100. Futurists anticipate major changes in demographics, climate, globalization, and technology that will alter the social fabric of this country and the world and have a tremendous effect on the health of the world's population. Some of these changes can be anticipated (e.g., aging of the population, increased global migration, better understanding and exploitation of the human genome and other technologic advances, and increased burdens on the world's natural resources). We have the tools to address many of these changes, and if we apply ourselves to the known and anticipated challenges, we will also be better prepared to address the inevitable unknown challenges.

At least 10 health priorities have been identified for the decades ahead, all of which have emerged over the last century and will continue to become more salient.[1] These priorities encompass fundamental changes in health-care systems, adaptation to demographic changes, elimination of health disparities, mitigation of the risks posed by our lifestyles and the environment, unraveling the mysteries of the brain and human behavior, and exploring new technologic frontiers. To position the nation for the century ahead, the medical, scientific, and public-health community must devote attention and resources to the following tasks.

Establish a New Paradigm in Health Care

The United States needs a health-care system that encompasses public health and clinical care and that balances equity, cost, and quality. The lack of health insurance for 45 million Americans[2] is just one symptom of an unnecessarily uneven distribution of health care. Similarly, the fact that half of the deaths that occur each year are from preventable causes[3] suggests that the health-care system has not exploited its potential to emphasize prevention as well as treatment of diseases, injuries, and disabilities. In late 2002, the Institute of Medicine released a report recommending a dramatic restructuring of clinical training that would require that public health practice be a primary element of competency for all physicians.[4] The application of evidence-based recommendations to both individual clinical care[5] and community-based practice[6] is an essential first step toward developing a rational approach to health.

Eliminate Health Disparities

Health disparities among racial and ethnic groups are reflected in differences in rates, severity, and treatment of several conditions (e.g., heart disease, cancers, diabetes, and human immunodeficiency virus [HIV]/acquired immunodeficiency syndrome [AIDS]).[7] Infant mortality rates, for example, are 2.5 times higher among African Americans than among whites. Eliminating these disparities in health requires improved access to quality health care and innovative and effective community-based interventions tailored to different racial and ethnic groups. Community-based participatory research that engages persons of all racial and ethnic groups in the setting of research priorities in their own communities is a crucial step in addressing health disparities.[8]

Focus on Children's Emotional and Intellectual Development

Attention to children's physical development must be matched with a focus on their emotional and intellectual development. Although vaccinations and other health advances have made infancy and childhood less perilous, the challenge remains to provide foster homes, preschools, and community environments that encourage positive interactions and relationships, permitting children to achieve their full potential. For example, public funded, center-based, comprehensive early childhood development programs designed for children aged 3–5 years from low-income families prevent developmental delay, improve grade retention, reduce teen pregnancy, and provide other long-term benefits.[9] Similarly, housing subsidy programs providing rental vouchers have been demonstrated to improve neighborhood safety and reduce low-income families' exposure to violence.[9]

Focus on Demographic Changes

In 1900, approximately one in 25 Americans was elderly (i.e., aged ≥65 years);[10] in 1990, the proportion was one in eight, or 10 times larger than in 1900. This trend will continue and accelerate as baby boomers age. By 2050, the number of elderly persons is expected to reach 79 million—a number twice that for the close of the twentieth century. The public health community must work not only to increase the life span of Americans, but to increase quality of life among elderly persons. Research findings from studies of healthy aging must be incorporated into practice, especially those findings that promote the lifelong dietary and physical activity habits that increase the chances of being healthy, active, and independent in the last years of life.

Because immigration has increased the racial and ethnic diversity in the United States, by 2050, Asians, non-Hispanic blacks, Hispanics, and American Indians together are expected to constitute 50% of the U.S. population.[11] The continuous integration of cultures and religions into the matrix of American life must be acknowledged by the health-care community, and U.S. clinical and public health practices must remain flexible and adapt to these influences.

Modify Activities of Daily Living Including Physical Activity and Healthy Eating

An obesity epidemic fueled by "supersized" portions, unhealthy diets, and lack of physical activity contributes to 300,000 premature chronic disease deaths each year.[3] Most alarmingly, the percentage of American children who are overweight has more than tripled since the 1960s, from 5% in 1964 to 16% in 2002,[16] making children more susceptible to diabetes and the precursors of heart disease and stroke. The reversal of these trends requires broad societal changes in views about eating habits and physical activity.

Protect the Environment

Progress in reducing pollution from cars and industries and in identifying and mitigating hazardous-waste sites has slowed. Smog alerts and polluted lakes and rivers (damaged by storm water runoff from our increasingly paved living areas) are warning signs that not enough attention has been given to balancing growth with environmental protection. The environment will be increasingly challenged by toxic exposures, disposal of radioactive materials, and continued urbanization. In addition, global warming trends in the face of an increasing population will increase the rates of disease and deplete the global food supply. Hence, better conservation of natural resources and greater use of environmentally enriching technologies are needed. The design and construction of communities should foster healthy lifestyles and improve the quality of life (e.g., safe and easy access to physical activity).

Respond to Emerging Infectious Diseases

During the past 30 years, at least 30 new viral, bacterial, and parasitic diseases have been classified as "emerging,"[12] meaning that they have newly appeared in a population or have suddenly increased their incidence or geographic scope. The devastating effects of HIV in the United States and around the world vividly document the impact of such emerging infections. Migration and travel, international trade, agricultural practices, and constant microbial adaptation are factors that help ensure that the United States will face more exotic and unusual diseases (e.g., West Nile virus in New York in 1999) and more antibiotic resistance in many pathogenic organisms. Although technology (e.g., a new multivalent childhood vaccine and more effective medication) are useful in preventing and treating disease, preparing state and local public health systems to detect and respond to emerging infections is crucial to the health of Americans. Such efforts will also simultaneously help prepare for the possibility of newly engineered bioterrorist agents. Unfortunately, preparing for and dealing with biologic, chemical, and radiologic terrorism may be an ongoing concern for the health sector into the twenty-first century.

Recognize and Address the Contributions of Mental Health to Overall Health and Well-Being

The impact of mental health on both physical health and productivity is underrecognized.[13] When the burden of disease is measured in disability-adjusted life years, mental illness becomes the second leading cause of disability and premature mortality in the United States and in other market economies.[1] Because the efficacy of mental-health treatments is well established and a range of treatments can be offered for most mental disorders, this disease burden could be reduced considerably. The challenges regarding mental health are to identify risk factors, improve access to effective treatment (including removing the stigma associated with seeking help), and promote good mental health in all communities. Specifically, in the current era of war and terrorism and recurring natural and manmade disasters, the importance of the prevention, recognition, and treatment of posttraumatic stress disorders must be addressed.

Reduce the Toll of Violence in Society

Homicide, suicide, and other forms of violence are public health issues for which risk factors and interventions should be further examined. In a national survey, 25% of women reported being raped or physically assaulted by an intimate partner at some time in their lives; 8% of men reported having had such an experience.[14] Half of all rapes occur among women aged less than 18 years, and 25% of these among girls aged less than 12 years.[14]

Public health approaches could include targeted interventions in communities, schools, workplaces, and churches and the use of mass media. Despite the popular opinion that violence has become ingrained in our society and glorified in every entertainment medium, this trend can be reversed. Only a few decades ago, another generally accepted societal norm, tobacco use, seemed similarly entrenched. However, tobacco companies are now banned from many advertising channels and are even required to contribute to antismoking campaigns. Social norms can and do change, but only after identification of the problem, development of effective interventions, and broad community support. Violence is increasingly being seen as a substantial public health problem, and support is being given to research designed (1) to determine underlying causes of violence and (2) to identify effective interventions to prevent death and injury result from violent behavior.

Appropriate Use of New Scientific Knowledge and Technologic Advances

The mapping of the human genome is an example of a novel technologic development that is full of potential. It is, however, only a beginning. (As one scientist observed, it creates the equivalent of a genetic dictionary full of letters and words, but most have not yet been given any meaning.[15]) This development holds promise for advancing health through sophisticated screening and targeted interventions, but like other breakthroughs, the challenge will be to apply this new knowledge equitably, ethically, and responsibly. The Internet and other technologic tools of information also provide new opportunities to promptly recognize public health problems and to educate the public in ways not previously possible. However, technology also can harm public health efforts. For instance, new technologies of convenience (e.g., the Segway scooter) could impose the same challenge to healthy lifestyles that television has over the last part of the twentieth century.

As we enter into a new century, the threat of international and domestic terror looms on the collective consciousness of the nation; concerns about national security historically have had an effect on health during both times of war and peace. The concern about war is not likely to disappear in the foreseeable future, and the widespread availability of weapons of mass destruction does not mitigate that concern.

In light of this tense climate in place at the start of the twenty-first century, four interrelated themes can be identified across the 10 priorities outlined in this chapter—themes that are not new, but that have a strong influence on how Americans view the future. First, globalization has reached into the daily lives of most Americans, not only through television and the media, but also through whom we meet, what we eat and wear, and what we think about. At the end of the twenty-first century, the United States likely will be the prototype of a global melting pot where peoples, cultures, religions, and diseases are brought into even greater proximity. A second theme, the concern for social equity, has always motivated public health efforts and fuels the concern about health disparities. A third theme is the fundamental principle that good medicine and good public health must be based on the use of the best available science, and that while the validity of social and political considerations must not be ignored, decisions based on inadequate or poor science inevitably lead to bad medicine and poor health. Fourth, we continue to struggle to translate good science into quality clinical and public health practice at the community level. Successful translation depends on a strong public health infrastructure integrated with quality, accessible clinical care, which requires community involvement in science, delivery of services, policy development, and implementation. Underlying this involvement is a better educated public and better communication of what is important and what works to those who will benefit from the health system of this new century.

In the twentieth century, public health professionals have demonstrated that they can use knowledge to improve health and quality of life and to affect individual behavior and the environment in which those behaviors occur. In the twenty-first century, public health professionals remain true to their primary mission, which is to constantly assess the major causes of death and disability and to identify the factors that place people at risk, develop and deliver effective interventions, and evaluate how well these tasks are accomplished. The causes of morbidity and mortality are likely to change over the next century; public health professionals must identify and anticipate these changes through the conduct of sound science and effective practice. New talent and potential must be tapped to achieve public health goals as the unfinished health priorities of the past century are reached and the new challenges that lie ahead are met head on.

References

1. Koplan JP, Fleming DW. Current and future public health challenges. *JAMA* 2000:284: 1696–98.
2. Kaiser Commission on Medicaid and the Uninsured. The Uninsured and Their Access to Health Care. Fact sheet. Washington, DC: The Henry J. Kaiser Family Foundation, 2000.
3. McGinnis JM, Foege WH. Actual causes of death in the United States. *JAMA* 1993:270: 2207–12.
4. Institute of Medicine. Who Will Keep the Public Healthy? Educating Public Health Professionals for the 21st Century. Washington, DC: National Academics Press, 2002.
5. U.S. Preventive Services Task Force. Guide to Clinical Preventive Services: An Assessment of the Effectiveness of 169 Interventions—Report of the U.S. Preventive Services Task Force. Baltimore, MD: Williams and Wilkins, 1989.
6. Task Force on Community Preventive Services. Introducing the guide to community preventive services: methods, first recommendations, and expert commentary. *Am J Prev Med* 2000:18(suppl 1):1–142.
7. Addressing Racial and Ethnic Disparities in Health Care. Fact sheet, February 2000. AHRQ publication no. 00-P041. Rockville, MD: Agency for Healthcare Research and Quality, 2000. Available at: www.ahrq.gov/research/diparit.htm. Accessed 14 September 2000.
8. Israel BA, Schulz AJ, Parker EA, Becker AB. Review of community based research: assessing partnership approaches to improve public health. *Ann Rev Public Health* 1998: 19:173–202.
9. Centers for Disease Control and Prevention. Community interventions to promote healthy social environments: early childhood development and family housing. *MMWR* 2002: 51:1–8.
10. U.S. Department of Commerce, Economics and Statistics Administration, Bureau of the Census. We the American Elderly. Washington, DC: Government Printing Office, 1993.

11. Council of Economic Advisors. Changing America: Indicators of Social and Economic Well-being by Race and Hispanic Origin. Washington, DC: Government Printing Office, 1998.
12. Morse SS. Factors in the emergence of infectious diseases. *Emerg Infect Dis* 1995:1:7–14.
13. Mental Health: A Report of the Surgeon General. Rockville, MD: U.S. Department of Health and Human Services, 1999.
14. Tjaden P, Thoennes N. Prevalence, Incidence and Consequences of Violence Against Women: Findings from the National Violence Against Women Survey. Research in brief. Washington, DC: U.S. Department of Justice, 1998.
15. Last lap in the genome race. *New York Times*, 26 July 2000, A20.
16. National Center for Health Statistics. Prevalence of Overweight Among Children and Adolescents: United States, 1999–2002. Available at: http://www.cdc.gov/nchs/products/pubs/pubd/hestats/overwght99.htm; Accessed 31 August, 2006.

Suggested Reading

Institute of Medicine. Future of the Public's Health in the 21st Century. Washington DC: National Academy Press, 2002.
Khoury MJ, Burke W, Thomson EJ. Genetics and Public Health in the 21st Century: Using Genetic Information to Improve Health and Prevent Disease. New York: Oxford University Press, 2000.

Index

CSTE (Council of State and Territorial
    Epidemiologists), 26
CTR (Council for Tobacco Research), 446, 450
Cultural obstacles, to occupational disease
    prevention, 222–223
Cutter Laboratories, vaccine-associated
    paralysis, 67
CVD. *See* Cardiovascular disease
Cyclospora infections, 32, 37

Dalkon Shield IUD, 260
DDT (dichlorodiphenyltrichloroethane), 23
Dean, H. Trendley, 308–309, 309*f*
Deaths. *See also* Infant mortality
    from cardiovascular disease, 381–383, 382*f*
    causes of, 3, 5*f*
    "deserved," 135
    from diabetes, 5*f*
    from heart disease, 381–385, 382*f*
    job-related, 209–210
    from lung cancer, 424–425, 438, 439–441
    maternal. *See* Maternal health, mortality
    motor-vehicle-related, 343–347, 344*f*, 345*f*,
        347*f*
    occupational-related, 211–212, 211*f*, 212*f*
    smoking-related, 424–425, 438, 439–441,
        452
DeBakey, Michael, 439–440
Decelerometer, 366
DeHaven, Hugh, 369–370
DeLee, Joseph, 110, 147–152
Demonstration clinics, 286–287
Dental caries
    in early to mid-1900s, 307
    prevention, water fluoridation and, 313
        effectiveness of, 316–317
        establishing mechanism of action, 314–315
        waterborne fluoride and, 310–311, 312*f*
Dentists, role in fluoridation campaigns, 332, 333
Department of Health and Human Services
        (Department of Health, Education and
        Welfare)
    family-planning projects, 263
    motor-vehicle trauma and, 352
    nutrition research and policy, 411, 412
    Secretary's Advisory Committee on Infant
        Mortality, 125
    tobacco-control interventions, 431
    WIC program and, 119
Department of Labor, Occupational Safety and
    Health Administration, 220
Developing nations, pesticide production in,
    226
DHEW. *See* Department of Health and Human
    Services

Diabetes deaths, 5*f*
Diaphragm, contraceptive, 256, 269*t*
Diarrhea
    deaths from, 3, 5*f*
    infant mortality and, 45, 136*f*, 137–138
Dichlorodiphenyltrichloroethane (DDT), 23
Dickinson, Robert Latou, 283
Diet/nutrition. *See also* Nutritional disorders
    atherosclerosis and, 404
    challenges for twenty-first century, 179
    changes, CVD death rates and, 391
    cholesterol-lowering, 407–408
    education, Food Administration and,
        176–177
    fadism/quackery, 406, 409
    feeding programs, school lunch programs,
        177–179
    health effects of, 401–402
    heart disease and, publicity about, 405–406
    improvements
        effect on mortality rates from infectious
            disease, 163
        height and, 163–164
    for infants. *See* Infant feeding
    pellagra and, 168
    progress, milestones in, 179, 180*t*–181*t*
Dietary Goals for the United States, 411
Dietary policy, 407–412
Diphtheria
    deaths from, 5*f*, 63–64
    outbreaks, historical, 73
Diphtheria-pertussis-tetanus vaccine (DPT), 9
Disease. *See also specific diseases*
    chronic
        infectious agents and, 13
        of lungs, deaths associated with, 5*f*
    foodborne. *See* Foodborne disease
    infectious. *See* Infectious disease
    prevention
        nutrition and. *See* Diet/nutrition
        in workplace, 218–219
    transmission, technology and, 14
    vaccine-preventable. *See* Vaccine-preventable
        disease
    workplace. *See* Occupational disease
Disease eradication concept, 9–10
DNA fingerprints, of bacterial strains, 36
Doe v. Bolton, 270
Dole, Elizabeth, 372
Doll, Richard, 441–442
Douche contraception method, 255
DPT (diphtheria-pertussis-tetanus vaccine), 9
Drinking age, minimum, 372
Driver education courses, effectiveness of,
    372–373